FETAL AND POSTNATAL CELLULAR GROWTH

FETAL AND POSTNATAL CELLULAR GROWTH

HORMONES AND NUTRITION

DONALD B. CHEEK, M.D., D.Sc.

Research Professor of Pediatrics
University of Melbourne
Director of the Royal Children's Hospital Research Foundation, Melbourne

previously

Professor of Pediatrics
The Johns Hopkins University School of Medicine
Baltimore, Maryland

with the assistance of collaborating investigators

A Wiley Biomedical-Health Publication

JOHN WILEY & SONS, New York • London • Sydney • Toronto

Copyright © 1975 by John Wiley & Sons, Inc.

All rights reserved. Published simultaneously in Canada.

No part of this book may be reproduced by any means,
nor transmitted, nor translated into a machine language
without the written permission of the publisher.

Library of Congress Cataloging in Publication Data:

Fetal and postnatal cellular growth.

  (A Wiley biomedical-health publication)
  Includes bibliographical references and index.

  1. Fetus—Growth. 2. Infants—Growth. 3. Hormones.
4. Nutrition. 5. Rhesus monkey. I. Cheek, Donald B.
[DNLM: 1. Fetus—Growth and development. 2. Hormones
—Growth physiology. 3. Infant, Newborn. 4. Nutrition. WQ210 C515f]

QP277.F47   612.6'47   75-5814
ISBN 0-471-15093-2

Printed in the United States of America

10 9 8 7 6 5 4 3 2 1

TO SUZANNE AND CECILIA

Contributors

Claude Bachmann, M.D.
Chemisches Zentrallabor Inselspital
Bern, Switzerland

Clarissa H. Beatty, Ph. D.
Scientist
Oregon Regional Primate Research
  Center
Beaverton, Oregon

Rose Mary M. Bocek, Ph.D.
Associate Scientist
Oregon Regional Primate Research
  Center
Beaverton, Oregon

James B. Brayton, D.V.M., M.P.H.,
  M.D.
Assistant Professor of Pediatrics and
  Laboratory Animal Medicine
The Johns Hopkins University School
  of Medicine
Baltimore, Maryland

Charles Chang, M.D.
Pediatric Neurology Fellow
St. Louis Children's Hospital
St. Louis, Missouri

Donald B. Cheek, M.D., D.Sc.
Research Professor of Pediatrics
  University of Melbourne
Director, Royal Children's Hospital
  Research Foundation
Parkville, Victoria, Australia

Ronald A. Chez, M.D.
Chief, Pregnancy Research Branch, NIH
National Institute of Child Health
Bethesda, Maryland

Robert E. Cooke, M.D.
Vice Chancellor for Health Services
Professor of Pediatrics
University of Wisconsin, Madison
Madison, Wisconsin

Gail Davila, B.A.
Research Associate
Fels Research Institute
Yellow Springs, Ohio

Louis Gluck, M.D.
Professor of Pediatrics
University of California, San Diego
La Jolla, California

Joan E. Graystone, M.Sc.
Research Officer
Royal Children's Hospital Research
  Foundation
Parkville, Victoria, Australia

Donald E. Hill, M.D., F.R.C.P.(C)
Assistant Professor, Department of
  Pediatrics
Program Director, Perinatal Growth and
  Development Research Institute
Hospital for Sick Children
Toronto, Canada

Alan B. Holt, A.A.I.M.T.
Chief Medical Technologist
Royal Children's Hospital Research
  Foundation
Parkville, Victoria, Australia

Mary Etta Hornbeck
Research Associate
Department of Pediatrics
University of California, San Diego
La Jolla, California

Clayton H. Kallman, B.S.
Statistician
Department of Pediatrics
Johns Hopkins University School
  of Medicine
Baltimore, Maryland

George R. Kerr, M.D.
Associate Professor of Nutrition
Department of Nutrition
Harvard School of Public Health
Boston, Massachusetts

Marie V. Kulovich, Ph.D.
Associate Research Biochemist
Department of Pediatrics
University of California, San Diego
La Jolla, California

Stanko Kulovich
Associate Specialist
Department of Pediatrics
University of California, San Diego
La Jolla, California

E. David Mellits, Sc.D.
Associate Professor, Department of
  Pediatrics, Johns Hopkins School of
  Medicine and Department of
  Biostatistics
Department of Pediatrics
Johns Hopkins School of Hygiene
  and Public Health
Baltimore, Maryland

William L. Nyhan, M.D., Ph.D.
Professor and Chairman
Department of Pediatrics
School of Medicine
University of California
San Diego, California

Adalberto Parra, M.D.
Head Protein Hormones Section
Instituto Mexicano del Seguro Social
Subdireccion General Medica
Jefatura de Ensenanze e Investigacion
Departamento de Investigacion
  Cientifica
Mexico City, Mexico

W. Ann Reynolds, Ph.D.
Professor of Anatomy
College of Medicine
Department of Anatomy
University of Illinois at the Medical
  Center
Chicago, Illinois

Alex F. Roche, M.D., Ph.D., D.Sc.
Senior Scientist
Fels Research Institute
Yellow Springs, Ohio

Jacques F. Roux, M.D.
Professor in Obstetrics and
  Gynaecology
Director, Perinatal Research Center
Cuyahoga County Hospital
Cleveland Metropolitan General
  Hospital
Cleveland, Ohio

Rachèl E. Scott, B.Sc.
Research Assistant
Department of Gynecology and
  Obstetrics
Johns Hopkins Hospital
Baltimore, Maryland

John J. White, M.D., C.M.
Associate Professor of Surgery
Department of Surgery
Division of Pediatric Surgery
The Johns Hopkins Hospital
Baltimore, Maryland

Robert G. Wyllie, M.B., B.S.
Assistant Professor of Pathology
Department of Pathology
Johns Hopkins Medical Institutions
Baltimore, Maryland

T. Yoshioka, M.D.
Okoyama Medical School
Department of Obstetrics and
  Gynecology
Okoyama, Japan

Foreword

As society becomes more sensitive to the ethical issues that arise in human experimentation, as science strives to improve the quality of human life, primate research acquires far greater importance than it has ever had before. It is no longer permissible to carry out nontherapeutic fetal research even before abortion, and research on the pregnant human must be sharply restricted in the interest of avoiding fetal injury. At the same time, through improved methods of contraception or more widespread use of abortion, the birthrate in developed countries is falling rapidly. As a consequence, the well-being of each newborn, particularly in terms of its freedom from defect, is considered to be of even greater significance than a generation ago.

If the full capability of biomedical research is to be brought to bear on problems of the pregnant human, the human fetus, and newborn, fetal research in higher animals must be augmented substantially. Although obvious species differences exist between *Homo sapiens* and *Macaca mulatta*, the differences are substantially less than between man and rodents, dogs, cats, sheep, and so on, particularly in relation to brain development. Controlled research on the effects of maternal undernutrition on fetal development, and particularly fetal brain development, is not possible in the human. Many unknown or uncontrollable factors, genetic, infectious, and behavioral, can influence brain development in addition to nutritional factors and prevent any clear-cut assignment of causality in prenatal or even early natal mental development.

By contrast, controlled dietary manipulation is possible in the monkey. In addition, a number of models of human disease in pregnancy, including placental insufficiency, diabetes, and other hormonal imbalances, have been established in the monkey and offer opportunities for the solution of grievously insoluble problems in fetal medicine.

Dr. Cheek's book is an important first step as an authoritative and precise description of the chemical anatomy of the normal fetal monkey and permits comparisons with similar human fetal data. The variations in this chemical anatomy with experimental alterations of the fetal environment suggest a number of important

explanations for human fetal aberrations that have heretofore been poorly understood.

This volume should initiate a series of investigative efforts in the primate that
will permit real progress in the conquest of fetal morbidity which still represents
the major cause of serious handicapping conditions for our society in terms of loss
of man-years of productivity and in terms of human sorrow.

ROBERT E. COOKE

Preface

In 1962, using our previous experience in the field of body composition, we began to assess growth from the viewpoint of cell size and cell number. These findings were discussed at a conference held by the New York Academy of Science (*Proceedings*, Vol. 110). An important role was suggested for growth hormone in cell multiplication and insulin in cytoplasmic growth, especially in muscle tissue. We became aware that the action of these hormones could be influenced by undernutrition and overnutrition. At a Ross Conference held in Baltimore in March 1965, we reported that growth hormone was necessary for nuclear replication in muscle in pituitary-insufficient humans, rats, and mice. William Daughaday, at the same Ross Conference, showed that the sulfation factor (eventually called somatomedin) was active in bone growth but it was only later that a relationship with cell multiplication in cartilage was demonstrated. Observations on cell replication in tissues were included in our first book which also reported the measurement and study of metabolically active and inactive tissues in postnatal, normal, and abnormal human growth.

Our interest in the role of insulin in human growth began when Professor John Waterlow visited Baltimore in 1966. He discussed changes in amino acid transport in muscle during protein deficiency. Regarding the status of insulin, fibrotic changes had long been known to exist in the pancreas, but it became clear that no satisfactory functional evaluation of hormone secretions had been made. Thus began our interest in insulin levels in marasmus of infants[1].

The present book is, to some extent, a sequel to our previous publication, *Human Growth*. However, attention has been directed almost exclusively to the prenatal growth of the primate (*Macaca mulatta*). Of interest has been the study of individual organs with the measurement in some tissues of cell number and cytoplasmic mass. The effect of hormones and nutrition on the growth process has been examined.

The brain has been the organ of central interest. Many coinvestigators contributed to our previous publication, *Human Growth*, and in this book once again it has been possible to present the work of our collaborators as well as the work of our own program. The progress of research over the last 12 years has given us some insight into factors that influence cell growth and has made us diffident concerning generalized dogma. We have learned, for example, of the great difference between patterns of growth in the rat and those of the primate.

Certain experimental techniques have produced alteration of hormonal or nutritional balance. However, questions answered represent only a small fraction of the problems presenting to the investigator interested in the perinatal period. This has also been stressed in the recent publication No. 540 of WHO (*Maturation of Fetal Body Systems*). Discussion of sex hormones and their influence on fetal and somatic growth has not been documented but can be found in the important papers of Alfred Jost[2].

We believe that future years will create a need for the use of a primate model since the field of perinatology is rapidly advancing. It is appreciated that fetal growth differs biologically and biochemically from postnatal growth and from eventual negative growth (senility). The last section of this book reviews postnatal growth in the human.

There are many aspects of fetal growth that remain unstudied (and not even mentioned in this book). There are other excellent works on the subject, for example the book by Dawes[3] and the recent publication of the centenary symposium for Sir Joseph Barcroft.[4] It is hoped that the present work when placed alongside such texts will help further the understanding of this important but relatively neglected field.

DONALD B. CHEEK

Parkville, Victoria, Australia
February 1975

REFERENCES

1. *Pediatr. Res.* **3**: 579, 1969; **4**: 135, 1970.
2. Jost, A.: *Harvey Lectures*, April 21, 1960 (p. 201).
3. Dawes, G. S.: *Foetal and Neonatal Physiology*. Yearbook, Chicago, 1968.
4. Comline, K. S., Cross, K. W., Dawes, G. S., and Nathanielsz, P. W. (Eds.): *Foetal and Neonatal Physiology* (*Proceedings of the Sir Joseph Barcroft Centenary Symposium, 1972*). Cambridge University Press, London and New York, 1973.

Acknowledgments

The research work reported in this book was made possible by Grant HD00126 of the National Institutes of Child Health and Human Development (a division of the National Institute of Health, Bethesda, Maryland). The time involved in the interpretation of these data and in the reporting of the information was made possible by a grant from the Royal Children's Hospital Research Foundation, Melbourne, Australia.

Grateful thanks are due to a large number of people without whose help this work would not have proceeded. In biochemistry the technical help of Rachel Scott, Elizabeth Higginbottom, Sara Lyles, and Julie Hildenbrand is acknowledged. For the care of primates and the experimental surgery undertaken; the help of Mr. William Bender and Mr. Jerry Harris, is acknowledged. Secretarial help was obtained from Ms. J. Humphries, L. Sprock, J. Lambert, J. Soutar, and C. Van Heurck.

Mr. Clayton Kallman undertook the extensive task of computer programming which was of central importance to the statistical evaluations of Dr. E. David Mellits. The advice of Dr. Edward Melby, Chief of the Division of Animal Medicine at the Johns Hopkins School of Medicine, is gratefully acknowledged. Mr. Adrian Daniel and his staff produced many of the charts and figures appearing in the book. We are grateful to Drs. William London, Jack Bieri, and John Sever of the National Institutes of Health for allowing us to refer to the preliminary experiments on restricted nutrition in the pregnant primate.

Acknowledgments by individual authors are given on the first page of each chapter.

The contributors and coinvestigators have all worked in association with our program, be they students or professors. Guest contributors present work that is related closely to our own. In this direction we have been privileged to have the thinking of Drs. Chez, Roux, and Reynolds, Beatty, Bozek and Gluck. Dr. Roche defines growth in the postpubertal period. All of these investigators have given generously in terms of time and expertise.

This book would never have been completed in the time allotted if it had not been for the superb editorial assistance of Dr. Margaret Sumner who so often provided clarity out of chaos.

D. B. C.

Contents

PART I

THE GROWTH OF THE BRAIN

CHAPTER 1

The Fetus

Donald B. Cheek

INTRODUCTION

In this introductory chapter our interests in fetal growth are outlined and an indication is given of those aspects elaborated on in subsequent chapters. The model chosen is the primate fetus and emphasis is placed on cell growth and particularly brain cell growth. Methods are described for the measurement of cell replication and protein synthesis and consideration is given to the role of the placenta in the delivery of nutrients and the effects of nutrients and hormones on the growth of the fetus. The conclusions from certain of our experiments elucidate these subjects to some extent. We have not investigated the role of sex hormones since the early experiments of Jost[1] have provided information on this aspect of fetal growth.

The growth of the fetus occurs by an increase in cell size and cell number, both processes occurring together in the primate. An understanding of methods for measuring these two parameters is therefore essential to these studies. The amount of deoxyribonucleic acid (DNA) in a tissue may be used as a measure of the cell number since the DNA per nucleus is constant in mammalian cells of the diploid class (about 6.2 pg per nucleus; see Enesco and Leblond[2] for review). Although this calculation has been known for some years its application, especially with respect to growth, was limited until the work of Mendes and Waterlow,[3] Enesco and Leblond,[2] Cheek,[4] and Winick and Noble[5] appeared in the late 1950s and early 1960s.

A measure of cell size may be obtained by relating the protein of the cytoplasm to the DNA and hence assessment of cytoplasmic growth is possible. The use of such an approach necessitates certain assumptions relating to the homogeneity of tissues. The presence of extracellular tissues (eg, collagen) is assumed to be minimal and the occurrence of polyploidy is considered to be associated with a commensurate increase of cytoplasm. The latter assumption holds true for liver cells.[6] The

3

Purkinje cells in brain are polyploid[7-9]* but they constitute only a small fraction of the cell population and little information is available on their cytoplasmic mass.

Cell proliferation may be accompanied by differentiation. An understanding of cellular differentiation will be achieved only when the factors that initiate transcription are elucidated; further discussion is not within the scope of this book. For some cells such as neurons, postnatal proliferation is minimal. At maturity a steady state of cell population exists where cell formation is precisely balanced by an equivalent cell loss. These considerations are dealt with in our previous book concerning postnatal human growth.[10]

Primate growth differs from nonprimate with respect to the growth of the soma and the brain, and therefore an understanding of human growth, normal and abnormal, necessitates the study of primates. Dawes[11] in 1968 recorded the relationship between fetal weight and gestational age in primates and nonprimates and noted that fetal growth rates were almost identical for the rhesus monkey (*Macaca mulatta*) and for man. It is known that the rate of growth of nonprimate mammals is much faster than is that of primates. Thus, using a log-log approach (which describes multiplicative growth), Payne and Wheeler showed in 1967 that the rate of fetal growth was slower for the primate.[12] Attention was drawn to the fact that the milk of primates contained a lower protein and caloric content.

In addition to differences in rates of growth, it can be shown that cellular events differ between rats (for example) and primates. In the rat, prenatal life is associated with cell multiplication without enlargement of cell size.[2,5] In postnatal life increments occur in cell size and cell number but after sexual maturation, cell size alone increases, and then only for a time.[2,5,10] A similar situation may pertain in the primate postnatally as shown by muscle growth.[13] For the primate fetus, however, it has become clear to us that by midgestation, cytoplasmic expansion and DNA replication are in full progress, growth in the macaque and human fetus occurring by increases in both cytoplasmic mass within individual cells and cell number. Mathematical expressions that take these factors into consideration should describe well the changes in fetal weight per age in the primate.[14]

These differences are particularly marked in the growth of the brain, and much of the data in this book relates to this organ. Attention is directed toward differences between the mode of growth of the primate and the nonprimate brains; these differences are of importance since so much of the available evidence on the effects of nutritional deprivation is derived from studies on the rat.

The remarkable similarity between human and subhuman primates with respect to the growth of chemical determinants of the brain is discussed later in this chapter and in Chapter 2. Chapter 4 documents the normal data relating to brain composition of the macaque. Essentially the data have been analyzed to determine the changes in composition in the cerebrum and cerebellum from midgestation into postnatal life, the equations being often cubic or quartic. Inspection of a slice of occipital cortex proved to be unrewarding as an index of cerebral composition.

MACACA MULATTA—THE MODEL

Many of the data presented in the following chapters are derived from experiments using *Macaca mulatta*. The gestational period for the fetus is 167 ± 5 days.[15-23]

---

* Setsuya Fujita (*J. Comp. Neurol.*, **155**:195, 1974) challenges the existence of polyploidy and claims nonspecific light loss (with the technique used) has led to incorrect conclusions.

Table 1.1　　　Weight gain in Macaca mulatta: perinatal
and postnatal period[15-23]

Male	Female
Regain birth weight in 2 weeks	Retain birth weight in 2 weeks
Double birth weight in 94 ± 29 days	Double birth weight in 94 ± 20 days
Weekly gain - 48 g	Weekly gain - 35 g
170 g/month the first year	140-170 g/month to 6/12 year
100 g/month the 2nd year	90-100 g/month $1\frac{1}{2}$ to 2 years
Growth spurt 220 g/month from $3\frac{1}{2}$ to 4 years, slows to 60-80 g/month at 5-6 years	Growth spurt to 140 g/month to $2\frac{1}{3}$ years, slows to 60-70 g/month to $4\frac{1}{2}$ years
Adult weight 9-12 kg	Adult weight 6-8 kg
Fertile 3-4 years	Fertile 3-4 years

The female is known to begin a menstrual cycle every 25 to 29 days, the histologic events and hormonal changes closely resembling those of the human, even to the extent that early cycles are irregular and anovulatory (Tables 1.1 and 1.2).

The pattern of growth for anthropometric measurement during the last trimester is said to be linear[16,19,20] while the average weight at full term is reported as 460 ± 60 g for the female and 480 ± 70 g for the male.[15-23] Infants born of primiparae are lower in weight by at least 50 g. In our own colony, only multiparae have been studied. The studies of Riopelle (personal communication) indicate that maternal protein intake influences the duration of pregnancy while a sex difference is again shown for birth weight. From 120 to 160 days of gestation the fetal weight can be given by the following equation, which includes our own data with the data of Behrman et al:[20]

$$\text{birth weight (grams)} = -522.115 + 6.308 \text{ (gestational age)}$$
$$\text{SD} = 49.5 \text{ g}$$
$$r = 0.84$$
$$n = 47$$

Table 1.2　　　　　　　　　　　　　　Food intake in Macaca mulatta

Age	Cals/kg/day
Day 2	120 ± 50
Day 6	290 ± 60
Day 35-120	240 ± 30
Day 360	200
Adult	80-100
Pregnant female (last trimester)	95-120

Protein intake for adults is estimated at 5g/kg/day

These predictions are in close agreement with those of Van Wagenen and Catchpole,[16] Fujikura and Niemann,[23] Dawes,[11] and Kerr et al.[22]

For the rhesus monkey the head size is already large at birth. The female monkey has a platypeloid type of pelvis; the human female does not have the ability to deliver such a relatively large head (possibly a cost of the complete upright posture). As will be discussed later, in the monkey, brain weight, cerebral cell number, and other components of growth are advanced at birth compared with the human.

CRITICAL PERIODS OF GROWTH

The rat is born with 20% of the expected brain cell number, and the multiplication of neurons continues up until birth.* In the rat by the fifth postnatal day a significant increase occurs in DNA polymerase activity which is followed by an increase in DNA, sulfate incorporation into myelin, and an escalation in carbonic anhydrase activity (present exclusively in neuroglial cells; Figures 1.1 and 1.2). By the 17th day the full complement of cells is reached. These additional cells developing postnatally are mainly neuroglial cells. The figures shown are based on the work of Brasel et al,[24] Chase et al,[25] and Millichap.[26]

Thus the period of 7th to 17th day is one of rapid growth for the rat brain and is considered by Dobbing[27] and Winick[28] to be a critical or vulnerable period when even mild insults to the brain (eg, nutritional restriction) will cause irreversible changes in brain chemistry, function, and structure. Experimental work and studies on nutritional deprivation support the concept of a critical period for brain growth in rats, as discussed in Chapter 6. However, the intensity and nature of the insult are also important. This can be illustrated by studies on the newborn rat during the first week of life, that is, outside the critical period described above. Nutritional deprivation produces no lasting effects but placing the rats in 12% oxygen from day 1 to day 7 can be shown to produce irreversible changes in weight, DNA, and protein content (Figure 1.3) in cerebrum and cerebellum at 5 weeks.[29]

The question arises as to whether critical periods exist for human brain growth. The data of Schulz et al[30] enable the calculation of weight gains for the human brain per unit time (Figure 1.4). Such a velocity curve indicates that spurts of growth for the human brain occur at 32 weeks of gestation and at 20 weeks postnatally. The earlier data of Coppoletta and Wolbach support this conclusion.[31]

If the data on DNA content for the human cerebrum (Figure 1.5) as obtained by Dobbing[31a] are related to age, a quadratic equation can be described. As recorded elsewhere, if the Mellits breaking line technique[10] is applied to this quadratic equation, one can describe the distribution of points as two straight lines, the intersection occurring at 32 weeks of gestation.[32] Here again there is indication of this period as being one of maximal growth. Dobbing has expressed his data as a fourth-order relationship with time, the sigmoid part of the curve indicating neuroblast proliferation.[33]

Winick has stated that "both animal experiments and human studies suggest that a critical period of brain growth may exist during which malnutrition even in a mild form and even for a short time, may produce irreversible damage".[28]

---

* By contrast, the human is born with 30% of expected brain cell number but neuronal division is complete by midgestation. (Dobbing, personal communication).

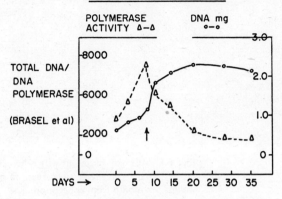

Fig. 1.1. The rise in DNA polymerase activity is shown to precede the accretion of whole brain DNA in the rat. The period between 8 and 10 days would appear to be critical. Curves are calculated from the data of Brasel et al.[24] Reprinted from Richardson (Ed.): "Brain and Intelligence" Copyright 1973 by National Educational Press, Hyattsville, Md.

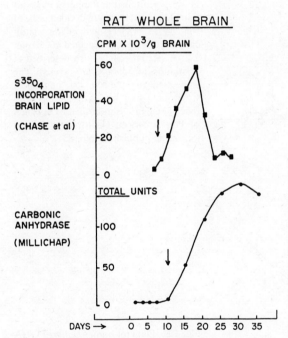

Fig. 1.2. The rise in carbonic anhydrase activity and $S^{35}O^4$ incorporation is seen to occur in the rat brain from the ninth postnatal day. Curves are calculated from the data of Millichap[26] and of Chase et al.[25] Again the period between 8 and 10 days would appear to be critical. Reprinted from Richardson (Ed.): "Brain and Intelligence" Copyright 1973 by National Educational Press, Hyattsville, Md.

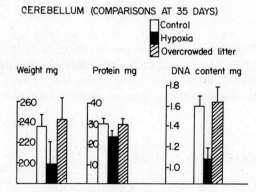

Fig. 1.3. This graph shows significant reduction in weight, protein, and DNA content in the cerebellum of 5-week-old rats exposed to hypoxia (12% oxygen) during the first week of life. The findings in the cerebellum of rats receiving protein restriction during the first week of life are also shown. The graph was constructed from the data in Cheek et al.[29]

7

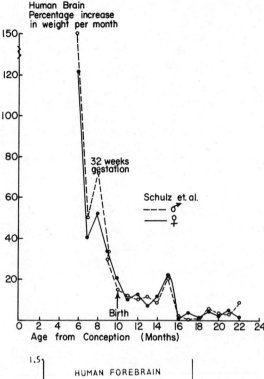

Human Brain Percentage increase in weight per month

32 weeks gestation

Schulz et. al.
--- ♂
— ♀

Birth

Age from Conception (Months)

Fig. 1.4. Human brain growth is expressed as the percentage of increase in weight per month from conception. The data are taken from the work of Schulz et al.[30] Note that at 8 months of gestation (32 weeks) there is a decided peak of velocity in brain growth. (The significance of this peak is discussed in Chapter 27). A second peak is also described at 5 months postnatally (20 weeks). The same peak may be found if the data of Coppoletta and Wolbach[31] are examined. The figure is published by courtesy of Pan American Health Organization (Scientific publication No. 251).

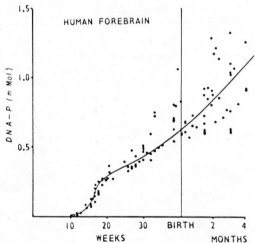

HUMAN FOREBRAIN

DNA-P (mMol)

WEEKS   MONTHS

Fig. 1.5. Data for human cerebral DNA during growth are recorded. (Reprinted from Dobbing et al: *Arch. Des Child.* **48**: No. 10, 1973, with the permission of the Editor.)

Dobbing had a similar message: "the possibility that under-nutrition in early life may permanently reduce the intellectual capacity of men and women has become increasingly recognized".[27] The evidence for such statements rests heavily on animal experiments and in particular on rat experiments. Such work has been critically reviewed elsewhere.[32, 58]

FETAL SUBSTRATE AND NUTRIENTS

Glucose is the main substrate utilized by the fetus; work by the Denver group[34] has demonstrated that amino acids also contribute to the fetal metabolic rate. Essentially the fetus receives a high carbohydrate, low fat "fuel supply." The quality and quantity of all of these nutrients may modify fetal growth. Enzymes are developed in the fetal liver to accommodate the metabolism of such substrates. In the neonatal rat, ketone bodies are utilized,[35,36] although no such information is available for the primate.

Mammals require essential amino acids in both prenatal and postnatal life. Clearly, the liver is one of the most important tissues for protein synthesis whereas liver, kidney, and muscle must account for much of the protein turnover. The liver plays an important role in regulating the incoming amino acids and can convert a large amount of amino nitrogen to urea prior to any further distribution of amino acids to other tissues.[37]

Our knowledge of the mechanisms of protein synthesis is incomplete. What is known has been reviewed by Munro.[38–40] It can be mentioned that 90% of liver cell RNA in the mature mammal is ribosomal[41] and aggregation of messenger RNA to ribosomes will only occur if the concentrations of all amino acids needed are optimal within the intracellular phase. Polysomal aggregation is the gauge of potential protein synthesis and is dependent on amino acid patterns.

Studies on the role of glucose, the secretion of insulin, and the role of the beta cell of the pancreas form an important portion of this book (Chapters 9 and 18). Data on plasma and tissue amino acids during development also form major chapters (10 and 20). The pattern of change of amino acids during normal and abnormal fetal growth is of great interest.

It is thought that the fatty acids and triglycerides in adipose tissue are derived from glucose conversion[42] since all the necessary enzymes are present in fetal adipose tissue.[43] In rats the fatty acid transport across the placenta is minimal or absent[44–48] but this is not the case for primates,[49,50] guinea pigs,[51–54] or sheep.[55] In the human the free fatty acid levels are far lower in the infant than in the mother, suggesting little placental transfer. However, lipoprotein lipase is present in placental tissue[56] so that lipolysis of the circulating esters may occur in the placenta with subsequent transfer of the free fatty acid to the fetus. If such is the case, then the low circulating level in the fetus may be due to rapid incorporation into adipocytes. It is probable that the fatty acids are transported and form a minor source of substrate.*

It has been pointed out by Sinclair[57] that the supply of substrates and nutrients to the fetus is necessary for three processes:

1. Maintenance—the chemical work or work of transport and concentration and the mechanical work required of each cell for its existence in a steady state.
2. Growth—the net formation of new cytoplasm.
3. Differentiation—or changing composition with characterization of specific tissue.

The process of growth requires the net input of energy for cell division and for cytoplasmic accretion, all of which is supplied by chemical energy.

Sinclair[57] has calculated the relationship between the resting oxygen consumption of human infants with gestational ages ranging from 25 to 42 weeks. Basically the measurement of resting oxygen consumption monitors the tissue mass of active cells. His results indicated a rate of increase of total metabolism of 10% per week or a doubling of the metabolic rate every 41 days from 24 to 42 weeks of gestation,

*Recent studies by Hull, D. B., Hudson, D., Elphick, M. C. and Saunders, R. R. (*Australian Paed. Assoc.*, 1975) concerning venous-arterial differences for FFA in human cord blood suggest that maternal fatty acids can make a major contribution to fetal fat stores.

while the rate of increase in cell number during the last trimester is about 10% per week. For *Macaca mulatta* basal metabolic rate and protein and calorie requirements are almost exactly double those of the human, so that a more rapid increase in cell number might be expected.

ATTAINMENT OF EXPECTED BRAIN SIZE AND CELL COMPLEMENT

With respect to brain cell numbers and conditions that may change the expected complement of cells, it is of importance to know what the expected normals and range of values are for the human.

The data concerning human brain DNA content are controversial. It has been pointed out[58] that the data of Winick[59-62] differ from the data of Dobbing and Sands[33] by two standard deviations (Figure 1.6). Moreover, the data of Howard et al[63] agree with those of Dobbing within the lower range of points. It would ap-

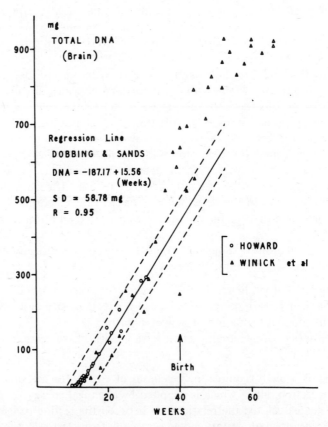

Fig. 1.6. The data of Dobbing and Sands[33] for whole brain DNA in the numan are expressed as a linear regression (the points are not shown but fall evenly around the line). One standard deviation around the line is shown by interrupted lines. Studies by Winick[59-61] are shown by triangles. The data of Howard et al[63] are shown by the open circles. These latter data agree with those of Dobbing. Reprinted from Richardson (Ed.): "Brain and Intelligence" Copyright 1973 by National Educational Press, Hyattsville, Md.

pear that the data of Dobbing are correct and that brain DNA content continues to increase until 2 years of age. Indeed, as pointed out elsewhere,[58] the concentration of DNA and protein in the brain differs in the various studies carried out by Winick.

Zamenhof and van Marthens[64] have reviewed their work on factors that influence the DNA content of the cerebral hemispheres of the rat and chicken. Findings in the chicken paralleled those in the rat; individual brain weight did not correlate with brain DNA content but on the average a higher number of neonatal brain cells was associated with a higher neonatal brain weight. The occasional rat, however, demonstrated an unusually high cerebral DNA content. Nutritional and hormonal influences could be demonstrated.

RELATIONSHIP OF BRAIN SIZE TO INTELLIGENCE

There are many reports in the literature of attempts to relate intelligence to various parameters of brain growth. However, there would seem to be no simple linear relationships between brain size, head circumference, and brain cell number, nor can any of these be related to intelligence. Neuroglial cells outnumber neuronal cells 10 to 1, so that variations in brain cell number may largely be a reflection of changes in glial cells and would not be expected to influence intelligence. Tobias[65] has discussed the relationship between head size and brain size and points out that Anatole France of Paris had a very small recorded brain size while the German philosopher Immanuel Kant, a mental giant, also had a very small brain.[66] Clearly, patients with gross microcephaly and a disproportionately small brain relative to body size represent an exceptional situation.

In our view, it cannot be too strongly emphasized that the finding of a reduced DNA content in the brain will have significance only if it can be related to the type of cell involved, the region of the brain concerned, and the functional consequences.

LIMITATION OF NUTRIENTS

In this book two approaches have been used to restrict nutrients to the fetus. The first has been to ligate the bridging vessels between the two placentas. A bidiscoid placenta is characteristic for *Macaca mulatta*; the secondary placenta constitutes up to 40% of total placental mass. By such an approach at 100 days of gestation, it is reasonable to believe that substrate supply would be restricted and at the same time a degree of hypoxia may also exist (Chapter 7).

The second approach (Chapter 6) has been to limit the protein and calorie intake in the maternal diet early in pregnancy. With both approaches, alterations in the growth and the biochemistry of brain have been found (particularly in the cerebellum). The obvious question is whether such changes or growth arrest would be reversible with adequate nutrition postnatally. Only future work will yield such answers.

The effect of restricted nutrition and/or of reduced placental blood supply is discussed later in this chapter and again in later chapters of this book. It can be mentioned here that restricted nutrition (8% protein) to the pregnant rat for 1 month prior to pregnancy and through gestation resulted in a reduced brain weight and reduced cerebral DNA content in the offspring; the protein per cell was 10% lower than expected. In another approach (tying off one of the uterine horns prior to mating so that only half of the normal fetuses developed), in those fetuses that developed there was a significant increase in cerebral DNA content. Extrapolation of these data would suggest that a single fetus could be produced with a 19% increase in brain DNA content.[64] When considering these results it must be remembered that during pregnancy the rate of accretion of tissues (protein) is much more rapid for the small mammal (Chapter 6). Restriction of maternal protein intake may therefore be more devastating for the rat than for the primate.[58]

It is clear from our own work (Chapter 6) that some growth arrest can be induced in the fetal primate by restriction of nutrients but whether, as in the guinea pig,[67] permanent cerebellar changes can be produced remains for further study. If the duration of insult continues from the fetal stage throughout childhood, such growth arrest would seem certain to produce brain dysfunction with mental aberration.

Experiments regarding maternal food restriction during pregnancy in the primate are of importance because, with widespread malnutrition existing in many areas of the world, this situation is common in the life of many humans.

Data for the human situation are sparse but the following observations are relevant. "Small for dates" babies contribute heavily to the group of children that have growth retardation with and without mental impairment.[68,69] In parabiotic twins, a transfusion syndrome may develop, the smaller fetus losing blood to the other through arteriovenous communication or "third circulation."[70,71] Although an extreme example, the smaller twin has the lower intelligence quotient.[67] Recent work by Lubchenco et al[72] shows that prematurity with a birth weight of less than 1500 g in the human accounts for a sizable number of mentally retarded children, especially if protein restriction is present in the early weeks of postnatal life. The information relating to the wartime starvation in Holland can be cited, when caloric intake fell to 400 per person per day. The newborn infants were retarded in growth.[73] The offspring (now 29 and 30 years old) were investigated by Stein and co-workers and no deficit in intelligence was found.[74]

Hypoxia may be of far greater significance than maternal food restriction in terms of subsequent brain damage in the offspring (Figure 1.3).[29] Windle[78] has shown that newborn rhesus monkeys exposed for short periods to hypoxia or asphyxia may appear to recover clinically but closer inspection reveals permanent structural brain damage. Neuropathology can be detected in brain stem centers, the inferior colliculus and ventrolateral thalamic nuclei being particularly susceptible. Asphyxia in monkeys has been shown to produce hypotonia of the muscles with difficulty in swallowing, sucking, or locomotion, lack of interest and of dexterity being characteristic. Prolonged asphyxia produces lesions of the cerebellar vermis, the globus pallidus, and in addition small areas of degeneration appear in the cerebral cortex.[79]

Interpretation of data for the human situation is difficult because it is possible that, in the human, other factors may operate. Intelligence is impaired if the environment includes complete emotional deprivation with lack of stimulation.[75–77]

However, there are clear indications that the growth and cell number in the brain can be modified during development by manipulation of the nutritional status of the fetus. Growth arrest can be produced or cell multiplication accelerated. Are these changes permanent? These questions are discussed in more detail in Chapters 6 and 7.

HORMONES

For some time a role for insulin as a major fetal growth hormone has been suspected. Our finding (Chapter 18) that ablation of fetal beta cells can produce a small-for-dates fetal monkey supports the argument. However, the problem is not simple since a normal-sized infant may present with enlargement of the adrenal gland. We consider this situation to result from reactive hyperplasia of the beta cells (or their progenitors). Ablation of maternal islet cells has produced the over-sized fetus with excess body fat and tissue growth (Chapter 18). Not only is there the expected visceromegaly and excess fat deposition but specific increases in cell cytoplasm including cerebral cells. It is difficult to escape the conclusion that insulin plays an important role in brain cell growth (Chapter 9).

Several workers consider that the fetal pancreas is inactive prior to birth.[80-82] Argument exists as to whether the pituitary shows changes in infants born of diabetic mothers[83, 84] but the pituitary per se is thought not to be responsible for the overgrowth of such fetuses. Of importance perhaps is the finding of an enlarged adrenal gland[84, 85] and the possibility exists that the hypothalamus and pancreas work together[86, 87] with the adrenal to modify fetal growth. Some of our data have been published elsewhere.[88-90]

Ablation of the fetal thyroid and the reduction of maternal thyroid function produce, we find, significant changes in fetal brain growth of the primate. The athyroid fetus is unable to synthesize protein effectively in the central nervous system (Chapter 8), while at the same time there is little evidence that DNA replication has been compromised in the cerebrum.[91] In this instance a similarity exists between the fetal primate and the neonatal rat, where the brain has been studied in animals in which thyroid ablation was carried out immediately after birth.[92-96] It is difficult to ascribe changes in the brain of these rats to a lack of thyroid hormone per se since growth hormone was also involved.[97-105] An association between thyroid hormone and growth hormone has often been suggested[106] and one might speculate that both hormones are required for proper brain development and protein synthesis. By contrast later in postnatal life (after infancy) it is also clear that thyroid hormone has little action with respect to protein synthesis.

Hypophysectomy in the fetal rhesus monkey has little effect on somatic growth[107-109] but an action on brain growth, especially in the case of the rat, cannot be discarded.[110-112]

Hypophysectomy of the pregnant rat on the 12th day of gestation, if combined with protein calorie restriction, produces a greater retardation in brain and somatic growth of the offspring than when food restriction alone is present[113]. In the latter situation Chow[114] considered that the pituitary gland was centrally involved since the growth hormone content of the pituitary in such offspring was reduced and the administration of growth hormone improved somatic growth. However, pituitary extract not containing growth hormone normalized behavioral changes. Thus some other hormone, perhaps thyroid stimulating hormone, may also be involved, in these rat experiments.

Thyroid hormone certainly influences fetal somatic growth as well as brain growth. Cytoplasmic growth or protein synthesis in the fetal lamb is reduced in the absence of the hormone[115]. Changes are thought to be similar to the effects of ablation of the fetal ovine pituitary[116].

BRAIN GROWTH: MACAQUE VERSUS HUMAN

In concluding this introduction it is appropriate to set the stage with a comparison of human growth versus that of a lower primate. With respect to the brain such a comparison is possible since Dr. John Dobbing and his co-workers have provided important information concerning human brain composition and Dr. Evelyn Howard has also published information on human growth up until the 30th week of gestation.

In Figure 1.7 is shown the similarity of growth in weight of the human brain versus that of the macaque. The weight scale of the macaque has been expanded 15-fold while the age scale has been expanded threefold. (This assumes that 1 day in the life of the monkey is equivalent to 3 days in the life of the human.)

The similarity in growth patterns is obvious (as will be noted for all primates in Chapter 2). The data for the human cerebrum and cerebellum[63] are compared with those of the macaque and considered against time (Figure 1.8). As pointed out by Dobbing[27] the event of birth seems of little significance in mammals when one considers brain growth. Brain weight follows a sigmoid curve in all mammals[14] with the event of birth occurring at different times on the curve. For the smaller mammals, such as the rat, the major spurt in brain growth is postnatal and growth rate is faster.

Brain weight is mainly accounted for by water and this water can be divided into a neuronal and nonneuronal space (Chapter 3).

The pattern of changes in percent water in the brain of the human versus that of the macaque is similar (Figure 1.9). Also, DNA values for man and monkey appear to be similar from birth and do not change with maturity (Figure 1.10). A difference exists between man and monkey insofar as cerebellar growth (the rate of cell number increase) is faster for macaque. Thus for the cerebellum the DNA concentration for the macaque reaches a peak just prior to birth (Figure 1.11). For the human the peak occurs in postnatal life. However, the values at maturity and the peak values are of similar order in both primates. The increase in cerebral cholesterol concentration (an indication of myelination) is similar in man and monkey throughout development and at maturity (Figure 1.12).

Thus, many aspects of growth and development are similar in the macaque and the human brain. For this reason, and because rodent brain growth shows many dissimilarities, we feel that extrapolations from primate models will probably have far greater predictive value for human growth than will those made from rodent models.

WHOLE BRAIN

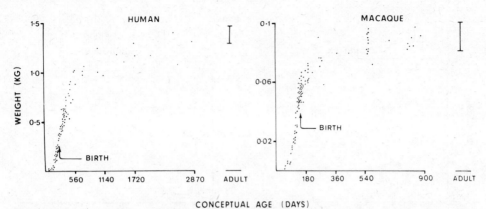

Fig. 1.7.   Growth of the human and macaque brain with the weight scale for the macaque expanded 15-fold thus giving adult macaque and human weights a similar scale of magnitude. The age scale for the macaque was then arbitrarily expanded until a pattern approximating the human brain curve was obtained. One could assume that with respect to brain growth, 1 day in the life of a monkey is equivalent to 3 days in the life of the human. The human data are derived from the work of Dobbing.[112] The macaque results are from data collected by us and additional data kindly provided by Dr. Oscar Portman of the Oregon Regional Primate Center.

Fig. 1.8.   A comparison of cerebral and cerebellar weights of the monkey and human during fetal life demonstrates the advanced development of the macaque brain in relation to time. Note that the macaque cerebrum weight plateaus after 140 days. The human data are taken from the work of Howard et al.[63]

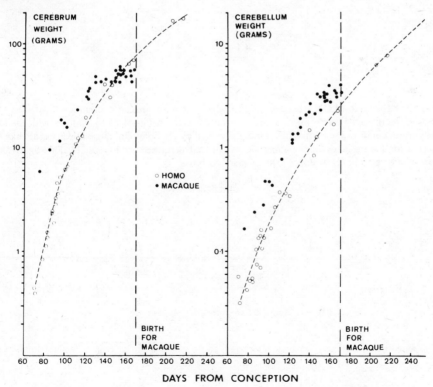

WHOLE BRAIN

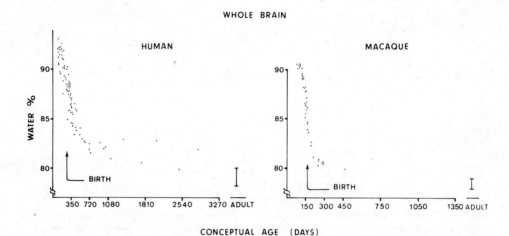

CONCEPTUAL AGE (DAYS)

Fig. 1.9. Water content in the human and macaque brain demonstrating a similarity in the magnitude and pattern of change of percent water exists in the human and macaque brain. The age scale has been adjusted for the macaque in a manner similar to that described for Figure 1.7. The human data are derived from the work of Dobbing.[112]

Fig. 1.10. The cerebral DNA concentration in the human and macaque brain is shown. The DNA values of the macaque cerebrum have been converted to DNA-P (μM/g) to conform with the DNA concentrating units of the human data kindly provided by Dr. John Dobbing. The age scale has been adjusted for the macaque in a manner similar to that described for Figure 1.7. This figure shows the rapid decrease in DNA concentration prior to birth.

CEREBRUM

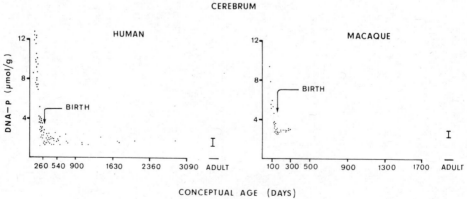

CONCEPTUAL AGE (DAYS)

16

CEREBELLUM

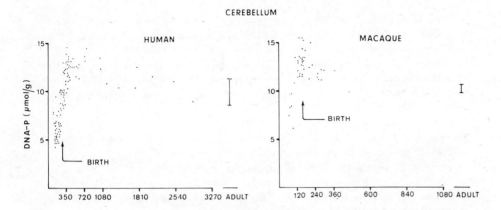

CONCEPTUAL AGE (DAYS)

Fig. 1.11. The cerebellar DNA concentration in the human and macaque brain is shown. The peak in cerebellar DNA concentration of the macaque has been made to coincide with that of the human by adjusting the relevant time scale. The DNA values of the macaque cerebellum have been converted to DNA-P (μM/g) to conform to the DNA concentration units of the human data kindly provided by Dr. John Dobbing. Note that the peak for the human is after birth and that of the macaque before.

Fig. 1.12. Cerebral cholesterol concentration is shown for the human and macaque brain. The age scale has been adjusted for the macaque in a manner similar to that described for Figure 1.7. The range of cerebral cholesterol concentrations appears to be similar in adult humans and macaques. The human data were kindly provided by Dr. John Dobbing.

CEREBRUM

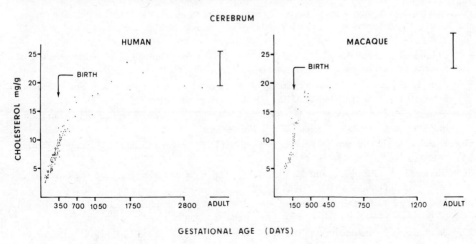

GESTATIONAL AGE (DAYS)

17

REFERENCES

1. Jost, A.: The role of fetal hormones in prenatal development. *Harvey Lect.* **55**:201, 1961.

2. Enesco, M., and Leblond, C.: Increase in cell number, as a factor in the growth of the organs and tissues of the young male rats. *J. Embryol. Exp. Morphol.* **10**:530, 1962.

3. Mendes, C. B., and Waterlow, J. C.: The effect of a low protein diet and refeeding on the composition of the liver and muscle in the weanling rat. *Br. J. Nutr.* **12**:74, 1958.

4. Cheek, D. B.: Cell growth and body composition. *Ann. N.Y. Acad. Sci.* **110**:865, 1963.

5. Winick, M., and Noble, A.: Quantitative changes in DNA, RNA and protein during prenatal and postnatal growth in the rat. *Dev. Biol.* **12**:451, 1965.

6. Epstein, C. J.: Cell size, nuclear content and the development of polyploidy in the mammalian liver. *Proc. Natl. Acad. Sci. U.S.A.* **57**:327, 1967.

7. Lentz, R. D., and Lapham, L. W.: A quantitative cytochemical study of the content of neurons of rat cerebellar cortex. *J. Neurochem.* **16**:379, 1969.

8. Herman, C. J., and Lapham, L. W.: Neuronal polyploidy. and nuclear volumes in the cat central nervous system. *Brain Res.* **15**:35, 1969.

9. Lentz, R. D., and Lapham, L. W.: Postnatal development of tetraploid DNA content in rat Purkinje cells: A quantitative cytochemical study. *J. Neuropathol. Exp. Neurol.* **29**:43, 1970.

10. Cheek, D. B.: Body composition, cell growth, energy and intelligence. In: Cheek, D. B. (Ed.): *Human Growth*. Lea & Febiger, Philadelphia, 1968.

11. Dawes, G. S.: The placenta and foetal growth. In: Dawes, G. S. (Ed.): *Foetal and Neonatal Physiology*. Yearbook, Chicago, 1968, pp. 42–59.

12. Payne, P. R., and Wheeler, E. F.: Comparative nutrition in pregnancy. *Nature* **215**:1134, 1967.

13. Cheek, D. B., Holt, A. B., Hill, D. E., and Talbert, J. L.: Skeletal muscle cell mass and growth: The concept of the deoxyribonucleic acid unit. *Pediatr. Res.* **5**:312, 1971.

14. Laird, A. K.: Evolution of the human growth curve. *Growth* **31**:345, 1967.

15. Van Wagenen, G., and Catchpole, H. R.: Physical growth of the rhesus monkey (*Macaca mulatta*). *Am. J. Phys. Anthropol.* **14**:245, 1956.

16. Van Wagenen, G., and Catchpole, H. R.: Growth of the fetus and placenta of the monkey (*Macaca mulatta*). *Am. J. Phys. Anthropol.* **23**:23, 1965.

17. Jacobson, H. M., and Windle, W. F.: Observations on mating, gestation, birth and postnatal development of *Macaca mulatta*. *Biol. Neonate* **2**:105, 1960.

18. Pickering, D. E.: Reproduction characteristics in a colony of laboratory confined macaque mulatta monkeys. *Folia Primatol.* **8**:169, 1968.

19. Kerr, G. R., Kennan, A. L., Waisman, H. A., and Allen, J. R.: Growth and development of the fetal rhesus monkey. I. Physical growth. *Growth* **33**:201, 1969.

20. Behrman, R. E., Seeds, E. A., Battaglia, F. C., Hellegers, A. E., and Bruns, P. D.: The normal changes in mass and water content in fetal rhesus monkey and placenta throughout gestation. *J. Pediatr.* **65**:38, 1964.

21. Valerio, D. A., Pallotta, A. J., and Courtney, K. D.: Experiences in large-scale breeding of simians for medical experimentations. *Ann. N.Y. Acad. Sci.* **162**:282, 1969.

22. Kerr, G. R., Scheffler, G., and Waisman, H. A.: Growth and development of infant *M. mulatta* fed a standardized diet. *Growth* **33**:185, 1969.

23. Fujikura, T., and Niemann, W. H.: Birth weight, gestational age and type of delivery in rhesus monkeys. *Am. J. Obstet. Gynecol.* **97**:76, 1967.

24. Brasel, J. A., Ehrenkranz, R. A., and Winick, M.: DNA polymerase activity in rat brain during ontogeny. *Dev. Biol.* **23**:424, 1970.

25. Chase, H. P., Dorsey, J., and McKhann, G.: The effect of malnutrition on the synthesis of myelin lipid. *Pediatrics* **40**:551, 1967.

26. Millichap, J. G.: Development of seizure patterns in newborn animals: Significance of brain carbonic anhydrase. *Proc. Soc. Exp. Biol. Med.* **96**:125, 1957.

27. Dobbing, J.: Undernutrition in the developing brain. *Am. J. Dis. Child.* **120**:411, 1970.

28. Winick, M.: Malnutrition and brain development. *J. Pediatr*. **74**:667, 1969.

29. Cheek, D. B., Graystone, J. E., and Rowe, R. D.: Hypoxia and malnutrition in newborn rats: Effects of RNA, DNA and protein in tissues. *Am. J. Physiol*. **217**:642, 1969.

30. Schulz, D. M., Gordiano, D. A., and Schulz, D. H.: Weights of organs of fetuses and infants. *Arch. Pathol*. **74**:244, 1962.

31. Coppoletta, J. M., and Wolbach, S. B.: Body length and organ weights of infants and children: Study of body length and normal weights of more important vital organs of body between birth and 12 years of age. *Am. J. Pathol*. **9**:55, 1933.

31a. Dobbing, J., and Sands, J.: Quantitative growth and development of human brain. *Arch. Dis. Child*. **48**:757, 1973.

32. Cheek, D. B., Holt, A. B., and Mellits, E. D.: Malnutrition and the nervous system. Symposium on nutrition, the nervous system and behaviour, Jamaica, January 10, 1972. *Pan American Health Organisation* **251**:3, 1972.

33. Dobbing, J., and Sands, J.: Timing in neuroblast multiplication in developing human brain. *Nature* **226**:639, 1970.

34. James, E. J., Raye, J. R., Gresham, E. L., Makowski, E. L., Meschia, G., and Battaglia, F. C.: Fetal oxygen consumption, carbon dioxide production and glucose uptake in a chronic sheep preparation. *Pediatrics* **50**: 361, 1972.

35. Hawkins, R. A., Williamson, D. H., and Krebs, H. A.: Ketone-body utilization by adult and suckling rat brain in vivo. *Biochem. J*. **122**:13, 1971.

36. Page, M. A., Krebs, H. A., and Williamson, D. H.: Activities of enzymes of ketone-body utilization in brain and other tissues of suckling rats. *Biochem. J*. **121**:49, 1971.

37. Elwyn, D.: In: Munro, H. N. (Ed.): *Mammalian Protein Metabolism*, Vol. IV. Academic Press, New York, 1970.

38. Munro, H. N.: A general survey of mechanisms regulating protein metabolism in mammals. In: Munro, H. N. (Ed.): *Mammalian Protein Metabolism*. Academic Press, New York, 1970.

39. Munro, H. N.: Free amino acid pools and their role in regulation. In: Munro, H. N. (Ed.): *Mammalian Protein Metabolism*, Vol. IV. Academic Press, New York, 1970, Chapter 34.

40. Munro, H. N.: Regulation of liver ribosome function in relation to amino acid supply. In: San Pietro, A., Lamborg, M. R., and Kenney, F. T. (Eds.): *Regulatory Mechanisms for Protein Synthesis in Mammalian Cells*. Academic Press, New York, 1968, p. 183.

41. Hirsch, C. A.: Quantitative determination of the ribosomal ribonucleic acid content of liver and Novikoff hepatoma from fed and from fasted rats. *J. Biol. Chem*. **242**:2822, 1967.

42. Pedersen, J., and Osler, M.: Hyperglycaemia as the cause of characteristic features of the fetus and newborn of diabetic mothers. *Danish Med. Bull*. **8**:78, 1961.

43. Villee, C. A., and Hagerman, D. D.: Effect of oxygen deprivation on the metabolism of fetal and adult tissues. *Am. J. Physiol*. **194**: 457, 1958.

44. Goldwater, W. H., and Stetten, D.: Studies in fetal metabolism. *J. Biol. Chem*. **169**:732, 1947.

45. Popjak, G.: The origin of fetal lipids. *Cold Spring Harbor Symp. Quant. Biol*. **19**:200, 1954.

46. Mueller, P. S., Solomon, F., and Brown, J. R.: Free fatty acid concentration in maternal plasma and fetal body fat content. *Am. J. Obstet. Gynecol*. **88**:196, 1964.

47. Fain, J. N., and Scow, R. O.: Fatty acid synthesis *in vivo* in maternal and fetal tissues in the rat. *Am. J. Physiol*. **210**:19, 1966.

48. Koren, Z., and Shafrir, E.: Placental transfer of free fatty acids in the pregnant rat. *Proc. Soc. Exp. Biol. Med*. **116**:411, 1964.

49. Portman, O. W., Behrman, R. E., and Soltys, P.: Transfer of free fatty acids across the primate placenta. *Am. J. Physiol*. **216**:143, 1969.

50. Szabo, A. J., and Grimaldi, R. D.: The effect of insulin on glucose metabolism of the incubated human placenta. *Am. J. Obstet. Gynecol*. **106**:75, 1970.

51. Hershfield, M. S., and Nemeth, A. M.: Placental transport of free palmitic and linoleic acids in the guinea pig. *J. Lipid Res*. **9**:460, 1968.

52. McBride, O. W., and Korn, E. D.: Uptake of free fatty acids and chylomicron glycerides by guinea pig mammary gland in pregnancy and lactation. *J. Lipid Res*. **5**:453, 1964.

53. Satomura, K., and Soderhjelm, L.: Deposition of fatty acids in the newborn in relation to the diet of pregnant guinea pigs: A preliminary report. *Texas Rep. Biol. Med.* **20**:671, 1962.

54. Kayden, H. J., Dancis, J., and Money, W. L.: Transfer of lipids across the guinea pig placenta. *Am. J. Obstet. Gynecol.* **104**:564, 1969.

55. Van Duyne, C. M., Parker, H. R., Havel, R. J., and Holm, L. W.: Free fatty acid metabolism in fetal and newborn sheep. *Am. J. Physiol.* **199**:987, 1960.

56. Paluszak, J., Wosicki, A., and Rakowski, W.: Studies on the lipolytic system of the human placenta. *Acta Med. Pol.* **7**:179, 1967.

57. Sinclair, J. C.: Energy metabolism and fetal development. In: Waisman, H. A., and Kerr, G. (Eds.): *Fetal Growth and Development.* McGraw-Hill, New York, 1970, p. 201.

58. Cheek, D. B.: Brain growth and nucleic acids: Effect of nutritional deprivation. In: Richardson, F. (Ed.): *Brain and Intelligence: Ecology of Child Human Development.* National Educational Press, Maryland, 1973, p. 237.

59. Winick, M., Rosso, P., and Waterlow, J.: Cellular growth of cerebrum, cerebellum, and brain stem in normal and marasmic children. *Exp. Neurol.* **26**:393, 1970.

60. Winick, M.: Changes in nucleic acid and protein content during growth of human brain. *Pediatr. Res.* **2**:352, 1968.

61. Winick, M., and Rosso, P.: The effect of severe early malnutrition on the human brain. *Pediatr. Res.* **3**:181, 1969.

62. Winick, M., Brasel, J. A., and Rosso, P.: Nutrition and cell growth. In: Winick, M. (Ed.): *Nutrition and Development.* Wiley, New York, 1972, p. 54.

63. Howard, E., Granoff, D., and Bujnovszky, P.: DNA, RNA and cholesterol increases in cerebrum and cerebellum during development of human fetuses. *Brain Res.* **14**:697, 1969.

64. Zamenhof, S., and van Marthens, E.: Hormonal and nutritional aspects of prenatal brain development. In: Pease, D. C. (Ed.): *Cellular Aspects of Neural Growth and Differentiation.* U.C.L.A. Forum in Medical Sciences, No. 14, 1971, p. 329.

65. Tobias, P. V.: Brain-size, grey matter and race—Fact or fiction? *Am. J. Phys. Anthropol.* **32**:3, 1970.

66. Hamburgh, M.: In: Zamenhof, S., and van Marthens, E.: Hormonal and nutritional aspects of prenatal brain development. In: Pease, D. C. (Ed.): *Cellular Aspects of Neural Growth and Differentiation.* U.C.L.A. Forum in Medical Sciences, No. 14, 1971, p. 355.

67. Chase, H. P., Dabiere, C. W., Welch, N. N., and O'Brien, D.: Intrauterine undernutrition and brain development. *Pediatrics* **47**:491, 1971.

68. Drillien, C. M.: Intellectual sequelae of "fetal malnutrition." In: Waisman, H. A., and Kerr, G. (Eds.): *Fetal Growth and Development.* McGraw-Hill, New York, 1970, Chapter 22.

69. Holley, W. L., and Churchill, J. A.: Physical and mental deficits of twinning. In: *Perinatal Factors Affecting Human Development.* Proceedings of the Special Session of the Eighth Meeting of PAHO Advisory Committee on Medical Research, October 1969, p. 24.

70. Naeye, R. L.: Structural correlates of fetal undernutrition. In: Waisman, H. A., and Kerr, G. (Eds.): *Fetal Growth and Development.* McGraw-Hill, New York, 1970, Chapter 19.

71. Benirschke, K., and Hoefnagel, D.: Structural development of the placenta in relation to fetal growth. In: Waisman, H. A., and Kerr, G. (Eds.): *Fetal Growth and Development.* McGraw-Hill, New York, 1970, Chapter 1.

72. Lubchenco, L. O., Delivoria-Papadopoulos, M., and Searls, D.: Long term follow up studies of prematurely born infants. II. Influence of birth weight and gestational age on sequelae. *J. Pediatr.* **80**:509, 1972.

73. Smith, C. A.: The effect of wartime starvation in Holland upon pregnancy and its product. *Am. J. Obstet. Gynecol.* **April**:559, 1947.

74. Stein, Z. A., Susser, M., Saenger, G., and Marolla, F.: Nutrition and mental performance. *Science* **178**:708, 1972.

75. Dobbing, J.: Lasting deficits and distortions of the adult brain following infantile undernutrition. Symposium on nutrition, the nervous system and behaviour, Jamaica, January 10, 1972. *Pan American Health Organisation* **251**:15, 1972.

76. Barnes, R. H.: Nutrition and man's intellect and behavior. *Fed. Proc.* **30**:1429, 1971.

77. Frisch, R. E.: Present status of the supposition that malnutrition causes permanent mental retardation. *Am. J. Clin. Nutr.* **23**:189, 1970.

78. Windle, W. F.: Asphyxial brain damage at birth, with reference to the minimally affected child. In: *Perinatal Factors Affecting Human Development*. Proceedings of the Special Session of the Eighth Meeting of PAHO Advisory Committee on Medical Research, October 1969, p. 215.

79. James, S.: Administration of oxygen, glucose, and alkali to mother and newborn. In: *Perinatal Factors Affecting Human Development*. Proceedings of the Special Session of the Eighth Meeting of PAHO Advisory Committee on Medical Research, October 1969, p. 239.

80. Baird, J. D., and Farquhar, J. W.: Insulin secreting capacity in newborn infants of normal and diabetic women. *Lancet* **1**:71, 1962.

81. Milner, D. E., Demoor, P., and Lukens, F. D. W.: Relation of purified pituitary growth hormone and insulin in regulation of nitrogen balance. *Am. J. Physiol.* **166**:354, 1951.

82. Schwartz, R.: Metabolic fuels in the fetus. *Proc. Roy. Soc. Med.* **61**:1231, 1968.

83. Naeye, R. L.: Infants of diabetic mothers. A quantitative morphologic study. *Pediatrics* **35**:980, 1965.

84. Gaunt, W. D., Bahn, R. C., and Hayles, A. B.: A quantitative cytological study of the anterior hypophysis of infants born of diabetic mothers. *Proc. Mayo Clin.* **37**:345, 1962.

85. Naeye, R. L.: New observations in erythroblastosis fetalis. *J.A.M.A.* **200**:281, 1967.

86. Han, P. W., Yu, Y. K., and Chow, S. L.: Enlarged pancreatic islets of tube-fed hypophysectomized rats bearing hypothalamic lesions. *Am. J. Physiol.* **218**:769, 1970.

87. Idahl, L.-A., and Martin, J. M.: Stimulation of insulin release by a ventro-lateral hypothalamic factor. *J. Endocrinol.* **51**:601, 1971.

88. Cheek, D. B., Brayton, J. B., and Scott, R. E.: Overnutrition, overgrowth and hormonal balance in the fetus and adolescent (the infant born of the diabetic mother). Burg Wartenstein Symposium No. 60, Nutrition and Malnutrition, Roche, A. F. and Falkner, F. (Eds.), *Advances in Experimental Medicine and Biology* **49**:47, 1974.

89. Cheek, D. B.: Insulin, early cell growth and excess adipose tissue. *Obesity/Barametric Med.* **2**:190, 1973.

90. Hill, D. E., and Cheek, D. B.: Studies on the cellular growth and substrate availability in the rhesus monkey fetus. XIII International Congress of Pediatrics, Wien, Osterreich, Aug. 29–Sept. 4, 1971.

91. Holt, A. B., Kerr, G. R., and Cheek, D. B.: Prenatal hypothyroidism and brain composition in the primate. *Nature* **243**:413, 1973.

92. Geel, S., and Timiras, P. S.: The influence of neonatal hypothyroidism and of thyroxine on the ribonucleic acid and deoxyribonucleic acid concentrations of the rat cerebral cortex. *Brain Res.* **4**:135, 1967.

93. Gomez, C. J., Ghittoni, N. E., and Dellacha, J. M.: Effect of L-thyroxine or somatotrophin on body growth and cerebral development in neonatally thyroidectomized rats. *Life Sci.* **5**:243, 1966.

94. Hamburgh, M.: An analysis of the action of thyroid hormone on development based on *in vivo* and *in vitro* studies. *Gen. Comp. Endocrinol.* **10**:198, 1968.

95. Clendinnen, B. G., and Eayrs, J. T.: The anatomical and physiological effects of prenatally administered somatotrophin on cerebral development in rats. *J. Endocrinol.* **22**:183, 1961.

96. Taurog, A., Tong, W., and Chaikoff, I. L.: Thyroid ^{131}I metabolism in the pituitary: The untreated, hypophysectomized rat. *Endocrinology* **62**:646, 1958.

97. Krawiec, L., Garcia Argiz, C. A., Gomez, C. J., and Pasquini, J. M.: Hormonal regulation of brain development. Effects of triodothyronine and growth hormone on the biochemical changes in the cerebral cortex and cerebellum of neonatally thyroidectomized rats. *Brain Res.* **15**:209, 1969.

98. Geel, S. E., and Timiras, P. S.: Influence of growth hormone on cerebral cortical RNA metabolism in immature hypothyroid rats. *Brain Res.* **22**:63, 1970.

99. Garcia, A., Pasquini, C. A., Kaplun, B., and Gomez, C. J.: Hormonal regulation of brain development. II. Effect of neonatal thyroidectomy on succinate dehydrogenase and other enzymes in developing cerebral cortex and cerebellum of the rat. *Brain Res.* **6**:635, 1967.

100. Pasquini, J. M., Kaplun, B., Garcia Argiz, C. A., and Gomez, C. J.: Hormonal regulation of brain development. I. The effect of neonatal thyroidectomy upon nucleic acids, protein and two enzymes in developing cerebral cortex and cerebellum of the rat. *Brain Res.* **6**:621, 1967.

101. Stone, B., Gregory, K. M., and Ehlert, J.: Regional failure of rat cortical development after early hypophysectomy. *Anat. Rec.* (*Abstr.*) **154**:428, 1966.

102. Gregory, K. M., and Diamond, M. C.: Effects of early hypophysectomy on brain morphogenesis in the rat. *Exp. Neurol.* **20**:394, 1968.

103. Diamond, M. C.: The effects of early hypophysectomy and hormone therapy on brain development. *Brain Res.* **7**:407, 1968.

104. Geel, S., Valcana, T., and Timiras, P. S.: Effect of neonatal hypothyroidism and of thyroxine of L-(^{14}C) leucine incorporation in protein *in vivo* and the relationship to ionic levels in the developing brain of the rat. *Brain Res.* **4**:143, 1967.

105. Gelber, S., Campbell, P. L., Deibler, G. E., and Sokoloff, L.: Effects of L-thyroxine on amino acid incorporation into protein in mature and immature rat brain. *J. Neurochem.* **11**:221, 1964.

106. Solomon, J., and Greep, R. O.: The effect of alterations in thyroid function on the pituitary growth hormone content and acidophil cytology. *Endocrinology* **65**:158, 1959.

107. Chez, R. A., Hutchinson, D. L., Salazar, H., and Mintz, D. H.: Some effects of fetal and maternal hypophysectomy in pregnancy. *Am. J. Obstet. Gynecol.* **108**:643, 1970.

108. Smith, P. E.: Continuation of pregnancy in rhesus monkeys (*Macaca mulatta*) following hypophysectomy. *Endocrinology* **55**:655, 1954.

109. Hutchinson, D. L., Westover, J. L., and Will, D. W.: The destruction of the maternal and fetal pituitary glands in subhuman primates. *Am. J. Obstet. Gynecol.* **83**:857, 1962.

110. Zamenhof, S., Mosley, J., and Schuller, E.: Stimulation of the proliferation of cortical neurons by prenatal treatment with growth hormone. *Science* **152**:1396, 1966.

111. Sara, V., and Lazarus, L.: The effect of maternal administration of pituitary growth hormone on progeny in rats. II. Learning ability. I.R.C.S. International Research Communication System (73-9) 15-13-7.

112. Dobbing, J.: The later development of the central nervous system and its vulnerability. In: Davis, J. A., and Dobbing, J. (Eds.): *Scientific Foundations of Paediatrics.* Heinemann, London, 1973.

113. Voyer, E. E.: Effect of maternal malnutrition superimposed to hypophysectomy on fetal growth in rats. *Medicina* **34**:39, 1974.

114. Chow, B. F.: Effect of maternal dietary protein on anthropometric and behavioral development of the offspring. In: *Nutrition and Malnutrition.* Roche, A. F. and Falkner, F. (Eds.), *Advances in Experimental Medicine and Biology* **49**,:183, 1974.

115. Erenberg, A., Omor, K., Menkes, J. H., Oh, W., and Fisher, D. A.: Growth and development of the thyroidectomized ovine fetus. *Pediatric Research* **8**:783, 1974.

116. Liggins, G. C., and Kennedy, F. C. Effects of electrocoagulation on the foetal lamb hypophysis on growth and development. *J. Endocrinol.* **40**:371, 1968.

CHAPTER 2

Brain Size and the Relation of the Primate to the Nonprimate

A. Barry Holt, Donald B. Cheek, E. David Mellits, and Donald E. Hill

INTRODUCTION

Brain size and brain growth relative to body size and body growth have been sub-jects of interest to biologists and anatomists for the past century. It is our purpose in this chapter to discuss how the subhuman primate—*Macaca mulatta*—compares with the human with respect to brain growth and anthropometry. Also we seek to explore whether this primate is more comparable with *Homo sapiens* than lower mammals or the usual laboratory animal (eg, the rat, rabbit, and guinea pig) in experimental situations that involve brain growth.

THE RELATION OF BODY WEIGHT AND BRAIN WEIGHT
(MATURE MAMMALS)

The relationship of brain weight to body weight has been given special consideration ever since the late nineteenth century. This interest was due to an attempt to develop a simple law that would relate the brain weight of animals to their "true" position on the phylogenetic or evolutionary scale.

Snell[1] in 1891 suggested that if an animal weighed x grams and its brain y grams, then the relationship between x and y could be expressed in the form

$$y = bx^k$$

where b and k are constants.

On theoretical grounds he suggested that the value of k should be somewhat more than two-thirds, that is,

$$y = bx^{0.68}$$

Seven years later, in 1897, Dubois,[2,3] closely followed by Lapicque,[4] empirically determined the value of k as 0.56 and adopted it as a universal constant—the phylogenetic constant.[5] The parameter b was termed the "cephalization coefficient," which later, according to Brummelkamp,[6,7] was an integral power of $\sqrt{2}$, that is,

$$\text{coefficient of cephalization } (b) = \frac{\text{brain weight}}{\text{body weight}^{0.56}}$$

Coefficient b seemed to classify mammals into a scheme that agreed with man's concept of animal's "intelligence." This simple theory of brain size, body mass, and intelligence, together with the derivation of k, gained wide support through the first three decades of this century. Brummelkamp was the greatest advocate. Lashly,[8] Goldstein,[9] and Head[10] had all considered that "intelligence" was related to the volume of brain cortex.

The Dubois-Lapicque-Brummelkamp theory was severely criticized by Sholl in 1947. Sholl,[11] with sound reasoning and strong evidence, showed conclusively that "the theory was untenable." However, the view that mammalian intelligence can be so equated still lingers in the minds of some. The recent example, although disguised in the form of a scaled ratio and said to relate to the "brightness" of an animal, is actually another form of the Dubois-Lapicque-Brummelkamp theory. Herschel[12] states that the ratio of the cube root of the body weight (x) over the square root of the brain weight (y) yields a ratio (f) that is a measure of "intellectual efficiency" which reflects the behavior of mammals; that is,

$$f = \frac{\sqrt[3]{x}}{\sqrt{y}}$$

which is equivalent to the form

$$y = bx^k \qquad \text{where} \quad k = 0.66 \quad \text{and} \quad b = \frac{1}{f^2}$$

In 1939 Von Bonin,[13] noting that Dubois had investigated a very limited number of species, collected all available brain and body weight data available at that time. He sought to define the relationship between brain weight and body weight for mammals at maturity. Using the logarithmic approach, a method made popular by Huxley,[14] he was able to express his data as a straight line, that is,

$$\text{brain weight} = b \text{ (body weight)}^k$$

is equivalent to the form

$$\log \text{brain weight} = \log b + k \text{ (log body weight)}$$

The correlation coefficient r was 0.83 for 120 different types of animals, showing that mammalian brain weight did indeed depend to a large extent on body weight.

Von Bonin came forward with values for b and k that gave an equation (expressed in grams) for adult mammals as

$$\text{brain weight} = 0.18(\text{body weight})^{0.655}$$

The exponent k was similar to that originally proposed in Snell's theorem of relative brain and body growth.[1] However, no claims were made concerning "intelligence."

The representative values for the adult are relatively easy to obtain in domestic animals, although problems do arise due to selective breeding and forced nutrition. Data for wild species are more difficult to obtain.

We have reviewed the data collected by Count[15] relating to adult mammals. His work collates the data of Crile and Quiring,[16] Brummelkamp,[6,7] and others.[17–20] These data have been evaluated and checked and are plotted on a log-log grid (Figure 2.1).

Allometric relationships of brain weight on body weight were calculated for (a) all Mammalia excluding man and the orders Cetacea and Proboscidea (b) all adult

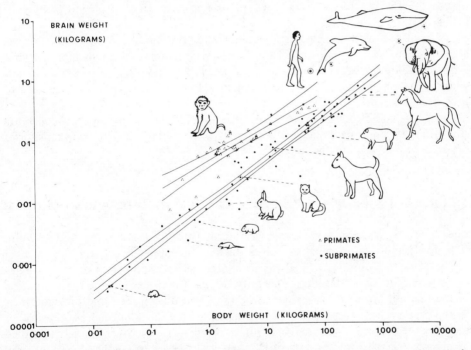

Fig. 2.1. This allometric (log-log) plot of brain weight on body weight of 103 species of mammals demonstrates that primates have relatively larger brains for body weight in comparison with lower mammals (Table 2.1). The lower extended line describes the relationship for subprimates (●). The plots of some common domestic and laboratory species are identified (ie, mouse, rat, guinea pig, rabbit, cat, dog, pig, and horse). The upper shorter line describes the relationship for subhuman primates (△). The position of *Macaca mulatta* is illustrated. Both lines are surrounded by confidence limits. The position of man is identified by an asterisk (*). The relative positions of mammals that have an absolute brain mass greater than man are also illustrated (ie, Cetacea, represented by the dolphin and the whale, and Proboscidea, represented by the elephant). The source of these data is given in the text.

primates excluding man, and (c) all other adult mammals excluding the orders Cetacea and Proboscidea.

Cetacea (whales, porpoises, and dolphins) were excluded from the calculation because of their high content of body fat and insufficient data. The data on the elephant (the only representative of the order Proboscidea) have also been excluded because of large brains. These two orders of Mammalia have a brain mass larger than that of man. Lilly[21] and Jerison[22] have discussed their survival and biological success.

Table 2.1 lists the three allometric relationships. Equation 1 shows that the relationships for Mammalia (excluding the subjects already noted) are similar to the relationships already reported by Von Bonin[13] and Jerison.[23] In the subprimate Mammalia (Equation 2) there is a marked reduction in variance, a downward displacement of the line in relation to Equation 1, and a significant increase in the correlation coefficient. Such an observation has already been made by Jerison.[23] The primate relationship (Equation 3) yields a line less well defined but with a greater intercept than for the other two lines. By analyses of covariance, the distribution of the points for the primate line is significantly different from that of the subprimate line. The slopes of the two regressions are also significantly different (Table 2.1).

It is well known that primates have relatively large brains. Animal models used commonly for the investigation of the effects of nutrition and/or hormones during growth include the lower subprimates (Equation 2). The position of these animals within the "mammalian group" is depicted in Figure 2.1. Clearly their pattern of growth is different.

Sacher[24] and Brody[25] have drawn attention to a relationship between brain size, life span, and metabolic rate, mammals with a smaller brain having a shorter life span and higher metabolic rate.

THE RELATION OF BRAIN WEIGHT AND BODY WEIGHT DURING GROWTH

The preceding discussion has dealt with adult values for brain and body weight. It is now important to consider values during development.

The work of Count[15] defined the first interspecies relationship of brain weight to body weight from fetal life to maturity. Figure 2.2 is a schematic representation of the relationship of brain weight to body weight during fetal and postnatal life. In the preparation of this figure the relationships for the subprimate species other than for the rabbit[26] were derived from photographs of growth curves published by many workers.[27-31] The data of Howard et al[32] concerning the human fetus fill an important need. (The specimens were obtained during surgical interruption of pregnancy and range in age from 10 to 30 weeks from conception. The general health of the mothers was considered by the authors as being such as to have not interfered with fetal growth. In addition, these workers reported fetal age and DNA contents of both the cerebrum and cerebellum. Where applicable these data are used for comparison with the monkey in this chapter.)

Our own data on the fetal macaque were supplemented with data from Dr. Oscar Portman of the Oregon Regional Primate Center. The limited data on the chimpanzee and Semnopithecus fetuses were recorded by Count.[15] Values for human

Table 2.1   Allometric relationships for Mammalia

Relationship	n	log y =	r	SE (log)
1. Mammalia (primates plus subprimates)	103	$-1.7885 + 0.6483 \log x$ ($y = 0.0163\, x^{0.6483}$)	0.91	0.3513
2. Subprimates only	73	$-2.0163 + 0.7065 \log x$ ($y = 0.0096\, x^{0.7065}$)	0.97	0.2273
3. Primates only	30	$-1.3219 + 0.5478 \log x$ ($y = 0.0477\, x^{0.5478}$)	0.87	0.1843

x = log body weight (kg)   y = log brain weight (kg)

Analysis of Covariance	Degrees freedom	F	P
Population difference	2, 99	73.4	less than 0.001
Slope difference	1, 99	26.4	less than 0.001

(Data exclude man, Cetacea, and Proboscidea)

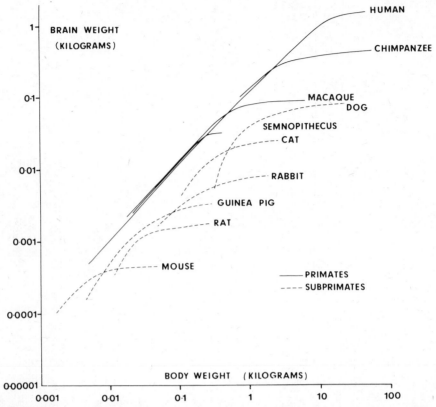

Fig. 2.2. This schematic allometric plot describes the relationship of brain weight to body weight from fetal life through development to adulthood for primates (Semnopithecus, macaque, chimpanzee, and man) and subprimates (mouse, rat, guinea pig, rabbit, cat, and dog). Note that all primate brains are relatively larger than those from subprimates during development. Primate brain growth is proportionate to body weight. The points fall along a common line until maturity is attained. The source of the data is given in the text.

brain weight from birth to adulthood were recorded by Schulz et al[33] and Mühlman.[34] The data of Michaelis[35] and Mikhailets[36] for the human fetus are not clearly defined and therefore have not been included.

In Figure 2.2, the uppermost solid lines represent the four primate species—Semnopithecus, macaque, chimpanzee, and man. The span is from the lowest to the highest weights for available data. In the case of Semnopithecus only the fetal points are plotted, while for the chimpanzee data are available beginning from around birth. The lines for all four primate species follow a common line until a critical body weight is reached. At that point the value for brain weight for each species departs and travels toward the ultimate value. With respect to time or chronological age the point of departure is prior to birth for Semnopithecus, approximately 150 days of gestation for the macaque, just after birth for the chimpanzee, and about 2 years of age postnatally for the human.

The interrupted lines in the figure illustrate the brain-to-body weight relationships for the common laboratory animals beginning with the mouse and moving upward

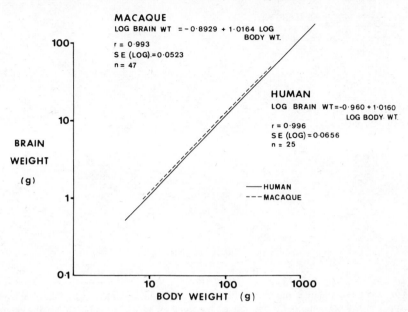

Fig. 2.3. This allometric figure illustrates the close similarity that exists between man and macaque for the relationship of body weight to brain weight: The slopes of both lines are essentially equal to unity, which indicates proportional growth during ontogenesis. The human line is derived from the data of Howard et al[32] while the macaque line was calculated from data collected by us and additional data kindly provided by Dr. Oscar Portman of the Oregon Regional Primate Center.

to the rat, guinea pig, rabbit, cat, and dog. No common line can be described for these animals which span a similar body weight range to that of the primate.

The brain of the primate during development is relatively larger than that of growing subprimates of similar weight. The figure shows that the primate brain grows proportionally to body weight along a single common line. This finding has not been shown by other workers. Throughout development the pattern of brain weight to body weight is unique for the primate but appears to be different for each lower mammal.

Figure 2.3 demonstrates the close, if not identical, relationship that exists between macaque and man when brain weight is plotted against body weight during fetal life. The slopes of both lines are essentially equal to unity, demonstrating proportional growth of the brain and the body weight during ontogenesis. Mikhailets[36] has stated that the rate of growth of the human brain during ontogenesis falls behind the rate of growth of the body weight. This is not in accord with our observations.

The relationship of cerebral weight or cerebellar weight to body weight is also of interest. For cerebral weight it can be shown that for the human and macaque points fall on a common line, the line being well above that for the rabbit (Figure 2.4). A 100-g rabbit would have a cerebrum of approximately 2 g, while a 100-g human or monkey fetus would have a cerebrum weighing 12 g. A close relationship of the cerebellar weight to body weight also exists for primates and subprimates, but lower mammals, while showing a similarity in early development, eventually show a lower ratio (Figure 2.5).

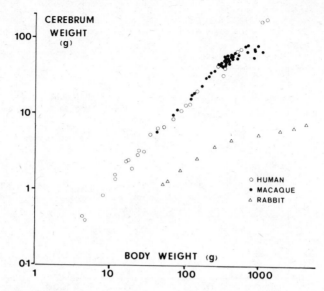

Fig. 2.4. Cerebral weight is plotted against body weight during ontogenesis. Note that points for the human[32] and macaque fall essentially on a common line while the points for the rabbit[26] fall well below.

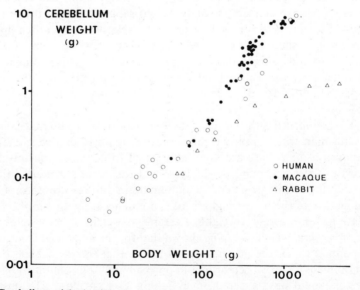

Fig. 2.5. Cerebellar weight is plotted against body weight during ontogenesis. Note that early in development the relationship of cerebellar weight to body weight is similar in the macaque, human, [32] and the subprimate represented by the rabbit.[26] Later in development the rabbit shows a smaller cerebellar : body-weight ratio.

BRAIN SIZE IN *MACACA MULATTA*

In Figures 2.6 to 2.11 the total brain weight and cerebrum weight are illustrated. The corresponding equations for these figures and the figures to be described later in this section are listed in Table 2.2. As expected, the total brain weight curves reflect those of the cerebrum since the cerebrum makes up the largest portion of the total brain weight. It is useful, however, to separate these two since much of the experimental data in both smaller mammals and humans have been separated into total brain weight, cerebrum, and cerebellum and brain stem.[37–40]

The brain stem was defined as the portion of whole brain remaining after transection at the foramen magnum, dissection from the cerebrum at the level of the upper pons (between inferior and superior colliculi) and separation from the cerebellum at the cerebellar peduncles (see Appendix I). The weight of the brain stem was 0.2, 0.9, and 2.1 g, respectively, at midgestation, birth, and maturity. As this portion of the brain is less than 3% of the total brain mass (containing a relatively small number of cells), no further consideration is given to this component.

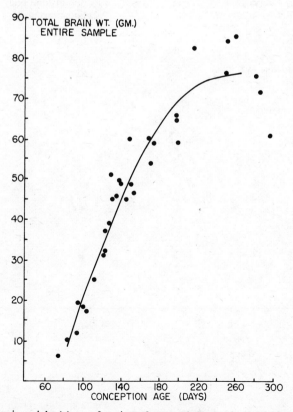

Fig. 2.6. Total brain weight (g) as a function of conception age (days) (Table 2.2, Equation 1).

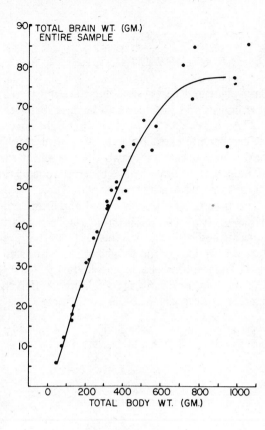

Fig. 2.7. Total brain weight (g) as a function of total body weight (g) (Table 2.2, Equation 2).

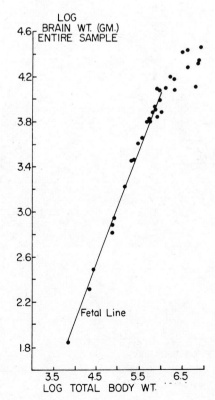

Fig. 2.8. Log brain weight (g) as a function of log total body weight (g) (Table 2.2, Equation 3).

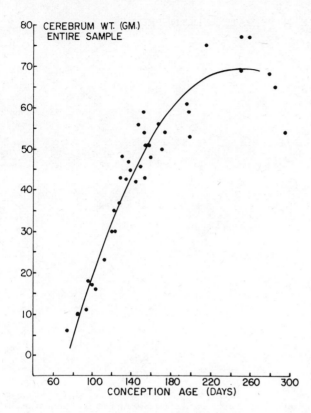

Fig. 2.9. Cerebral weight (g) as a function of conception age (days) (Table 2.2, Equation 4).

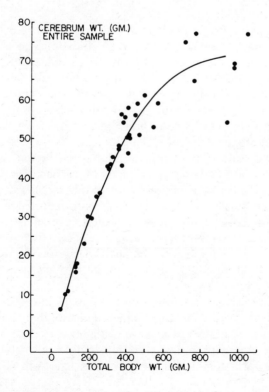

Fig. 2.10. Cerebral weight (g) as a function of total body weight (g) (Table 2.2, Equation 5).

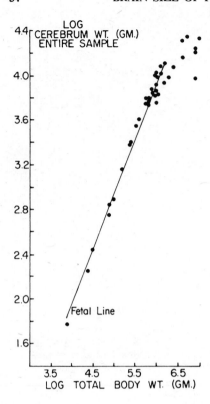

Fig. 2.11. Log cerebral weight (g) as a function of log total body weight (g) (Table 2.2, Equation 6).

The curves shown relating brain weight to either conception age or body weight are best expressed over the entire sample by convex quadratic curves, probably representing exponential or asymptotic growth patterns. Of particular interest are the figures for the log-log conversions of brain weight to total body weight and cerebrum weight to total body weight during the fetal period. As pointed out by both Huxley[14] and Needham,[41] the conversion to a log-log basis allows a comparison of relative growth rates. In both the total brain and cerebrum the value for the slope in these graphs is approximately unity. This indicates that the brain and body weight are increasing at essentially the same rate; that is, the brain is growing in constant proportion to the total body weight. This is of particular interest in trying to assess the influence of adverse conditions *in utero* that might affect body growth or brain growth or both. It is known from previous work reported by us and others[42–44] that in most instances of intrauterine insult the brain is relatively spared. This suggests to us that there is some basic protective or selective mechanism at work. A similar argument can be applied to the heart. These two organs may occupy a selective place in blood flow or have other protective mechanisms that allow growth under conditions of adversity.

If the data for the postnatal period are plotted on a log-log grid (brain weight versus body weight), a gradient of 0.3 is obtained which indicates that the rate of brain growth decreases to one-third of the rate *in utero*. Data for the human indicate a lesser gradient or rate of brain growth for late gestation, and the postnatal period the gradient is greater than 0.3 which indicates a lesser change in growth rate.[32, 46]

Table 2.2   Equations describing brain and head size in Macaca mulatta

	Time span	n	Y units	X units	Equation Y =	SD	Fit
1.	80 days CA to 120 days PN	33	Total brain weight (g)	CA (days)	$-78.287 + 1.2297 (X) - 0.0024455 (X)^2$	5.85	0.001 quadratic
2.	" " "	33	"	Total body weight (g)	$-3.6797 + 0.18415 (X) - 0.00010367 (X)^2$	5.19	0.001 quadratic
3.	80 days CA to birth	20	Log brain weight (g)	Log body weight (g)	$-2.1094 + 1.0220 (X)$	0.072	0.001 linear r = 0.99
4.	80 days CA to 120 days PN	39	Cerebrum weight (g)	CA (days)	$-73.531 + 1.1696 (X) - 0.0023938 (X)^2$	5.38	0.001 quadratic
5.	" " "	39	"	Total body weight (g)	$-2.6273 + 0.16981 (X) - 0.00098606 (X)^2$	4.72	0.001 quadratic
6.	80 days CA to birth	26	Log cerebrum weight (g)	Log body weight (g)	$-1.9942 + 0.9875 (X)$	0.0811	0.001 linear r = 0.99
7.	80 days CA to 120 days PN	39	Cerebrum weight (g)	Body length (cm)	$-58.758 + 4.9246 (X) - 0.042882 (X)^2$	5.76	0.01 quadratic
8.	80 days CA to birth	26	Log cerebrum weight (g)	"	$0.47787 + 0.11844 (X)$	0.138	0.001 linear r = 0.98

Table 2.2 continued

	Time span	n	Y units	X units	Equation Y =	SD	Fit
9.	80 days CA to 120 days PN	39	Cerebellum weight (g)	CA (days)	$2.2217 - 0.081424 (X) + 0.00081407 (X)^2 - 0.0000016803 (X)^3$	0.342	0.01 cubic
10.	80 days CA to birth	26	Log cerebellum weight (g)	CA (days)	$-4.3427 + 0.03586 (X)$	0.193	0.001 linear $r = 0.98$
11.	80 days CA to birth	26	Log cerebellum weight (g)	Log body weight (g)	$-7.7493 + 1.4559 (X)$	0.162	0.001 linear $r = 0.98$
12.	80 days CA to 120 days PN	17	Head circumference (cm)	CA (days)	$-2.33078 + 0.19672 (X) - 0.00039618 (X)^2$	0.624	quadratic
13.	"	17	Cerebrum plus cerebellum weight (g)	Head circumference (cm)	$33.2654 - 6.4830 (X) + 0.38677 (X)^2$	3.895	quadratic
14.	"	17	Head circumference (cm)	Body length (cm)	$-3.2328 + 1.1257 (X) - 0.012524 (X)^2$	0.405	0.001 quadratic
15.	"	17	Total brain DNA (mg)	Head circumference (cm)	$115.3324 - 15.59 (X) + 0.74947 (X)^2$		0.001 quadratic

Key: CA = Days from conception; PN = Postnatal days; SD = Standard deviation; n = Number of subjects

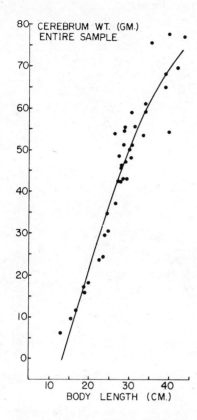

Fig. 2.12. Cerebral weight (g) as a function of body length (cm) (Table 2.2, Equation 7).

The brain of macaca reaches 60% of adult size before birth and is more advanced in development than the human.[40, 42, 46]

In Figures 2.12 and 2.13 cerebral weight is related to body length. The points for the entire sample describe a slightly convex quadratic line. As expected, when only the fetal period is examined, the log of the cerebral weight is linearly related to body length. These relationships become important when one is attempting to define proportional or disproportional changes in fetal growth. The information is of interest where somatic growth is affected more than brain growth. It is likely that using these curves one could predict with great accuracy the deficit in body length relative to the log of cerebral weight.

When cerebellar weight is expressed as a function of conception age the curve approaches a sigmoid shape, since the growth of the cerebellum does not become rapid until midgestation, progesses very rapidly through late gestation, and is nearly finished shortly after birth (Figure 2.14). The logarithmic transformation of the entire sample would linearize this curve. Focusing again on the fetal period, the log of cerebellar weight is linearly related to the conception age, as seen in Figure 2.15. In order to examine growth of the cerebellum relative to total body weight, the log of cerebellar weight as a function of the log of total body weight is seen in Figure 2.16. The slope of this curve is approximately 1.5 as contrasted with a slope of approximately 1 for the cerebrum and the brain as a whole. This accelerated growth enables the cerebellum to achieve well in excess of three-fourths of its total organ size at the time of birth as opposed to a brain size of only about 60% of its final adult weight. Postnatally this slope drops to about 0.66.

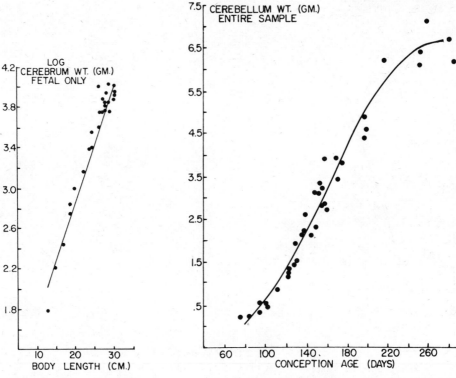

Fig. 2.13. Log cerebral weight (g) as a function of body length (cm) (Table 2.2, Equation 8).

Fig. 2.14. Cerebellar weight (g) as a function of conception age (days) (Table 2.2, Equation 9).

Studies of Dobbing and Sands,[47] Chase et al,[48] and our own work[42] have shown that the cerebellum is the portion of the brain most involved in abnormal growth patterns following either intrauterine or postnatal insults. Changes are in total weight and reductions occur in DNA and protein. Since the cerebellum is growing faster than the cerebrum in the latter part of pregnancy, the cerebellum is more vulnerable when, for example, nutritional insults are involved.

BRAIN WEIGHT AND HEAD CIRCUMFERENCE IN *MACACA MULATTA*

Head circumference has been used as a measure of brain growth during the first year of life in the human. This assumes that head circumference reflects cranial volume which in turn is related to the volume or weight of the brain it contains.

Although our data for *Macaca mulatta* are limited, we can describe an inverted quadratic relationship for head circumference on age from 80 days after conception to 120 days after birth (Table 2.2, Equation 12). Using head circumference as the dependent variable, one can predict the sum of the cerebral weight plus the cerebellar weight from another quadratic equation over the same age range (Table 2.2, Equation 13). Figure 2.17 illustrates the relationship between head circumference of the entire sample as a function of body length, and is described by a

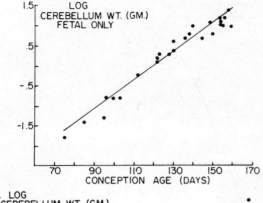

Fig. 2.15. Log cerebellar weight (g) as a function of conception age (days) (Table 2.2, Equation 10).

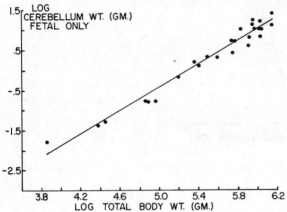

Fig. 2.16. Log cerebellar weight (g) as a function of log total body weight (g) (Table 2.2, Equation 11).

convex quadratic line. It is included here only to indicate that, in the rhesus monkey, the relationship of head growth to body length is similar to that of the human. The reader is referred to Duterloo and Enlow's recent comparative study of cranial growth in man and the macaque.[49] These workers, while describing a number of distinct similarities in the growth and remodeling processes, pointed to several marked differences between the two species. These differences generally related to the cranial floor and appeared to be associated with the differences in size, configuration, and disposition of the brain in the two species.

A NOTE ON CEREBRAL CELL POPULATION VERSUS BODY SIZE

The demonstration of differences in the ratios of the brain weight to body weight in primates versus nonprimates, together with the finding that the ratio is the same for all primates considered, leads one to wonder whether these relationships are reflected in the mode of growth of cell numbers. Figure 2.18 records the DNA content of the cerebrum for the human, macaque, and rabbit. (The only data available of this nature for the lower mammals pertain to the rabbit.) A curvilinear relationship is seen for the human when cerebral DNA content is plotted against body weight during development. The points would appear to be described by two inter-

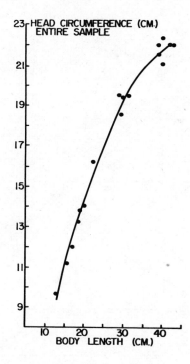

Fig. 2.17. Head circumference (cm) as a function of body length (cm) (Table 2.2, Equation 14).

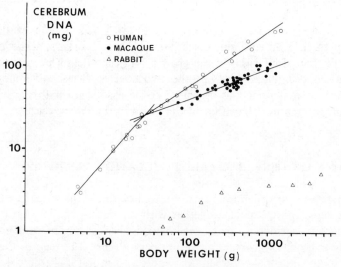

Fig. 2.18. The relationship of cerebral DNA to body weight during ontogenesis is seen to be curvilinear for the human when cerebral DNA is plotted against body weight.[32] The points appear to be described by two lines that intersect at about 35 g of body weight. The cerebral DNA of the rabbit[26] is shown for comparison.

secting lines, the intersection occurring at a body weight of about 35 g (94 days of gestation). Of interest is the finding that the points for the macaque DNA content fall away from and below the human data in a linear fashion. However, on extrapolation back to the human line the intersection is again at 35 g. No comment in the literature has ever been made regarding growth and this point in time except for the observation of Weinbach[50] who considered that human growth and its mathematical expression moved forward from a point in time that for the human began at 95 days. He showed the identity between the human and chimpanzee with respect to somatic growth. Thus, 35 g in weight for the primate may be a landmark. Only further research will show the significance of the point, which may represent the end of embryological and organogenetic growth and the beginning of true fetal growth. On examination of the existing data on the protein plus water contents of the human fetus (as shown in our previous book[51]), a quadratic relationship unfolds that begins to sweep upward or to depart from the horizontal at 13 weeks of gestation (93 days).

As expected, the cell population of the rabbit cerebrum falls well below that of the primate even when the same body weight pertains.

Winick and Rosso[52] have suggested that total brain DNA is linearly related to the change in head circumference during human infancy. Although no direct comparison can be made between man and monkey in this situation, it can be suspected that this is not the case in the monkey (Figure 2.19). This relationship of total brain DNA to head circumference is best fitted by a quadratic expression (Table 2.2, Equation 15).

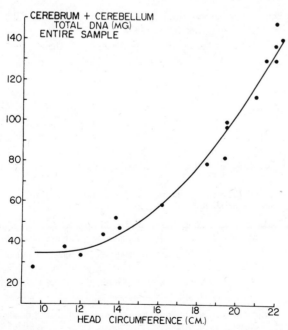

Fig. 2.19. The relationship of total brain DNA to head circumference is quadratic (Table 2.2, Equation 15). This is in contrast to the human infant where a linear relationship has been reported.[52]

CONCLUSION

The brain development of the rodent is far removed from that of the human. The significance of this fact has often been neglected. To quote one example, considerable concern has arisen regarding the deleterious effects of restricted protein intake on subsequent brain growth. Pertinent data have been derived from brain analyses of small lower mammals subjected to protein deprivation and these data have been extrapolated to the primate. There is no evidence that such extrapolation is justified.

While recognizing that some differences exist between primates with respect to brain growth, the evidence presented in this chapter gives ample reason to justify the use of primates in animal experimentation when answers are to be obtained which will relate to human brain development. The common relationships for primates in the ratio of brain weight to body weight promise to assist our knowledge concerning problems of development.

REFERENCES

1. Snell, O.: Die Abhängigkeit des Hirngewichts von dem Körpergewicht und den geistigen Fähigkeiten. *Arch. Psychiatr.* **23**(2): 12, 1891.
2. Dubois, E.: De verhouding van het gevicht der hersenen tot de groote van het lichaam bij zoogdieren. *Arch. Kon. Akad. Wet., Amsterdam* **5**:10, 1897.
3. Dubois, E.: Über die Abhängigkeit des Hirngewichtes von der Körpergrösse. *Arch. Anthropol.* **25**:1, 1898.
4. Lapicque, L.: Sur la relation du poids de l'encéphale au poids du corps (chez le chien). *C. R. Soc. Biol. Paris* **50**:62, 1898.
5. Dubois, E.: On the relation between the quantity of brain and the size of the body in vertebrates. *Verh. Kon. Akad. Wet., Amsterdam* **16**:647, 1913.
6. Brummelkamp, R.: Das Wachstum der Gehirnmasse mit kleinen Cephalisierungssprünger (sog. $\sqrt{2}$ − sprünger) bei den Rodentiern. *Acta Neerlandica Morphol. Norm. Pathol.* **2**:188, 1939.
7. Brummelkamp, R.: Das Wachstum der Gehirnmasse mit kleinen Cephalisierungssprüngen (sog. $\sqrt{2}$ − sprüngen) bei den Ungulaten. *Acta Neerlandica Morphol. Norm. Pathol.* **2**:260, 1939.
8. Lashley, K. S.: *Brain Mechanisms and Intelligence.* University of Chicago Press, Chicago, 1929, pp. xiv and 186.
9. Goldstein, K.: Die Lokalisation in der Grosshirnrinde. *Handb. Norm. Pathol. Physiol.,* **10**:600, 1927.
10. Head, H.: *Aphasia and Kindred Disorders of Speech,* Vol. I. Cambridge University Press, London and New York, 1926, pp. 431 and 498.
11. Sholl, D.: The quantitative investigation of the vertebrate brain and the applicability of allometric formulae to its study. *Proc. Roy. Soc. London Ser. B* **135**:243, 1948.
12. Herschel, J.: A scaled ratio of body weight to brain weight as a comparative index for relative importance of brain size in mammals of widely varying body mass. *Psychol. Rep.* **31**:84, 1972.
13. Von Bonin, G.: Brain-weight and body-weight of mammals. *J. Gen. Psychiatr.* **16**:379, 1937.
14. Huxley, J.: *Problems of Relative Growth.* Methuen, London, 1932.
15. Count, E. W.: Brain and body weight in man: Their antecedents in growth and evolution. *Ann. N.Y. Acad. Sci.* **46**:Art. 10, 1947.
16. Crile, G. W., and Quiring, D. P.: A record of the body weight and certain organ and gland weights of 3,690 animals. *Ohio J. Sci.* **40**(5):219, 1940.

17. Hrdlicka, A.: Brain weight in vertebrates. *Smithsonian Misc. Coll.* **48**(1582):89, 1905.

18. Hrdlicka, A.: Weight of the brain and of the internal organs in American monkeys. *Am. J. Phys. Anthropol.* **8**(2):201, 1925.

19. Spitzka, E. A.: Brain weights of animals with special reference to the weight of the brain in the macaque monkey. *J. Comp. Neurol.* **13**:9, 1903.

20. Herre, W., and Thiede, U.: Studien an Gehirnen südamerikanischer Tylopoden. *Zool. Jahrb. Aft. II* **825**:155, 1965.

21. Lilly, J. G.: *Man and Dolphin.* Doubleday, Garden City, New York, 1961.

22. Jerison, H. J.: Interpreting the evolution of the brain. *Human Biol.* **35**:263, 1963.

23. Jerison, H. J.: Brain to body ratios and the evolution of intelligence. *Science* **121**:449, 1955.

24. Sacher, G. A.: Relation of life span to brain weight and body weight in mammals. In: Wolstenholme, G. E. N., and O'Connor, M. (Eds.): *Ciba Foundation Colloquia on Ageing*, Vol. 5. *The Life Span of Animals.* Churchill, London, 1959, p. 115.

25. Brody, S.: *Bioenergetics and Growth.* Van Nostrand-Reinhold, Princeton, New Jersey, 1945.

26. Harel, S., Watanabe, K., Linke, I., and Schain, R. J.: Growth and development of the rabbit brain. *Biol. Neonate* **21**:381, 1972.

27. Agrawal, H. C., Davis, J. M., and Himwich, W. A.: Developmental changes in mouse brain: Weight, water content and free amino acids. *J. Neurochem.* **15**:917, 1968.

28. De Souza, S. W., and Dobbing, J.: Cerebral edema in developing brain. I. Normal water and cation content in developing rat brain and post mortem changes. *Exp. Neurol.* **32**:431, 1971.

29. Dobbing, J., and Sands, J.: Growth and development of the brain and spinal cord of the guinea pig. *Brain Res.* **17**:115, 1970.

30. Agrawal, H. C., Davis, J. M., and Himwich, W. A.: Water content of developing kitten brain. *J. Neurochem.* **14**:179, 1967.

31. Agrawal, H. C., Davis, J. M., and Himwich, W. A.: Water content of dog brain parts in relation to maturation of the brain. *Am. J. Physiol.* **215**:846, 1968.

32. Howard, E., Granoff, D., and Bujnovszky, P.: DNA, RNA and cholesterol increases in cerebrum and cerebellum during development of the human fetus. *Brain Res.* **14**:697, 1969.

33. Schulz, D. M., Giordano, D. A., and Schulz, D. H.: Weights of organs of fetuses and infants. *Arch. Pathol.* **74**:244, 1962.

34. Mühlman, L.: Die Abhängigkeit des Hirngewichtes von Körpergewicht, Körperlänge und Körperbautypen. Inaug.-Diss. Munich, 1957.

35. Michaelis, P.: Altersbestimmungen menschlicher Embryonen und Foeten auf Grund von Messungen und von Daten der Anamnese. *Arch. Gynäkol.* **78**:267, 1906.

36. Mikhailets, V. Ya: Increase in weight of the brain during the intrauterine development of man. *Mauch. Zap. Uzhgorodsk. Gos. Univ.*, **5**. *Sb. Stud. Rabot. Uzhgorod* **2**:47, 1952.

37. Winick, M., Rosso, P., and Waterlow, J.: Cellular growth of cerebrum, cerebellum, and brain stem in normal and marasmic children. *Exp. Neurol.* **26**:393, 1970.

38. Chase, H. P.: The effects of intrauterine and postnatal under-nutrition on normal brain development. *Ann. N.Y. Acad. Sci.* **205**:231, 1973.

39. Dobbing, J., and Sands, J.: Timing of neuroblast multiplication in developing human brain. *Nature* **226**:639, 1970.

40. Portman, O. W., Alexander, M., and Illingworth, D. R.: Changes in brain and sciatic nerve composition with development of rhesus monkey (*Macaca mulatta*). *Brain Res.* **43**:197, 1972.

41. Needham, J.: *Chemical Embryology*, Vol. 3. Cambridge University Press, London and New York, 1931, p. 1496.

42. Hill, D. E., Myers, R. E., Holt, A. B., Scott, R. E., and Cheek, D. B.: Fetal growth retardation produced by experimental placental insufficiency in the rhesus monkey. II. Chemical composition of the brain, liver, muscle and carcass. *Biol. Neonate* **19**:68, 1971.

43. Wigglesworth, J. S.: Experimental growth retardation in the foetal rat. *J. Pathol.* **88**:1, 1964.

44. Roux, J. M., Tordet-Caridroit, C., and Chanex, C.: Studies on experimental hypotrophy in the rat. I. Chemical composition of the total body and some organs in the rat fetus. *Biol. Neonate* **15**:342, 1970.

45. Dobbing, J., and Smart, J. L.: Early undernutrition, brain development and behaviour. In: Barnett, S. A. (Ed.): *Clinics in Developmental Medicine*, No. 47. Heinemann, London, 1973.

46. Kerr, G., and Waisman, H. A.: Fetal biology of the rhesus monkey. *Medical Primatology, 1970. Proc. 2nd Conf. Exp. Med. Surg. Primates, N.Y. 1969.* Karger, Basel, 1971, pp. 590–602.

47. Dobbing, J., and Sands, J.: Vulnerability of the developing brain: IX. The effect of nutritional growth retardation on the timing of the brain growth spurt. *Biol. Neonate* **19**:363, 1972.

48. Chase, H. P., Lindsley, W. F. B., and O'Brien, D.: Undernutrition and cerebellar development. *Nature* **221**:554, 1969.

49. Duterloo, H. S., and Enlow, D. H.: A comparative study of cranial growth in Homo and Macaca. *Am. J. Anat.* **127**:357, 1970.

50. Weinbach, A. P.: The human growth curve: I. Prenatal. *Growth* **5**:217, 1941.

51. Cheek, D. B. In: Cheek, D. B. (Ed.): *Human Growth.* Lea & Febiger, Philadelphia, 1968, p. 301.

52. Winick, M., and Rosso, P.: Head circumference and cellular growth of the brain in normal and marasmic children. *J. Pediatr.* **74**:774, 1969.

CHAPTER 3

Morphological and Biochemical
Correlates in Brain

A. Barry Holt, Donald E. Hill, and Donald B. Cheek

INTRODUCTION

The mathematical relationships with time of certain biochemical determinants in the brain of the rhesus monkey are described in the next chapter. The present discussion defines more clearly some of these components and aims to clarify their biological significance.

Growth, including brain growth, occurs by increments in cell number and cell size along with accretion of protein, fat, electrolyte, water and carbohydrate. Growth of the brain is ahead of that of many other organs and maintains a rate comparable with that of the cardiovascular system[1,2] and body size. Neuronal growth precedes neuroglial development.[3] During development of the nervous system,[3,4] neuroblast migration occurs together with spongioblast proliferation, so that neuronal and glial populations escalate. Axonal and dendritic development occurs in a predetermined sequence. Finally synaptic connections are made and organization is achieved. Total myelination of neuronal processes is the last phenomenon to occur.

While the chemical approach is generally nonspecific, some identity can be given to certain components. DNA and lipids in brain tissue have been the subject of detailed study and have served as a base line for evaluating development. A reduction of water concentration is characteristic of developing tissue; this, together with an increment in protein, has been used to monitor brain growth.

These estimations, however, do not define the nature of the cell population, for instance whether the cells involved are neuroglial or neuronal. Clearly, enzyme systems and other "marker" substances indicative of specific histological structures must also be used if functions or functional changes within the nervous system are to be defined. The following is a description of some of the methods selected to monitor changes in the structure of tissue during the development of the monkey brain.

METHODS USED TO MONITOR CHANGES

DNA

Heller and Elliott in 1954 assessed the DNA per cell nucleus in diploid cells in brain tissue as being about 7 pg.[5] Although the majority of glial and neuronal cells are diploid, in the cerebellar cortex the Purkinje cells show polyploidy.[6–8] The number of Purkinje cells is small, however, so that the DNA content of the cerebellum divided by DNA per nucleus gives a close approximation of cell number.* The cellular heterogeneity of brain tissue may be thought to restrict the usefulness of this measure. However, in view of the different timing of multiplication of the different cell types in both cerebrum and cerebellum, valuable data on the number of cells can be obtained.

Protein to DNA

Our definition of "cell size" is that one unit of DNA (or nucleus) has jurisdiction over a finite amount of protein (or cytoplasm). In brain tissue, because of the disproportion in the number and mass of glial cells in relation to neurons and their processes, this ratio must indicate an integrated cell size.

RNA

RNA is found in large amounts in the neuronal cytoplasm (eg, in the Nissl granules) and less abundantly in the cytoplasm of neuroglia.[9] It has been suggested that regional variations in RNA concentration in brain tissue reflect the volume distribution of neuronal cell bodies and large dendrites.[10]

Gangliosides (Lipid N-Acetylneuraminic Acid, NANA)

Gangliosides, although considered as characteristic lipids of the nervous system, also exist in the spleen and red cells.[11] These lipids are hydrophilic and are associated with the transport of cations and the maintenance of the excitable state of nervous tissue.

It has been shown that gangliosides occur predominantly in areas of brain tissue that are rich in neurons.[12] Studies at the cellular and subcellular level indicate that neuronal cell bodies contain relatively little ganglioside[13] while high concentrations of this lipid are observed in microsomal fractions of brain tissue that contain

---

* Setsuya Fujita (*J. Comp. Neurol.*, **155**:195, 1974) challenges the existence of polyploidy and claims nonspecific light loss (with the technique used) has led to incorrect conclusions.

dendrites and nerve endings.[14] Synaptic membranes are particularly rich in this class of lipid.[13] However, this distribution is not exclusive as they have also been demonstrated in purified myelin in small but definite amounts.[15,16]

On the basis of this evidence, we, like other workers,[10,12] have selected lipid NANA (a measure of ganglioside) as an index of dendritic and axonal plasma membranes and synapses.

Sodium Potassium ATPase

The stimulatory effect of sodium and potassium on magnesium-dependent ATPase in the brain was first described in 1957 by Hess and Pope[17] although at the time they did not associate the enzyme with active cation transport.

Four years later Bonting et al,[18] Deul and McIlwain,[19] and Jarnefelt[20,21] described the presence of $Na^+K^+ATPase$ in the brains of various mammalian species. Bonting and co-workers[18] demonstrated that cortical gray matter contained by far the highest activity of this enzyme when compared with other areas of the brain and indeed other somatic tissues of the cat. Subsequently Fahn and Côté[22] demonstrated similar activities and distribution of this enzyme in the rhesus monkey brain.

This uniquely high activity of $Na^+K^+ATPase$ in gray matter raised the question of its role in central nervous system function. Correlation between ouabain-sensitive cation transport and $Na^+K^+ATPase$ activity in brain and other tissues has been established.[23] While this enzyme is essential in all cells in the maintenance of intracellular osmotic pressure, nerve cells require, in addition, an active sodium pump to maintain the ionic gradients across the cell membrane that determine their excitability.[24] It is estimated that 40% of the respiration of brain tissue *in vitro* is utilized for the active transport of sodium and potassium.[25]

Cellular fractionation studies on brain tissue indicate high activities of Na^+K^+ ATPase in the neuronal unit and much lower activities in glial cells and capillaries.[26] It was estimated that the activity per astroglial cell in an implanted astrocytoma was 1% of the activity found in an average cell of the upper layers of rat cortex, where the predominant cell is a neuron.[27] This difference in activity between neuroglia and neurons must be considered relative in brain tissue; glial cell $Na^+K^+ATPase$ activity is similar to that of striated muscle tissue, which has considerable sodium pump activity.[27]

Neuronal cell bodies seem to be almost devoid of $Na^+K^+ATPase$ activity[28] (as they are of ganglioside), indicating that the bulk of enzyme is associated with dendrites and synaptic membranes. This is confirmed by subcellular fractionation studies demonstrating that the nerve ending fraction contains a substantial proportion of the enzyme found in whole brain.[29,30]

Of interest is the fact that $Na^+K^+ATPase$ has a subcellular distribution similar to that of gangliosides,[14] which also occur predominantly in neuronal plasma membranes. The appearance of $Na^+K^+ATPase$ activity during maturation has been shown to be closely linked with appearance of electroencephalographic activity,[31] dendritic formation, and the increase in metabolism.[32]

On the basis of the evidence presented, we have used the estimation of Na^+K^+ ATPase (or more specificially ouabain-sensitive ATPase) activity in brain tissue as a measure of neuronal nerve endings and dendrites.

Carbonic Anhydrase

Carbonic anhydrase was first demonstrated in the nervous system by Van Goor in 1940.[33] Ashby et al investigated the distribution of this enzyme in human and animal tissues.[34] Until 1962 its localization and physiological role in brain were still unknown.

Giacobini[35, 36] demonstrated by the Cartesian diver technique (a sensitive micromethod for determining the carbonic anhydrase activity in a single cell) that glial cells have 120 to 250 times more carbonic anhydrase activity than do neuronal cells. The presumed localization of carbonic anhydrase activity to glial cells has recently been discussed by Tower and Young.[37] The regional distribution of this enzyme has been determined in human brain[38] while changes in activity have been demonstrated for the rat brain during postnatal development.[39, 40] The available evidence suggests that changes in carbonic anhydrase activity will largely reflect changes occurring in glial cells.

Cholesterol

Cholesterol is the only significant sterol and one of the most prominent lipids found in the mature nervous system.[41] Approximately 70 to 80% of cholesterol in adult brain is found in myelin where it is the most abundant lipid.[42] It is on this evidence that cholesterol has often been used as a chemical marker for the myelination process.

Many workers [10, 13, 43, 44] consider cerebroside levels to be a more appropriate indicator of myelination because approximately 90% of the amount present in the mature brain is found in the myelin. However, although accumulation of cerebroside generally parallels the rate of myelin deposition, this may not be the case during early development.[13, 45] It has been shown that in the early myelination of rat brain an initial peak of cholesterol deposition occurs, preceding the deposition of cerebroside and sulfatide.[46, 47] This peak is maximal and of relatively short duration and coincides with a rapid increase in brain weight.[46] A later, less intense, but sustained increase in cholesterol accretion accompanies the peak rate in cerebroside accumulation.[46] Biochemical evidence suggests that a high percentage of cholesterol in the brain is synthesized prior to myelination, followed by a redistribution of the sterol into myelin as myelination proceeds.[45] Histological evidence indicates that even when myelination is established morphologically, unexpectedly small amounts of cerebrosides are found.[46] Further aspects of the chemical development of the myelin sheath are discussed by Davison.[45]

It has been our experience that the levels of cerebroside are more variable biologically and that their estimation is technically less reliable than is the case for cholesterol in fetal and mature monkey brain. This is confirmed by the recently published data of lipid profiles in developing monkey brain. Kerr and co-workers were unable to detect cerebrosides consistently in fetal monkey brain.[48] Furthermore, in adult monkey samples the coefficients of variation for the concentration of cerebroside and cholesterol were 33 and 9%, respectively. Similarly, the data of Portman et al[49] showed a much greater scatter in concentration of cerebroside compared with cholesterol during the development of the pons of mature monkeys, the cholesterol concentrations ranging from 40 to 50 mg/g, and for cerebroside from approximately 22 to 65 mg/g.

Although we concur that cerebroside is theoretically most representative of mature myelin, we do not believe that it is the best practical index for determining the progress of myelination, at least in the monkey. This becomes apparent during the initiation of myelination when there is morphological evidence of myelination with little or no cerebroside deposition. It is this period that constitutes a known vulnerable period in the development of the rat brain.[50] We have therefore used cholesterol content as an index of myelination.

In the present studies cholesterol has been determined by a method that makes no distinction between demosterol or esterified cholesterol. Both these sterol components could be present in relatively small amounts in fetal newborn brain tissue. Paoletti and his co-workers have discussed these components and changes in sterol metabolism of developing brain in a recent review.[41]

The Chloride and Nonchloride Space of Brain

It is accepted that the fluid space of skeletal muscle measured by chloride distribution provides a measure of the extracellular compartment.[51,52] In brain, evidence based on electrical and chemical measurements in the past indicated no fundamental difference in the nature of the extracellular space from that in other tissues. However, electron microscopic examination of nervous tissue failed to demonstrate a substantial extracellular compartment.[53,54]

Until recently this controversy has led to much speculation of the role that neuroglia may play as a functional extracellular space. The finding of high chloride content in glial tissue tended to support the argument.[55,56] Glial swelling in cerebral edema[57,58] and the demonstration of a low membrane resistance measured in astrocytes cultured in vitro[59] also added to the evidence that glial cells acted as a functional extracellular medium for neurons in the absence of a morphological extracellular space.

Vernadakis and Woodbury[60] studied the distribution of ^{36}Cl in the cerebral cortex of nephrectomized rats and suggested that chloride distributed into three spaces: interstitial space, glial cells, and neurons. However, the total space measured in this way was approximately 35 to 50% higher than was the chloride space measured by endogenous chloride in the cerebral cortex of normal growing rats studied earlier by the same workers.[61] Plasma chloride values for nephrectomized rats have been published by Ferguson and Woodbury.[62] Using these together with the chloride content in the cerebral cortex of the nephrectomized rats described above, the endogenous chloride space in the cerebral cortex of nephrectomized rats can also be calculated. These derived values, although elevated with respect to the normal rat, fail to agree with the chloride space calculated from the ^{36}Cl estimations.[60] These data are illustrated in Figure 3.1.

The data from the nephrectomized rats should therefore be accepted with caution in view of the physiological insult received, the difference in chloride space when compared to normal, and the apparent failure of agreement when chloride space is calculated from the distribution of endogenous chloride and ^{36}Cl.

During water intoxication, glial cells and other nervous tissue elements show considerable intracellular swelling at the expense of the extracellular space.[57,58] There is a definite reduction in the activity of $Na^+K^+ATPase$ of glial cells after experimental water intoxication which indicates no doubt an intracellular shift of water.[63] Such a situation may conceivably occur in the nephrectomized rat.

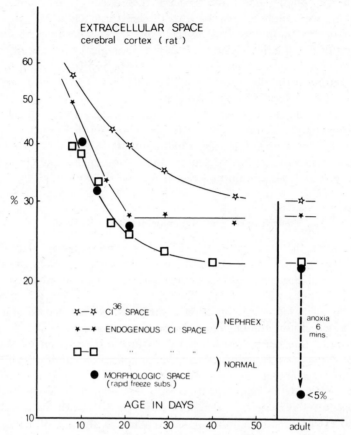

Fig. 3.1. Estimates of the chloride space in developing rat cerebral cortex are taken from the data of Vernadakis and Woodbury.[60,61] The space is expressed as a percentage of cerebral cortical weight and is plotted on a semilog grid against age. The ^{36}Cl space obtained in rat cerebral cortex 24 hours after nephrectomy (NEPHREX) is shown (open stars). The endogenous chloride space in NEPHREX animals (closed stars) was calculated from the chloride content of the cerebral cortex and the plasma water chloride concentrations obtained in nephrectomized rats by Ferguson and Woodbury.[62] The endogenous chloride space in NORMAL rat cerebral cortex[61] is shown (open squares). The disparity in size of these chloride spaces is discussed in the text. Estimates of the extracellular space in normal rat cerebral cortex determined stereologically[69] from electron micrographs following rapid freeze-substitution fixation are also illustrated (closed circles). These values are in close agreement with the endogenous chloride space in NORMAL rat cerebral cortex.[61] The effect of anoxia during delayed fixation on the extracellular space determined histologically is shown by the hatched arrow for the adult sample. The significance of this change is explained in the text.

Van Harreveld and co-workers,[64] using a rapid freeze substitution fixation technique, were able to demonstrate in brain tissue a morphological extracellular space of large magnitude that agreed with extracellular space measurements made by chemical and electrical impedance[66] methods. It is suggested that the conventional fixation techniques employed to prepare tissues for electron microscopy have failed to prevent uptake of extracellular fluid into the cells due to Donnan forces, especially into glial cells. Arrest of active transport mechanisms either by tissue anoxia[67] or by chemical means (eg, ouabain)[68] can cause cell swelling in any tissue, and in brain this process is extremely rapid.[64,67] As a Donnan equilibrium will never be reached, swelling will continue until virtually no extracellular space is left.

Bondareff and Pysh[69] have estimated the extracellular space of rat cerebral cortex by the rapid freeze-substitution fixation technique. When these data are compared with those of Vernadakis and Woodbury[61] in cerebral cortex of normal rats using endogenous chloride distribution, these estimates are in close agreement. The data of Bondareff and Pysh[69] are also shown in Figure 3.1.

We believe that the evidence reconciles the previous disparity between the morphological and the physiological findings although further confirmatory data are required. Thus in this text the chloride and nonchloride spaces, respectively, have been used to describe the extracellular space and the intracellular space (neurons plus neuroglia) of cerebrum and cerebellum.

CONCLUSION

A description has been given of biochemical "marker" substances that have been used as indicators of the morphological character of the developing monkey brain. Their use in the study of primate brain growth is the subject of the following chapter.

Although the information obtained by this approach is valuable, it is limited as to its specificity. With a computer-oriented approach to quantitative histology, it may now be possible to define further the complexities of the brain.[70,71] New techniques in tissue fixation[64] and instrumentation such as an image analyzing computer[72,73] and a laser-illuminated screening interferometer[74,75] are now available for a more sophisticated approach to growth and development of the brain.

REFERENCES

1. Timiras, P. S.: Summary of main events of embryonic and fetal growth and development in man. In: Timiras, P. S. (Ed.): *Developmental Physiology and Aging.* MacMillan, New York, 1972, p. 63.
2. Timiras, P. S.: Fetal circulation and metabolism. In: Timiras, P. S. (Ed.): *Developmental Physiology and Aging.* MacMillan, New York, 1972, p. 115.
3. Davison, A. N., and Dobbing, J.: The developing brain. In: Davison, A. N., and Dobbing, J. (Eds.): *Applied Neurochemistry.* Davis, Philadelphia, 1968, p. 253.
4. Timiras, P. S.: Development and plasticity of the nervous system. In: Timiras, P. S. (Ed.): *Developmental Physiology and Aging.* MacMillan, New York, 1972, p. 129.

5. Heller, I. H., and Elliott, K. A. C.: Desoxyribonucleic acid content and cell density in brain and human brain tumors. *Can. J. Biochem. Physiol.* **32**:584, 1954.

6. Lentz, R. D., and Lapham, L. W.: A quantitative cytochemical study of the DNA content of neurons of rat cerebellar cortex. *J. Neurochem.* **16**:379, 1969.

7. Lapham, L. W., and Lentz, R. D.: Postnatal development of tetraploid DNA content in rat Purkinje cells: A quantitative cytochemical study. *J. Neuropathol. Exp. Neurol.* **29**:43, 1970.

8. Herman, C. J., and Lapham, L. W.: Neuronal polyploidy and nuclear volumes in the cat central nervous system. *Brain Res.* **15**:35, 1969.

9. Hyden, H., and Lange, P. W.: Differences in metabolism of oligodendroglia and nerve cells in the vestibular area. In: Kety, S. S., and Elkes, J. (Eds.): *Regional Neurochemistry*. Pergamon Press, Oxford, 1961, p. 190.

10. Hess, H. H., and Thalheimer, C.: Microassay of biochemical structural components in nervous tissues—1. Extraction and partition of lipids and assay of nucleic acids. *J. Neurochem.* **12**:193, 1965.

11. Svennerholm, L.: The gangliosides. *J. Lipid Res.* **5**:145, 1964.

12. Lowden, J. A., and Wolfe, L. S.: Studies on brain gangliosides. (iii) Evidence for the location of gangliosides specifically in neurones. *Can. J. Biochem.* **42**:1587, 1964.

13. Davison, A. N.: Lipids and brain development. In: Pease, D. C. (Ed.): *Cellular Aspects of Neural Growth and Differentiation*. U.C.L.A. Forum in Medical Sciences, No. 14, 1951, p. 365.

14. De Robertis, E., and Rodriguez de Lores A. G.: Structural components of the synaptic region. In: *Handbook of Neurochemistry*, Vol. 2, Plenum Press, New York, 1969, p. 365.

15. Suzuki, K., Poduslo, S. E., and Norton, W. T.: Gangliosides in the myelin fraction of developing rats. *Biochim. Biophys. Acta* **144**:375, 1967.

16. Suzuki, K., Poduslo, J. F., and Poduslo, S. E.: Further evidence for a specific ganglioside fraction closely associated with myelin. *Biochim. Biophys. Acta* **152**:576, 1968.

17. Hess, H. H., and Pope, A.: Effect of metal cations on adenosinetriphosphatase activity of rat brain. *Fed. Proc.* **16**:196, 1957.

18. Bonting, S. L., Simon, K. A., and Hawkins, N. M.: Studies on sodium-potassium-activated adenosine triphosphatase. 1. Quantitative distribution in several tissues of the cat. *Arch. Biochem. Biophys.* **95**:416, 1961.

19. Deul, D. H., and McIlwain, H.: Activation and inhibition of adenosine triphosphatases of subcellular particles from the brain. *J. Neurochem.* **8**:246, 1961.

20. Jarnefelt, J.: Properties of sodium-stimulated adenosine triphosphatase in microsomes from rat brain. *Exp. Cell Res.* **21**:214, 1960.

21. Jarnefelt, J.: Sodium-stimulated adenosine triphosphatase in microsomes from rat brain. *Biochim. Biophys. Acta* **48**:104, 1961.

22. Fahn, S., and Côté, L. J.: Regional distribution of sodium-potassium activated adenosine triphosphatase in the brain of the rhesus monkey. *J. Neurochem.* **15**:433, 1968.

23. Bonting, S. L., Caravaggio, L. L., and Hawkins, N. M.: Studies on sodium-potassium activated adenosine-triphosphatase. IV. Correlation with cation transport sensitive to cardiac glycosides. *Arch. Biochem. Biophys.* **98**:413, 1962.

24. Bonting, S. L.: Sodium-potassium activated adenosinetriphosphatase and cation transport. In: Bittar, E. E. (Ed.): *Membranes and Ion Transport*, Vol. 1. Wiley-Interscience, New York, 1970, p. 289.

25. Whittam, R.: The dependence of the respiration of brain cortex on active cation transport. *Biochem. J.* **82**:205, 1962.

26. Cummins, J., and Hyden, H.: ATP levels and ATPases in neurons, glia and neuronal membranes of the vestibular nucleus. *Biochim. Biophys. Acta* **60**:271, 1962.

27. Shein, H., Britva, A., Hess, H., and Selkoe, D.: Isolation of hamster brain astroglia by *in vitro* cultivation and subcutaneous growth, and content of cerebroside, ganglioside, RNA and DNA. *Brain Res.* **19**:497, 1970.

28. Medzihradsky, F., Sellinger, O. Z., Nandhasri, P. S., and Santiago, J. C.: ATPase activity in glial cells and in neuronal perikarya of rat cerebral cortex during early postnatal development. *J. Neurochem.* **19**:543, 1972.

29. Rodriguez de Lores, A. G., Alberici, M., and De Robertis, E.: Ultrastructural and enzymatic studies of cholinergic and non cholinergic synaptic membranes isolated from brain cortex. *J. Neurochem.* **14**:215, 1967.

30. Kurokawa, M., Sakamoto, T., and Kato, M.: Distribution of sodium-plus-potassium-stimulated adenosine-triphosphatase activity in isolated nerve-ending particles. *Biochem. J.* **97**:833, 1965.

31. Abdel-Latif, A. A., Brody, J., and Ramahi, H.: Studies on sodium-potassium adenosine triphosphatase of the nerve endings and appearance of electrical activity in developing rat brain. *J. Neurochem.* **14**:1133, 1967.

32. Samson, F. E., and Quinn, D. J.: Na$^+$-K$^+$-activated ATPase in rat brain development. *J. Neurochem.* **14**:421, 1967.

33. Van Goor, H.: Carbonic anhydrase, its properties, distribution and significance for carbon dioxide transport. *Enzymologia* **13**:73, 1948.

34. Ashby, W., Garzoli, R. F., and Schuster, E. M.: Relative distribution patterns of three brain enzymes, carbonic anhydrase, cholinesterase and acetylphosphatase. *Am. J. Physiol.* **170**:116, 1952.

35. Giacobini, E.: A cytochemical study of the localisation of carbonic anhydrase in the nervous system. *J. Neurochem.* **9**:169, 1962.

36. Giacobini, E.: Metabolic relations between glia and neurons studied in single cells. In: Cohen, M. M., and Snider, R. S. (Eds.): *Morphological and Biochemical Correlates of Neural Activity*. Harper (Hoeber), New York, 1964, p. 15.

37. Tower, D. B., and Young, O. M.: The activities of butyrylcholinesterase and carbonic anhydrase, the rate of anaerobic glycolysis, and the question of a constant density of glial cells in cerebral cortices of various mammalian species from mouse to whale. *J. Neurochem.* **20**:269, 1973.

38. Nishimura, T., Tanimukai, H., and Nishinuma, K.: Distribution of carbonic anhydrase in human brain. *J. Neurochem.* **10**:257, 1963.

39. Millichap, J. G.: Development of seizure patterns in newborn animals. Significance of brain carbonic anhydrase activity. *Proc. Soc. Exp. Biol. Med.* **96**:125, 1957.

40. Nair, V., and Bau, D.: Effects of prenatal X-irradiation on the ontogenesis of acetylcholinesterase and carbonic anhydrase in rat central nervous system. *Brain Res.* **16**:383, 1969.

41. Paoletti, R., Grossi-Paoletti, E., and Fumagalli, R.: Sterols. In: Lajtha, A. (Ed.): *Handbook of Neurochemistry*, Vol. 1. Plenum Press, New York, 1969, p. 195.

42. Norton, W. T., and Antilio, L. A.: The lipid composition of purified bovine brain myelin. *J. Neurochem.* **13**:213, 1966.

43. Shein, H. M., Britva, A., Hess, H. H., and Selkoe, D. J.: Isolation of hamster brain astroglia by *in vitro* cultivation and subcutaneous growth, and content of cerebroside, ganglioside, RNA and DNA. *Brain Res.* **19**:497, 1970.

44. Wells, M. A., and Dittmer, J. C.: A comprehensive study of the postnatal changes in the concentration in lipids of developing rat brains. *Biochemistry* **6**:3169, 1967.

45. Davison, A. N.: The biochemistry of the myelin sheath. In: Davison, A. N., and Peters, A. (Eds.): *Myelination*. Thomas, Springfield, Illinois, 1970, p. 80.

46. Cuzner, M. L., and Davison, A. N.: The lipid composition of rat myelin and subcellular fractions during development. *Biochem. J.* **106**:29, 1968.

47. Davison, A. N., and Gregson, N. A.: The physiological role of cerebron sulphuric acid (sulphatide) in the brain. *Biochem. J.* **85**:558, 1962.

48. Kerr, G. R., Helmuth, A. C., and Waisman, H. A.: Growth and development of the fetal rhesus monkey. IV. Fractional lipid analysis of the developing brain. *Growth* **37**:41, 1973.

49. Portman, O. W., Alexander, M., and Illingworth, D. R.: Changes in brain and sciatic nerve composition with development of the rhesus monkey (*Macaca mulatta*). *Brain Res.* **43**:197, 1972.

50. Dobbing, J.: Vulnerable periods in developing brain. In: Davison, A. N., and Dobbing, J. (Eds.): *Applied Neurochemistry*. Davis, Philadelphia, 1968, p. 287.

51. Barlow, J. S., and Manery, J. F.: The changes in electrolytes, particularly chloride, which accompany growth in chick muscle. *J. Cell. Comp. Physiol.* **43**:165, 1954.

52. Cotlove, E.: Mechanism and extent of distribution of inulin and sucrose in chloride space of tissues. *Am. J. Physiol.* **176**:396, 1954.

53. Donahue, S., and Pappas, G. D.: The fine structure of capillaries in the cerebral cortex of the rat at various stages of development. *Am. J. Anat.* **108**:331, 1961.

54. Pappas, G. D., and Purpura, D. P.: Electron microscopy of immature human and feline neocortex. In: Purpura, D. P., and Schade, J. P. (Eds.): *Progress in Brain Research*, Vol. 4: *Growth and Maturation of the Brain*. Elsevier, Amsterdam, 1964, p. 176.

55. Koch, A., Ranck, J. B., Jr., and Newman, B. L.: Ionic content of neuroglia. *Exp. Neurol.* **6**:186, 1962.

56. Katzmann, R.: Electrolyte distribution in mammalian central nervous system. Are glia high sodium cells? *Neurology* **11**:27, 1961.

57. Gerschenfeld, H. M., Wald, F., Zadunaisky, J. A., and De Robertis, E. D.: Function of astroglia in the water-ion metabolism of the central nervous system. *Neurology* **9**:412, 1959.

58. Luse, S. A., and Harris, B.: Electron microscopy of the brain in experimental edema. *J. Neurosurg.* **17**:439, 1960.

59. Hild, W., and Tasaki, I.: Morphological and physiological properties of neurons and glial cells in tissue culture. *J. Neurophysiol.* **25**:277, 1962.

60. Vernadakis, A., and Woodbury, D. M.: Cellular and extracellular spaces in developing brain. *Arch. Neurol.* **12**:284, 1965.

61. Vernadakis, A., and Woodbury, D. M.: Electrolyte and amino acid changes in rat brain during maturation. *Am. J. Physiol.* **203**:748, 1962.

62. Ferguson, R. K., and Woodbury, D. M.: Penetration of ^{14}C-inulin and ^{14}C-sucrose into brain, cerebrospinal fluid and skeletal muscle of developing rats. *Exp. Brain Res.* **7**:181, 1969.

63. Medzihrudsky, F., Sellenger, O. Z., Nandhasri, P. S., and Santiago, J. C.: Adenosine triphosphatase activity in glial cells and in neuronal perikarya of edematous rat brain. *Brain Res.* **67**:133, 1974.

64. Van Harreveld, A., Crowell, J., and Malhotra, S. K.: A study of extracellular space in central nervous tissue by freeze substitution. *J. Cell Biol.* **25**:117, 1965.

65. Koch, A., and Woodbury, D. M.: Carbonic anhydrase inhibition and brain electrolyte composition. *Am. J. Physiol.* **198**:434, 1960.

66. Van Harreveld, A.: Extracellular space in the central nervous system. *Kon. Nederl. Akad. van Wet. Ser. C* **69**:17, 1966.

67. Van Harreveld, A.: *Brain Tissue Electrolytes*. Butterworth, London, 1966.

68. Renkawek, K., Palladini, G., and Ieradi, L. A.: Morphology of glia cultured *in vitro* in presence of ouabain. *Brain Res.* **18**:363, 1970.

69. Bondareff, W., and Pysh, J. J.: Distribution of the extracellular space during postnatal maturation of rat cerebral cortex. *Anat. Rec.* **160**:773, 1968.

70. Glaser, E. M., and Van der Loos, H.: A semi-automatic computer-microscope for the analysis of neuronal morphology. *IEEE Trans. Biomed. Eng.* **12**:22, 1965.

71. Dudley, A. W., Jr.: Computer analysis of neurones. *J. Neuropathol. Exp. Neurol.* (*Abstr.*) **29**:145, 1970.

72. Jesse, A.: Quantitative image analysis in microscopy—A review. *The Microscope* **19**:87, 1971.

73. Mawdesley-Thomas, L. E., and Healey, P.: Automated analysis of cellular change in histological sections. *Science* **163**:1200, 1969.

74. Smith, F. H.: A laser-illuminated screening interferometer for determining the dry mass of living cells. *The Microscope* **20**:153, 1972.

75. Barer, R., and Smith, F.: Microscope for weighing bits of cells. *New Sci.*, 380, 24 August 1972.

CHAPTER 4

Mathematical Appraisal
of Biochemical Determinants
# of Brain Growth

Donald B. Cheek, David E. Mellits, Donald E. Hill, and A. Barry Holt

INTRODUCTION

This chapter deals with curve fitting, by the polynomial regression approach, to data obtained from brain analyses. Initially, each set of data has been analyzed sequentially for a group of equations starting from a simple first-order or linear equation and concluding with a fifth-order polynomial expression. The equation that most adequately describes the data mathematically has been objectively selected by assessing the reduction of variance around the fitted line by the "F test." As it is always possible to fit accurately n points with an $(n - 1)$-degree polynomial expression, the equation showing the best fit statistically has also been inspected to see that it coincides with the biological description of the data. The equations listed in the following four tables satisfy both the biological and statistical criteria.

Documentation of a minimum of five significant figures for each coefficient, especially in high-order equations, is mandatory if high-accuracy predictions are required. This fact is emphasized as many workers who are not accustomed to the use of high-order equations, may well wonder why the quartic term is expressed (for example) as $0.00000049999(CA)^4$.

EXPLANATION OF TABLES AND FIGURES

Tables

The headings on tables are described from left to right.

Time Span

Time span is the time in days over which the data are described. *CA* indicates the age from conception while *PN* (postnatal age) indicates the age from birth. Birth is considered to occur in the macaque at 165 ± 5 days from conception. The actual conception age (CA) at birth for each animal can be ascertained from Appendix II.

n

n indicates the number of subjects in each age bracket used to derive the equation.

Y

Y is the value to be predicted from the equation for an age *within* the time span designated. The *units* for each *Y* value are also given. For example, for the first equation in Table 4.1 the predicted value *Y* would be the cerebral weight expressed in grams.

Equation

In the main, we have considered the period from midgestation up until birth, but where the growth pattern appears to be continuous into the perinatal period (up to 30 days) we have given the full or complete expression and included these points for the first postnatal month. On occasion, the overall equation up until 120 days postnatally can also be given (ie, from midgestation to 120 days postnatally).

It is emphasized that the equations are based on *conceptual age (CA)*. Relationships pertaining only to the postnatal period are, of course, expressed in terms of *postnatal days (PN)*.

SD

SD is the standard deviation around the fitted line.

Fit

The decimalized figure for each equation represents the probability value *P*.

When *linear* equations are documented, the *P* value indicating the significance level of an F test was used to test the existence of regression. In the case of linear equations the correlation coefficient *r* is also given.

In the case when higher order expressions are used (ie, *quadratic*, *cubic*, and *quartic* equations), the *P* value indicates the significance level of an F test used to test the improvement (ie, reduction in variance) from fitting the listed equation over the immediate lower order polynomial equation.

Figures

The majority of the figures in this section and later chapters describing the data derived from our study of macaque have been constructed in a discontinuous manner. This has been done to describe most adequately our findings with a minimum of illustrations.

Each figure has been arbitrarily divided at the "birth" line, which is equivalent to 170 days from conception or approximately to the accepted upper limit of birth (ie, 165 ± 5 days).

All points that fall to the left of this line are derived from animals that were delivered by cesarean section prior to natural birth. This area has been given the title "gestational days" on the abscissa and is synonymous with conceptual age (CA).

All the points that fall to the right of the "birth" line are animals that have been naturally born and allowed to live for 12 hours to 120 days after birth. This postnatal area is titled "postnatal days" and originates from the "birth" line where "birth" equals zero postnatal days. The scale on the abscissa is the same for "gestational days" and "postnatal days."

The mean birth age of the 14 animals included in the postnatal subseries is 166 ± 5 days. Therefore in terms of age of conception the mean displacement of points on the right side of the "birth" axis is 4 days to the right. However, when the postnatal points are considered individually, displacement could be an extreme of 6 days to the left (animal born at 176 days from conception) or 13 days to the right (animal born at 157 days). In essence, the graphs will still essentially illustrate the patterns and changes to be described. Workers wishing to adjust the information to their benefit are referred to the data in Appendix II.

Therefore where equations have been calculated for both fetal and infant monkeys, the age from conception for animals designated PN has been calculated by summing the "gestational days" and the "postnatal days."

The term *mature* on the figure refers to sexually mature or adolescent monkeys of approximately $2\frac{1}{2}$ years of age.

In general, it will become apparent that for the cerebrum and cerebellum when we consider the changes in concentration of a particular determinant, a "tight-fitting" relationship usually is described, whereas when the total amount is considered, the relationship is not so precise due to variation of the weight of the brain at any particular time. The greatest variation in brain weight is seen after the first month of postnatal life; here our data are inadequate.

THE CEREBRUM

Changes in Total Amounts (Table 4.1)

Mass

It will be recalled that the weight of the cerebrum rose from 5 g in midgestation directly to 50 to 55 g at birth. From 80 days of gestation to birth a cubic equation was defined (Equation 1). To determine the total amount of most determinants a large mass is multiplied by a small concentration. Thus the weight of the cerebrum has a large effect on the distribution of the data. However, only total amounts have been considered where the concentration of any determinant varies significantly with time (see below).

The variation of cerebral weight between 30 and 120 postnatal days causes considerable scatter in terms of total amount. Since further information regarding this period is unavailable, these data are not always included. The values can be obtained from Appendix II.

Table 4.1   Equations for components of cerebrum (total amounts)

	Time span	n	Y = units	Equation	SD	Fit
1.	80 days CA to 160 days CA	26	Cerebral weight g	$215.04699 - 6.4643\,(CA) + 0.062688\,(CA)^2 - 0.00017946\,(CA)^3$	4.219	0.05 cubic
2.	80 days CA to birth	26	H_2O ml	$195.89877 - 5.9098\,(CA) + 0.057585\,(CA)^2 - 0.00016628\,(CA)^3$	3.819	0.05 cubic
3.	80 days CA to 30 days PN	28	Non-chloride space ml	$29.82404 - 1.1059\,(CA) + 0.011731\,(CA)^2 - 0.000031283\,(CA)^3$	1.80	0.01 cubic
4.	80 days CA to birth	22	Chloride space ml	$- 6.75096 + 0.18275\,(CA)$	3.514	0.001 linear $r = 0.75$
5.	80 days CA to 30 days PN	32	Protein g	$7.80961 - 0.22707\,(CA) + 0.0020910\,(CA)^2 - 0.000049999\,(CA)^3$	0.292	0.001 cubic
6.	80 days CA to 30 days PN	32	Protein g (Lowry)	$7.70156 - 0.22209\,(CA) + 0.0020268\,(CA)^2 - 0.0000048294\,(CA)^3$	0.292	0.001 cubic
7.	80 days CA to birth	26	RNA mg	$- 104.44771 + 1.39283\,(CA)$	10.19	0.001 linear $r = 0.96$
8.	80 days CA to 30 days PN	32	RNA mg	$103.72178 - 3.8695\,(CA) + 0.043388\,(CA)^2 - 0.00011746\,(CA)^3$	10.45	0.01 cubic

No.	Age period	n	Variable	Equation	Value	p	Type
9.	80 days CA to birth	26	Phospholipid mg	$327.18265 - 11.343 (CA) + 0.10815 (CA)^2$	101.62	0.01	quadratic
10.	80 days CA to birth	26	Cholesterol mg	$184.34876 - 5.99 (CA) + 0.051179 (CA)^2$	35.54	0.001	quadratic
11.	80 days CA to 30 days PN	32	Cholesterol mg	$1402.09058 - 37.698 (CA) + 0.31643 (CA)^2 - 0.00071598 (CA)^3$	48.22	0.01	cubic
12.	80 days CA to 30 days PN	32	Lipid NANA mg	$80.00721 - 2.6472 (CA) + 0.025828 (CA)^2 - 0.000063331 (CA)^3$	6.18	0.05	cubic
13.	80 days CA to 30 days PN	31	$Na^+ K^+$ ATPase Total units	$5676.704 - 218.65 (CA) + 1.791 (CA)^2$	2851	0.001	quadratic
14.	80 days CA to 120 days PN	38	$Na^+ K^+$ ATPase Total units	$86363.31 - 2009.1 (CA) + 14.183 (CA)^2 - 0.026858 (CA)^3$	3670	0.001	cubic
15.	80 days CA to birth	26	Carbonic anhydrase Total units	$1785.27868 - 48.206 (CA) + 0.33537 (CA)^2$	420.7	0.05	quadratic
16.	80 days CA to 120 days PN	39	Carbonic anhydrase Total units	$18754.23883 - 417.8 (CA) + 2.8056 (CA)^2 - 0.0050101 (CA)^3$	714.3	0.001	cubic
17.	80 days CA to birth	26	DNA mg	$-77.36415 + 1.7903 (CA) - 0.0056015 (CA)^2$	5.6236	0.05	quadratic
18.	80 days CA to 30 days PN	32	DNA mg	$-31.55925 + 0.99585 (CA) - 0.0023251 (CA)^2$	6.14	0.01	quadratic
19.	80 days CA to 30 days PN	32	Non-protein dry solid g	$-2.81149 + 0.03464 (CA)$	0.236	0.001	linear r = 0.98

Table 4.1 continued

	Time span	n	Y = units	Equation	SD	Fit
20.	80 days CA to 30 days PN	32	Non-protein dry solid g (Lowry)	$-2.97298 + 0.03717 (CA)$	0.255	0.001 linear r = 0.98
21.	80 days CA to birth	26	RNA to DNA mg/mg	$-1.02458 + 0.01759 (CA)$	0.134	0.001 linear r = 0.96
22.	Birth to 120 days PN	13	RNA to DNA mg/mg	$1.73571 - 0.0036 (PN)$	0.0786	0.001 linear r = -0.90
23.	80 days CA to 120 days PN	39	RNA to DNA mg/mg	$2.45203 - 0.088456 (CA) + 0.0011473 (CA)^2 - 0.0000050804 (CA)^3 + 0.0000000073455 (CA)^4$	0.139	0.001 quartic
24.	80 days CA to birth	26	Protein to DNA mg/mg	$5.09847 - 0.16302 (CA) + 0.0035069 (CA)^2$	4.30	0.05 quadratic
25.	80 days CA to 120 days PN	39	Protein to DNA mg/mg	$176.26141 - 5.3403 (CA) + 0.057783 (CA)^2 - 0.00022778 (CA)^3 + 0.0000000030343 (CA)^4$	4.79	0.001 quartic
26.	80 days CA to 120 days PN	39	Protein to DNA mg/mg (Lowry)	$180.01709 - 5.4589 (CA) + 0.058839 (CA)^2 - 0.00023277 (CA)^3 + 0.0000000031079 (CA)^4$	5.22	0.001 quartic

Key: CA = Days from conception;   PN = Postnatal days;   SD = Standard deviation;   n = Number of subjects

60

In midgestation, the cerebral weight increases rapidly with a slight inflection from 80 days and a less rapid increase toward 160 days (Figure 4.1). The point of maximum inflection is about 120 days or three-fourths of the way through pregnancy. Thus, the period around 120 days in gestation may represent a critical period for fetal growth where insults may be expected to produce the most change or growth arrest. The period could be compared with 32 weeks of gestation for the human since we have indicated that this is a critical time (Chapter 1).

Water

Water is the largest mass component of the brain and represents 90% of the cerebral weight in midgestation and 85% at birth. The curve for total water (Figure 4.2) is similar to the curve for cerebral weight, and can be described by a cubic equation for the fetal period (Equation 2). As will be noted for so many cerebral components, there appears to be a steady increase postnatally up to 90 days followed by a decrease toward "mature" values. Whether this apparent decrease represents a fall in brain water or is an artifact must await further investigation.

Nonchloride Space (Total Water Minus Chloride Space)

Chloride ion in the brain is most probably distributed through the extracellular fluid (Chapter 3). Thus subtraction of the chloride space from the cerebral water in effect gives some measure of the intracellular space. As can be seen from Figure 4.3, this space rises from 2.5 ml in midgestation to 25 ml at birth, again a ten-fold increase (same as weight increment). Whether or not perinatal subjects are included, a well-defined cubic equation can be defined (Equation 3). Thus the pattern is essentially similar to those for cerebral weight and water. Postnatally, it would appear that mature values are attained by 60 days.

Chloride Space

The changes with growth are different here. During fetal life there is a five-fold increase from 5 to 25 ml while postnatally there is a progressive decrease (Figure 4.4), suggesting either that the nonchloride space is still enlarging at the expense of the chloride space or that the loss of water with time is from the chloride space. The linear relationship for the fetal period is given by Equation 4.

Protein

The data points (Figure 4.5) can be described by a linear function or by a quadratic equation. If the data points for the perinatal subjects are included, a cubic relationship unfolds (Equation 5). A maximum is reached about 90 days postnatally. The pattern again follows that of cerebral weight, water, and nonchloride space, except that the steepest part of the curve is attained later, after 120 days, not before. Protein determined by the Lowry method yields very similar information (Equation 6).

RNA

For the fetal period a linear relationship can be described (Figure 4.6, Equation 7). However, the exact relationship is most likely cubic and again the addition of points in the perinatal period yields this equation (Equation 8). The points excluded from

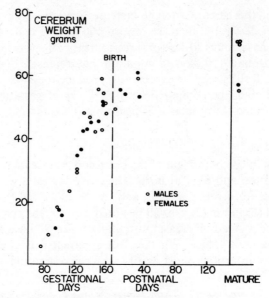

Fig. 4.1. The change in cerebral weight with age in the macaque.

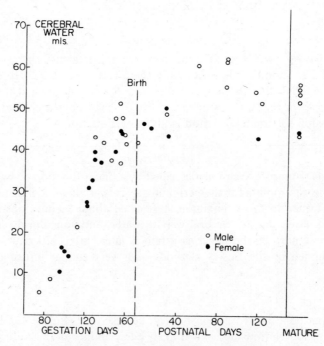

Fig. 4.2. The change in cerebral water content with age in the macaque.

62

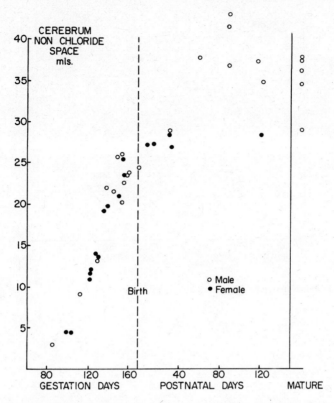

Fig. 4.3. The change in cerebral nonchloride space with age in the macaque.

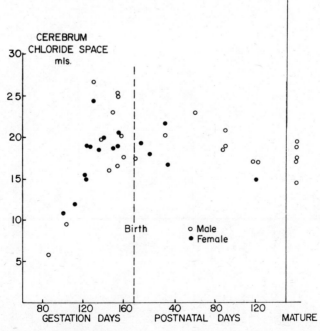

Fig. 4.4. The change in cerebral chloride space with age in the macaque.

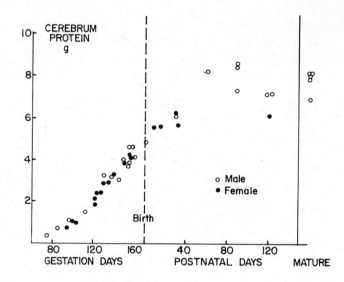

Fig. 4.5. The change in cerebral protein content with age in the macaque.

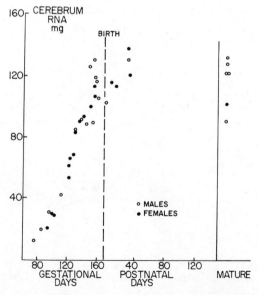

Fig. 4.6. The change in cerebral RNA content with age in the macaque.

the figure (from 30 to 120 postnatal days) suggest that total RNA continues to increase after 30 days then decreases after 90 days to levels comparable with those
found in the mature monkey. Further work is needed.

Phospholipid

Phospholipid is also a major component of brain and increases steadily from midgestation until birth and continuing on into the postnatal period (Figure 4.7). It is
possible that mature levels are not reached for some time, although the limited data
suggest that at 90 postnatal days levels comparable with those in the mature monkey
are obtained. The points for fetuses fall on a quadratic line (Equation 9). The addition of points for the perinatal period (30 days) allows a quadratic or cubic expression. A cubic equation would obtain if all points up to 120 days were included.

Cholesterol

The increase in cerebral cholesterol content (Figure 4.8) is well described through
the fetal period by a quadratic equation (Equation 10). The inclusion of the points
from birth to 30 days alters the relationship to a cubic function (Equation 11). A
comparison of the content at 30 days with the content for $2\frac{1}{2}$-year-old rhesus monkeys emphasizes that cholesterol accretion (and therefore myelination) is a continuous process in early postnatal life. Thus the pattern of growth for cholesterol
resembles that for water, nonchloride space, RNA, and protein, where a linear or
quadratic equation can be used for fetal growth and where inclusion of the points
for perinatal subjects allows the use of a cubic equation. However, as with phospholipid, cholesterol is well below mature levels at birth.

Lipid N-Acetylneuraminic Acid (NANA)

The points for increments in the cerebral lipid NANA (or ganglioside) content of
the fetus can be described by a linear equation while inclusion of the perinatal
data again allows for the use of a cubic equation (Equation 12). The points at
birth are close to expected values for the mature cerebrum (Figure 4.9), suggesting
that this aspect of neuronal structure (nerve endings and dendrites) is well developed at birth.

$Na^+K^+ATPase$-Neuronal Enzyme

After 120 days the increments in total activity of this enzyme are steep and continue
through 30 days postnatally (Figure 4.10). Values at birth are below the expected
mature levels. At 90 days postnatally, a maximum in activity is reached. This enzyme
which predominates in the synaptic membranes (Chapter 3), is possibly not fully
functional at birth but appears to reach its full potential at about 90 postnatal days.
The points up to 30 days are described by a quadratic relationship (Equation 13)
and the overall relationship is cubic (Equation 14).

Carbonic Anhydrase-Neuroglial Enzyme

The total activity of this enzyme present in neuroglial cells is expressed by the
points in Figure 4.11. A quadratic equation describes the fetal period (Equation 15).
At birth the value is one-third to one-quarter that in a mature cerebrum. An overall
cubic equation (Equation 16) can be used to express all points from midgestation
to 120 days postnatally.

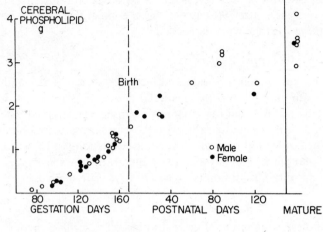

Fig. 4.7. The change in cerebral phospholipid content with age in the macaque

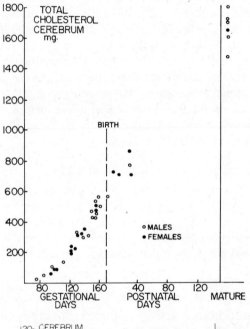

Fig. 4.8. The change in cerebral cholesterol content with age in the macaque.

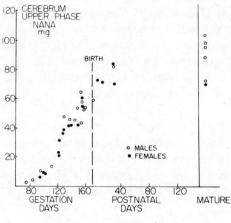

Fig. 4.9. The change in cerebral N-acetylneuraminic acid content with age in the macaque.

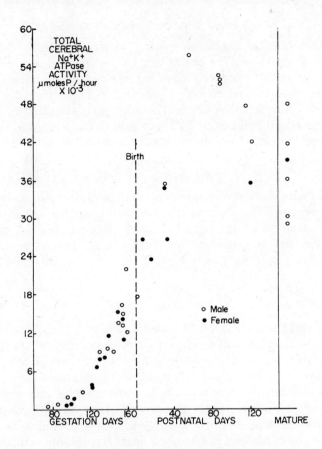

Fig. 4.10. The change in cerebral $Na^+K^+ATPase$ activity with age in the macaque.

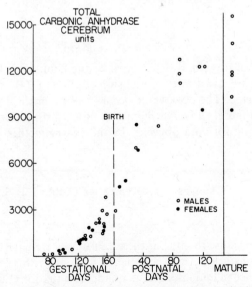

Fig. 4.11. The change in cerebral carbonic anhydrase activity with age in the macaque.

Cerebral DNA-Index of Cell Number

Figure 4.12 illustrates the increase in cerebral DNA content from 30 to 70 mg during the last half of gestation. The points can be described by a quadratic equation (Equation 17). Consideration of the additional points in the perinatal area would yield another quadratic relationship somewhat different from the previous one (Equation 18). Thus the DNA accumulation is slower than that of the other components, suggesting that the addition of new cells to the cerebrum is relatively slow. Clearly, the period prior to midgestation is the period of more rapid growth.

Nonprotein Dry Solid

The dry solid content of the cerebrum other than protein defines mainly the total lipid and mucopolysaccharide. This relationship is linear for the fetus ($r = 0.97$) and the addition of points for the infants up until 120 days does not distort this relationship (Equation 19). Consideration of the protein content (and the nonprotein dry solid content) from the Lowry method yields very similar information (Equation 20).

RNA: DNA Ratio

It is recalled that the total DNA increased slowly with time from midgestation to birth while the RNA increased rapidly. It will be shown below that the concentration of cerebral DNA is decreasing while that of RNA (and protein) is increasing. Clearly, these two components are changing at different rates and it is possible that RNA:DNA may be a measure of the potential protein accretion per cell. The changes in the ratio are shown in Figure 4.13. There is an increase during fetal growth that can be described by a simple line with time (Equation 21). Similarly, the postnatal points can be described by a linear relationship with a negative slope since the ratio decreases (Equation 22). The fourth-order equation (Equation 23) describes the overall relationship. Thus a peak is reached around birth and the intersection of the lines for prenatal and postnatal periods occurs at approximately 160 days of gestation.

Protein: DNA Ratio

The concentration of protein as determined by the Dumas method relative to DNA can be described as a quadratic relationship (Equation 24) or as linear with time during the fetal period. The peak value occurs around birth. Postnatally, a constant value is reached (Figure 4.14). All points do fit a fourth-order relationship (Equation 25). Information for data obtained by the Lowry method is similar (Equation 26).

Changes in Concentration (Table 4.2)

Percentage of Water

Protein accounts for close to 10% of the cerebrum by weight at birth while water is the other major constituent, with a value of 85% at birth. Water comprises 90% of the brain substance in midgestation. A quadratic equation (Equation 27) describes

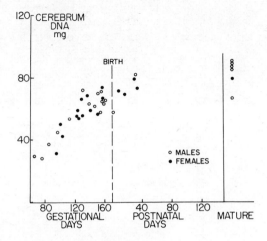

Fig. 4.12. The change in cerebral DNA content with age in the macaque.

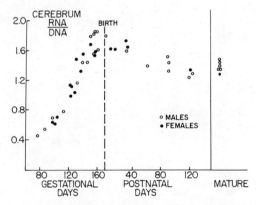

Fig. 4.13. The change in the cerebral RNA:DNA ratio with age in the macaque.

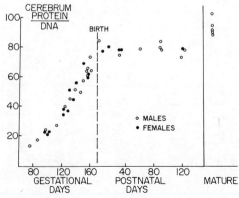

Fig. 4.14. The change in the cerebral protein:DNA ratio with age in the macaque.

Table 4.2   Equations for components of cerebrum (concentrations and ratios)

	Time span	n	Y = units	Equation	SD	Fit
27.	80 days CA to birth	26	H_2O g/100 g	$82.69550 + 0.16842 \, (CA) - 0.00091662 \, (CA)^2$	0.483	0.001 quadratic
28.	Birth to 120 days PN	13	H_2O g/100 g	$84.6391 - 0.080601 \, (PN) + 0.00039446 \, (PN)^2$	0.254	0.001 quadratic
29.	80 days CA to 120 days PN	39	H_2O g/100 g	$55.85235 + 0.91838 \, (CA) - 0.0081004 \, (CA)^2 + 0.000027152 \, (CA)^3 - 0.000000031455 \, (CA)^4$	0.53875	0.001 quartic
30.	80 days CA to birth	22	Non-chloride space ml/g	$0.02246 + 0.00289 \, (CA)$	0.0338	0.001 linear r = 0.88
31.	80 days CA to 120 days PN	35	Non-chloride space ml/g	$-0.07843 + 0.0049905 \, (CA) - 0.0000099554 \, (CA)^2$	0.0313	0.001 quadratic
32.	80 days CA to 120 days PN	35	Chloride space ml/g	$1.10977 - 0.0064024 \, (CA) + 0.000012073 \, (CA)^2$	0.0311	0.001 quadratic
33.	80 days CA to birth	26	Protein mg/g	$127.64250 - 1.3280 \, (CA) + 0.0066629 \, (CA)^2$	3.991	0.001 quadratic
34.	80 days CA to 120 days PN	39	Protein mg/g	$336.39082 - 7.2892 \, (CA) + 0.065331 \, (CA)^2 - 0.00022989 \, (CA)^3 + 0.0000028289 \, (CA)^4$	4.44	0.001 quartic
35.	80 days CA to 120 days PN	39	Protein mg/g (Lowry)	$322.85251 - 7.1657 \, (CA) + 0.065264 \, (CA)^2 - 0.00023339 \, (CA)^3 + 0.0000029024 \, (CA)^4$	4.61	0.001 quartic

		n			SD	
36.	80 days CA to 120 days PN	39	RNA mg/g	$8.45281 - 0.17480\,(CA) + 0.0016193\,(CA)^2 - 0.0000061267\,(CA)^3 + 0.0000000081111\,(CA)^4$	0.105	0.001 quartic
37.	80 days CA to 120 days PN	38	Phospholipid mg/g	$45.49977 - 0.76585\,(CA) + 0.0056973\,(CA)^2 - 0.00001075\,(CA)^3$	3.23	0.001 cubic
.38.	80 days CA to birth	26	Cholesterol mg/g	$-21.99502 + 0.73331\,(CA) - 0.0066311\,(CA)^2 + 0.000020735\,(CA)^3$	0.550	0.05 cubic
39.	Birth to 120 days PN	13	Cholesterol mg/g	$12.24646 + 0.05637\,(\dot{P}N)$	0.957	0.001 linear r = 0.94
40.	80 days CA to birth	26	Lipid NANA mg/g	$4.06585 - 0.10518\,(CA) + 0.00097324\,(CA)^2 - 0.0000027073\,(CA)^3$	0.072	0.05 cubic
41.	80 days CA to birth	26	DNA mg/g	$14.32636 - 0.17327\,(CA) + 0.00057561\,(CA)^2$	0.174	0.001 quadratic
42.	Birth to 120 days PN	13	DNA mg/g	$1.25867 + 0.00145\,(PN)$	0.0533	0.001 linear r = 0.78
43.	80 days CA to 120 days PN	38	Na$^+$ K$^+$ ATPase μmoles P/g/hr	$778.92488 - 18.245\,(CA) + 0.13991\,(CA)^2 - 0.00027079\,(CA)^3$	47.7	0.001 cubic
44.	80 days CA to birth	26	Carbonic anhydrase units/g	$-26.77634 + 0.45971\,(CA)$	9.144	0.001 linear r = 0.79
45.	Birth to 120 days PN	13	Carbonic anhydrase units/g	$82.10253 + 0.85971\,(PN)$	16.64	0.001 linear r = 0.92

Key: CA = Days from conception; PN = Postnatal days; SD = Standard deviation; n = Number of subjects

71

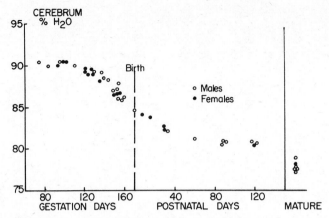

Fig. 4.15.   The change in cerebral water concentration with age in the macaque.

the changes for water concentration in the fetal period (Figure 4.15) while a quadratic equation in the opposite direction describes the postnatal period (Equation 28). These two equations are continuous and a fourth-order expression describes the overall relationship from midgestation up until 120 days postnatally (Equation 29).

Nonchloride Space and Chloride Space

The nonchloride space (an index of the intracellular space) when considered as milliliters per gram of fresh brain (Figure 4.16) rises linearly from midgestation (Equation 30) while the overall relationship for prenatal and postnatal points is quadratic (Equation 31). The chloride space (milliliters per gram) shows an inverse relationship with a steady decrease during fetal life and a more gradual fall during the postnatal period. The overall fit for points is quadratic (Equation 32).

Protein

For assessment of change in protein concentration with growth we have chosen the Dumas method as the best assessment (see Appendix I) but very similar findings with the Lowry method are also documented. From 80 days of gestation to birth the points define a true quadratic equation (Equation 33) with the lowest point at about 100 days (Figure 4.17). Here again, if all points are considered up to 120 days postnatally a very strong fourth-order equation can be recorded (Equation 34), which suggests that the events taking place in the cerebrum in fetal life continue on in a smooth fashion into postnatal life. Application of the Lowry Technique (which does not account for amino acid nitrogen) gave lower values (Equation 35).

RNA

As shown in Figure 4.18, the relationship with time for RNA concentration during fetal life is rather irregular. Possibly there is an initial (midgestation) decrease rather than an increase. The overall points (up to 120 days postnatally) yield a fourth-order relationship (Equation 36).

Phospholipid

The concentration of phospholipid shows a steep rise in late gestation (150 days). This elevation is only sustained until birth, then there must be a gradual increase in

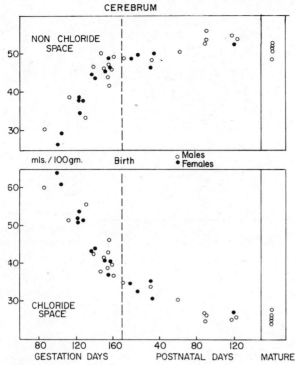

Fig. 4.16. The change with age of chloride and nonchloride spaces expressed per unit weight of the macaque cerebrum.

phospholipid concentration over a sustained period (Figure 4.19). At 120 days postnatally levels are lower than those of the mature monkey. The overall expression is a cubic equation (Equation 37).

Cholesterol

A cubic (Equation 38) or quadratic relationship describes the change in cerebral cholesterol concentration for the fetal period, while a simple linear relationship can be used to define the postnatal period (Equation 39). Clearly, the concentration postnatally is still below the expected level for mature monkeys (see Fig. 4.20).

Lipid NANA

The concentration of ganglioside (as reflected by the upper phase NANA) rises sharply at about 120 days of gestation (Figure 4.21) for only a short period, then this component increases more slowly so that the fetal points are well described by a cubic equation (Equation 40). Shortly after birth a constant concentration is reached.

DNA

In Figure 4.22 it is seen that from midgestation until about 130 days there is a rapid fall in DNA concentrations and a quadratic fit (Equation 41) can be applied to the points for DNA concentration through the fetal period. Clearly, the mature value is reached at the time of birth. In the postnatal period a linear relationship can be described with a positive slope (Equation 42).

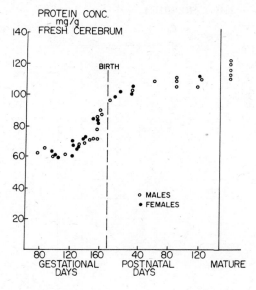

Fig. 4.17. The change in protein concentration with age in the macaque cerebrum.

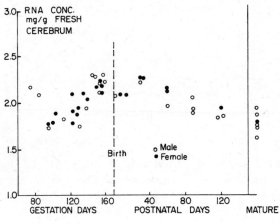

Fig. 4.18. The change in RNA concentration with age in the macaque cerebrum.

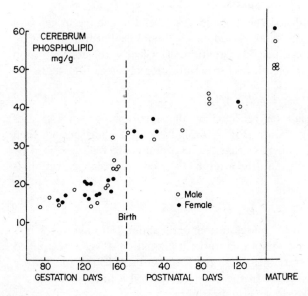

Fig. 4.19. The change in phospholipid concentration with age in the macaque cerebrum.

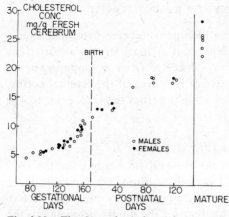

Fig. 4.20. The change in cholesterol concentration with age in the macaque cerebrum.

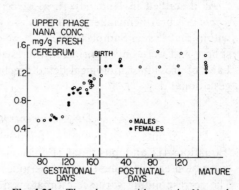

Fig. 4.21. The change with age in *N*-acetylneuraminic acid concentration in the macaque cerebrum.

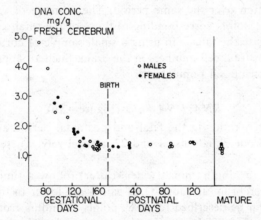

Fig. 4.22. The change in DNA concentration with age in the macaque cerebrum.

$Na^+K^+ATPase$ Activity

The activity of this enzyme per unit weight of tissue increases rapidly from 120 gestational days and continues this rate until 30 days postnatally where mature levels are reached (Figure 4.23). Combined fetal and postnatal points fit a cubic equation (Equation 43).

Carbonic Anhydrase Activity

The enzyme carbonic anhydrase (Figure 4.24) shows a steady increase in activity per unit weight of tissue during fetal life which can be described as a linear function (Equation 44) or as a semilog relationship. The sudden increase in activity during the time of birth and the immediate perinatal period, allows the use of a distinctly new linear relationship postnatally (Equation 45).

Comparisons with Occipital Cortex

In this section values for discrete samples of occipital cortex (O.C.) are compared with cerebral values.

As described in Appendix I, most cerebral components were determined on a *whole* cerebral hemisphere and thus are independent of local structural variations within that tissue. Samples of O.C. were always dissected from the opposing hemisphere and were only considered representative of that area of the cerebral cortex. Lack of gross morphological detail precluded sampling from the O.C. prior to 110 gestational days.

DNA Concentration (Figure 4.25)

All O.C. points are elevated in relation to the cerebral predictions for the fetal (Equation 41) and postnatal (Equation 42) periods. Although an inverse linear expression can describe the fetal period, it has a low predictive value ($r = -0.66$). The corresponding variance estimate is double that for the points belonging to the fetal cerebrum.

No significant regression can be established for the postnatal O.C. points. However, the average value is approximately 0.6 mg/g higher in comparison with cerebral concentration over the same period. The estimate of variance is 20-fold greater than for the points corresponding to those of the total cerebrum.

The data emphasize the fallacy in using a small sample of cortex or brain tissue to predict values for total cell numbers in the brain. Such an approach will lead to gross overestimation of cell populations.

RNA:DNA Ratio (Figure 4.26)

Cerebral RNA:DNA ratios in the fetal and postnatal period are represented by line plots derived from Equations 21 and 22, respectively. These lines intersect at 160 days of gestation.

The O.C. points (exhibiting much wider scatter) follow a similar shape to that described for the cerebrum although O.C. values are lower in the fetal period. A linear expression can be described for O.C. points extending from 110 gestational days to 30 days postnatally. It is suggested that a peak ratio occurs 4 to 6 weeks after birth. The reason for this apparent time difference in peak values between the cortical and cerebral samples is unknown at the present time.

THE CEREBELLUM

Changes in Total Amounts (Table 4.3)

Weight

The weight of the cerebellum (Figure 4.27) is measured only in milligrams in mid-gestation but the weight rises steeply from 100 days of gestation (0.5 g) to a weight of 4 g at birth. The weight then has to double before mature values are reached. It will be recalled that the points for weight against time fit a cubic equation (Equation 46). Water, of course, makes up the major component. It is again cautioned that calculation of the total amount of a constituent is heavily influenced by the weight of the cerebellum.

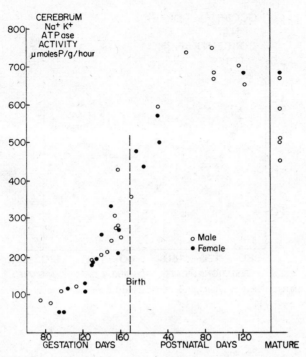

Fig. 4.23. The change with time of Na⁺K⁺ATPase activity per unit weight of macaque cerebrum.

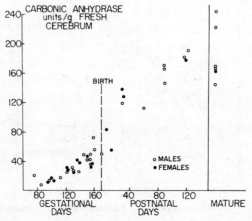

Fig. 4.24. The change with time of carbonic anhydrase activity per unit weight of macaque cerebrum.

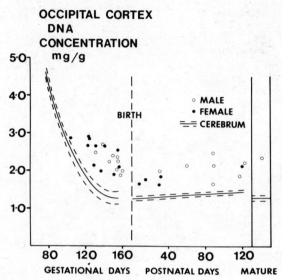

Fig. 4.25. A comparison between occipital cortical and cerebral concentrations of DNA during development in the macaque.

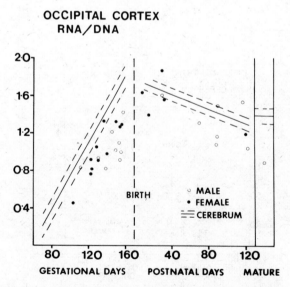

Fig. 4.26. A comparison between occipital cortical and cerebral RNA:DNA ratios during development in the macaque.

Table 4.3

Equations for components of cerebellum (total amounts)

	Time span	n	Y = units	Equation	SD	Fit
46.	80 days CA to 30 days PN	32	Weight g	$8.11719 - 0.22638 \,(CA) + 0.0019475 \,(CA)^2 - 0.00000004516 \,(CA)^3$	0.296	0.01 cubic
47.	80 days CA to birth	26	H_2O ml	$0.83044 - 0.030909 \,(CA) + 0.00027265 \,(CA)^2$	0.258	0.01 quadratic
48.	80 days CA to 30 days PN	32	H_2O ml	$6.36124 - 0.1809 \,(CA) + 0.001589 \,(CA)^2 - 0.0000037496 \,(CA)^3$	0.25	0.01 cubic
49.	80 days CA to 30 days PN	28	Non-chloride space ml	$7.33524 - 0.18967 \,(CA) + 0.0015283 \,(CA)^2 - 0.0000035194 \,(CA)^3$	0.157	0.01 cubic
50.	80 days CA to 30 days PN	28	Chloride space ml	$-0.7183 + 0.01081 \,(CA)$	0.129	0.001 linear r = 0.92
51.	80 days CA to 30 days PN	32	Protein g	$1.22253 - 0.031786 \,(CA) + 0.00025249 \,(CA)^2 - 0.00000055033 \,(CA)^3$	0.032	0.001 cubic
52.	80 days CA to 30 days PN	32	Protein g (Lowry)	$1.40038 - 0.035583 \,(CA) + 0.00027807 \,(CA)^2 - 0.0000061351 \,(CA)^3$	0.035	0.001 cubic
53.	80 days CA to 30 days PN	32	RNA mg	$30.28252 - 0.87139 \,(CA) + 0.0076967 \,(CA)^2 - 0.000019001 \,(CA)^3$	1.095	0.001 cubic
54.	80 days CA to 30 days PN	25	Phospholipid mg	$804.4144 - 18.38 \,(CA) + 0.1319 \,(CA)^2 - 0.00028227 \,(CA)^3$	14.2	0.05 cubic

Table 4.3 continued

	Time span	n	Y = units	Equation	SD	Fit
55.	80 days CA to 30 days PN	26	Cholesterol mg	$324.65567 - 7.3151 \,(CA) + 0.051557 \,(CA)^2 - 0.00010766 \,(CA)^3$	6.23	0.05 cubic
56.	80 days CA to 30 days PN	27	Lipid NANA mg	$2.05459 - 0.049159 \,(CA) + 0.00031488 \,(CA)^2$	0.353	0.001 quadratic
57.	80 days CA to 30 days PN	32	DNA mg	$67.4132 - 1.8569 \,(CA) + 0.015713 \,(CA)^2 - 0.000036804 \,(CA)^3$	2.15	0.001 cubic
58.	80 days CA to 120 days PN	29	Na$^+$ K$^+$ ATPase Total units	$6035.53975 - 128.48 \,(CA) + 0.81647 \,(CA)^2 - 0.0014313 \,(CA)^3$	344	0.001 cubic
59.	80 days CA to 120 days PN	32	Carbonic anhydrase Total units	$3113.73865 - 61.298 \,(CA) + 0.37139 \,(CA)^2 - 0.00062985 \,(CA)^3$	165.6	0.05 cubic
60.	80 days CA to 120 days PN	39	Non-protein dry solid g	$0.52798 - 0.012967 \,(CA) + 0.000095484 \,(CA)^2 - 0.0000001771 \,(CA)^3$	0.0236	0.001 cubic
61.	80 days CA to 120 days PN	39	Non-protein dry solid g (Lowry)	$0.51361 - 0.013045 \,(CA) + 0.0000009895 \,(CA)^2 - 0.00000018316 \,(CA)^3$	0.037	0.001 cubic

No.	Age	n	Measure	Equation	SD	p
62.	Birth to 120 days PN	13	RNA to DNA mg/mg	$0.43333 - 0.00083 \, (PN)$	0.03	0.001 linear r = - 0.79
63.	80 days CA to 30 days PN	32	Protein to DNA mg/mg	$23.57378 - 0.17327 \, (CA) + 0.00076307 \, (CA)^2$	1.77	0.01 quadratic
64.	Birth to 120 days PN	13	Protein to DNA mg/mg	$17.2472 + 0.03059 \, (PN)$	1.29	0.01 linear r = 0.74
65.	80 days CA to 30 days PN	32	Protein to DNA mg/mg (Lowry)	$26.089 - 0.22637 \, (CA) + 0.00092135 \, (CA)^2$	2.16	0.01 quadratic

Key: CA = Days from conception;   PN = Postnatal days;   SD = Standard deviation;   n = Number of subjects

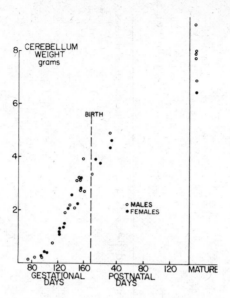

Fig. 4.27. The increase in the cerebellar weight with time in the macaque.

Water

The points fit a quadratic equation (Equation 47) for the fetal period, and the addition of points in the postnatal period (up to 30 days) yields a cubic relationship (Equation 48). Figure 4.28 illustrates the relationship of cerebellar water to age.

Nonchloride Space

The volume of the nonchloride space (Figure 4.29) rises sharply from midgestation to birth. At that time, the volume is only 50% of the mature value. All points fit a quadratic equation but the period from midgestation to 30 days postnatally is also given by a cubic equation (Equation 49).

Chloride Space

The points for the fetal and perinatal period form a linear relationship (Equation 50). From 100 days of gestation there is a steady increment. After 30 days postnatally, there is slower expansion of volume. All points can be described by a quadratic equation (Figure 4.30).

Protein

A quadratic equation can be used to describe the points for total protein in the fetal period (Figure 4.31). If the points for the perinatal period are added in, the expression becomes cubic (Equation 51). The points from 40 to 120 days, which are not shown, suggest that mature levels for cerebellar protein are not reached by 120 days. Postnatal points yield a quadratic relationship. Similar information is obtained when the Lowry method is used for protein determination (Equation 52). The accretion of protein in the cerebellum does not gain impetus until after 120 days of gestation.

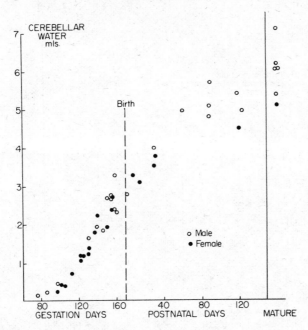

Fig. 4.28. The change in total cerebellar water with time in the macaque.

RNA

The increase in cerebellar RNA content starts earlier than that for protein (as one might expect) and by 100 days of gestation the content increases linearly. Figure 4.32 shows the distribution of points in the fetal and perinatal periods. A cubic equation can be described (Equation 53). For the period 40 to 120 postnatal days, three out of seven points fall above the values shown for mature monkeys, suggesting that first an increase then a decrease in RNA content may occur. More data are needed to verify the statement.

Phospholipid

The elevation in phospholipid content does not begin until after 120 days of gestation (Figure 4.33) but accumulation continues well into the postnatal period where values are still below those for mature primates. The inclusion of the points for the first 30 days of the postnatal period allows the documentation of a cubic equation (Equation 54).

Cholesterol

The increment in total cholesterol content is also delayed until about 140 days (Figure 4.34). At birth, the value is only 20% of that expected for the mature primate. The fetal points and those up to 30 days can be described by a cubic equation (Equation 55).

Lipid NANA (Ganglioside)

A steady rise in upper phase NANA content can be deduced from inspection of Figure 4.35. This elevation is sustained through the perinatal period. A quadratic

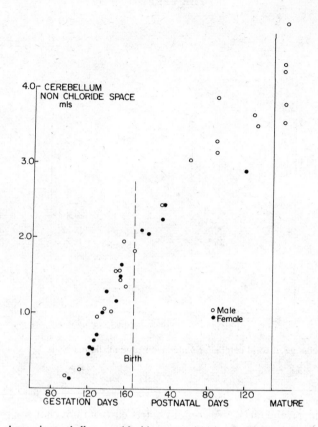

Fig. 4.29. The change in cerebellar nonchloride space with time in the macaque.

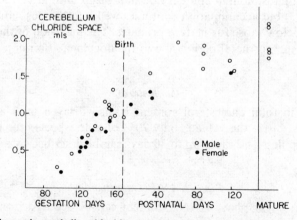

Fig. 4.30. The change in cerebellar chloride space with time in the macaque.

84

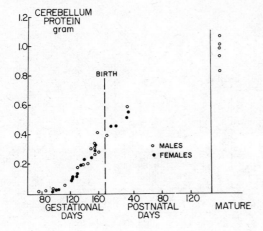

Fig. 4.31. The change in cerebellar protein content with time in the macaque.

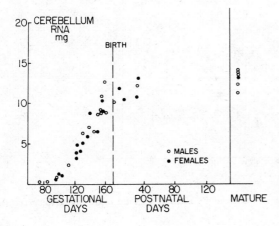

Fig. 4.32. The change in cerebellar RNA content with time in the macaque.

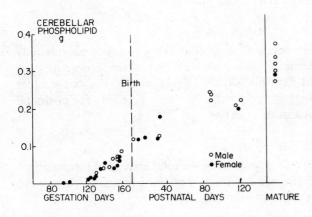

Fig. 4.33. The change in cerebellar phospholipid content with time in the macaque cerebellum.

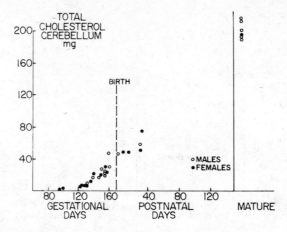

Fig. 4.34.   The change in cholesterol content with time in the macaque cerebellum.

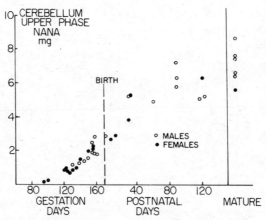

Fig. 4.35.   The changes in *N*-acetylneuraminic acid content with time in the macaque cerebellum.

equation describes the relationship (Equation 56). All points could be described by a cubic equation since after 80 postnatal days a decrease in ganglioside content may occur. Further work is indicated to clarify this finding.

DNA

From 100 days of gestation, the content of cerebellar DNA rises appreciably only to lose velocity shortly after birth (Figure 4.36). A cubic equation describes the points from midgestation to 30 days postnatally (Equation 57). Points for older infant monkeys (30–120 days) suggest that mature levels are reached. The postnatal points can be described by a quadratic equation.

$Na^+ K^+ ATPase$

The points indicate (Figure 4.37) a dramatic rise in the total activity of this neuronal enzyme just prior to birth. The increase is sustained into the postnatal period. All points are well described by a cubic equation (Equation 58).

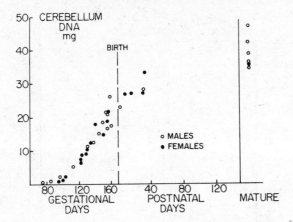

Fig. 4.36. The change in DNA content with time in the macaque cerebellum.

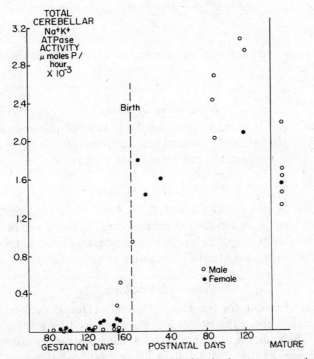

Fig. 4.37. The change in Na^+K^+ATPase activity with time in the macaque cerebellum.

Carbonic Anhydrase

As with the neuronal enzyme, the activity of this neuroglial enzyme also shows a remarkable increase just prior to birth (Figure 4.38). This increase is sustained into the postnatal period. The points can all be described by a cubic equation (Equation 59).

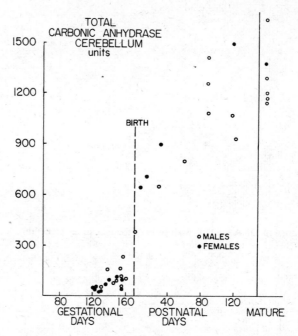

Fig. 4.38. The change in carbonic anhydrase content with time in the macaque cerebellum.

Nonprotein Dry Solid

A cubic equation can be used to describe the growth of this component (mainly composed of lipids) in fetal and postnatal life (Equations 60 and 61) or, alternatively, a separate quadratic relationship can be used for each period.

RNA: DNA Ratio

Inspection of the figures for DNA and RNA contents in the cerebellum during fetal life reveals somewhat similar patterns of change, hence the ratio is constant and no mathematical fit is applicable. For the postnatal period a definite slope can be defined and a linear relationship is indicated (Equation 62).

Protein: DNA Ratio

The distribution of points for the ratio of protein (Dumas method) to DNA resembles a "teacup," hence the points are described well by a quadratic equation (Equation 63). The addition of points up to 30 days postnatally changes this quadratic equation only slightly. Postnatally a linear relationship holds (Equation 64). Information obtained from the Lowry method is essentially similar (Equation 65).

Changes in Concentration (Table 4.4)

Water

In Figure 4.39 it can be seen that the percentage of water begins to decrease at about 100 days of gestation and continues to do so at a steady rate until about 30

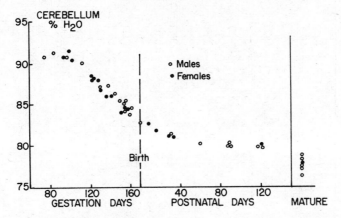

Fig. 4.39. The changes in water concentration with time in the macaque cerebellum.

days postnatally when constancy is soon reached. The points for the fetal period through the first 30 days fit a cubic expression very well (Equation 66) and all points fit a fourth-order equation (Equation 67). As with the cerebrum, the percentage of water is about 90 in midgestation and 85 at birth.

Nonchloride and Chloride Space

The volume per gram for the nonchloride space shows a sigmoid curve for the fetal period with a value almost at the mature level at birth (Figure 4.40). The points (all points) fit a fourth-order equation (Equation 68) but can be well expressed also by a cubic equation that does not take into account the "dip" in the postnatal period.

The plot of the chloride space tends to be a mirror image of the above with a decreasing value up until birth. The fit for these points can be expressed by a cubic equation (Equation 69).

Protein

The protein concentration appears to remain constant from 80 to 100 days, then increases steadily to birth and shortly afterwards reaches a constant value (Figure 4.41). The points in the fetal period plus or minus those in the perinatal period (first 30 days) yield a cubic equation (Equation 70). The remaining postnatal period can be expressed as a mean $\pm$SD. The Lowry method for protein determination gave similar data.

RNA

Figure 4.42 demonstrates the rapid increase in RNA concentration in the cerebellum during fetal life. The concentration reaches a zenith at about 120 days of gestation, then there follows a gradual decrease in RNA concentrations. The fetal relationship can be described by a quadratic equation (Equation 71) while a linear relationship (Equation 72) pertains for the postnatal period. This is an instance where a breaking line relationship exists, with the break around 120 days. Thus the period from 80 to 120 days is represented by one line and the period from 120 days prenatally to 120 days postnatally can be represented by another.

Table 4.4

Equations for components of cerebellum (concentrations)

	Time span	n	Y = units	Equation	SD	Fit
66.	80 days CA to 30 days PN	32	H_2O g/100 g	$69.23965 + 0.62238\,(CA) - 0.0053537\,(CA)^2 + 0.000012718\,(CA)^3$	0.533	0.001 cubic
67.	80 days CA to 120 days PN	39	H_2O g/100 g	$63.70769 + 0.85398\,(CA) - 0.008697\,(CA)^2 + 0.00003267\,(CA)^3 - 0.0000000041959\,(CA)^4$	0.512	0.001 quartic
68.	80 days CA to 120 days PN	35	Non-chloride space ml/g	$45.45469 - 1.4267\,(CA) + 0.016468\,(CA)^2 - 0.000083392\,(CA)^3 + 0.0000001562\,(CA)^4$	0.0187	0.01 quartic
69.	80 days CA to 120 days PN	35	Chloride space ml/g	$2.14649 - 0.024819\,(CA) + 0.00010948\,(CA)^2 - 0.00000016\,(CA)^3$	0.028	0.001 cubic
70.	80 days CA to 30 days PN	32	Protein mg/g	$211.0157 - 4.3409\,(CA) + 0.037854\,(CA)^2 - 0.000092166\,(CA)^3$	3.93	0.001 cubic
71.	80 days CA to birth	26	RNA mg/g	$-6.15795 + 0.13238\,(CA) - 0.00046677\,(CA)^2$	0.284	0.001 quadratic
72.	Birth to 120 days PN	13	RNA mg/g	$2.96933 - 0.0085\,(PN)$	0.163	0.001 linear r = - 0.92
73.	80 days CA to 30 days PN	25	Phospholipid mg/g	$-15.3516 + 0.2443\,(CA)$	3.8	0.001 linear r = 0.87

90

	Period	n	Measure (units)	Equation	SD	p / Type
74.	80 days CA to 30 days PN	26	Cholesterol mg/g	$107.44413 - 2.3258\,(CA) + 0.016589\,(CA)^2 - 0.00003656\,(CA)^3$	1.55	0.01 cubic
75.	80 days CA to 120 days PN	34	Lipid NANA mg/g	$0.32402 + 0.00242\,(CA)$	0.136	0.001 linear $r = 0.70$
76.	80 days CA to 30 days PN	32	DNA mg/g	$-4.18886 + 0.13068\,(CA) - 0.0003876\,(CA)^2$	0.642	0.001 quadratic
77.	80 days CA to 120 days PN	39	DNA mg/g	$-0.43814 + 0.07373\,(CA) - 0.00018348\,(CA)^2$	0.672	0.001 quadratic
78.	80 days CA to 120 days PN	29	$Na^+\ K^+$ ATPase μmoles P/g/hr	$883.85163 - 19.282\,(CA) + 0.1286\,(CA)^2 - 0.00023426\,(CA)^3$	93.7	0.05 cubic
79.	80 days CA to 120 days PN	32	Carbonic anhydrase Units/g	$-116.19791 + 1.15545\,(CA)$	39.9	0.001 linear $r = 0.84$

Key: CA = Days from conception; PN = Postnatal days; SD = Standard deviation; n = Number of subjects

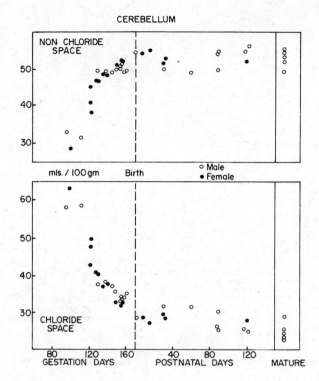

Fig. 4.40. The changes with time of chloride and nonchloride space per unit weight of macaque cerebellum.

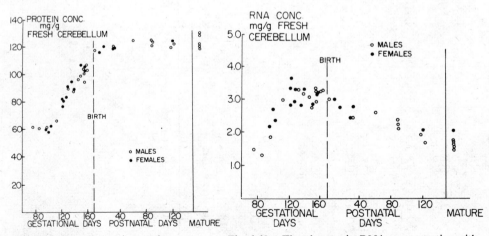

Fig. 4.41. The changes in protein concentration with time in the macaque cerebellum.

Fig. 4.42. The changes in RNA concentration with time in the macaque cerebellum.

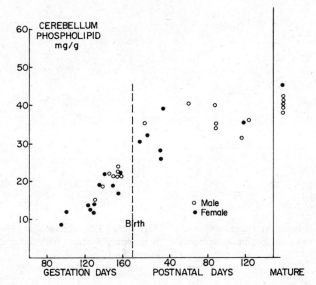

Fig. 4.43.   The changes in phospholipid concentration with time in the macaque cerebellum.

Phospholipid

Figure 4.43 shows a linear rise for the fetal points for phospholipid concentration. This linearity persists into the perinatal period and the equation is given (Equation 73).

Cholesterol

The concentration of cholesterol increases during fetal life from 120 days until after birth. These points, including those from the first 30 days postnatally, fit a cubic equation (Equation 74). After this period, a mean value can be defined (Figure 4.44) that is still considerably lower than that for the mature monkey.

Lipid NANA (Ganglioside)

The points for upper phase NANA concentrations are shown in Figure 4.45. There is no fit for the fetal points as the change in concentration is slight. There is the suggestion that toward the prenatal period a rise does occur.

A linear equation of low predictive value ($r = 0.70$) can be defined for all points (Equation 75). Here, then, is an example where the increased content of a constituent is mainly a reflection of increase in cerebellar weight.

DNA

The concentration of DNA rises from midgestation until birth in the cerebellum (Figure 4.46) and the distribution of points is described by a quadratic equation. The same equation continues into the postnatal period up to 30 days (Equation 76). Clearly, cell proliferation is rapid in the fetal cerebellum prior to birth. For all points an overall quadratic equation (Equation 77) can be used, since at or shortly after birth the DNA concentration decreases. This pattern of change of the DNA concentration (or cell density) during the fetal period is in contrast to that observed in the cerebrum (Figure 4.22).

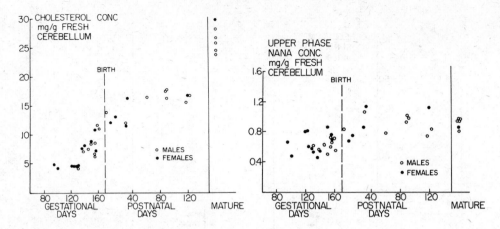

Fig. 4.44. The changes in cholesterol concentration with time in the macaque cerebellum.

Fig. 4.45. The changes in *N*-acetylneuraminic acid concentration with time in the macaque cerebellum.

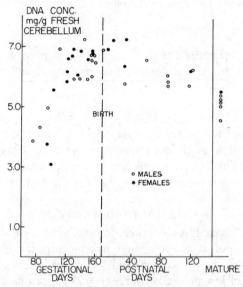

Fig. 4.46. The changes in concentration of DNA with time in the macaque cerebellum.

Na⁺K⁺ATPase

The activity per unit weight of tissue of this enzyme shows a marked increase just prior to birth and postnatally appears to reach levels above that found in the mature monkey (Figure 4.47). All points up to 120 postnatal days can be described by a cubic equation (Equation 78).

Carbonic Anhydrase

A steep rise in the activity per unit weight of tissue occurs around birth (Figure 4.48). The points can only be described by an overall linear equation (Equation 79), which in fact is really joining two discrete groups of points and may not be meaningful. The fourfold rise in activity of prenatal versus postnatal values becomes clear.

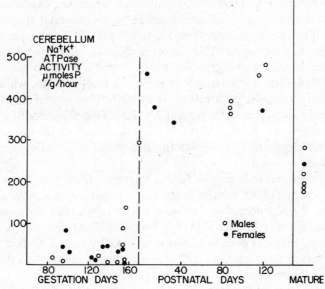

Fig. 4.47. The changes with time of the activity of $Na^+K^+ATPase$ per unit weight of macaque cerebellum.

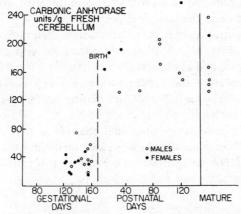

Fig. 4.48. The changes with time of the activity of carbonic anhydrase per unit weight of macaque cerebellum.

GENERAL SUMMARY

The findings presented on normal brain growth can now be summarized.

Cerebrum

The weight of the cerebrum increases steeply from a value of 5 g at midgestation (80 days) to a value of 52 g at birth (160 days) where almost stable values are reached, the mature weight of a macaque cerebrum being 66 ± 7 g in our series. In midgestation, water represents 90% of the weight and at birth 85%. Similarly, there are steep increases in the nonchloride space, total phospholipid, cholesterol, protein, and RNA from midgestation, and the data points are expressed by a linear relationship or a quadratic equation. Inclusion of the perinatal subjects (up to 30 days postnatally) yields a cubic equation for RNA, protein, or phospholipid content and for the nonchloride space. RNA, protein, NANA, and nonchloride space, as well as DNA content, are at mature or almost mature levels 30 days postnatally. The protein:DNA ratio is also nearly at a mature level at birth, while the RNA: DNA ratio shows a definite peak just prior to birth. The increments in cholesterol, NANA, carbonic anhydrase activity, and $Na^+K^+ATPase$ (indices of neuronal and neuroglial function) are well below mature levels, indicating the continued growth or functional development of neuronal and neuroglial cells in the cerebrum in the postnatal period.

By contrast, neuronal cells may be further ahead in development when compared to glial cells since the NANA content is already at a mature level. As already pointed out, the DNA, RNA, and protein content are at levels close to those present at maturity. However, the finding that the $Na^+K^+ATPase$ activity (present in the membranes and synapses) does not increase markedly until 120 days of gestation and reaches levels at birth less than half of mature levels, emphasizes that functional development of the neuronal unit is far from complete.

The water content of the cerebrum follows the general curve shown for cerebral weight. This statement is also true for the nonchloride space (an index of intracellular volume). By contrast, the chloride space (extracellular volume) shows a sharp rise from 5 ml (midgestation) to 20 to 25 ml at birth, following which there appears to be a decrease in the postnatal period.

Inspection of concentration changes indicates increased rates of protein and RNA synthesis from 120 days of gestation and increased deposition of ganglioside (NANA), phospholipid, and cholesterol (myelination). Of particular interest is the fact that from midgestation the concentration of DNA is falling (in contrast to what happens in the cerebellum). Stable and mature levels are reached at birth. The striking escalation of carbonic anhydrase and of $Na^+K^+ATPase$ activity around and after birth, indicates considerable functional changes at that time.

Occipital cortex values generally show greater variability than the corresponding cerebral sample and DNA concentrations are considerably higher. Cortical samples do not therefore reflect cerebral cell populations.

Cerebellum

Certain components of the cerebellum do not show accelerated growth until 100 days of gestation (DNA, RNA, protein, water, and NANA). For these components the velocity of growth increases almost linearly until birth, at which time mature levels are nearly reached for DNA and RNA. The values for protein, water, phospholipid, and NANA content are below mature levels. If extension is made into the perinatal period, the growth of DNA, RNA, protein, phospholipid, and water can be well expressed by cubic equations.

The rises in cholesterol content and of total carbonic anhydrase and Na^+K^+ ATPase activity do not occur until toward the end of gestation (130–150 days). At birth cholesterol, carbonic anhydrase activity, and ATPase are only 25% of the mature values. Thus the functional activity within the neuroglial and neuronal cells is still immature and below that suggested for these cells in the cerebrum. This conclusion is reinforced for neuronal cells by the finding that Na+K+ATPase activity does not accelerate until about 150 days of gestation. At birth the nonchloride space is only 50% of the eventual or final level. Furthermore, the weight of the cerebellum at birth is less than half the mature value (ie, 3.2 g at birth versus 7.7 g at $2\frac{1}{2}$ years).

Unlike the cerebral DNA concentration, cerebellar DNA concentration is increasing during fetal growth. Cell multiplication must be rapid during the last third of gestation and a stable cell number is reached soon after birth. RNA concentration rises steeply until 120 days of gestation and then begins to decrease. The activity in cell multiplication and in DNA and protein synthesis is reflected in the steep upward slope of protein concentration from 120 days to birth. Moreover, while the nonchloride space increases with time up until birth, the chloride space diminishes.

In a general comparison of cerebrum and cerebellum it appears that the rates of deposition of phospholipid and ganglioside are similar for both. The rate of growth of the cerebellum accelerates from midgestation, the increase in cell number and DNA accumulation being 10 times faster than for the cerebrum. A similar figure applies to cholesterol content. Protein accretion is five times faster for the cerebellum. The conclusion is that the rate of growth of the cerebellum is relatively delayed until midgestation. This would lead us to suggest that insults to the fetus in the last trimester would be much more likely to affect cerebellar growth than cerebral growth.

CHAPTER 5

Cerebral Zinc Content During Normal Development and the Effects of Altered Protein Synthesis

Charles Chang and Rachel E. Scott

Zinc was found to be essential for the growth of *Aspergillus niger* by Raulin over 100 years ago.[1] In 1926, Somner and Lipman[2] demonstrated the essential role of zinc in higher plants. The significance of zinc in animal nutrition was suspected early by Birckner,[3] but it was only in 1934 that Todd and his coworkers[4] first showed growth retardation caused by zinc deficiency in the rat. It had been thought that naturally occurring zinc deficiency did not exist due to the ubiquitous nature of zinc; however, Tucker and Salmon[5] clearly established that porcine parakeratosis resulted from a lack of zinc and that zinc supplementation of the diet cured the disease. Since then, zinc deficiency has been either experimentally produced or naturally observed in other animal species including man. [6–12]

Zinc deprivation leads to growth retardation or failure, inanition, bone disorders, dermal lesions, and impaired reproductive function. The severity of these symptoms as well as the order of their appearance depends on the degree and duration of the deficiency imposed and on the age and sex of the animal.[13] In addition, Hurley[14–16] has demonstrated severe congenital malformations in the offspring of zinc-deficient rats; marginally zinc-deficient female rats placed on severely zinc-deficient diets on day 0 of gestation showed a high rate of fetal resorption (54% of implanted sites). Of those fetuses that reached term, 98% were grossly malformed. The pregnant rat is apparently unable to mobilize zinc stores to meet the needs of the developing fetus. Because the offspring of zinc-deficient rats contained less tissue zinc, it has been suggested that the teratogenic effect of maternal zinc deprivation is a direct

Table 5.1   Equations for zinc in the cerebrum

	Time span	n	Y units	Equation Y =	SD	Fit
1.	80 days CA to 30 days PN	32	Total Zn μg	$639.98297 - 18.487\,(CA) + 0.17027\,(CA)^2 - 0.00038991\,(CA)^3$	26.187	0.01 cubic
2.	80 days CA to 30 days PN	32	Zn μg/g	$11.69434 - 0.10487\,(CA) + 0.00051977\,(CA)^2$	0.664	0.001 quadratic
3.	80 days CA to 30 days PN	32	Zn to DNA μg/mg	$16.61425 - 0.42332\,(CA) + 0.0036795\,(CA)^2 - 0.0000088658\,(CA)^3$	0.513	0.01 cubic
4.	80 days CA to 120 days PN	39	Zn to RNA μg/mg	$3.05861 - 0.0049771\,(CA) + 0.000069492\,(CA)^2$	0.517	0.01 quadratic

Key: CA = Days from conception;   PN = Postnatal days;   SD = Standard deviation;   n = Number of subjects

Table 5.2　　　　　　Equations for zinc in cerebrum

	Time span	n	Y units	X units	Equation Y =	SD	Fit
1.	80 days CA to 30 days PN	32	Zn μg/g	Protein mg/g (Dumas)	$11.40694 - 0.18823\,(X) + 0.0017587\,(X)^2$	0.490	0.01 quadratic
2.	80 days CA to 120 days PN	39	Carbonic anhydrase Units/g	Zn μg/g	$-111.37421 + 20.58155\,(X)$	20.393	0.001 linear $r = 0.93$

Key:　CA = Days from conception;　PN = Postnatal days;　SD = Standard deviation;　n = Number of subjects

result of low levels in the fetus rather than a change in some aspect of metabolism in the mother. Previous studies in chickens concerning the influence of maternal dietary zinc on prenatal development yielded similar findings.[17–19]

The metabolic fate of zinc and the consequences of zinc deficiency have been studied [13, 20–23] but the exact metabolic role of zinc is still a matter of debate. Most efforts to study zinc have been hampered by difficulty in experimental design as discussed by Mills and Chesters.[24] Nevertheless, the accumulated evidence suggests that altered nucleic acid metabolism (particularly RNA) leads to altered protein metabolism which in turn may lead to the clinical manifestations of zinc deficiency. In general the concentration of zinc follows the concentration of protein. Holt et al[21] were able to demonstrate a close linear relationship between zinc and RNA in the liver of normal, hypophysectomized, and calorie-restricted rats. Some investigators have suggested that zinc is vital to DNA replication.[25–28]

Data on the level of zinc in normal tissues are available,[12] but little work has been done on the changes in tissue zinc during fetal development and in postnatal life. Widdowson and Spray[29] determined zinc content in the human fetus at different ages; however, their analyses, done prior to the development of atomic absorption spectrophotometry, were limited to total body zinc concentrations. Cheek et al[30] studied variations in manganese, zinc, and copper levels of rat muscle and liver during the first 6 weeks of postnatal life in thyroid- and pituitary-insufficient rats as well as normal rats. Zinc content per unit DNA in normal controls showed a steady decrease in liver and a steady increase in muscle over the 6 weeks. The thyroid- or pituitary-insufficient rats differed from controls in that their tissues at any given age contained concentrations of metal that would be found in much younger rats.

This chapter presents further data on the levels of zinc in normal tissue. The zinc content has been measured in the cerebrum of the rhesus monkey during the last trimester of gestation and the early neonatal period. The relationships between zinc levels and other measurable parameters of growth have been studied in the hope that the metabolic role of zinc in growth might be elucidated. The concentration of zinc was also measured in the muscle and liver during this period of development. Also, zinc in the cerebrum has been examined under circumstances where protein synthesis is altered during hypothyroidism and in the infant born of the diabetic mother.

The tissues used in this study were obtained from fetal rhesus monkeys of known gestational age. In the postnatal period studies were made at approximately 30, 60, 90, and 120 days. Tissue was dried, ground to powder, and used for protein and zinc analyses. The zinc analyses involved dry ashing 250-mg aliquots of powdered tissue in a muffle furnace. The ash residue was dissolved in 0.6 ml of concentrated HCl, and then diluted to an appropriate volume for zinc determination using a Perkin-Elmer Model 303 atomic absorption spectrophotometer. DNA, RNA, protein, and carbonic anhydrase activity were determined simultaneously on fresh tissue.

The total zinc content in the cerebrum increased linearly in relation to the conceptual age of the animal from the earliest fetal period studied through to the first month of postnatal life (Figure 5.1). However, the line fitting the points is best described by a cubic equation (Table 5.1, Equation 1). Thereafter, tissue zinc values were scattered but for mature monkeys the mean value for the total amount of zinc was 895 μg (SD ± 150 μg).

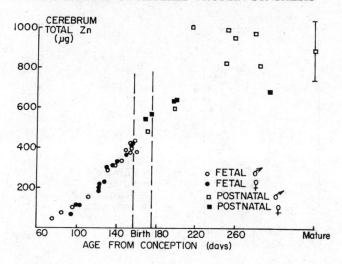

Fig. 5.1.   The zinc content of the cerebrum is plotted against the age from conception for prenatal and postnatal macaques. For mature monkeys a mean value and standard deviation are shown.

Zinc concentration in the fetal cerebrum, on the other hand, remained relatively constant until about 130 days from conception and then increased linearly with age throughout the first postnatal month. A constant level approaching that for mature tissue was reached 120 days postnatally (Figure 5.2). A quadratic equation described the distribution of the data points to 30 days postnatally (Table 5.1, Equation 2). Since zinc concentration was constant up to 130 days of gestation, the linear relationship over the same period for zinc content appears to be a reflection of increasing cerebral weight rather than concurrent variations in cerebral weight and zinc concentration. The concentration of zinc in mature tissue was 13.2 $\mu g/g$ (SD $\pm$ 1.2 $\mu g/g$).

The concentration of zinc also increased linearly with the protein concentration in the cerebrum. Protein concentration varied directly with zinc concentration ($r = 0.934$) throughout fetal life and until the end of the first postnatal month of life (Table 5.2, Equation 2). In animals older than 1 month the cerebral zinc and protein concentrations were generally higher but not directly related.

No significant relationship could be found between the concentration of zinc and DNA in the cerebrum. Comparison of the cerebral zinc:DNA ratio with time revealed a cubic relationship (Figure 5.3, Table 5.1, Equation 3) up until 30 days postnatally. Cerebral zinc:RNA ratio versus conceptual age showed no change during fetal life up until 140 days from conception. Thereafter the ratio showed an increment until 120 days postnatally when stable values were reached (Figure 5.4, Table 5.1, Equation 4).

An effort was made to correlate zinc concentration with zinc metalloenzyme activity.[32,33] Points for carbonic anhydrase concentration in the cerebrum fitted best a linear regression ($P < 0.001$) when plotted against zinc concentration in the same tissue in the overall situation (Figure 5.5, Table 5.2, Equation 2).

In contrast, the concentration of zinc in fresh muscle was 28.0 $\mu g/g$ (SD $\pm$ 4.3 $\mu g/g$) and 175 μg (SD $\pm$ 76 $\mu g/g$) in fresh liver. These values remained constant over the prenatal and postnatal periods and agree with other data.[31]

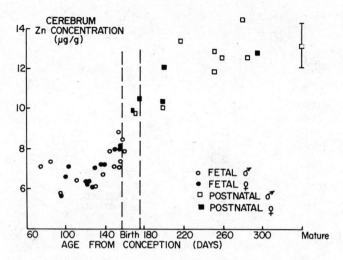

Fig. 5.2. The increase in cerebral zinc concentration with age from conception is presented. The relationship is described mathematically as Equation 2 in Table 5.1. The mean zinc concentration for mature monkeys is shown together with the standard deviation.

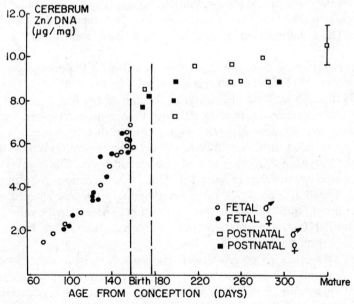

Fig. 5.3. The zinc:DNA ratio in cerebral tissue is plotted against the age from conception for pre-natal and postnatal macaques. The mean value for mature monkeys is also shown together with the standard deviation.

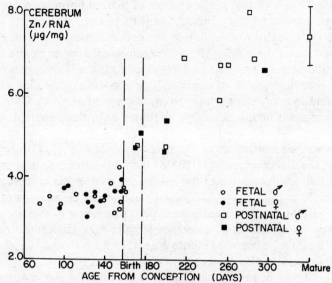

Fig. 5.4. Cerebral zinc:RNA ratio is plotted against the age from conception for pretanal and postnatal macaques. The relationship is described mathematically as Equation 4 in Table 5.1. The mean value for mature monkeys is also shown together with the standard deviation.

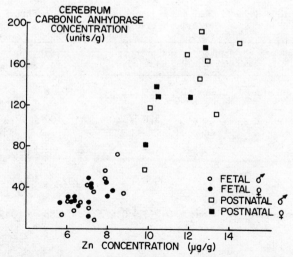

Fig. 5.5. The activity of the zinc-containing metalloenzyme carbonic anhydrase is plotted against the concentration of zinc in the cerebrum.

It is shown in Chapter 8 that in the absence of thyroid hormone protein synthesis does not progress in the fetal cerebrum. Attention to zinc, magnesium, and manganese in this tissue revealed a reduction in the concentration and total amounts for magnesium and zinc (Table 5.3). The data again emphasize the close relationship between zinc and protein synthesis and in this context the finding of a reduction in magnesium concentrations is of interest, this ion being essential in ribosomal organization and in many steps related to protein synthesis.[34, 35] DNA replication was not compromised in this situation; carbonic anhydrase content was reduced by 40%.

In the opposite circumstances of increased cytoplasmic growth as seen in the infant born of the diabetic monkey (IBDM) the amount of zinc in the cerebrum is increased. Figure 5.6 demonstrates the values for zinc in the cerebrum of IBDM compared with 20 normal infants in the same age range. By analysis of covariance the values for IBDM are significantly increased. Inspection of the zinc:DNA ratio showed an even more significant difference (Figure 5.7). Concentration of zinc in the cerebrum was also increased (Figure 5.8). It will be shown elsewhere that the carbonic anhydrase was also increased in the cerebral tissue.

In conclusion it may be said that if growth of the rat fetus shows any similarity to that of the primate, then maternal zinc deprivation could yield offspring with growth retardation and congenital abnormalities that may affect the central nervous system as well as the soma. It is only necessary to restrict zinc intake during the period of organogenesis (8th–14th day for the rat) to produce such pathology.[40]

Only recently has definitive evidence accumulated that zinc deficiency can occur in man and presumably in other primates. Much of the knowledge concerning zinc metabolism has been recently reviewed by Halsted and his colleagues in a monograph (containing 330 references) on zinc requirements for man.[36] The work of Hambidge et al[37] indicates that analysis of hair is a reliable index of zinc deficiency. Roman[38] has found the level of urinary zinc excretion in normal adult subjects to be 400 to 600 μg in 24 hours, while Cheek et al in earlier work showed that from infancy to adolescence 100 to 400 μg was excreted.[39]

Table 5.3   The metal ion content of the cerebrum
                in hypothyroid fetal macaques

		Control (n = 6)	Hypothyroid (n = 6)
Magnesium	Conc. μg/g	*119.9 ± 4.9	**104.6 ± 2.4
	Total μg	5870 ± 440	** 5100 ± 410
Zinc	Conc. μg/g	7.95 ± 0.33	** 6.83 ± 0.67
	Total μg	389.6 ± 27.5	**325.2 ± 22.7
Manganese	Conc. μg/g	0.257 ± 0.051	0.288 ± 0.047
	Total μg	12.6 ± 2.5	13.8 ± 2.5

* Values are mean ± SD   ** P = less than 0.01

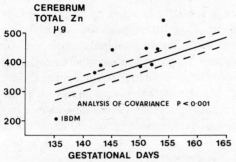

Zn = 639·98297 − 18·487 (CA) + 0·17027 (CA)² − 0·00038991 (CA)³
SD = 26·187 µg   n = 32

Fig. 5.6. Cerebral zinc content in fetal macaques born of diabetic monkeys (IBDM). The content of zinc in the cerebrum for 32 normal macaque fetuses from 140 to 160 days of gestation is shown by a single regression line with one standard deviation on either side.

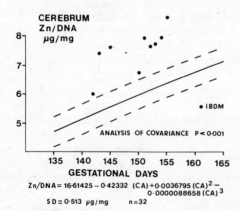

Zn/DNA = 16·61425 − 0·42332 (CA) + 0·0036795 (CA)² − 0·0000088658 (CA)³
SD = 0·513 µg/mg   n = 32

Fig. 5.7. The ratio of zinc:DNA in the cerebrum of fetal macaques born of diabetic monkeys (IBDM) are compared with the regression line for normal macaque fetuses from 140 to 160 days of gestation

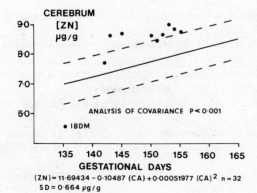

(ZN) = 11·69434 − 0·10487 (CA) + 0·00051977 (CA)²   n = 32
SD = 0·664 µg/g

Fig. 5.8. The concentration of zinc in the cerebrum is shown for normal fetuses and compared with points from fetal macaques born of diabetic monkeys (IBDM).

Attention to the role of zinc in the brain is a matter of importance since zinc is involved in at least 18 metalloenzymes,[33] one of the foremost of which is carbonic anhydrase with widespread representation in the brain. In mammals zinc is heavily represented in the hippocampus associated with axons and mossy fibers projecting from the granule cells in the fascia dentata to the apical dendrites of the pyramidal cells. The work of Crawford and Connor[41] suggests that zinc is involved in the maturation and function of the mossy fiber pathway. At the same time zinc is important to nucleic acid metabolism and to the synthesis of brain protein.[25] The study of zinc metabolism is therefore of importance in any consideration of factors affecting fetal and perinatal growth, especially growth of the brain.*

REFERENCES

1. Raulin, J.: Etudes clinique sur la vegetation. *Ann. Sci. Nat. Bot. Biol. Veg.* **11**:93, 1869.
2. Somer, A. L., and Lipman, C. B.: Evidence of the indispensable nature of zinc and boron for higher green plants. *Plant Physiol.* **1**:231, 1926.
3. Birckner, V.: The zinc content of some food products. *J. Biol. Chem.* **38**:191, 1919.
4. Todd, W. R., Elvehjem, C. A., and Hart, E. B.: Zinc in the nutrition of the rat. *Am. J. Physiol.* **107**:146, 1934.
5. Tucker, H. F., and Salmon, W. D.: Parakeratosis or zinc deficiency disease in pigs. *Proc. Soc. Exp. Biol. Med.* **88**:613, 1955.
6. O'Dell, B. L., and Savage, J. E.: Potassium, zinc and distillers' dried solubles as supplement to a purified diet. *Poultry Sci.* **36**:459, 1957.
7. Legg, S. P., and Sears, L.: Zinc sulfate treatment of parakeratosis in cattle. *Nature* **186**:1061, 1960.
8. Prasad, A. S., Halstead, J. A., and Nadimi, M.: Syndrome of iron deficiency anemia, hepatosplenomegaly, hypogonadism, dwarfism, and geophagia. *Am. J. Med.* **31**:532, 1961.
9. Miller, J. K., and Miller, W. J.: Development of zinc deficiency in Holstein calves fed a purified diet. *J. Dairy Sci.* **43**:1854, 1960.
10. Robertson, B. T., and Burns, M. J.: Zinc metabolism and the zinc deficiency syndrome in the dog. *Am. J. Vet. Res.* **24**:997, 1963.
11. Ott, E. A., Smith, W. H., Stob, M., and Deeson, W. M.: Zinc deficiency syndrome in young lambs. *J. Nutr.* **82**:41, 1964.
12. Fox, M. R. S., and Harrison, B. N.: Zinc deficiency and plasma proteins. In: Prasad, A. S. (Ed.): *Zinc Metabolism*. Thomas, Springfield, Illinois, 1966, p. 187.
13. Underwood, E. J.: *Trace Elements in Human and Animal Nutrition*. Academic Press, New York, 1970, p. 208.
14. Hurley, L. S., and Swenerton, H.: Congenital malformations resulting from zinc deficiency in rats. *Proc. Soc. Exp. Biol. Med.* **123**:692, 1966.
15. Hurley, L. S., Swenerton, H., and Growan, J.: Zinc levels in the maternal fetal organism under teratogenic conditions of zinc deficiency. *Fed. Proc.* **27**:484, 1968.
16. Hurley, L. S., Dreosti, I. E., Swenerton, H., and Growan, J.: The movement of zinc in maternal and fetal rat tissues in teratogenic zinc deficiency. *Teratology* **1**:216, 1968.
17. Turk, D. E., Sunde, M. L., and Hoekstra, W. G.: Zinc deficiency experiments with poultry. *Poultry Sci.* **38**:1256, 1959.
18. Blamberg, D. L., Blackwood, U. B., Supplee, W. C., and Combs, C. F.: Effect of zinc deficiency in hens on hatchability and embryonic development. *Proc. Soc. Exp. Biol. Med.* **104**:217, 1960.

* Recent work by Fosmire et al. and by Halas and Sandstead (*Pediat.* **9:** pp. 89–97, 1975) indicates that for rats zinc is essential to the development of the brain.

19. Kienholz, E. W., Turk, D. E., Sunde, M. L., and Hoekstra, W. G.: Effects of zinc deficiency in the diet of hens. *J. Nutr.* **75**:211, 1961.

20. Vallee, B. L.: Zinc. In: Comar, C. L., and Drenner, F. (Eds.): *Mineral Metabolism*, Vol. II, Part B. Academic Press, New York, 1962, p. 443.

21. Holt, A. B., Mellits, E. D., and Cheek, D. B.: Comparisons between nucleic acids, proteins, zinc, and manganese in rat liver: A relation between zinc and ribonucleic acid. *Pediatr. Res.* **4**:157, 1970.

22. Price, C. A.: Control of processes sensitive to zinc in plants and micro-organisms. In: Prasad, A. S. (Ed.): *Zinc Metabolism*. Thomas, Springfield, Illinois, 1966, p. 69.

23. Mills, C. F., Quarterman, J., Chesters, J. K., Williams, R. B., and Dalgarno, A. C.: Metabolic role of zinc. *Am. J. Clin. Nutr.* **22**:1240, 1969.

24. Mills, C. F., and Chesters, J. K.: Problems in the execution of nutritional and metabolic experiments with trace elements deficient animals. In: Mills, C. F. (Ed.): *International Symposium on Trace Element Metabolism in Animals*. Livingstone, Edinburgh, 1970, p. 39.

25. Sandstead, H. H., Gillespie, D. D., and Brady, R. N.: Zinc deficiency: Effect on brain of the suckling rat. *Pediatr. Res.* **6**:119, 1972.

26. Sandstead, H. H., and Rinaldi, R. A.: Impairment of deoxyribonucleic acid synthesis by dietary zinc deficiency in the rat. *J. Cell. Physiol.* **73**:81, 1969.

27. Stephan, J. K., and Hsu, J. M.: Effect of zinc deficiency and wounding on DNA synthesis in rat skin. *J. Nutr.* **103**:548, 1973.

28. Prasad, A. S.: Metabolism of zinc and its deficiency in human subjects. In: Prasad, A. S. (Ed.): *Zinc Metabolism*. Thomas, Springfield, Illinois, 1966, p. 250.

29. Widdowson, E. M., and Spray, C. M.: Chemical development *in utero*. *Arch. Dis. Child.* **26**:205, 1951.

30. Cheek, D. B., Powell, G. K., Reba, R., and Feldman, M.: Manganese, copper, and zinc in rat muscle and liver cells and in thyroid and pituitary insufficiency. *Bull. Johns Hopkins Hosp.* **118**:338, 1966.

31. Macapinlac, M. P., Barney, G. H., Pearson, W. N., and Darby, W. J.: Production of zinc deficiency in the squirrel monkey. *J. Nutr.* **93**:499, 1967.

32. Lutwak-Mann, C., and McIntosh, J. E. A.: Zinc and carbonic anhydrase in the rabbit uterus. *Nature* **221**:1111, 1969.

33. Parisi, A. F., and Vallee, B. L.: Zinc metalloenzymes: Characteristics and significance in biology and medicine. *Am. J. Clin. Nutr.* **22**:1222, 1969.

34. Valcana, T., and Timiras, P. S.: Effect of hypothyroidism on ionic metabolism of Na—K activated ATP phosphohydrolase activity in the developing rat brain. *J. Neurochem.* **16**:935, 1969.

35. Petermann, M. L.: *The Physical and Chemical Properties of Ribosomes*. Elsevier, Amsterdam, 1964.

36. Halstead, J. A., Smith, J. C. Jr., and Irwin, M. I.: Monograph. A conspectus of research on zinc requirements of man. *J. Nutr.* **104**:345, 1974.

37. Hambidge, K. M., Hambidge, C., Jacobs, M., and Baum, J. D.: Low levels of zinc in hair, anorexia, poor growth, and hypogeusia in children. *Pediatr. Res.* **6**:868, 1972.

38. Roman, W.: Zinc in porphyria. *Am. J. Clin. Nutr.* **22**:1290, 1969.

39. Cheek, D. B., Reba, R. C., and Woodward, K.: Cell growth and the possible role of trace metals. In: Cheek, D. B. (Ed.): *Human Growth*. Lea & Febiger, Philadelphia, 1968, Chapter 30, p. 424.

40. Hurley, L. S., and Mutch, P. B.: Prenatal and postnatal development after transitory gestational zinc deficiency in rats. *J. Nutr.* **103**:649, 1973.

41. Crawford, I. L., and Connor, J. D.: Zinc in maturing rat brain: Hippocampal concentration and localisation. *J. Neurochem.* **19**:1451, 1972.

CHAPTER 6

Maternal Nutritional Restriction and Fetal Brain Growth

Donald B. Cheek

INTRODUCTION

This chapter reviews the subject of malnutrition and the nervous system in mammals and primates. Emphasis is placed on the prenatal situation and the influence of the maternal diet during pregnancy.

Concern has arisen throughout the world relating to whether restricted nutrition, particularly with respect to protein intake, may cause lasting and permanent effects on the mentality of the unborn child. If protein deprivation is present during infancy and childhood, will subsequent intellectual ability be compromised? The writings of Dobbing[1] and Winick[2] warn that undernutrition in early life will permanently reduce intellectual capacity of men and women. Both of these workers have pointed to the existence of critical periods in animals and man when the growth rate of the brain is at a maximum and "when malnutrition even in a mild form or for a short time will produce irreversible damage."

Such provocative statements have had considerable impact on governments and nutritional biochemists as well as on the medical profession and medical research in general, which is to be expected since there are vast areas of the world subjected to undernutrition. The major evidence rests with rat studies (see Table 6.1) and uncontrolled postnatal human studies. The consensus of opinion is that malnutrition induces mental retardation.

Recently an attempt has been made to evaluate the evidence concerning food restriction, particularly that relating to protein deprivation and brain development.[3] Cheek, at the opening of the Mailman Kennedy Institute in Miami in March 1971, reviewed the evidence and considered that the phenomenon was mainly one concerning nonprimates, particularly small mammals such as rats.[4] Cheek

111

considered that the incapacitation caused in these animals by early, particularly prenatal, protein deficiency, would not be remarkable in the primate since growth and cell multiplication are slower and protein requirement is less. A temporary growth arrest of the brain might be the only effect. This view, which is contrary to the consensus, was again expressed at another meeting on *Nutrition, the Nervous System, and Behavior* sponsored by the Pan American Health Organization and held in Jamaica in January 1972[5]. In a more recent meeting concerning the *Swedish Symposium on Malnutrition and Behavior*, Riopelle[6] presented information on protein deprivation in pregnant primates and the effect on the offspring which supported the thinking.

Clearly a conflict exists but the vast majority of workers accept the thesis of brain damage following in the wake of malnutrition. Table 6.1 documents much of the available data and it is pertinent to present briefly the arguments that tend to challenge the climate of opinion.

TABLE 6.1. UNDERNUTRITION: MOUSE—BRAIN

Method	Findings	Reference
1. Remove litter from dam (2–16 days) then refeed ad lib to 9/12 (DNA, protein, cholesterol)	Cerebrum, cerebellum weight reduced. DNA reduced (14% cerebrum, 22% cerebellum). No behavioral changes	Howard and Granoff: *J. Nutr.*, **95**: 111, 1968
2. Explant cerebellum from animals exposed to altered nutritional environment (8% protein) and normals (27% protein) grown under optimal conditions for 30 days	Developmental patterns of cultures suggest that differentiation of both oligodendroglia and neurons retarded. Delay in myelinogenesis	Allerand: *Nature (New Biol.)* **239**: 257, 1972
3. Perinatal malnutrition and overcrowding of litter. Effect on catecholamines and biogenic amine metabolism and enzymes. Malnourished groups fed gluten diets. Animals killed at 2–3 months of age	High incorporation of tyrosine C^{14} into brain of progeny of malnourished mothers or mice from overcrowded litters. Contents of norepinephrine and dopamine depressed in mice raised from malnourished mothers. No difference in crowded or infected litters. Growth hormone (GH) treatment of malnourished mothers did not improve weight gain during pregnancy but helped retain weight during lactation. Progeny of malnourished mothers treated with GH corrected tyrosine hydroxylase activity and catecholamine content, both *reduced* in untreated progeny	Lee and Dubos: *J. Exp. Med.* **136**: 1031, 1972

TABLE 6.1—CONTINUED

UNDERNUTRITION: RAT, FETAL ONLY—BRAIN

Method	Findings	Reference
1. Reduced maternal intake to 8% protein	Reduced DNA, protein in brain at birth	Zamenhof et al.: *Science* **160**: 322, 1968
2. Reduced maternal intake to 6% protein	Reduced DNA, protein in brain at birth	Zeman and Stanborough: *J. Nutr.* **99**: 274, 1969
3. Maternal starvation for 3 days beginning from 12, 14, 16, or 18 days of gestation. Delivered by cesarean. Water ad lib	Development of β-hydroxybutyrate dehydrogenase activity in brain accelerated. Capacity to utilize ketones after 17 days of gestation	Thaler: *Nature* **236**: 140, 1972
4. Reduced maternal intake to one-third of normal caloric value (protein normal amount) from 10–20 days pregnancy. Mothers treated with growth hormone or untreated	Without GH, cerebral weight, DNA, and protein contents decreased. With GH, these decreases did not usually occur	Zamenhof et al.: *Science* **174**: 954, 1971
5. IUGR (intrauterine growth retardation)—Wigglesworth technique (ligation of uterine artery of one horn). Examined at birth for incorporation of labeled thymidine into DNA (*in vivo*)	No significant differences in DNA-thymidine incorporation between controls and IUGR	Roux: *Biol. Neonate* **18**: 463, 1971
6. Reduced maternal intake 8%. Female offspring maintained on normal diet from birth and at maturity mated with normal males. Second generation analyzed	Second generation infants exhibited significantly lower brain weights and DNA contents despite normal nutrition	Zamenhof et al: *Science* **172**: 850, 1971
7. Protein-free diet given for varying periods during pregnancy (i.e. 0–10, 10–15, 13–18, 15–20 or 10–20 days), rest of time on "normal" protein diet (20.5%). Offspring examined at birth	In all groups—significant decrease in body weight, cerebral DNA, and protein of offspring. This is despite the fact that up to day 15 the rat fetus has insignificant protein requirement of mother. Placental deficiency of nutrient is proposed	Zamenhof et al: *J. Nutr.* **101**: 1265, 1971

113

TABLE 6.1—CONTINUED

UNDERNUTRITION: RAT, FETAL PLUS POSTNATAL—BRAIN

Method	Findings	Reference
1. Reduced maternal intake to birth (6% protein). Offspring suckled on control dam from birth until 21 days. From 7 days half of the litters reduced to 4 while rest suckled as 8	Reduced DNA, RNA, protein in brain at birth. Refeeding failed to restore to normal values in litters of 8. Litters of 4 showed full restoration in comparison to paired control	Zeman: *J. Nutr.* **100:** 530, 1970
2. Reduced maternal intake (8% protein) from last week of gestation until investigated in perinatal period, 12, 24 days PN	Body weight reduced 60 and 70% of normal at 12 and 24 days, respectively. Cortical weight reduced 20%. Synaptosomal fractions showed greater recovery of protein, acetylcholinesterase, and so on, than controls. Morphology of synaptosomal fractions not different	Gambetti et al: *Brain Res.* **47:** 477, 1972
3. Maternal intake reduced to 50% of normal from fifth gestational day through birth and subsequent lactation. Fetal brain analyzed at 21 days of age	Greatest growth retardation in cerebellum. Retardation of cholesterol in cerebrum, cerebellum, and brain stem. Lipid NANA concentration reduced in cerebrum and brain stem. Rehabilitation to 140 days—failures for complete recovery	Dickerson and McAnulty: *Resuscitation* **1:** 61, 1972
4. Reduced maternal intake (5% protein) from 8–14 days of gestation and all lactation. Cerebral protein metabolism monitored during lactation	Reduced cerebral weight, DNA, and protein contents. Protein synthesis assessed (*in vitro*) to be low (ie, labeled amino acid into ribosomal protein)	Enwonwu and Glover: *J. Nutr.* **103:** 61, 1973
5. Reduced maternal intake from midgestation to birth and also during the whole of lactation	Malnourished rat brains contained only 75% of norepinephrine of controls. Also malnutrition suppressed accumulation of dopamine. Paradoxical *increase* in activity of tyrosine hydroxylase	Shoemaker and Wurtman: *Science* **171:** 1017, 1971

TABLE 6.1—CONTINUED

UNDERNUTRITION: RAT, FETAL PLUS POSTNATAL—BRAIN—CONTINUED

Method	Findings	Reference
6. Reduced maternal intake (50% of normal intake) 7 days of gestation to birth. Litters reduced to 8 at birth. Similar rations used during lactation until weaning. Offspring on reduced or normal rations until 12th week when analyzed	Body weight deficit 65% of controls (maln). Rehab 84%. Cerebellum affected most. Demonstration that acetylcholinesterase activity for region reduced (maln < rehab < control). Activity per gram reversed pattern. ATPase not significantly affected. Rehabilitated rats also show deficiency	Adlard and Dobbing: *Br. J. Nutr.* **28**: 139, 1972
7. Plan as directly above. However, animals rehabilitated to 16 weeks	Rehabilitated rats have body and brain weight deficiency. High acetylcholinesterase activity per gram. Total activity same as controls	Adlard and Dobbing: *Brain Res.* **30**: 198, 1971
8. Combination of maternal diet restriction (fetal life) and overcrowded litter 1–14 days of lactation	Ultimate deficit in adult brain weight resulting from mild growth retardation during growth spurt of brain is explained on chronological age, not developmental age. The brain has a once-only opportunity to grow correctly. Mild developmental restriction can result in true microencephaly	Dobbing and Smart: *Biol. Neonate* **19**: 363, 1971
9. Reduced maternal intake (50% of normal intake) 7 days of gestation to birth. Litter reduced to 8 at birth. Similar rations to mother during lactation. Prior offspring analyzed at 21 days of age	Reduced activities of mitochondrial acetylcholinesterase (unit/g) in malnourished brain, therefore less per region. Cerebellum most affected (compare with 6 and 7 above). Brain nonprotein solids reduced	Adlard and Dobbing: *Pediatr. Res.* **6**: 38, 1972
10. Reduced maternal intake (50% of normal intake) 7 days of gestation to birth. Litter reduced to 8 at birth. Similar rations to mother during lactation period. Offspring observed between 0–21 days postnatally	Two out of three physical features delayed. Four out of eight reflexes delayed. Characteristics that usually appear later were delayed. Behavior—exploratory behavior retarded	Smart and Dobbing: *Brain Res.* **28**: 85, 1971

TABLE 6.1 CONTINUED

UNDERNUTRITION: RAT, FETAL PLUS POSTNATAL—BRAIN—CONTINUED

Method	Findings	Reference
11. As above. Compare 9 above—similar	Enzyme maturation restricted, for example, succinate dehydrogenase, fructose diphosphate aldolase, and acetylcholinesterase, 21, 14, and 11%, respectively. Brain weight deficit 27%. β-N-Glucosaminidase (lysosomal enzyme) unaffected	Adlard and Dobbing: *Brain Res.* **28**: 97, 1971
12. As above, plus cross-fostering experiment between control and malnourished mother. Compare 10 above—similar	Nutritional deprivation during gestation on reflex ontogeny and physical features negligible. Exploratory behavior mildly affected. Animals undernourished after day 10 of postnatal life showed highly significant changes regarding reflexes and behavior	Smart and Dobbing: *Brain Res.* **33**: 303, 1971
13. As 10 above	Na^+K^+ stimulated Mg^{2+} dependent ATPase in cerebrum significantly reduced (14% reduction) as concentration ($\mu M/g/hr$). [Na] [K] not significantly changed. However, ratio was significant. Percentage of water elevated. 68% reduction in weight. 18% reduction in brain weight	Adlard, De Sousa, and Dobbing: *Pediatr. Res.* **7**: 494, 1973

UNDERNUTRITION: RAT, POSTNATAL ONLY—BRAIN

Method	Findings	Reference
1. Overcrowded litter 1–21 days, then refed (weight, lipids, cholesterol, phospholipid only)	Values 80% of normal at 21 days, return to normal with refeeding	Benton et al: *Pediatrics* **38**: 801, 1966
2. Overcrowded litter 1–21 days or 1–9 days, then refed (DNA, RNA, protein)	Reduction in DNA, RNA, protein persists if undernutrition is continued to 21 days. Changes in cerebellum only after 1–9 days insult—reversed by refeeding	Winick and Noble: *J. Nutr.* **89**: 300, 1966; **95**: 4, 1968

Method	Findings	Reference
3. Restricted diet from weaning (3 weeks) to 11 weeks, then refed (weight, cholesterol, phospholipid only)	Return to normal composition at 19th week	Dobbing and Widdowson: *Brain* **88**: 357, 1965
4. Restricted diet from weaning (3 weeks) to 11 weeks (DNA, cholesterol, protein)	No reduction in DNA, cholesterol, protein	Dickerson and Warmsley: *Brain* **90**: 897, 1967
5. Reduced suckling time (DNA, protein, cholesterol, cerebroside, phospholipid)	Restriction up to 17 days. Brain did not recover. Cerebellum affected most	Culley and Lineberger: *J. Nutr.* **96**: 375, 1968
6. Overcrowded litter and removed dams. Refed 21–35 days (somatosensory cortex DNA, RNA, protein, lipid NANA, histology)	Decrease in RNA and lipid NANA per cell. Failure of cell migration. Recovery poor. Decreased myelination due to damaged glial cell precursors is postulated	Bass, Netsky, and Young: *Arch. Neurol.* **23**: 290, 303, 1970
7. Overcrowded litter 1–18 days (DNA, protein)	Cerebellum: reduced DNA, protein at 18 days	Chase, Lindsley, and O'Brien: *Nature* **221**: 554, 1969
8. Overcrowded litter vs undercrowded litter 1–21 days. One from each litter housed together until maturity. Killed at 30 weeks (histology)	Considered mild restriction. Selective permanent reduction of weight and DNA of cerebellum. Histology—permanent reduction in numbers of cerebral cortex neurons and neurons in granular layer of cerebellum. Seems to be preliminary study	Dobbing, Hopewell, and Lynch: *Exp. Neurol.* **32**: 439, 1971
9. Overcrowded litter, dam fed suboptimal protein diet (12% protein)—21 days. Rehabilitated extra 21 days. DNA, carbonic anhydrase activity	20–25% reduction in net CA activity and DNA content (parallel effect). Concluded that reduction in cell numbers due to reduction in glial cell fraction	Muzzo, Bassi, and Winick: *Pediatr. Res.* (*Abstr.*) **7**: 314, 1973
10. Undernutrition to weaning (28 days). Based on time of feeding rather than litter size. Brain chemistry and psychological performance	No effect found in either brain composition, psychological performance, or further growth. Rats studied in small numbers. Weights of control animals seem to be very low	Rajalakshmi et al: *J. Neurochem.* **14**: 29, 1967

117

TABLE 6.1—CONTINUED

Method	Findings	Reference
11. Overcrowded litter to weaning, when analyzed. Cerebrum only	Decreased DNA content, protein:DNA lower but not significant. Enzyme : DNA not affected and total enzyme activity reduced	Swaiman et al: *J. Neurochem.* **17**: 1387, 1970
12. Overcrowded litter to weaning, then fed ad lib to 110 days. Cerebrum only	Retain decreased DNA content although protein:DNA and enzyme activity:DNA normal at 110 days. Data indicates that prime effect of malnutrition is interference with cell replication process during preweaning period	Swaiman: *Brain Res.* **43**: 296, 1972
13. Overcrowded litter vs undercrowded litter until weaning (ie, 16 pups vs 4 pups). Effect on cerebellar development. Histology	Animals rehabilitated from weaning to 50 days of age. Vermis shown to be the primary area of cerebellum affected, that is, wet weight, DNA, and protein—persistent in rehabilitated adult animals. Greater density of Purkinje cells in undernourished weanling until adulthood despite rehabilitation	Neville and Chase: *Exp. Neurol.* **33**: 485, 1971
14. Various forms of protein and calorie restriction tested on rats from conception, birth, or weaning until 13 weeks old. Rehabilitation for 5 weeks. Psychological testing	Study suggests malnourished rats generally perform not as well as well-nourished ones (Hebb-Williams test). Protein-deficient diet more harmful than calorie deficient. Effect on behavior (learning) persists after 5 weeks of rehabilitation	Baird, Widdowson, and Cowley: *Br. J. Nutr.* **25**: 391, 1971
15. Overcrowded (18 per litter), undercrowded (4 per litter), and control (9 per litter) compared for brain glycolipids during lactation. Avoidance conditioning tested in animals 120 days old	Reduction in glycoproteins and gangliosides at weaning (20 days) in both over- and undercrowded litters. ? Defect neural membrane. Lower scores in both under- and overnutrition groups suggesting impairment	Di Benedetta and Cioffi: *Bibl. Nutr. Diet.* **17**: 69, 1972
16. Overcrowded litter to 21 days or 7 weeks on restricted diet. Synaptic cortical development. Histology	40% reduction in neuronal connectivity. Density of neuronal bodies increased 20–30% due to reduction in	Cragg: *Brain* **95**: 143, 1972

TABLE 6.1—CONTINUED

UNDERNUTRITION: RAT, FETAL ONLY—BRAIN—CONTINUED

Method	Findings	Reference
16. Continued	neuropil development (eg, neuroglia). Visual and frontal cortex only. No qualitative abnormalities of synaptic or neuronal structure	

UNDERNUTRITION: GUINEA PIG—BRAIN

Method	Findings	Reference
1. Restricted maternal diet from 35 days of gestation. Analyzed at birth	Brain weight, DNA, protein, cholesterol, cerebroside, and sulfatide all reduced at birth	Chase et al: *Pediatrics* **47**: 491, 1971
2. Restricted maternal diet from 35 days of gestation. Normal diet from birth to adulthood	No changes seen in cerebrum of adult animal restricted when *in utero*. However, cerebellar weight and DNA reduced	*Ibid.*

UNDERNUTRITION: RABBIT—BRAIN

Method	Findings	Reference
1. Newborn animals starved for 2 days after birth. Matched with controls for birth weight. Brain analyzed at 60 days for DNA, RNA, protein, cholesterol	Fasted animals at 12 days, their body weight 25% less than controls. They showed significant reduction in chemical components at 60 days. Cholesterol affected to a greater extent. Fasted animals with body weights that were essentially normal at 12 days showed no brain differences. Results indicate that the degree of catchup of body weight will affect subsequent brain development. Authors attach relevance of this study to body weight "catchup" of very low birth weight human infants. Cerebral effects appear to be more definite than cerebellar effects (eg, RNA, DNA)	Schain, Watanabe, and Harel: *Pediatrics* **51**: 240, 1973

TABLE 6.1 CONTINUED

UNDERNUTRITION: DOG—BRAIN

Method	Findings	Reference
1. Combination of dietary manipulations during growth, pregnancy, and lactation	Offspring of protein-calorie malnourished (PCM) mothers given low protein diets show 1. Abnormal gait 2. Run and follow less readily 3. Tire more easily 4. Frequency of athetoid movements of head and neck when compared with animals born of normal mothers 5. Exercise exacerbates abnormalities, for example, convulsive seizures. Intensity of abnormalities 2–3 months of age 6. ECG changes *Rehabilitation:* Offspring of normal mothers subjected to a period of PCM after weaning show marked recovery although often obese. Gestationally malnourished puppies tend to remain small and full recovery does not occur	Platt and Stewart: *Dev. Med. Child Neurol.* **10**: 3, 1968

UNDERNUTRITION: PIG—BRAIN

Method	Findings	Reference
1. Protein-free diet to mother during pregnancy	Borderline reduction in RNA in brain in young adult. DNA of cerebrum or cerebellum not permanently affected	Pond et al: *J. Nutr.* **99**: 61, 1970
2. Selection of runts and these compared with large littermates. DNA, protein, cholesterol, lipid NANA	Brains from runts weighed less than those from littermates but were heavier than brains of fetuses of similar body weight. Brains of runts were less highly developed than their better nourished littermates	Dickerson, Merat, and Widdowson: *Biol. Neonate* **19**: 354, 1971

TABLE 6.1—CONTINUED

UNDERNUTRITION: PIG—BRAIN—CONTINUED

Method	Findings	Reference
3. Protein-deficient diet 3–17 weeks after birth	Changes in neurons and neuroglia not reversed by refeeding	Lowrey et al: *J. Nutr.* **78**: 245, 1962
4. Restricted food intake 2 weeks to 1 year, then refed for additional 2 years	Brain DNA reduced in spite of refeeding	Dickerson and Dobbing: *Proc. Roy. Soc. B,* **166**: 396, 1967
5. Miniature swine weaned at 7 weeks, 19% protein to 9 weeks, then fed 40% or control diet. Examined 13–41 weeks at 4-week intervals	Brain weight and indices of myelination appeared unaffected during later brain development, although grossly malnourished from 9 to 41 weeks PN ($\simeq$0.2-kg weight gain). Controls gained 0.55 kg over same period	Fishman et al: *Am. J. Clin. Nutr.* **25**: 7, 1972

UNDERNUTRITION: MACAQUE—BRAIN

Method	Findings	Reference
1. Reduction of maternal protein:calorie intake to one-third during pregnancy. Pilot study 1	Cerebrum not affected. Significant reduction in protein, cholesterol concentration, protein:DNA, and elevation of % H_2O of the cerebellum	Cheek, Severs, London et al: In progress
2. Reduction of maternal protein, calorie, or protein-plus-calorie intake to one-half during pregnancy. Pilot study 11	Cerebrum and cerebellum showed no significant differences from control during restriction	*Ibid.*
3. Removal of secondary disc of placenta at 100 days of gestation. Offspring analyzed at birth	Reduced protein, DNA, weight in cerebellum (RNA borderline deficit). Cerebrum reduction in weight. No decrease in DNA and protein	Hill et al: *Biol. Neonate* **19**: 68, 1971
4. Diet of 3% protein from 3 to 9 months	Sparing of brain in relation to other organs. 13% lower than animals on high and standard diets. Borderline significance	Ordy et al: *Proc. Soc. Exp. Biol. Med.* **135**: 680, 1970
5. Infants of 1 month fed 25% of normal protein intake until 7 months. Normal diet 7 months to 1 year on	Brain weight not reduced. Head circumference normal. Psychologically normal (Dr. Peggy Harlow)	Kerr et al: *Am. J. Clin. Nutr.* **23**: 739, 1970

TABLE 6.1—CONTINUED

UNDERNUTRITION: MACAQUE—BRAIN—CONTINUED

Method	Findings	Reference
6. Normal rhesus separated from mother 110–180 days. PN on normal diet with social experience. Then deficient diet 3% protein (age 9–13 months) or control diet (age 6–8 months)	Psychological study. Animals on low protein diet showed retarded curiosity, manipulation, and social motivation	Zimmermann and Strobel: Proc. 77th Ann. Convention A.P.A., 1969, p. 241.
7. Diet of 3% protein from 3 to 9 months (see 4 above). DNA, RNA, protein, acetylcholinesterase, and biogenic amines	Low protein group—inferior in acquisition and reversal of usual discrimination problems. Low RNA:DNA ratios in hippocampus. Reduced concentration of norepinephrine and serotonin in hypothalamus. Electron microscopy showed differences in ribosomes of hippocampal neurons and concentration of vesicles of synaptic structures in hypothalamus	Ordy and Samorajski: *Anat. Rec.* **166**: 357, 1970

UNDERNUTRITION: HUMAN, FETAL ONLY—BRAIN

Method	Findings	Reference
1. Study of birth weights of Dutch infants during German occupation. Mothers—low calorie intake. Test IQ, and so on, 20 years later	Reduced growth of fetus	Smith: *Am. J. Obstet. Gynecol.* **55**: 599, 1947
	Normal to superior intelligence	Stein et al: *Science* **178**: 708, 1972
2. Small-for-dates infants—EEG status	Great proportion showed abnormal EEG patterns. Occurred in absence of hypoxia or hypoglycemia	Schulte, Hinze, and Schrempf: *Neuropaediatrie* **2**: 439, 1971
3. Small-for-dates infants—Compared with appropriate weight-for-age infants. Samples taken from autopsy material. Control infants obviously abnormal	Small-for-dates infants show cerebellum to be most affected by IUGR. Reduction in weight, DNA, cerebrosides, and sulfatide. Lipid NANA, cholesterol, and phospholipids not affected. Number small, sample biased	Chase et al: *Pediatrics* **50**: 403, 1972

TABLE 6.1 CONTINUED

UNDERNUTRITION: HUMAN, FETAL ONLY—BRAIN—CONTINUED

Method	Findings	Reference
4. Small - for - dates infants— Compared with appropriate weight-for-age	Eight-year follow-up showed that children born small for dates had an abnormal distribution of head circumference skewed to the left (smaller). Evidence indicates that relatively minor undernutrition could result in a permanent deficit in the ultimate size of the brain	Davies and Davis: *Lancet* Dec. 12, 1216, 1970

UNDERNUTRITION: HUMAN, POSTNATAL—BRAIN

Method	Findings	Reference
1. Analysis of brains from deceased marasmic infants	Lipid, cholesterol, and other myelin compounds all reduced in brain	Fishman, Prensky, and Dodge: *Nature* **221**: 553, 1969
2. Analysis of brains from deceased marasmic infants (gestational history not known)	DNA, RNA, protein reduced	Ulrith and Rosio: *Pediatr. Res.* **3**: 18, 1969
3. Analysis of brain from deceased marasmic infants. Low protein, calorie intake	Gross reduction in DNA, RNA, and protein of cerebrum and cerebellum	Winick, Russo, and Waterlow: *Exp. Neurol.* **26**: 393, 1970

NUTRITION AND BRAIN GROWTH

Small Mammals

Rats restricted of nutrition and fed 6 to 8% protein during pregnancy deliver offspring with reduced brain size, behavioral changes,[7] reductions in brain DNA (cell number), protein, enzymes, and cholesterol content.[8-10] (See Cheek et al[5] for review.) The early experiments of Widdowson et al[11,12] showed that more severe effects arose if restriction extended from 1 to 21 days. By contrast, defects in myelination or reduction of DNA content produced by restriction of nutrients after weaning[13,14] were shown to be reversible, and restriction from 1 to 7 days was found by Cheek et al[15] and Winick et al[16] to cause no persistent chemical changes. If the insult is continued through the weaning period,[17-20] particularly from the 7th to the 17th day, irreversible changes in DNA, lipid, and cerebroside content occur. Cell histology, especially that relating to the somatosensory area, is abnormal.[21]

Culley and Lineberger's data[22] indicate that the 17th day is the end of the critical period.

In Chapter 1 the eighth to the ninth day was shown to be a time when the cell number of the rat brain increased rapidly, when sulfate was incorporated into myelin (myelination), and when carbonic anhydrase activity escalated (neuroglial function). Cell number became constant at the 17th day. Neuroblast formation continued in the rat up to the end of pregnancy. (In the human it is almost complete at the end of the first trimester and a growth spurt of the brain occurs at the 32nd week of gestation.) Neuronal increase is minimal at birth in the human.

Thus in the rat, the period of 7 to 17 days is a critical period of maximal cell multiplication, but the significance of this critical period is not completely clear. In Chapter 1 it was mentioned that hypoxia (12% oxygen) for the first 1 to 7 days in rats can cause irreversible changes in the brain. Both the nature and intensity of the insult are of consequence.

The rat is born at a very immature stage. While the human is born with only 30% of brain cells and the rat 20%, the neuroblast:neuroglial ratio is entirely different and so is the degree of brain development and cell migration. In a sense the process of birth is only an incident in the history of brain development, all mammals being born at different stages. Therefore the existence of behavioral defects in the offspring as a result of maternal protein restriction might be expected to vary from mammal to mammal, since the length of pregnancy varies for each species. Chow[7] considered that food restriction for rats during lactation brought about growth stunting, but no decrease in learning ability. This conclusion would agree with that of the earlier work of Howard and Granoff[23] on mice.

The combination of restriction during gestation and into the postnatal period (a double insult) clearly produces irreversible chemical and behavioral changes (Table 6.1). The somatosensory area of the cortex may be seriously affected. Allard and Dobbing[24] find that sustained changes in certain enzyme activities persist, which led them to suspect that during the rapid growth period of the brain with the formation of interneuronal connections, a deficit of nerve ending particles may eventuate.

Larger Mammals

Of concern to us has been the suitability of the rat as an experimental model. In Table 6.2, it can be seen that the rate of accretion of new fetal tissue for the rat is 5 times faster than for the human and 100 times faster than for the elephant.

Chase et al[25] restricted the nutrition of pregnant guinea pigs from the 35th day of gestation and while the chemical determinants were reduced in the offspring at birth, in the adult only cerebellar weight and DNA were reduced.

Platt et al[26] demonstrated an abnormal gait (behavioral changes with athetoid movements) in the offspring of pregnant dogs that had been subjected to restriction of protein and calories. Early refeeding did not reverse the changes.

Pond et al[27] gave pregnant pigs a protein-free diet but offered the litter an adequate diet postnatally. Only borderline reductions in cerebral RNA were found and while at first behavioral changes were identified, it was found subsequently that these were heavily influenced by environmental factors.[28] The pig at birth weighs only 2.5 kg but the adult weighs at least 100 kg, which represents a 40-fold increase; hence postnatal nutritional deprivation should exert profound

Table 6.2   Accretion of weight (offspring) per unit of
                   mother's pre-pregnant weight per day of
                   gestation

Species	Mother Wt. in kg (A)	Offspring Wt. in kg (B)	Gestation In days (C)	$\frac{(B)}{(A)} \times \frac{1}{(C)}$	Relative rate*
Mouse	0.04	0.014 (10 in litter)	22	0.0159	7.6
Rat	0.20	0.045 (10 in litter)	22	0.0102	4.9
Rabbit	1.90	0.400 (7 in litter)	32	0.0066	3.1
Guinea pig	0.97	0.371 (4 in litter)	66	0.0057	2.7
Macaca	6	0.45	164	0.0046	2.2
Human	58	3.2	267	0.0021	1.0
Pig	100	12.5 (5 in litter)	112	0.0011	0.5
Elephant	3,600	200	600	0.0001	0.05

* Rates using human as standard = 1

Reprinted from Richardson (Ed.): "Brain and Intelligence" Copyright
1973 by National Education Press, Hyattsville, Md.

effects. The DNA in the forebrain, cerebellum, and cord increases maximally just
before birth, whereas cell multiplication continues until 12 weeks postnatally.[29]

If one restricts food intake for the entire first year of life and then refeeds for
an additional 2 years, a reduction in cellular content can be shown in the brain.[30]
A protein-deficient diet given to pigs 3 to 12 weeks in postnatal life produces changes
in neurons and neuroglial cells despite refeeding,[31] while studies by Fishman
et al[32] concerning restricted feeding in the postnatal period did not reveal changes
in brain weight or myelination.

One is left with the impression that it is difficult to produce changes in the fetal
brain of the pig by gestational deprivation but in the postnatal period growth arrest
can be induced, and if the insult is prolonged, permanent changes result.

Primates

During recent years we have been associated with the National Institute of Neurological Disease and Stroke, a division of the NIH, in work relating to protein and/or
calorie deprivation during gestation in *Macaca mulatta*. This work has been done
in association with Drs. London, Sever, and Bieri. In a preliminary study two
groups of animals were studied—controls and those receiving a reduced protein

Table 6.3   Macaca mulatta: Brain composition in maternal
nutrition study

	Normal	Restricted
Cerebrum		
% water	86.0	86.8
DNA mg/g	1.24	1.27
Protein mg/g	88	84
Protein:DNA	71	66
Cholesterol mg/g	10.2	9.5
Cerebellum		
% water	83.4	*84.5
DNA mg/g	6.97	7.67
Protein mg/g	114	*107
Protein:DNA	16.4	**13.9
Cholesterol mg/g	10.6	**9.1

Significance   * P = less than 0.025; ** P = less than 0.01

plus calorie intake. The experimental group was only allowed to gain the weight expected for growing nonpregnant females. In other words, no weight gain relative to pregnancy was allowed. The fetuses were taken by cesarean section at 158 days. There were changes in the cerebellum, a reduction in the protein and cholesterol concentrations, elevation of water content, and reduction of the protein:DNA ratio suggesting reduced cerebellar cytoplasmic growth (Table 6.3).

A further study, in which the level of maternal protein and/or calorie intake was reduced to about one-half of the ideal during pregnancy, involved 20 mothers. The fetuses were again taken by cesarean section at 158 days (see Table 6.4). The fetuses did not reveal changes in the cerebrum or cerebellum with respect to DNA, RNA, protein, lipids, NANA, carbonic anhydrase, $Na^+K^+ATPase$, water, chloride space, or organ weight. However, as recorded in Chapters 10 and 20 it was clear that amino acid patterns in the cerebrum and cerebellum were different whether the mother was subjected to protein-calorie deprivation or protein or calorie deprivation per se. It appears that considerable reduction in food intake can be inflicted on the maternal macaque without remarkable chemical changes in the fetal brain. Our current work relates to a fully designed experiment where protein restriction is even more severe (1 g/kg/day). It can be pointed out that with respect to cell numbers, the cerebellum achieves rapid growth from about midgestation (80 days) and continues to grow beyond the period of birth, while the concentration of DNA per gram is increasing up until birth (Chapter 4). This is in contrast to the cerebrum where the DNA concentration is decreasing during the last trimester. This phenomenon is present in other mammals and the fact the cell multiplication is accelerating in the cerebellum may account for the greater growth arrest that can be produced in that organ by nutritional restriction.

Riopelle, Hill, and Li of Baton Rouge, Louisiana, have recently completed important studies on 45 pregnant primates and the effect of protein restriction and

Table 6.4   Primate maternal nutrition study

Experimental conditions

	Protein (gm) (per kg body weight)	Calories	Maternal weight gain during pregnancy
Diet 1	4.2	100*	Normal
Diet 2	2.1	100*	Normal
Diet 3	4.2	50	Zero
Diet 4	2.1	50	Zero

Animals studied were of zero parity. Animals fed Diets 1 and 2 fed additional calorie pellets (*) to maintain standard weight gain during pregnancy - 30% increase over pre-pregnancy weight at term. Animals fed Diets 3 and 4 controlled to a maximum of 500 gm weight gain during pregnancy (minimal requirement of extra calories).

have generously given us access to their information prior to publication. Dietary intake was reduced to as low as 0.5 g/kg/day in one group while the calorie intake approached 120 cal/kg/day. Remembering that the protein requirement of the monkey is double that of the human, the level reached for protein is indeed low. They found the following:

1. Reduced protein intake affects the nonpregnant female more than the pregnant female.
2. Protein intake influences the duration of pregnancy, a low intake extending pregnancy, a high intake (eg, 4 g/kg/day) shortening it.
3. No differences were found between groups for body size, plasma proteins, or bone length.
4. Neonatal period behavioral testing revealed no differences.

They have concluded tentatively that a single primate fetus works in conjunction with the mother to monitor length of gestation; while protein intake, climate, and sex of the fetus all influence the situation. By contrast in the rodent litter, some fetuses are big and some are small; some are viable and some nonviable, so no sensitive feedback occurs between the mother and offspring. These workers are inclined to agree with our original view, that since the rate of growth of the rat is so rapid, the induction of brain damage is more likely to occur with maternal deprivation in the small mammal.

Data are available on the immediate postnatal period in the macaque. Kerr et al[33] reduced the protein intake of 1-month-old macaque infants to one-quarter of the normal up until the seventh month. Some of the subjects died. After refeeding, head circumference returned to normal. Harlow and Deets (personal communication) were not able to detect psychological changes.

In contrast, other workers have reported some psychological changes. Ordy et al (Table 6.1) have reported that a 3% protein intake from 3 to 9 months produces psychological changes, changes in brain chemistry (RNA : DNA ratio and catechols), and histological evidence of neuronal changes.

Zimmerman (cited by Riopelle[6]) restricted dietary protein in the macaque to 2% but found (as have other workers) that calorie intake remained satisfactory. (If a rat is given a low protein diet of 6%, for example, the animal voluntarily refuses to take calories.) Zimmermann and co-workers studied the macaque after 4 years of protein deprivation that began at the 120th or 210th day of postnatal life. The animals showed patterns of behavior that differed from those of control animals maintained in otherwise equivalent circumstances but fed a high protein diet (see also Table 6.1). Their sexual and grooming behavior was diminished, but with respect to learning ability, no differences could be found. Riopelle discusses the complexity and difficulties in evaluating the significance of the findings and the limitations of behavioral testing.

Our own data and those of Portman et al[34] are relevant to these findings. It was demonstrated that the cerebrum reached full growth prior to 120 days postnatally, that is, before the period of nutritional restriction used in the study of Zimmermann. If it is conceded that periods of growth represent vulnerable periods, the timing of the insult was such that behavioral changes would not be expected. Alternatively, a change in environmental factors may have been concomitant with a change in diet and may be an equally important factor in determining the results. With respect to the human situation, conflicting results are again present. The studies of Zena Stein and co-workers[35] on the effects of starvation (400 cal/day) on pregnant Dutch women during the Nazi occupation show that their offspring (now 28–29 years) have normal or superior intelligence quotients. Also the careful studies of Hansen's group in South Africa[36] do not indicate psychological differences between infants with kwashiorkor during the postnatal period.

In the human situation it has been suggested that enrichment of the environment is of equal importance to reduced protein intake. Numerous studies can be produced (see Proceedings of Jamaica Conference) to show that infants living in a non-enriched environment together with reduced nutrition have growth arrest of the brain with chemical changes similar to those found in lower mammals. Transfer of a deprived child into a foster home or an enriched environment can be shown to cause remarkable catchup growth and escalation of intelligence.[37]

Moreover, infants with fibrocystic disease but with a satisfactory environment show no subsequent reduction in learning ability even though their nutritional intake may be poor in the first year of life.[38] In conclusion, the statement that protein restriction per se can cause mental retardation in the human infant would appear to be unproven. It is possible that the duration of the insult might have to extend not only through gestation but also well into the postnatal period and that an un-enriched environment is a necessary ingredient.

In mammals the size of the litter and the rate of growth vary inversely with the size of the mammal.[39] This is especially so for small rodents in which protein restriction does produce growth arrest in the brain, hormonal aberrations, and behavioral changes, all of which would appear to be permanent. Since the rate of growth of the primate brain is much slower[40] it may well be that maternal protein restriction during pregnancy produces only a temporary growth arrest in the fetal brain.

A NOTE ON MATERNAL FOOD RESTRICTION AND HORMONAL CHANGES

A disturbance in catechol metabolism was established by the work of Sereni[41] and later by Shoemaker and Wurtman,[42] changes in serotonin and norepinephrine being found in the brain stem of offspring of mothers deprived of protein. A disturbance in neurotransmitters or of their precursors (tryptophan) and an increase in tyrosine hydroxylase has been reported by one group[42] but denied by Lee and Dubos[43] who found low levels of tyrosine hydroxylase and low levels of dopamine and norepinephrine. Catecholamines influence the release of hypothalamic hormones.

Chow, in the early part of 1960s,[7] demonstrated that the offspring of restricted pregnant rats grew toward normal if given growth hormone in postnatal life. Later work by Stephan et al[44] showed that the growth hormone content of the pituitary and the activity of the pituitary gland were reduced in such offspring.

Growth hormone either directly or indirectly may influence brain growth, even neuronal growth,[45–47] and elsewhere in this book evidence is brought forward to show that insulin and thyroid hormone are also important to brain growth. Insulin release falls during protein restriction. It is perhaps not surprising that Lee[9] and Dubos,[43] while investigating the effects of insulin and growth hormone on mice subjected to protein deprivation during gestation or early postnatal life, were able to correct the high rate of turnover of catechols, and partially to correct the depression of body weight. There was restoration of the biosynthesis of brain protein and ribonucleic acid to normal levels. They argued[9] according to our previous work[48] that insulin is important for cytoplasmic growth and growth hormone is important for DNA replication.

Clearly protein restriction cannot be divorced from hormone imbalance but the changes in homeostasis could all be reversible.

REFERENCES

1. Dobbing, J.: Undernutrition in the developing brain. *Am. J. Dis. Child.* **120**:411, 1970.
2. Winick, M.: Malnutrition and brain development. *J. Pediatr.* **74**:667, 1969.
3. Eichenwald, H. F., and Fry, P. C.: Nutrition and learning. *Science* **163**:644, 1969.
4. Cheek, D. B.: Brain growth and nucleic acids, the effect of nutritional deprivation. In: Richardson, F. (Ed.): *Brain and Intelligence*, National Educational Press, Maryland, 1973, p. 237.
5. Cheek, D. B., Holt, A. B., and Mellits, E. D.: Malnutrition and the nervous system. In: *Nutrition, the Nervous system, and Behaviour: Proceedings of the Seminar on Malnutrition in Early Life and Subsequent Mental Development, Mona, Jamaica, January 10–14, 1972.* Scientific Publication No. 251, Pan American Health Organization, Washington, 1972, p. 3.
6. Riopelle, A. J.: Attention deficiencies in malnourished monkeys. Paper presented before Swedish Symposium on Malnutrition and Behaviour, December 1973. Almovist and Wiksell Tryckeri AB, Uppsala, Sweden.
7. Chow, B. F.: Effects of protein in the maternal diet on anthropometric and behavioral developments of the offspring. In: Roche, A. F., and Falkner, F. (Eds.): *Nutrition and Malnutrition*, Advances in Experimental Medicine and Biology, Volume 49: Plenum Press, New York, 1974, p. 183.
8. Zeman, F. J.: Effect of protein deficiency during gestation on postnatal cellular development in the young rat. *J. Nutr.* **100**:530, 1970.

9. Lee, C.-J.: Biosynthesis and characteristics of brain protein and ribonucleic acid in mice subjected to neonatal infection or undernutrition. *J. Biol. Chem.* **245**:1998, 1970.

10. Zamenhof, S., Mosley, J., and Schuller, E.: Stimulation of the proliferation of cortical neurons by prenatal treatment with growth hormone. *Science* **152**:1396, 1966.

11. Widdowson, E. M., Dickerson, J. W. T., and McCance, R. A.: Severe undernutrition in growing and adult animals. 4. The impact of severe undernutrition on the chemical composition of the soft tissues of the pig. *Br. J. Nutr.* **14**:457, 1960.

12. Widdowson, E. M., and McCance, R. A.: The effect of finite periods of undernutrition at different ages on the composition and subsequent development of the rat. *Proc. Roy. Soc. London (Biol.)* **158**:329, 1963.

13. Dobbing, J., and Widdowson, E. M.: The effect of undernutrition and subsequent rehabilitation on myelination of rat brain as measured by its composition. *Brain* **88**:357, 1965.

14. Dickerson, J. W., and Walmsley, A. L.: The effect of undernutrition and subsequent rehabilitation on the growth and composition of the central nervous system of the rat. *Brain* **90**:897, 1967.

15. Cheek, D. B., Graystone, J., and Rowe, R. D.: Hypoxia and malnutrition in newborn rats: Effects on RNA, DNA, and protein in tissues. *Am. J. Physiol.* **217**:642, 1969.

16. Winick, M., Fish, I., and Rosso, P.: Cellular recovery in rat tissues after a brief period of neonatal malnutrition. *J. Nutr.* **95**:623, 1968.

17. Winick, M., and Noble, A.: Cellular response in rats during malnutrition at various ages. *J. Nutr.* **89**:300, 1966.

18. Guthrie, H. A., and Brown, M. L.: Effect of severe undernutrition in early life on growth, brain size and composition in adult rats. *J. Nutr.* **94**:419, 1968.

19. Culley, W. J., and Mertz, E. T.: Effect of restricted food intake on growth and composition of pre-weanling rat brain. *Proc. Soc. Exp. Biol. Med.* **118**:233, 1965.

20. Chase, H. P., Dorsey, J., and McKhann, G. M.: The effect of malnutrition on the synthesis of a myelin lipid. *Pediatrics* **40**:551, 1967.

21. Bass, N. H., Netsky, M. G., and Young, E.: Effect of neonatal malnutrition on developing cerebrum. 2. Microchemical and histologic study of myelin formation in the rat. *Arch. Neurol.* **23**:303, 1970.

22. Culley, W. J., and Lineberger, R. O.: Effect of undernutrition on the size and composition of the rat brain. *J. Nutr.* **96**:375, 1968.

23. Howard, E., and Granoff, D. M.: Effect of neonatal food restriction in mice on brain growth, DNA, and cholesterol, and on adult delayed response learning. *J. Nutr.* **95**:111, 1968.

24. Allard, B. P. F., and Dobbing, J.: Vulnerability of developing brain. V. Effects of fetal and postnatal undernutrition on regional brain enzyme activities in 3 week old rats. *Pediatr. Res.* **6**:38, 1972.

25. Chase, H. P., Dabiere, C. S., Welch, N. N., and O'Brien, D.: Intrauterine undernutrition and brain development. *Pediatrics* **47**:491, 1971.

26. Platt, B. S., Heard, C. R. C., and Stewart, R. J. C.: Experimental protein calorie deficiency. In: Munro, H. N., and Alison, J. B. (Eds.): *Mammalian Protein Metabolism*, Vol. II. Academic Press, New York, 1964, Chapter 21.

27. Pond, W. G., Strachan, D. N., Sinha, Y. N., Walter, E. F., Dunn, J. A., and Barnes, R. H.: Effect of protein deprivation of swine during all or part of gestation on birth weight, postnatal growth rate, and nucleic acid content of brain and muscle of progeny. *J. Nutr.* **99**:61, 1970.

28. Barnes, R. H.: Nutrition and man's intellect and behavior. *Fed. Proc.* **30**:1429, 1971.

29. Dickerson, J. W. T., and Dobbing, J.: Prenatal and postnatal growth and development of the central nervous system of the pig. *Proc. Roy. Soc. B* **166**:384, 1967.

30. Dickerson, J. W. T., Dobbing, J., and McCance, R. A.: The effect of undernutrition on the postnatal development of brain and cord in pigs. *Proc. Roy. Soc. B* **166**:396, 1967.

31. Lowrey, R. S., Pond, W. G., Barnes, R. H., Krook, L., and Loosli, J. K.: Influence of caloric level and protein quality on the manifestations of protein deficiency in the young pig. *J. Nutr.* **78**:245, 1962.

32. Fishman, M. A., Prensky, A. L., Tumbleson, M. E., and Daftari, B.: Relative resistance of the later phase of myelination to severe undernutrition in miniature swine. *Am. J. Clin. Nutr.* **25**:7, 1972.

33. Kerr, G. R., Allen, J. R., Scheffler, G., and Waisman, H. A.: Malnutrition studies in the rhesus monkey. I. Effect of physical growth. *Am. J. Clin. Nutr.* **23**:739, 1970.

34. Portman, O. W., Alexander, M., and Illingworth, D. R.: Changes in brain and sciatic nerve composition with development of the rhesus monkey (*Macaca mulatta*). *Brain Res.* **43**:197, 1972.

35. Stein, Z., Susser, M., Saenger, G., and Marolla, F.: Nutrition and mental performance. *Science* **178**:708, 1972.

36. Evans, D. E., Moodie, A. D., and Hansen, J. D. L.: Kwashiorkor and intellectual development. *S. A. Med. Tydskr.* **71**:1413, 1971.

37. Graham, G. G., and Adrianzen, B.: Growth, inheritance, and environment. *Pediatr. Res.* **5**:691, 1971.

38. Studies presented at the International Congress of Nutrition, Mexico City, Sept. 3, 1972.

39. Dawes, G. S.: *Foetal and Neonatal Physiology.* Yearbook, Chicago, 1968, p. 15.

40. Payne, P. R., and Wheeler, E. F.: Comparative nutrition in pregnancy. *Nature* **215**:1134, 1967.

41. Sereni, F., Principi, N., Perletti, P., and Piceni-Sereni, L.: Undernutrition and the developing rat brain. I. Influence on acetylcholinesterase and succinic acid dehydrogenase activities and on norephinephrine and 5-OH-tryptamine tissue concentrations. *Biol. Neonate* **10**:254, 1966.

42 Shoemaker, W. J., and Wurtman, R. J.: Perinatal undernutrition: Accumulation of catecholamines in rat brain. *Science* **171**:1017, 1971.

43. Lee, C.-J., and Dubos, R.: Lasting biological effects of early environmental influences. VIII. Effects of neonatal infection, perinatal malnutrition, and crowding on catecholamine metabolism of brain. *J. Exp. Med.* **136**:1031, 1972.

44. Stephan, J. K., Chow, B., Frohman, L. A., and Chow, B. F.: Relationship of growth hormone to the growth retardation associated with maternal dietary restriction. *J. Nutr.* **101**:1453, 1971.

45. Zamenhof, S., Mosley, J., and Schuller, E.: Stimulation of the proliferation of cortical neurons by prenatal treatment with growth hormone. *Science* **152**:1396, 1966.

46. Sara, V. R., Lazarus, L., Stuart, M., and King, T.: The physiological mechanism of pituitary growth hormone action on fetal brain growth. I.R.C.S. International Research Communications System (73-9) 15-13-8, 1973.

47. Sara, V. R., and Lazarus, L.: The effect of maternal administration of pituitary growth hormone on progeny in rats. II. Learning ability. I.R.C.S. International Research Communications System (73-9) 15-13-7, 1973.

48. Cheek, D. B., Brasel, J. A., and Graystone, J. E.: In: Cheek, D. B. (Ed.): *Human Growth.* Lea & Febiger, Philadelphia, 1968, p. 322.

CHAPTER 7

Placental Insufficiency
and Brain Growth of the Fetus

Donald E. Hill

Growth of the normal human fetus is regulated by the interaction of numerous factors including maternal size and nutrition, placental size and function, and the genetic and metabolic potential of the fetus. When the factors known to influence fetal growth adversely, such as low maternal weight,[1] congenital anomalies,[2] intrauterine infections,[3, 4] toxemia,[5, 6] placental insufficiency,[7] maternal vascular disease,[8] and others[1, 9] are recognized, the etiology is still unknown in 60 to 70% of cases. In addition, it is apparent that the timing of the insult to the fetus is crucial in the final morphology and appropriate classification of the infant.

In spite of the difficulties in the recognition of homogeneous subgroups within the larger groups of growth-retarded infants, some attempts have been successful.[10–12] In many of the surviving infants somatic growth is chronically impaired,[13–15] and the incidence of poor mental performance is higher than in appropriate weight control infants.[16, 17] Attention has been focused on the changes in brain growth in an attempt to explain the poor mental performance.

Chase et al,[18] in a recent report, detailed the chemistry of the brain in a group of small-for-gestational-age infants and a control group of infants of appropriate weight for gestational age. The changes in the cerebrum and brain stem portion of the brain were limited to a significant reduction in weight when compared with the appropriate weight infants. However, the deficits in both weight and total DNA content were significant in the cerebellum. The brain lipids were reported as combined figures, and there were significant reductions in the total lipid and myelin lipids (cerebroside and sulfatide). There was no change in cell size in the cerebrum or cerebellum. These results should be interpreted with caution since the numbers are small and the cause of the intrauterine growth failure was not known. It is probable that the deficits in the cerebellum were related to the fact that the period between 34 and 40 weeks is the time of maximum growth rate of the cerebellum and when it would most likely be vulnerable to a growth-retarding influence. It is not known at the present time whether the deficits in DNA and lipid could be recovered during the period of postnatal brain growth.

Most experimental data relevant to the problem of intrauterine growth retardation and brain growth have followed from two designs. A number of investigators using rats,[19, 20] guinea pigs,[21] and sheep[22] have recorded retarded fetal growth following restricted maternal nutrition during pregnancy. In each of these experiments, the brain was least affected in terms of weight deficit. However, specific deficits were reported in brain DNA and protein content in rats [19, 20] and DNA and lipids in guinea pigs.[21] In the latter experiments, the cerebellum was more affected than the cerebrum, and although there was postnatal recovery of the cerebral deficit, the cerebellar deficit persisted. It is important to reemphasize the concept postulated by Dobbing[23] that the timing and duration of the insult in relation to the maximum growth spurt of the brain have a significant influence on the outcome of such experiments. During prenatal life the rat brain grows only to 15 to 20% of its adult size at birth, whereas guinea pig brain is some 60% of its adult size at birth. It is reasonable, therefore, that brain growth impairment (weight, DNA, lipid content) in rats is more severe in postnatal malnutrition experiments[24–26] than in prenatal studies.

These studies can be contrasted with the second approach to the problem, which has been to reduce the vascular supply to the fetus by compromising the uterine and/or placental circulation. Wigglesworth,[27] Roux et al,[28] and Oh and Guy[29] studied the effects of uterine artery ligation on body composition and brain chemistry of rats. The latter authors found no reduction in brain weight, DNA, or RNA content, while the former two authors reported reductions in total brain weight. The deficits in body weight were of a similar order to that produced by maternal undernutrition. These data suggest that, at least in the rat, the effects of vascular impairment are not similar to those produced by maternal undernutrition.

In sheep, the placental vascular supply has been compromised by embolization with carbonized microspheres, and preferential sparing of the brain, heart, and kidneys was noted in terms of a weight deficit.[30] Chemical analyses were not reported, and we have no basis for comparison with other studies.

In our work[31,32] fetal growth retardation has been induced in rhesus monkeys by compromising the placental circulation. This was accomplished by the ligation of intraplacental bridging vessels at 100 to 110 days of gestation and allowing the fetuses to continue to near term (158 days). The data concerning anthropometric changes and body composition are discussed in Chapter 17. The brain growth changes are of interest here.

This form of placental insufficiency produced a severe deficit in body weight, but only a minimal reduction in total brain weight, the brain being the least affected of any of the body organs (Figure 7.1). The pattern of organ involvement is similar to that seen in infants and has been described by Naeye[33] and Gruenwald.[7] Although the weight of the cerebrum in the intrauterine growth-retarded group was significantly less than that in control animals, the total DNA was not significantly reduced, and the DNA concentration in milligrams per gram was in fact significantly increased (Figure 7.2). In the cerebellum, the wet weight, the DNA concen-

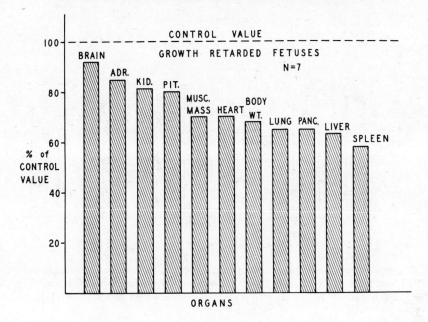

Fig. 7.1. The effect of placental insufficiency in the macaque on the mean body weight and organ weights. The brain is least affected. (Reprinted from Myers et al: *Biol. Neonate* **18**: 379, 1971, with the permission of S. Karger A.G., Basel.)

tration, and the total DNA content were significantly below that of control animals (Figure 7.3). Other changes in brain composition (Table 7.1) consisted of a minimal reduction in total water in the cerebrum, and a reduction in the total RNA, total protein, and total water in the cerebellum. These findings are similar to those mentioned earlier in the human growth-retarded fetus and suggest a similar pattern of involvement. The ligations of intraplacental vessels in the monkey were performed at a time when the brain, particularly the cerebellum, was growing at a maximal rate (see Chapter 4). It is not surprising, therefore, to find the greatest deficit in the cerebellum. The major difference between the growth of the macaque brain and that of the human is that the monkey brain reaches 60% of its adult size by birth, whereas the human is only 25 to 30% of its adult size at birth. To obtain a strict comparison, therefore, we would have to move back to approximately mid-gestation in the monkey and impose the nutrient or vascular insult at that stage.

The question remains as to whether the deficit in the cerebellum and other organs can be recovered with time and adequate nutrition. To this end, we have repeated the ligation experiments using a slightly different technique to minimize the perturbation of the fetus. The interplacental bridging vessels were identified by transillumination[34] and ligated without entering the amniotic sac. Preliminary results of this group of growth-retarded fetuses confirm the previous observations (Table 7.2). One-half of a similar growth-retarded group will be studied during a year of adequate nutrition and postnatal growth to determine if specific behavioral anomalies can be identified and correlated with changes in brain chemistry. The brains

CEREBRUM

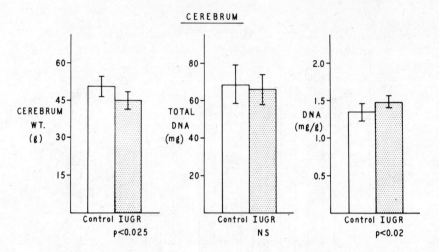

Fig. 7.2.   The effect of placental insufficiency in the macaque on fetal cerebrum weight, total DNA, and DNA concentration. Results are shown for control and intrauterine growth-retarded (IUGR) animals. (Reprinted from Hill et al: *Biol. Neon.*, **19,** 68, 1971 with permission of S. Karger A.G., Basel.)

CEREBELLUM

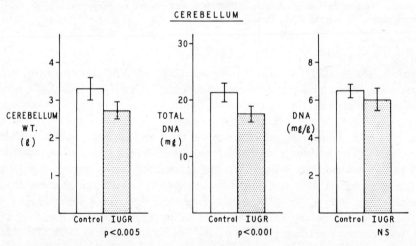

Fig. 7.3.   The effect of placental insufficiency in the macaque on cerebellum weight, total DNA, and DNA concentration. Results are shown for control and intrauterine growth-retarded (IUGR) animals. (Reprinted from Hill et al: *Biol. Neon.*, **19,** 68, 1971 with permission of S. Karger A.G., Basel.)

of these animals will have reached 95% of their adult size by the end of 1 year, and at that time we will examine similar brain constituents to determine the extent of catchup growth. We should then be able to provide some answers with respect to a species somewhat closer to humans than most of the previous studies.

    It is clear from these studies, where experimental placental insufficiency has produced a reduction in the available placental mass and probably an overall reduction

Table 7.1   The effect of placental vessel ligation on brain
composition (intra-amniotic experiments)

	(a) Controls (N = 6)	(b) IUGR (N = 7)	a vs. b
Cerebrum			
Wet weight, g	50.4 ± 3.4	45.0 ± 3.5	P = less than 0.025
RNA, mg/g	2.09 ± 0.07	2.14 ± 0.18	NS
Total RNA, mg	105.7 ± 4.6	96.4 ± 10.4	P = 0.05
Protein, mg/g	85.9 ± 3.6	84.3 ± 5.6	NS
Total protein, mg	4164 ± 411	3799 ± 423	NS
Prot/DNA	64.4 ± 8.1	57.6 ± 6.5	NS
H_2O, %	85.6 ± 0.4	85.8 ± 0.5	NS
Total H_2O, g	43.21 ± 3.14	38.7 ± 3.02	P = less than 0.025
Cerebellum			
Wet weight, g	3.3 ± 0.3	2.7 ± 0.2	P = less than 0.005
RNA, mg/g	2.87 ± 0.12	3.00 ± 0.46	NS
Total RNA, mg	9.53 ± 1.01	8.18 ± 1.38	P = 0.05
Protein, mg/g	108 ± 3.4	105 ± 4.11	NS
Total protein, mg	356 ± 31	286 ± 22	P = less than 0.001
Prot/DNA	16.5 ± 0.7	17.3 ± 1.8	NS
H_2O, %	83.4 ± 0.4	83.2 ± 0.7	NS
Total H_2O, g	2.75 ± 0.25	2.26 ± 0.19	P = less than 0.005

NS = Non-significant   IUGR = Intra-uterine growth retardation

(Taken from Hill et al: *Biol. Neon.*, **19**, 68, 1971 with permission of S. Karger A.G., Basel.)

in nutrient and oxygen supply, that cerebral growth as we measured it was not particularly impaired. It has been suggested that relative sparing of the brain may arise through altered cerebral blood flow, and this might be induced on a basis of hypoxia.[29,30] We have no direct evidence on fetal oxygen levels following ligation of interplacental bridging vessels. It is likely, however, that a transient period of hypoxia related to the reduced blood flow and sudden change in blood volume might occur with these ligations.

It is difficult, as pointed out earlier, to mimic even these minimal brain changes by restriction of the maternal food intake during pregnancy (see Chapter 6). Further experiments will be required to determine whether the final common pathway in the production of intrauterine growth retardation by placental insufficiency is an overall reduction in the nutrient supply to the fetus or whether hypoxia plays an important role.

Table 7.2   The effect of placental vessel ligation on brain composition (extra-amniotic experiments)

	(a) Controls (N = 5)	(b) IUGR (N = 8)	a vs. b
Cerebrum			
Wet weight g	51.8 ± 4.9	46.6 ± 2.5	P = less than 0.05
H_2O %	86.0 ± 0.6	86.8 ± 2	NS
Total DNA mg	64.1 ± 8.2	55.8 ± 6.6	NS
Total RNA mg	115 ± 13.3	105 ± 12.9	NS
Total protein g	4.14 ± 0.97	3.05 ± 0.39	NS
Cerebellum			
Wet weight g	3.14 ± 0.18	2.68 ± 0.3	P = less than 0.005
H_2O %	83.7 ± 0.61	86.2 ± 1.6	P = less than 0.025
Total DNA mg	21.5 ± 3.3	18.8 ± 2.9	P = less than 0.05
Total RNA mg	7.87 ± 0.44	5.84 ± 1.9	P = less than 0.05
Total protein mg	318 ± 31	238 ± 50	P = less than 0.005

NS = Non-significant   IUGR = Intra-uterine growth retardation

REFERENCES

1. Scott, K. E., and Usher, R.: Fetal malnutrition: Its incidence, causes, and effects. *Am. J. Obstet. Gynecol.* **94:** 951, 1966.
2. Warkany, J., Munroe, B. B., and Sutherland, B. S.: Intrauterine growth retardation. *Am. J. Dis. Child.* **102:** 249, 1961.
3. Sever, J. L., Nelson, K. B., and Gilkeson, M. R.: Rubella epidemic, 1964: Effect on 6000 pregnancies. *Am. J. Dis. Child.* **110:** 395, 1965.
4. Gregg, N.: Congenital cataracts following German measles in the mother. *Trans. Ophthalmol. Soc. Aust.* **3:** 54, 1941.
5. Naeye, R. L.: Abnormalities in infants of mothers with toxemia of pregnancy. *J. Obstet. Gynecol.* **95:** 276, 1966.
6. Woodhill, J. M., van den Berg, A. S., Burke, B. S., and Stare, F. J.: Nutrition studies of pregnant Australian women. Part I. Maternal nutrition in relation to toxemia of pregnancy and physical condition of the infant at birth. *Am. J. Obstet. Gynecol.* **70:** 987, 1955.
7. Gruenwald, P.: Chronic fetal distress and placental insufficiency. *Biol. Neonate* **5:** 215, 1963.

8. Browne, J. C. M., and Veall, N.: The maternal placental blood flow in normotensive and hypertensive women. *J. Obstet. Gynecol. Br. Commonw.* **60**: 142, 1953.

9. Cassady, G.: Body composition in intrauterine growth failure. *Pediatr. Clin. North Am.* **17**: 79, 1970.

10. Lubchenco, L., Hansman, M., and Boyd, E.: Intrauterine growth in length and head circumference as estimated from live births at gestational ages from 26–42 weeks. *Pediatrics* **37**: 403, 1966.

11. Urrusti, J., Yoshida, P., Velasco, L., Frenk, S., Rosado, A., Sosa, A., Morales, B. S., Yoshida, T., and Metcoff, J.: Human fetal growth retardation: I. Clinical features of sample with intrauterine growth retardation. *Pediatrics* **50**: 547, 1972.

12. Miller, H. C., and Hassanien, K.: Diagnosis of impaired fetal growth in newborn infants. *Pediatrics* **48**: 511, 1971.

13. Lubchenco, L. O., Horner, F. A., Reed, L., Hix, I., Metcalf, D., Cohig, R., Elliott, H., and Bourg, M.: Sequelae of premature birth. *Am. J. Dis. Child.* **106**: 101, 1963.

14. Drillien, C. M.: *The Growth and Development of the Prematurely Born Infant*. Livingstone, Edinburgh, 1964, p. 77.

15. Fitzhardinge, P. M., and Steven, E. M.: The small-for-date infant. I. Later growth patterns. *Pediatrics* **49**: 671, 1972.

16. Drillien, C. M.: Intellectual sequelae of "fetal malnutrition." In: Waisman, H. A., and Kerr, G. R. (Eds.): *Fetal Growth and Development*. McGraw-Hill, New York, 1970.

17. Fitzhardinge, P. M., and Steven, E. M.: The small-for-date infant. II. Neurological and intellectual sequelae. *Pediatrics* **50**: 50, 1972.

18. Chase, H. P., Welch, N., Dabiere, C. S., Vasan, N. S., and Butterfield, L. J.: Alterations in human brain biochemistry following intrauterine growth retardation. *Pediatrics* **50**: 403, 1972.

19. Zamenhof, S., van Marthen, E., and Margolis, F. L.: DNA (cell number) and protein in the neonatal brain: Alteration by maternal dietary restriction. *Science* **160**: 322, 1968.

20. Zeman, F. J., and Stanbrough, E. C.: Effect of maternal protein deficiency on cellular development in the fetal rat. *J. Nutr.* **99**: 274, 1969.

21. Chase, H. P., Dabiere, C. S., Welch, N. N., and O'Brien, D.: Intrauterine undernutrition and brain development. *Pediatrics* **47**: 491, 1971.

22. Wallace, L. R.: The effect of diet on fetal development. *J. Physiol.* **104**: 34, 1945.

23. Dobbing, J.: Vulnerable periods in developing brain. In: Davidson, A. N., and Dobbing, J. (Eds.): *Applied Neurochemistry*. Davis, Philadelphia, 1968, p. 287.

24. Winick, M., and Noble, A.: Cellular response in rats during malnutrition at various ages. *J. Nutr.* **89**: 300, 1966.

25. Dobbing, J., Hopewell, J. W., and Lynch, A.: Vulnerability of developing brain VII. Permanent deficit of neurons in cerebral and cerebellar cortex following early mild undernutrition. *Exp. Neurol.* **32**: 439, 1971.

26. Chase, H. P., Lindsley, W. F. B., and O'Brien, D.: Undernutrition and cerebellar development. *Nature* **221**: 554, 1969.

27. Wigglesworth, J. S.: Experimental growth retardation in the foetal rat. *J. Pathol. (Bacteriol.)* **88**: 1, 1964.

28. Roux, J. M., Tordet-Caridroit, C., and Chanez, C.: Studies on experimental hypotrophy in the rat I. Chemical composition of the total body and some organs in the rat fetus. *Biol. Neonate* **15**: 342, 1970.

29. Oh, W., and Guy, J. A.: Cellular growth in experimental intrauterine growth retardation in rats. *Nutrition* **101**: 1631, 1971.

30. Creasy, R. K., Barrett, C. T., Swiet, M., Kahanp, K. V., and Rudolph, A. M.: Experimental intrauterine growth retardation in the sheep. *Am. J. Obstet. Gynecol.* **112**: 566, 1972.

31. Myers, R. E., Hill, D. E., Cheek, D. B., Holt, A. B., Scott, R. E., and Mellits, E. D.: Fetal growth retardation produced by experimental placental insufficiency in the rhesus monkey I. Body weight, organ size. *Biol. Neonate* **18**: 379, 1971.

32. Hill, D. E., Myers, R. E., Holt, A. B., Scott, R. E., and Cheek, D. B.: Fetal growth retardation produced by experimental placental insufficiency in the rhesus monkey II. Chemical composition of the brain, liver, muscle, and carcass. *Biol. Neonate* **19**: 68, 1971.

33. Naeye, R. L.: Malnutrition. Probable cause of fetal growth retardation. *Arch. Pathol.* **79**: 284, 1965.

34. Reynolds, S. R. M., Paul, W. M., and Huggett, A. St. G.: Physiological study of the monkey monkey fetus *in utero*: A procedure for blood pressure recording, blood sampling, and injection of the fetus under normal conditions. *Bull. Johns Hopkins Hosp.* **95**: 256, 1954.

CHAPTER 8

Prenatal Hypothyroidism
and Brain Composition

A. Barry Holt, George R. Kerr, and Donald B. Cheek

INTRODUCTION

There is ample clinical and experimental evidence that thyroid hormones play an essential role in the regulation of the maturational processes of the central nervous system both in animals and in man. [1–5]

Clinical observations in man clearly define the effects of thyroid dysfunction arising in infancy or childhood through to adulthood.[2] The neurological symptoms seen in thyroid diseases of later childhood and the adult can be corrected by appropriate thyroid therapy.[2] On the other hand, irreversible mental retardation may be the outcome when severe thyroid dysfunction is found during infancy.[2–5]

At birth, most hypothyroid infants are of normal length and appear normal although their birth weight tends to be excessive.[5] Therefore it has not been generally accepted by clinicians that this condition could orginate during fetal life. The assumption has been made that the fetus receives sufficient thyroid hormone from the mother for fetal growth during uterine life. Doubt has been cast on the role of thyroid deficiency *in utero* as the cause of mental retardation. The neurological disorders have been attributed either to a delay in diagnosis and therapy after birth or to additional disorders or complications.[3, 4, 6]

The neonatal rat has been used as a convenient extrauterine "fetal" model to investigate the effects of thyroid hormone or thyroid ablation on the developing nervous system.[2] This animal is born in an immature state with the major proportion of brain growth occurring after birth.[7, 8] The study of the rat (neonatally thyroidectomized) has yielded extensive and valuable information in terms of morphology,[9–11] biochemistry,[12–24] electrophysiology,[3, 25] and behavior.[3, 4] However, it is obvious that this model is unsuitable for the investigation of the effects of fetal-maternal interaction of thyroid hormone during brain development which is the key to understanding the human situation.

Osorio and Myant in 1960[26] remarked on the paucity of information concerning the effects of removing the thyroid from the fetus *in utero*. They emphasized that no one had studied the effects of thyroidectomy *in utero* or of fetal thyroid deficiency on the subsequent development of tissues postnatally, particularly tissues influenced by thyroid hormone (e.g, the central nervous system and skeleton). It is only recently that the question has been studied.[27-29]

In Chapter 4 it was established that brain development of the rhesus monkey is predominantly prenatal. Furthermore, Pickering[30-32] in his extensive and excellent studies of thyroid gland development of the fetal macaque has demonstrated that this animal has a functional thyroid gland prior to midgestation. These essential prerequisites make the fetal macaque a suitable animal in which to investigate the effects of intrauterine thyroid ablation on brain development.

In the course of our studies the importance of reducing the supply of thyroid hormones from both the maternal and fetal thyroid gland was recognized so that base-line data could be obtained for comparison with data from neonatally thyroidectomized rats. It has not been our purpose at this time to investigate the differential effects of maternal hormone versus fetal hormone on fetal brain development.

Thyroid ablation *in utero* was performed by one of us (G.K.) and his co-workers at the Department of Pediatrics and the Regional Primate Research Center of the University of Wisconsin. The details of the procedure are described elsewhere,[28] together with details on physical growth, skeletal maturation, and serum hormone levels. A brief summary is included here.

Pregnant female rhesus monkeys were injected intravenously with 2 mCi of radioactive sodium iodide per kilogram of body weight between 71 and 88 days of gestation. Each pregnancy was allowed to continue until 150 days when the fetuses were delivered by cesarean section. A similar number of untreated pregnant females was delivered by cesarean section at 150 days.

Fetuses delivered from the mothers with thyroid ablation weighed slightly less than expected for gestational age and exhibited reduced respiratory movements and cretinoid faces. Thyroid hormone levels (Table 8.1) were low in both the mother and the fetus, although the mothers showed no apparent clinical symptoms of hypothyroidism during pregnancy. Both macroscopic and microscopic examination of the fetuses exposed to ^{131}I showed complete ablation of the thyroid gland. No parathyroid tissue was identified although there was no evidence of clinical parathyroid dysfunction in the pregnant mothers or fetuses who were treated with the radioisotope. The thyroid gland of the mothers treated with ^{131}I was not examined.

The brain, considered either as a whole or as separate parts, did not differ in weight when compared with controls (Table 8.2). The pituitary was enlarged. The thymus in the experimental fetuses was significantly smaller than that obtained from controls. The weights of the spleen, liver, adrenals, pancreas, and placenta were within expected limits. Skeletal maturation was markedly retarded in the primate cretins. Epiphyseal ossification centers revealed a developmental age appropriate for fetuses of less than 125 days of gestation.

The shape of the skull was disproportionately wide in relation to its length when compared with a normal fetus (Table 8.3).

Table 8.4 presents the chemical analysis of both cerebrum and cerebellum for DNA, RNA, and protein. Cerebral DNA content was unchanged. There was an

Table 8.1   Thyroid hormone levels at time of study

		Maternal plasma	Fetal plasma
P.B.I. μg %	Control	7.2 ± 1.2	7.3 ± 0.5
	I^{131}	4.6 ± 1.4	4.7 ± 0.4
T_4 μg %	Control	9.6 ± 2.3	7.2 ± 2.1
	I^{131}	2.3 ± 0.9	0.6 ± 0.8

Table 8.2   Fetal brain weights (g) after thyroid ablation during pregnancy

		Control	I^{131}
Whole brain	$M \pm SD$	52.71 ± 3.3	51.36 ± 3.34
	Range	$47.62 - 55.63$	$47.42 - 53.60$
Cerebrum	$M \pm SD$	49.01 ± 3.08	47.79 ± 3.27
	Range	$43.74 - 51.52$	$43.98 - 52.34$
Cerebellum	$M \pm SD$	2.67 ± 0.32	2.38 ± 0.12
	Range	$2.09 - 2.99$	$2.23 - 2.58$
Pontine stem	$M \pm SD$	1.03 ± 0.22	1.19 ± 0.23
	Range	$0.83 - 1.43$	$0.99 - 1.52$

Table 8.3   Effect of thyroid ablation during pregnancy on the dimensions of the fetal skull, data of Kerr[28]

		Control	I^{131}
Length cm	M	6.54	6.26
	SD	0.15	0.26
	n	12	12

Difference = 0.28, t = 3.233, P = less than 0.005

		Control	I^{131}
Width cm	M	4.82	5.01
	SD	0.20	0.09
	n	12	12

Difference = 0.19, t = 3.004, P = less than 0.01

Table 8.4   The effect of thyroid ablation during pregnancy on brain composition in the macaque fetus (content of nucleic acids and protein)

	Control	I^{131}
Cerebrum		
DNA, mg	62.94 ± 4.53	63.50 ± 1.61
RNA, mg	104.28 ± 7.42	*87.59 ± 3.04
Protein, g	3.973 ± 0.275	*3.295 ± 0.170
RNA:DNA	1.662 ± 0.141	*1.370 ± 0.084
Protein:DNA	63.27 ± 4.7	*51.57 ± 3.75
Cerebellum		
DNA, mg	23.24 ± 3.57	20.39 ± 0.82
RNA, mg	7.64 ± 0.98	*6.23 ± 0.22
Protein, g	0.277 ± 0.035	*0.211 ± 0.007
RNA:DNA	0.330 ± 0.019	*0.306 ± 0.013
Protein:DNA	12.19 ± 0.58	*10.8 ± 0.09

Values are mean ± SD
* Significantly different from controls, P = less than 0.01

apparent 10% reduction in the content of DNA within the cerebellum; this result was not statistically significant. The content of RNA and protein in both cerebrum and cerebellum was reduced significantly. Table 8.5 shows definite depression of the RNA:DNA ratio and the ratio of protein to DNA (mean cell size). DNA concentration remained unchanged while significant reductions in the concentration of RNA and protein were found in the cerebrum and cerebellum of the hypothyroid primates.

Table 8.5   The effect of thyroid ablation during pregnancy on brain composition in the macaque (nucleic acid and protein concentrations)

		Control	I^{131}
Cerebrum			
DNA	mg/g	1.286 ± 0.082	1.344 ± 0.091
RNA	mg/g	2.128 ± 0.093	*1.839 ± 0.125
Protein	mg/g	81.1 ± 2.2	* 69.1 ± 3.3
Cerebellum			
DNA	mg/g	8.70 ± 0.46	8.60 ± 0.45
RNA	mg/g	2.87 ± 0.14	* 2.62 ± 0.12
Protein	mg/g	105.9 ± 4.1	* 92.5 ± 3.9

Values are mean ± SD
* Significantly different from controls, P = less than 0.01

The percentage of water in the hypothyroid cerebrum and cerebellum was elevated in comparison with controls, although the total water content of both cerebrum and cerebellum remained within normal limits (Table 8.6). The chloride space was unchanged in both cerebrum and cerebellum although there was a trend for the relative expansion of this space per unit weight. On the other hand, the nonchloride space (an index of neuronal volume) was reduced in both the cerebrum and cerebellum.

The plasma sodium and potassium concentrations were unchanged while the total plasma proteins were depressed significantly (Table 8.7). Significantly high concentrations of sodium were found in the cerebrum and cerebellum with little or no increase in total content. Partitioning of the sodium into extra- and intracellular compartments failed to show any difference when compared with brains from control fetuses. The concentration of potassium was significantly low in the cerebrum and cerebellum. On calculation it was found that there was a deficit of potassium of 17 and 22% for cerebrum and cerebellum, respectively. There was a significant elevation of chloride concentration in the cerebellum only.

As was discussed in Chapter 5 the content and concentration of zinc and magnesium in the cerebrum were reduced. The ratios of magnesium or zinc to RNA or protein remained unchanged, however. (Manganese, on the other hand, showed no change in concentration or total content.) Thus the reductions in zinc and magnesium emphasized once again the retarded protein synthesis.

Table 8.6   The effect of thyroid ablation during pregnancy on water content and distribution in the fetal macaque

		Controls	I^{131}
Cerebrum			
% water		87.09 ± 0.27	*88.88 ± 0.41
Total water	ml	42.68 ± 2.68	42.48 ± 3.04
Chloride space	ml	20.06 ± 1.97	**21.79 ± 3.49
	ml/kg	409 ± 17	** 454 ± 42
Non-chloride space	ml	22.62 ± 0.91	*20.69 ± 0.96
	ml/kg	462 ± 16	435 ± 40
Cerebellum			
% water		84.55 ± 0.50	*86.37 ± 0.56
Total water	ml	2.25 ± 0.27	2.05 ± 0.10
Chloride space	ml	0.86 ± 0.10	0.96 ± 0.14
	ml/kg	324 ± 15	* 401 ± 36
Non-chloride space	ml	1.39 ± 0.19	* 1.10 ± 0.06
	ml/kg	521 ± 16	463 ± 40

Values are Mean ± SD
P = not more than * 0.01, or ** 0.05

Table 8.7   The effect of thyroid ablation during pregnancy
on plasma and brain electrolyte composition

		Control	I^{131}
Plasma			
Sodium	mEq/L	138 ± 5.5	140 ± 4.2
Chloride	mEq/L	110 ± 3.1	110 ± 3.2
Protein	g/100 ml	5.01 ± 0.25	* 4.3 ± 0.34
Cerebrum			
Sodium	mEq/kg	57.9 ± 2.1	* 67.8 ± 3.5
	mEq total	2.84 ± 0.24	** 3.25 ± 0.38
Potassium	mEq/kg	72.8 ± 2.0	* 61.8 ± 2.3
	mEq total	3.57 ± 0.2	* 2.95 ± 0.21
Chloride	mEq/kg	49.9 ± 3.0	54.7 ± 5.9
	mEq total	2.45 ± 0.28	2.63 ± 0.41
Cerebellum			
Sodium	mEq/kg	53.4 ± 5.7	* 61.5 ± 0.146
	mEq total	0.142 ± 0.021	0.146 ± 0.016
Potassium	mEq/kg	88.6 ± 3.9	* 77.4 ± 3.2
	mEq total	0.236 ± 0.237	*0.184 ± 0.016
Chloride	mEq/kg	39.6 ± 2.7	* 48.2 ± 3.5
	mEq total	0.105 ± 0.013	0.115 ± 0.014

Values are Mean ± SD

Significant difference from controls: * P = less than 0.01
                                   ** P = less than 0.05

Sodium-potassium-activated magnesium-dependent ATPase, a measure of neuronal nerve-ending function, was found to have reduced activity in the cerebellum and cerebrum of the hypothyroid fetuses (Table 8.8). The activity in relation to DNA, RNA, and protein was found to be depressed in these tissues. Total activity in the cerebrum and cerebellum was reduced 34 and 30%, respectively. Carbonic anhydrase (found in glial cells) showed similar results. Total activity was reduced 43 and 48%, respectively, for cerebrum and cerebellum.

Two classes of cerebral lipids were measured in the cerebrum and cerebellum (Table 8.9). Cholesterol, which is a component of biological membranes (found extensively in myelin), was reduced in content and total amount. Cholesterol in relation to DNA was reduced while the relationship of cholesterol to RNA and protein remained unchanged. Ganglioside (lipid NANA) showed a reduced concentration and a depressed ratio in relation to DNA, the total content being also reduced. The ratio of lipid NANA to RNA and protein remained unchanged.

Table 8.10 shows that the weight of the pituitary in the hypothyroid fetuses tended to be larger than normal. When the weight of the gland was calculated relative to body weight, a significant increase was observed. The pituitaries from the hypothyroid fetuses showed a definite reduction in the concentration of growth hormone. There was a trend toward a reduction in the total amount.

Table 8.8   The effect of thyroid ablation during pregnancy on enzyme levels in fetal macaque brain

	Control	I^{131}
Cerebrum		
[1] ATPase		
units/g	315 ± 38	$*215 \pm 23$
Total units x 10^2	15.48 ± 2.39	$*10.26 \pm 1.11$
[2] Carbonic anhydrase		
units/g	51.8 ± 11.1	$*30.7 \pm 4.9$
Total units x 10^3	2.53 ± 0.49	$*1.45 \pm 0.50$
Cerebellum		
ATPase		
units/g	334 ± 21	$*264 \pm 25$
Total units x 10^2	0.90 ± 0.16	$*0.63 \pm 0.06$
Carbonic anhydrase		
units/g	125.7 ± 22.6	$*72.8 \pm 13.8$
Total units x 10^3	0.336 ± 0.080	$*0.174 \pm 0.041$

Values are Mean $\pm$ SD

1 ATPase = Na^+ K^+ activated Mg^{++} dependent ATPase, unit = μmoles P/hour

2 Carbonic anhydrase - for definition of units see Chapter 3.

* Significantly different from controls. P = Less than 0.025

Table 8.9   The effect of thyroid ablation during pregnancy on cholesterol and lipid NANA in fetal cerebrum and cerebellum

	Control	I^{131}
Cerebrum		
Cholesterol		
mg/g	9.14 ± 0.39	$* 7.94 \pm 0.39$
Total mg	448 ± 32	$* 379 \pm 31$
Lipid NANA		
mg/g	0.93 ± 0.05	$* 0.79 \pm 0.05$
Total mg	45.5 ± 1.8	$* 37.7 \pm 2.7$
Cerebellum		
Cholesterol		
mg/g	10.68 ± 0.91	$* 8.56 \pm 0.46$
Total mg	28.3 ± 2.2	$* 20.3 \pm 1.1$
Lipid NANA		
mg/g	0.60 ± 0.09	$* 0.47 \pm 0.06$
Total mg	1.61 ± 0.37	$* 1.11 \pm 0.14$

Values are mean $\pm$ SD   * P = less than 0.25

Table 8.10   Effect of thyroid ablation during pregnancy on weight and growth hormone content of the fetal pituitary

	Control	I^{131}
Weight (mg)	16.6 ± 2.3	$*20.9 \pm 4.5$
Pituitary (mg per 100 g body weight)	3.8 ± 0.8	$** 5.3 \pm 1.0$
Growth hormone (μg/mg)	3.6 ± 0.7	$** 2.2 \pm 0.3$
Total growth hormone (μg)	60.0 ± 11	$*47.0 \pm 11$

Values are Mean $\pm$ SD

*P = less than 0.05   ** P = less than 0.001

DISCUSSION

These data reveal that the total number of cells and cellular density (as indicated by total DNA and DNA concentration, respectively) in the cerebrum and cerebellum of the ^{131}I-treated fetuses are similar to normal fetuses of the same gestational age. Similarly, the weight of the cerebrum and cerebellum was also essentially normal. On the other hand, total RNA, total protein, and the activity of two functionally important enzymes were significantly suppressed, strongly suggesting that RNA and/or protein synthesis had been affected. The nonmorphologic measures of mean cell size (protein:DNA ratio) and cell volume (nonchloride space) support these findings.

Many of the changes that are described for the athyroid fetal macaque have been previously observed in young rats that received thyroid ablation 7 days after birth (Table 8.11).

Balázs et al[12,13] have reported that cerebral DNA is not affected by neonatal hypothyroidism of the rat, whereas cerebral weight, cholesterol, protein, and RNA contents are all reduced. The amount of ganglioside (measured as lipid NANA) was not changed. Brasel and Winick[14] have reported normal DNA content of the whole brain of hypothyroid rats with reduced brain weight and RNA content; in their series, however, there was only a small deficit in total protein.

Pasquini et al[23] examined the effect of neonatal thyroidectomy upon nucleic acid and protein of the cerebral cortex and cerebellum of the rat and cerebral weight was 10 to 15% lower than for controls from 20 days of age. The cerebellum showed a weight reduction after 40 days. DNA concentration was elevated in the cortex whereas cerebellar DNA concentration was only affected during the early stages of development. Close inspection of their data indicates that the total amount of DNA of cerebrum and cerebellum was not reduced. The concentration of RNA in the cortex was similar to that for controls but a reduced concentration was observed for the cerebellum. The ratio of RNA to DNA was consistently reduced. Similar reductions were demonstrable for protein concentrations and the ratio of protein to DNA. Geel and Timiras[16] also studied the effect of neonatal hypothyroidism

TABLE 8.11.   THE EFFECT OF THYROIDECTOMY ON THE
MACAQUE AND THE RAT

	Fetal Macaque*		Neonatal Rat†	
		Ref.		Ref.
Body weight ⎱	Within normal limits	28	Reduced	12–14, 16, 19, 23
Brain weight ⎰			Reduced	12–14, 19, 23
Skull length/width	Reduced	28	Reduced	9
Skeletal development	Retarded	28	Retarded	42
Pituitary	Enlarged	28	Enlarged	43
Other organ weights	Thymus only reduced	28	Many organs reduced	14
Brain composition				
Cell density	Normal‡		Elevated	12, 16, 19, 23
Cell population (total DNA)	Normal		Normal	14, 23
Cell size (protein:DNA)	Reduced		Reduced	12, 16, 23
RNA:DNA	Reduced		Reduced	12, 14, 16, 19, 23
%H_2O	Elevated		Elevated	16, 17, 24
Potassium	Reduced		Reduced	17, 24
Sodium	Elevated		Elevated	17, 24
Chloride	Elevated		Elevated	17, 24
Magnesium	Reduced		Reduced	24
Nonchloride space	Reduced		Indication of reduction	24
Neuronal markers				
a. $Na^+K^+ATPase$	Reduced		Reduced	17, 24
b. Lipid NANA	Reduced		Reduced	44
Neuroglial markers				
a. Carbonic anhydrase	Reduced		—	—
b. Cholinesterase	—		Reduced	18
c. Cholesterol	Reduced		Reduced	12, 13

* Thyroidectomized at 71–89 days, brain studied at 150 days.
† Thyroidectomized at birth to 7 days, brain studied at 15–35 days.
‡ The findings that follow in this column are from this study.

in rats on RNA and DNA concentrations in the cortex. These workers demonstrated an increased DNA concentration, a reduced RNA:DNA ratio, and an elevated concentration of water.

Valcana and Timiras[24] have described reductions in $Na^+K^+ATPase$ activity, increased percentage of water, and data suggestive of intracellular volume change in both cerebral cortex and cerebellum in the young athyroid rat. Garcia Argiz et al[15] have also described a similar depression of $Na^+K^+ATPase$ in the cortex and cerebellum. The depression, in terms of activity per gram, was greater in the cortex than in the cerebellum. A similar pattern is found in the macaque brain in the absence of thyroid function.

Carbonic anhydrase, an enzyme found exclusively in glia,[33] was greatly reduced in cerebrum and cerebellum of our athyroid fetuses. The activity of this enzyme has not been inspected in the hypothyroid rat brain. However, the activity of cholinesterase, another enzyme that predominates in glial cells, has been found to be decreased in hypothyroid rats.

It is emphasized that the reduction in cerebral weight and elevation in cerebral DNA concentrations, described for young rats deprived of thyroid function, were not observed in the hypothyroid fetal macaque.

Gangliosides are found concentrated in the gray matter of the central nervous system and are associated with maintenance of electrical activity and ion transport.[34] Subcellular fractionation studies show gangliosides to be present in the microsomal fraction, presumably with fragments of dendrites and nerve endings.[34,35] $Na^+K^+ATPase$ has a similar distribution [34–37] and is closely associated with appearance of cerebral electrical activity.[38]

Brain $Na^+K^+ATPase$ activity and ganglioside content[44] are depressed in hypothyroidism of both species. An earlier report of a normal content of ganglioside in the hypothyroid rat cerebrum[12] is unexpected in view of the diminution of dendritic arboration described by the same workers.[9] Recent evidence for the reduction of synaptic terminals has also been documented in hypothyroid rats.[39]

The work of Gelber et al[40,45] suggests that thyroid hormones influence protein synthesis *only* in the immature brain. Most workers[12,14,16,19,23] who have used the neonatal thyroidectomized rat in their studies agree that the retarded brain maturation is caused by an impairment in protein synthesis. However, it is not yet understood whether the thyroid hormones affect brain development in a direct or indirect way. Aberrations in amino acid transport[17] and alteration of ionic environment[24] have been suggested as a cause of retarded protein synthesis. On the contrary, Balázs et al[12] claimed that derangement of protein synthesis is at the level of translation whereas others suggested a probable effect at the transcriptional level.[41]

Influence of the thyroid state on the maturation of the pituitary gland may play an important part in the symptomatology of both thyroid deficiency and thyroid hormone treatment. Protein synthesis is also depressed in the pituitary gland by neonatal thyroidectomy in the rat.[41,19] It is obvious from our results that growth hormone is compromised in the monkey fetus with thyroid ablation.

The effects of growth hormone on brain growth in the neonatally thyroidectomized rat have been intensively studied. The results are still controversial and inconclusive. Eayrs[9] and Hamburgh[42] have observed only marginal improvement after treatment, Geel and Timiras[19] have described partial rectification of brain pathology, while Krawiec et al[22] claim reversals that are in many respects akin to those of thyroid treatment alone. Therefore, while it has been demonstrated that thyroid hormone must be of importance to the development of the fetal primate brain, one cannot exclude the relevance of growth hormone in this situation.

Finally, it can be stated that these changes are essentially specific for the athyroid primate fetus. Concurrent studies (Chapter 6) indicate that fetal malnutrition exerts minimal effects on fetal primate brain composition.

CONCLUSION

Overall RNA and protein synthesis is reduced in the fetal monkey brain in the absence of thyroid hormone. The data indicate that both neuronal and neuroglial cell populations are functionally affected in the cerebrum and cerebellum. Modification of this fetal primate model should advance the understanding of the role of fetal thyroid and pituitary hormones in the development of the brain.

REFERENCES

1. Hamburgh, M., and Barrington, E. J. W. (Eds.): *Hormones in Development*. Appleton-Century-Crofts, New York, 1971.
2. Rall, J. E., Robbins, J., and Lewallen, C. G.: The thyroid. In: Pincus, G., Thimann, K. V., and Astwood, E. B. (Eds.): *The Hormones*, Vol. 5. Academic Press, New York, 1964, p. 358.
3. Eayrs, J. T.: Thyroid and central nervous development. In: *The Scientific Basis of Medicine Annual Reviews*. British Postgraduate Medical Federation, Oxford University Press (Athlone), London and New York, 1966, p. 317.
4. Eayrs, J. T.: Development relationships between brain and thyroid. In: Michael, R. P. (Ed.): *Endocrinology and Human Behaviour*. Oxford University Press, London and New York, 1968, p. 239.
5. Andersen, H. J.: Nongoitrous hypothyroidism. In: Gardner, L. I. (Ed.): *Endocrine and Genetic Diseases of Childhood*. Saunders, Philadelphia, 1969, p. 216.
6. Smith, D. W., Blizzard, R. M., and Wilkins, L.: The mental prognosis in hypothyroidism of infancy and childhood. *Pediatrics* **19**: 1011, 1957.
7. Davison, A. N., and Dobbing, J.: The developing brain. In: Davison, A. N., and Dobbing, J. (Eds.): *Applied Neurochemistry*. Davis, Philadelphia, 1968, p. 253.
8. Brasel, J. A., Ehrenkranz, R. A., and Winick, M.: DNA polymerase activity in rat brain during ontogeny. *Dev. Biol.* **23**: 424, 1970.
9. Eayrs, J. T.: Protein anabolism as a factor ameliorating the effects of early thyroid deficiency. *Growth* **25**: 175, 1961.
10. Legrand, J.: Comparative effects of thyroid deficiency and undernutrition on maturation of the nervous system and particularly on myelination in the young rat. In: Hamburgh, M., and Barrington, E. J. W. (Eds.): *Hormones in Development*. Appleton-Century-Crofts, New York, 1971, p. 381.
11. Mitskevich, M. S., and Koskovkin, G. N.: Some effects of thyroid hormone on the development of the central nervous system in early ontogenesis. In: Hamburgh, M., and Barrington, E. J. W. (Eds.): *Hormones in Development*. Appleton-Century-Crofts, New York, 1971, p. 437.
12. Balázs, R., Kovács, S., Teichgräber, P., Cocks, W. A., and Eayrs, J. T.: Biochemical effects of thyroid deficiency on the developing brain. *J. Neurochem.* **15**: 1335, 1968.
13. Balázs, R., Brooksbank, B. W. L., Davison, A. N., Eayrs, J. T., and Wilson, D. A.: The effect of neonatal thyroidectomy on myelination in the rat brain. *Brain Res.* **15**: 219, 1969.
14. Brasel, J. A., and Winick, M.: Differential cellular growth in the organs of hypothyroid rats. *Growth* **34**: 197, 1970.
15. Garcia Argiz, C. A., Pasquini, J. M., Kaplun, B., and Gomez, C. J.: Hormonal regulation of brain development. II. Effect of neonatal thyroidectomy on succinate dehydrogenase and other enzymes in developing cerebral cortex and cerebellum of the rat. *Brain Res.* **6**: 635, 1967.
16. Geel, S. E., and Timiras, P. S.: The influence of neonatal hypothyroidism and of thyroxine on the ribonucleic acid and deoxyribonucleic acid concentrations of rat cerebral cortex. *Brain Res.* **4**: 135, 1967.
17. Geel, S. E., Valcana, T., and Timiras, P. S.: Effect of neonatal hypothyroidism and of thyroxine on L-(^{14}C) leucine incorporation in protein *in vivo* and the relationship to ionic levels in the developing brain of the rat. *Brain Res.* **4**: 143, 1967.

18. Geel, S. E., and Timiras, P. S.: Influence of neonatal hypothyroidism and of thyroxine on the acetylcholinesterase and cholinesterase activity in the developing central nervous system of the rat. *Endocrinology* **80**: 1069, 1967.

19. Geel, S. E., and Timiras, P. S.: Influence of growth hormone on cerebral cortical RNA metabolism in immature hypothyroid rats. *Brain Res.* **22**: 63, 1970.

20. Gomez, C. J., and Ramirez De Guglielmone, A. E.: Influence of neonatal thyroidectomy on glucose-amino acids interrelations in developing rat cerebral cortex. *J. Neurochem.* **14**: 1119, 1967.

21. Gomez, C. J., Ghittoni, N. E., and Dellacha, J. M.: Effect of L-thyroxine or somatotrophin on body growth and cerebral development in neonatally thyroidectomized rats. *Life Sci.* **5**: 243, 1966.

22. Krawiec, L., Garcia Argiz, C. A., Gomez, C. J., and Pasquini, J. M.: Hormonal regulation of brain development. III. Effects of triiodothyronine and growth hormone on the biochemical changes in the cerebral cortex and cerebellum of neonatally thyroidectomized rats. *Brain Res.* **15**: 209, 1969.

23. Pasquini, J. M., Kaplun, B., Garcia Argiz, C. A., and Gomez, C. J.: Hormonal regulation of brain development. I. The effect of neonatal thyroidectomy upon nucleic acids, protein and two enzymes in developing cerebral cortex and cerebellum of the rat. *Brain Res.* **6**: 621, 1967.

24. Valcana, T., and Timiras, P. S.: Effect of hypothyroidism on ionic metabolism and Na-K activated ATP phosphohydrolase activity in the developing rat brain. *J. Neurochem.* **16**: 935, 1969.

25. Meisami, E., Valcana, T., and Timiras, P. S.: Effects of neonatal hypothyroidism on the development of brain excitability in the rat. *Neuroendocrinology* **6**: 160, 1970.

26. Osorio, C., and Myant, N. B.: The passage of thyroid hormone from mother to foetus and its relation to foetal development. *Br. Med. Bull.* **16**: 159, 1960.

27. Erenberg, A., Omori, K., Oh, W., and Fisher, D. A.: The effect of fetal thyroidectomy on growth of the ovine fetus. *Pediatr. Res.* **6**: 77, 1972.

28. Kerr, G. R., Tyson, I. B., Allen, J. R., Wallace, J. H., and Scheffler, G.: Deficiency of thyroid hormone and development of the fetal rhesus monkey. *Biol. Neonate* **21**: 282, 1972.

29. Holt, A. B., Cheek, D. B., and Kerr, G. R.: Prenatal hypothyroidism and brain composition in a primate. *Nature* **243**: 413, 1973.

30. Pickering, D. E., Settergren, K. F., and Kontaxis, N. E.: Thyroid function in the foetus of the macaque monkey (*Macaca mulatta*). I. The quantitative estimation of the iodinated components of the thyroid gland. *J. Endocrinol.* **23**: 261, 1961.

31. Pickering, D. E., and Kontaxis, N. E.: Thyroid function in the foetus of the macaque monkey (*Macaca mulatta*). II. Chemical and morphological characteristics of the foetal thyroid gland. *J. Endocrinol.* **23**: 267, 1961.

32. Pickering, D. E.: Thyroid physiology in the developing monkey fetus (*Macaca mulatta*). *Gen. Comp. Endocrinol.* **10**: 182, 1968.

33. Giacobini, E.: A cytochemical study of the localisation of carbonic anhydrase in the nervous system. *J. Neurochem.* **9**: 169, 1962.

34. De Robertis, E., and Rodriguez de Lores Arnaiz, G. Structural components of the synaptic region *Handb. Neurochem.* **2**: 365, 1969.

35. Seminario, L. M., Hren, N., and Gomez, C. J.: Lipid distribution in subcellular fractions of the rat brain. *J. Neurochem.* **11**: 197, 1964.

36. Bonting, S. L., Simon, K. A., and Hawkins, N. M.: Studies on sodium-potassium-activated adenosine triphosphatase. I. Quantitative distribution in several tissues of the cat. *Arch. Biochem. Biophys.* **95**: 416, 1961.

37. Kurokawa, M., Sakamoto, T., and Kato, M.: Distribution of sodium-plus-potassium-stimulated adenosine-triphosphatase activity in isolated nerve-ending particles. *Biochem. J.* **97**: 833, 1965.

38. Abdel-Latif, A. A., Brody, J., and Ramahi, H.: Studies on sodium-potassium adenosine triphosphatase of the nerve endings and appearance of electrical activity in developing rat brain. *J. Neurochem.* **14**: 1133, 1967.

REFERENCES

39. Nicholson, J. L., and Altman, J.: Synaptogenesis in the rat cerebellum: Effects of early hypo- and hyperthyroidism. *Science* **176**: 530, 1972.

40. Gelber, S., Campbell, P. L., Deibler, G. E., and Sokoloff, L.: Effects of L-thyroxine on amino acid incorporation into protein in mature and immature rat brain. *J. Neurochem.* **11**: 221, 1964.

41. Szijan, I., Kalbermann, L. E., and Gomez, C. J.: Hormone regulation of brain development. IV. Effect of neonatal thyroidectomy upon incorporation "*in vivo*" of (3H)-phenylalanine into proteins of developing rat cerebral tissues and pituitary gland. *Brain Res.* **27**: 309, 1971.

42. Hamburgh, M.: An analysis of the action of thyroid hormone on development based on *in vivo* and *in vitro* studies. *Gen. Comp. Endocrinol.* **10**: 198, 1968.

43. Solomon, J., and Greep, R. O.: The effect of alterations in thyroid function on the pituitary growth hormone content and acidophil cytology. *Endocrinology* **65**: 158, 1959.

44. Faryna de Raveglia, I., Gomez, C. J., and Ghittoni, N. E.: Hormonal regulation of brain development. V. Effect of neonatal thyroidectomy on lipid changes in cerebral cortex and cerebellum of developing rats. *Brain Res.* **43**: 181, 1972.

45. Sokoloff, L.: The mechanism of action of thyroid hormones on protein synthesis and its relationship to the differences in sensitivities of mature and immature brain. In: *Protein Metabolism of the Nervous System*, Lajtha, A. (Ed.) Plenum Press, New York, 1970, Chapter 18.

CHAPTER 9

Changes in Growth in the Fetal Brain After Ablation of the Pancreatic Beta Cells

Donald B. Cheek, Donald E. Hill, James Brayton, and Rachel E. Scott

INTRODUCTION

The role of insulin as a "growth promoting" hormone has not been extensively investigated in fetal or postnatal life. Salter and Best[1] injected long-acting protamine zinc insulin into weanling hypophysectomized rats and reported significant skeletal and visceral growth, but Wagner and Scow[2] claimed that tube-feeding hypophysectomized rats produced similar effects. However, Cheek and Graystone[3, 4] repeated and expanded the work of Salter and Best and confirmed the specific growth-promoting effect of insulin in hypophysectomized and intact rats.

Much of the available data is derived from clinical situations and particularly from studies on the infant born of the diabetic mother (IBDM).

In 1826 Bennewitz[5] was the first to record the unusual features of the infant born of the diabetic mother and there is now extensive information (see Farquhar[6] for review). Prior to the use of insulin the incidence of conception in diabetic women was low, but today pregnancy is as frequent in diabetic women as in normal women. The infants have a high mortality and morbidity, they are oversized with size incompatible with gestational age, and they appear plethoric and have a peculiar facial appearance akin to that seen in Cushing's syndrome. The face and body are erythematous and appear somewhat edematous, although it has been shown that edema is not present.[7] Such infants have in fact a reduced extracellular and intracellular volume in various tissues.[7-9] The work of Fee and Weil[9] using direct analysis of deceased infants demonstrated the very high fat content, the visceromegaly, and the increase in lean body mass. They demonstrated that there was a reduction of total chloride and sodium with a trend toward an increase in body potassium in viscera and muscle. The latter finding is of interest since we have

155

postulated that, in these infants, there is excess cytoplasmic growth. Fee and Weil drew attention to the fact that not all infants born of diabetic mothers are oversized. If vascular degeneration is present in the mother and in the placenta, placental insufficiency will result with reduced development of the fetus.

In review articles by Hoet[10] and De Gasparo and Hoet[11] the role of insulin in fetal growth was stressed. The large infants of diabetic mothers were contrasted with the small-for-dates infants of diabetic mothers who had vascular complications. In the large infant there was hyperplasia of the islet cells and hyperinsulinemia secondary to chronic material hyperglycemia[12-14] associated with increased accumulation of body fat and protein.[9] In addition, Naeye[15] reported an increase in the number of cell nuclei and cytoplasmic mass in various organs. In contrast, the small-for-dates infant has a smaller mass of islet tissue and a reduced total pancreatic mass[10,16] associated with reduced amounts of body protein, fat, and glycogen.[15,17] Similarly, in infants with transient neonatal diabetes, the beta-cell maturation is delayed[18,19] and they are frequently small for gestational age. These findings suggest a regulatory role for insulin in the growth of the fetus. Laron et al[20] have reviewed the clinical conditions in which hypoinsulinemia or hyperinsulinemia occurs and concluded that insulin should be regarded as a growth-promoting hormone.

We have employed two approaches to investigate the role of insulin as a fetal growth hormone in the primate, using the drug streptozotocin which ablates beta cells in the pancreas and produces diabetes in rats, dogs, and monkeys.[21-23]

In the first approach, steptozotocin was administered to the maternal primate at midgestation. It produced a moderate to mild diabetes in the maternal monkey, as shown by Mintz et al.[24] In our experiments, a single dose of glucose in a streptozotocin-treated monkey produced a large rise in blood sugar 1 hour later (Figure 9.1). The circulating plasma insulin was depressed.

The second series of experiments formed a separate study undertaken by one of us (D.E.H.). Streptozotocin was administered to the fetus *in utero*. The placenta appears to be a complete barrier to insulin crossover in sheep[25] and in rats.[26] While limited permeability may be present in monkeys and man,[27-29] the consensus of opinion is that the placenta in man is impermeable to insulin in early and late gestation.[30-32] With the view that insulin did not cross the placenta to the fetus in any appreciable amount, streptozotocin was administered to ablate beta-cell function in the fetal rhesus monkey. In this way, the effect of insulin on the cellular and somatic growth of the fetus could be determined.[33,34]

The effect of these two procedures on the growth of the fetal brain is the subject of this chapter. The effect on somatic growth is described in Chapter 18.

METHODS

Injection of Streptozotocin into the Mother

Nine pregnant females were given a single intravenous injection of streptozotocin (50 mg/kg) towards midgestation (60–70 days). The fetuses were taken either by elective cesarean section or allowed to deliver normally between 143 and 155 days. The 9 fetuses were compared with 22 normal fetuses delivered by cesarean section from 140 to 160 days of gestation.

EFFECT OF GLUCOSE LOAD

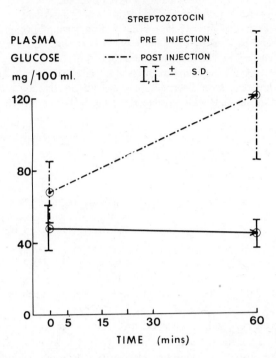

Fig. 9.1. The level of plasma glucose after a glucose load is shown for pregnant monkeys before receiving streptozotocin and after beta-cell ablation with streptozotocin.

Injection of Streptozotocin into the Fetus

Twenty-four pregnant rhesus monkeys (*Macaca mulatta*) with known gestational ages formed the experimental group. Nine normal animals served as unoperated controls, and 10 sham operations were performed at 110 days of gestation. The normal gestation is 165 ± 5 days. The animals were fasted overnight and presedated with 0.2 mg of atropine and 0.5 mg/kg of phencyclidine hydrochloride (*Sernylan*®). They were then intubated and maintained on a mixture of halothane, oxygen, and air, and ventilation was controlled with an Amerson respirator. The right maternal femoral vein was exposed and a catheter inserted to provide samples of maternal blood. The abdomen was prepared and a midline or paramedian incision was used to expose the gravid uterus. A fetal leg was identified by gentle palpation and then manipulated into a region of thin myometrium and held against the surface. The leg was then exposed through a small incision and gently eased through the incision to allow access to the fetal saphenous vein.

A fetal weight estimate was obtained from previous data, and 75 mg/kg of freshly prepared streptozotocin (pH 4.5) was given by way of the fetal saphenous vein. The fetal leg was immediately replaced in the uterus and the incision closed. Blood samples were taken from the mother at 0-, 5-, 10-, and 20-minute intervals following the injection. The abdominal incision was closed, the monkeys were allowed to recover, and near term (158 days) the surviving fetuses were delivered by cesarean section. The sham-operated animals underwent a similar procedure except that saline was injected in place of the streptozotocin.

Following delivery, the animals were immediately exsanguinated by the umbilical vessels. Total body weight, sex, crown-heel length, crown-rump length, and head circumference were recorded. The fetuses were then quickly dissected and tissue samples were taken according to the protocol described in Appendix I. Deoxyribonucleic acid (DNA), ribonucleic acid (RNA), and protein were determined by the methods also described in Appendix I. Water and fat contents in the tissues and whole carcass were determined by gravimetric methods.

Plasma insulin was measured by immunoassay.[35] Pancreatic insulin was extracted with acid alcohol and measured by the same immunoassay procedure. Histologic sections of the pancreas were prepared by using hematoxylin and eosin and aldehyde fuchsin stains. Fetal and maternal glucose levels were determined by the glucose oxidase method, and streptozotocin was assayed in the maternal plasma according to the method of Forist.[36]

RESULTS

Maternal Beta-Cell Ablation

Most of the fetuses born of diabetic mothers were oversized with visceromegaly. The pituitary gland was heavier than normal (16.0 ± 1.2 versus 13.3 ± 2.1 mg for controls). The adrenal glands were also increased in the IBDM (330 ± 96 versus 240 ± 81 mg). These increments were significant ($P < 0.001$ in the case of the pituitary and $P = 0.02$ for the adrenals). Discussion of these somatic differences is given in Chapter 18.

The cerebrum and cerebellum showed no increase in weight. While the weights were not changed, the concentration of water (percent water) was reduced in both tissues (Figures 9.2 and 9.3). The protein content tended to increase in cerebral tissues. Figure 9.4 illustrates increased protein:DNA ratio in cerebral cells, indicating that cytoplasmic growth was clearly increased. The change in ratio was partly because of a reduction in DNA (Figure 9.5). Hence fewer than expected cerebral cells were present but the cells had a larger than normal cytoplasmic growth.

In the cerebellar cells, the DNA content tended to increase (Figure 9.6) but not significantly so, while the concentration of protein was significantly elevated (Figure 9.7). Thus there was an increase in protein in cerebellar tissue without a significant change in cell number.

It was shown in Chapter 5 that in the cerebrum of IBDM there was an increase in the concentration and content of zinc as well as in the zinc:DNA ratio. Zinc was not measured in the cerebellum of the IBDM. We have previously emphasized that zinc is important to protein synthesis and these findings are consistent with the view that in IBDM an increase in protein accretion occurs (Figure 9.7). The association of zinc with carbonic anhydrase has also been discussed. The concentration of this latter enzyme (which is exclusive to neuroglial cells) was significantly elevated in the cerebrum and the total amount was increased in the cerebellum (Figures 9.8 and 9.9). The finding is consistent with an expansion of growth or function of neuroglial cells. Cholesterol concentration increased in the cerebrum (Figure 9.10) and in the cerebellum there was also a tendency toward an increase (Figure 9.11). The reduction of water content was not enough to explain the observed rise in cholesterol, hence the evidence suggests that myelination is advanced. By contrast, the phospholipid concentration of the cerebrum was reduced, indicating a retardation of growth with respect to this important component (Figure 9.12). Thus the changes in brain growth present a complex picture. Some aspects such as myelination and protein

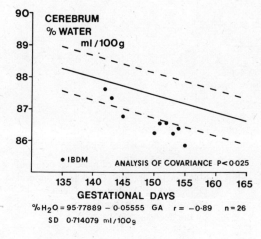

Fig. 9.2. The decrease in water content of the cerebrum in primate fetuses is shown after the mother has received beta-cell ablation.

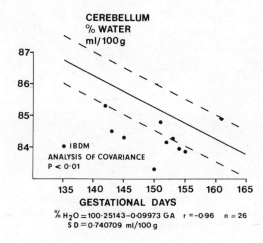

Fig. 9.3. The decrease in water content of the cerebellum in primate fetuses is shown after beta-cell ablation in the mother.

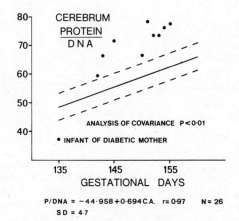

Fig. 9.4. The effect of maternal beta-cell ablation in the primate on fetal cerebral growth. The earlier development of cytoplasmic growth is suggested by the increase in protein: DNA ratio.

159

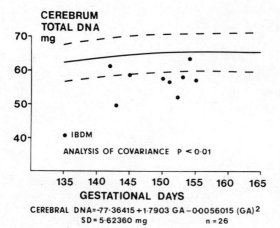

Fig. 9.5. The effect of maternal beta-cell ablation in the primate on fetal cerebral DNA levels. A slowing of cell multiplication in the fetal cerebrum is indicated by the decreased DNA.

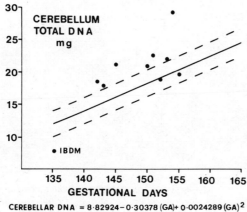

Fig. 9.6. The effect of maternal beta-cell ablation in the primate on fetal cerebellar DNA levels. (Not significant.)

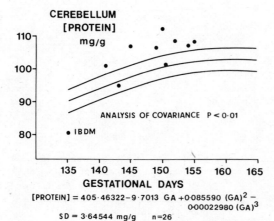

Fig. 9.7. The effect of maternal beta-cell ablation in the primate on the fetal cerebellar protein concentration. The concentration of protein in the cerebellum is greater than that in control animals.

160

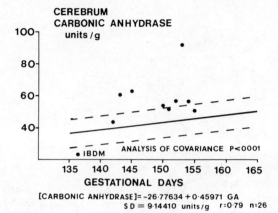

Fig. 9.8. The effect of maternal beta-cell ablation on cerebral carbonic anhydrase concentration in the fetus. There is a significant increase in concentration.

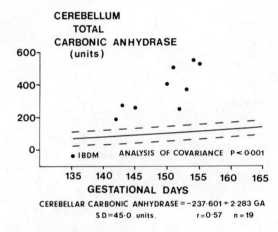

Fig. 9.9. The effect of maternal beta-cell ablation on fetal cerebellar carbonic anhydrase content.

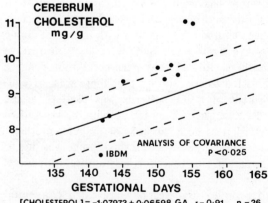

Fig. 9.10. The effect of maternal beta-cell ablation on cholesterol concentration in the fetal cerebrum. An increase in the cholesterol concentration is shown for the IBDM, suggesting that myelination is advanced in terms of time.

161

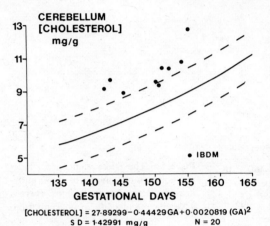

[CHOLESTEROL] = 27·89299 − 0·44429 GA + 0·0020819 (GA)^2
SD = 1·42991 mg/g   N = 20

Fig. 9.11. The effect of maternal beta-cell ablation on cholesterol concentration in the fetal cerebellum.

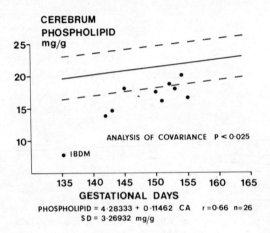

PHOSPHOLIPID = 4·28333 + 0·11462 CA   r = 0·66 n = 26
SD = 3·26932 mg/g

Fig. 9.12. The effect of maternal beta-cell ablation on the concentration of phospholipid in the fetal cerebrum. A reduction in phospholipid is produced.

accretion are advanced. In other respects brain growth is retarded as shown by the reduction in phospholipid and DNA content of the cerebrum.

Data are available concerning the human infant born of a diabetic mother. A decrease in brain weight has been reported for human infants born of diabetic mothers[37] and a disturbance in hydration has been suspected. Such dehydration might help to explain the hyperexcitability and occasional convulsions that occur. Immature behavior during sleep has been claimed,[38] together with increased clonic spinal motor neuron activity.[39] The investigations of Schulte et al[40] into nerve conduction in infants of diabetic mothers showed that peripheral motor nerve conduction velocity was increased. This led to speculation that there was "irregularity in myelination." Visual assessment of EEG patterns was used to assess maturity of dendritic arborization and axodendritic synaptic activity. It was shown that bioelectric brain activity was retarded in some infants of diabetic mothers, although, of course, it was not possible to determine whether this change was due to delay in formation of axodendritic synapses or due to abnormal humoral influences. Hypoglycemia was not responsible.

Experiments employing alloxan to produce diabetes have revealed congenital abnormalities in the brain of rabbits born of diabetic mothers.[41] Alloxan, unlike streptozotocin, attacks cells other than beta cells. Congenital abnormalities (including brain) are most frequent in human infants born of diabetic mothers. Barashnev[41] has concluded that 39% of such infants have psychoneurological abnormalities while 11% show serious retardation of mental development. Clearly, one should separate the large overgrown infant from the one that is reduced in size due to prematurity and vascular disease in the placenta.

Churchill et al[42] found that the IQ was reduced in infants of diabetic mothers if ketosis was present during pregnancy. They speculated that the occurrence of ketoacidosis may represent a state of metabolism in which amino acids are being catabolized instead of being converted to protein within the brain.

There is little doubt that the infant born of the diabetic mother has increased insulin release and hyperplasia of the islet cells[43] (see Farquhar[6] for review). The mode of induction of the hyperplasia is not proven but it has been suggested that the hyperglycemia of the mother is reflected in the fetal circulation and this in turn causes pancreatic stimulation.[44] Such stimulation to the rat pancreas can easily be produced by glucose.[45] Mintz et al[24] suggest that the increased levels of amino acids may play an equally important role. It is possible that the stimulus for increased insulin release and pancreatic hyperplasia comes from the effect of substrate on the hypothalamus, since the latter is known to contain cells capable of inducing insulin release from the pancreas.[46, 47]

Testicular interstitial cell hyperplasia or formation of luteinized ovarian cysts is found in infants of diabetic mothers[37] and is thought to arise from fetal chorionic gonadotropin. While excess insulin secretion in the fetus seems very probable, it is possible that other hormones such as growth hormone or cortisol are also being secreted in excess.

The finding of increased cytoplasmic growth in cerebrum (with some evidence of the same situation developing in the cerebellum) may be related to the excessive secretion of insulin. In Chapter 18 data are presented concerning increased cytoplasmic growth in muscle where the action of insulin on protein accretion is conspicuous. The increased carbonic anhydrase activity in cerebrum and cerebellum might well suggest that neuroglial cells are affected. In any event the circumstantial evidence indicating a role for insulin in brain growth is strong. To what extent the changes in cholesterol can be related to insulin is difficult to predict, as indeed is the reduction in phospholipid.

In the cerebrum, cell population was reduced, which draws attention to factors responsible for cell multiplication. Certain biochemical determinants of the brain were advanced (protein, Zn, water, cholesterol) while others (phospholipid, DNA) were delayed. Thus a deviation in development is demonstrated.

Fetal Beta-Cell Ablation

While fetal losses were great, it appeared that in surviving fetuses either runting resulted (three fetuses) through beta-cell ablation or, alternatively, progenitor cells were stimulated (we believe) to give rise to beta-cell hyperplasia. In this latter situation adrenal enlargement presented. Excessive insulin may have been released from the pancreas in these fetuses (histological evidence) with a trend to overgrowth. Thus in seven fetuses excessive growth of the adrenal gland (relative to body weight or time of gestation) presented and in these seven body weight was above the expected mean. The findings in the cerebrum and cerebellum for these seven fetuses are given in Tables 9.1 and 9.2 and are compared with nine comparable controls.

There was no change in the weight of the cerebrum when the controls were compared with the fetuses having elevated adrenal body weight ratio. There were minimal changes in the composition of the cerebrum (Table 9.1). However, the decrease in the percentage of water in the cerebrum and the borderline increases in the DNA concentration, protein concentration, total DNA, and total protein were similar to the changes seen in the cerebrum of the infants of the diabetic mothers described earlier. The protein:DNA ratio was unchanged in all groups, suggesting that DNA and protein were increasing in a parallel fashion.

Table 9.1   The effect of injection of streptozotocin on the cerebral composition in the primate fetus.

	Controls (n=9)	SZ* (n=7)	t p <	Analysis of Covariance p <
Weight g	51.0±4.9	51.5±3.6	NS	NS
Water %	86.7±0.78	85.8±0.58	0.02	NS
DNA mg/g	1.28±0.08	1.38±0.10	0.05	0.025
Protein mg/g	81.8±6.6	87.9±4.1	=0.05	NS
Total protein g	4.15±0.33	4.53±0.34	0.05	NS

Values are means ± SD.   *SZ = Streptozotocin treated fetuses with increased adrenal:body weight ratios (see text). NS = not significant.

Changes in the cerebellum were similar but more definite than those in the cerebrum and are summarized in Table 9.2. Of particular interest was the increase in carbonic anhydrase, both in activity and in total amount. There was also a significant increase in the ratio of protein to DNA, indicating that protein content increased to a greater extent than the DNA content. There was no change in the DNA content in the group compared with the controls.

Thus the overall information derived from the study of maternal diabetes and from the direct interference of the fetal pancreatic cells leads to the following conclusions. Insulin influences brain growth of the fetus and augments protein accretion with coincidental reduction in water content; stimulation of neuroglial growth occurs as evidenced by the change in carbonic anhydrase. The three runted fetuses showed growth retardation in all aspects and it is suspected that they had poor insulin secretion (histological evidence).

Table 9.2   The effect of injection of
streptozotocin on the cerebellar
composition in the primate fetus.

	Controls (n=9)	SZ* (n=7)	t p <	Analysis of Covariance p <
Weight g	3.0±0.45	3.3±0.33	NS	
Carbonic anhydrase units	112±56	272±75	0.001	0.01
Carbonic anhydrase units/g	36.5±14.6	81.6±18.6	0.001	0.01
Water %	84.6±0.64	83.8±0.58	0.02	NS
Protein mg/g	102.3±4.0	109.4±5.2	0.01	0.05
Protein g	0.31±0.05	0.36±0.05	0.05	NS
Protein to DNA	15.7±0.54	17.8±0.88	0.001	0.001

Values are means ± SD.   *SZ = Streptozotocin
treated fetuses with increased adrenal:body weight
ratios (see text).   NS = not significant.

REFERENCES

1. Salter, J., and Best, C. H.: Insulin as a growth hormone. *Br. Med. J.* **2**: 353, 1953.
2. Wagner, E. M., and Scow, R. O.: Effect of insulin on growth in force-fed hypophysectomized rats. *Endocrinology* **61**: 419, 1957.
3. Cheek, D. B., and Graystone, J. E.: The action of insulin, growth hormone, and epinephrine on cell growth in liver, muscle, and brain of the hypophysectomized rat. *Pediatr. Res.* **3**: 77, 1969.
4. Graystone, J. E., and Cheek, D. B.: The effects of reduced caloric intake and increased insulin-induced caloric intake on the cell growth of muscle, liver, and cerebrum, and on skeletal collagen in the post-weanling rat. *Pediatr. Res.* **3**: 66, 1969.
5. Bennewitz, H. G.: In: *Osann, Jahresberichte des koeniglichen poliklinischen Institutes der Universitaet zu Berlin 1823–1825*, Vol. 12. G. Remier, Berlin, 1826, p. 23.
6. Farquhar, J. W.: In: Gairdner, D. (Ed.): *Recent Advances in Paediatrics*. Churchill, London, 1965, Chapter 6.
7. Cheek, D. B., Maddison, T. G., Malinek, M., and Coldbeck, J. H.: Further observations on the corrected bromide space of the neonate and investigation of water and electrolyte status in infants born of diabetic mothers. *Pediatrics* **28**: 861, 1961.
8. Osler, M., and Pedersen, J.: The body composition of newborn infants of diabetic mothers. *Pediatrics* **26**: 985, 1960.
9. Fee, B., and Weil, W. B. Jr.: The body composition of infants of diabetic mothers by direct analysis. *Ann. N.Y. Acad. Sci.* **110**: 869, 1963.

10. Hoet, J. J.: Normal and abnormal foetal weight gain. In: Wolstenholme, G. E. W., and O'Connor, M. (Eds.): *Foetal Autonomy*, a Ciba Foundation Symposium. Churchill, London, 1969, p. 186.

11. De Gasparo, M., and Hoet, J. J.: Normal and abnormal foetal weight gain. In: Rodriguez, R. R., and Vallance-Owen, J. (Eds.): *Diabetes*. Excerpta Medica, The Netherlands, 1971, p. 667.

12. Baird, J. D.: Some aspects of carbohydrate metabolism in pregnancy with special reference to the energy metabolism and hormonal status of the infant of the diabetic woman and the diabetogenic effect of pregnancy. *J. Endocrinol.* **44**: 139, 1969.

13. Cardell, B. S.: Infants of diabetic mothers, a morphological study. *J. Obstet. Gynaecol. Br. Commonw.* **60**: 834, 1953.

14. Steinke, J., and Driscoll, S.: The extractable insulin content of pancreas from fetuses and infants of diabetic and control mothers. *Diabetes* **14**: 573, 1965.

15. Naeye, R. L.: Infants of diabetic mothers. A quantitative morphologic study. *Pediatrics* **35**: 980, 1965.

16. Kyle, G. C.: Diabetes and pregnancy. *Ann. Intern. Med.* **59**: 1, 1963, Suppl. 3–4.

17. Shelley, H. J., and Neligan, G. A.: Neonatal hypoglycemia. *Br. Med. Bull.* **22**: 34, 1966.

18. Ferguson, A. W., and Milner, R. D. G.: Transient neonatal diabetes mellitus in sibs. *Arch. Dis. Child.* **45**: 80, 1970.

19. Milner, R. D. G., Barson, A. J., and Ashworth, M. A.: Human foetal pancreatic insulin secretion in response to ionic and other stimuli. *J. Endocrinol.* **51**: 323, 1971.

20. Laron, Z., Karp, M., Pertzelan, A., and Kauli, R.: Insulin, growth, and growth hormone. *Isr. J. Med. Sci.* **8**: 440, 1972.

21. Rakieten, N., Rakieten, M. L., and Nadkarni, M. V.: Studies on the diabetogenic action of streptozotocin (NSC-37917). *Cancer Chemother. Rep.* **29**: 91, 1963.

22. Junod, A., Lambert, A. E., Orci, L., Pictet, R., Gonet, A. E., and Renold, A. E.: Studies of the diabetogenic action of streptozotocin. *Proc. Soc. Exp. Biol. Med.* **126**: 201, 1967.

23. Pitkin, R. M., and Reynolds, W. A.: Diabetogenic effects of streptozotocin in rhesus monkeys. *Diabetes* **19**: 85, 1970.

24. Mintz, D. H., Chez, R. A., and Hutchinson, D. L.: Subhuman primate pregnancy complicated by streptozotocin-induced diabetes mellitus. *J. Clin. Invest.* **51**: 837, 1972.

25. Alexander, D. P., Britton, H. G., Cohen, N. M., Nixon, D. A., and Parker, R. A.: Insulin concentration in the foetal plasma and foetal fluids of the sheep. *J. Endocrinol.* **40**: 389, 1968.

26. Goodner, C. J., and Freinkel, N.: Carbohydrate metabolism in pregnancy. IV. Studies on the permeability of the rat placenta to I^{131} insulin. *Diabetes* **10**: 383, 1961.

27. Josimovich, J. B., and Knobil, E.: Placental transfer of I^{131} insulin in the rhesus monkey. *Am. J. Physiol.* **200**: 471, 1961.

28. Mintz, D. H., Chez, R. A., and Horger, E. O.: Fetal insulin and growth hormone metabolism in the subhuman primate. *J. Clin. Invest.* **48**: 176, 1969.

29. Gitlin, D., Kumate, J., and Morales, C.: On the transport of insulin across the human placenta. *Pediatrics* **35**: 65, 1965.

30. Adam, P. A. J., Teramo, K., Raiha, N., Gitlin, D., and Schwartz, R.: Human fetal insulin metabolism early in gestation. Response to acute elevation of the fetal blood glucose concentration and placental transfer of human insulin-I^{131}. *Diabetes* **18**: 409, 1969.

31. Buse, M. G., Roberts, W. J., and Buse, J.: The role of the human placenta in the transfer and metabolism of insulin. *J. Clin. Invest.* **41**: 29, 1962.

32. Wolff, H., Sabata, V., Frerichs, H., and Stubbe, P.: Evidence for the impermeability of the human placenta for insulin. *Horm. Metab. Res.* **1**: 274, 1969.

33. Hill, D. E., and Cheek, D. B.: Studies on the cellular growth and substrate availability in the rhesus monkey fetus. XIII International Congress of Pediatrics, Wien, Oesterreich. September 1971, p. 33.

34. Hill, D. E., Holt, A. B., Reba, R., and Cheek, D. B.: Alterations in the growth pattern of fetal rhesus monkeys following the *in utero* injection of streptozotocin. *Pediatr. Res.* (*Abstr.*) **6**: 336, 1972.

35. Herbert, V., Lau, K. S., Gottlieb, C. W., and Bleicher, S. J.: Coated charcoal immunoassay of insulin. *J. Clin. Endocrinol.* **25**: 1375, 1965.

36. Forist, A. A.: Spectrophotometric determination of streptozotocin. *Anal. Chem.* **36**: 1338, 1964.

37. Driscoll, S. G., Benirschke, K., and Curtis, G. W.: Neonatal deaths among infants of diabetic mothers. Postmortem findings in ninety-five infants. *Am. J. Dis. Child.* **100**: 818, 1960.

38. Schulte, F. J., Albert, G., and Michaelis, R.: Brain and behavioural maturation in newborn infants of diabetic mothers. Part III: Motor behaviour. *Neuropaediatrie* **1**: 44, 1969.

39. Schulte, F. J., Lasson, U., Parl, U., Nolte, R., and Juergens, U.: Brain and behavioural maturation in newborn infants of diabetic mothers. Part II: Sleep cycles. *Neuropaediatrie* **1**: 36, 1969.

40. Schulte, F. J., Michaelis, R., Nolte, R., Albert, G., Parl, U., and Lasson, U.: Brain and behavioural maturation in newborn infants of diabetic mothers. Part I: Nerve conduction and EEG patterns. *Neuropaediatrie* **1**: 24, 1969.

41. Barashnev, Y. L.: Malformation of fetal brain resulting from alloxan diabetes in mother. *Ark. Patol.* **26**(5): 63, 1964.

42. Churchill, J. A., Berendes, H. W., and Nemore, J.: Neuropsychological deficits in children of diabetic mothers. *Am. J. Obstet. Gynecol.* **105**: 257, 1969.

43. Isles, T. E., Dickson, M., and Farquhar, J. W.: Glucose tolerance and plasma insulin in newborn infants of normal and diabetic mothers. *Pediatr. Res.* **2**: 198, 1968.

44. Pedersen, J., Bojsen-Moller, B., and Poulsen, H. E.: Blood sugar in newborn infants of diabetic mothers. *Acta Endocrinol.* **15**: 33, 1954.

45. Woerner, C. A.: The effects of continuous intravenous injection of dextrose in increasing amounts on the blood sugar level, pancreatic islets, and liver of guinea pigs. *Anat. Rec.* **75**: 91, 1939.

46. Idahl, L. A., and Martin, J. M.: Stimulation of insulin release by a ventro-hypothalamic factor. *J. Endocrinol.* **51**: 1, 1971.

47. Han, P. W., Yu, Y. K., and Chow, S. L.: Enlarged pancreatic islets of tube-fed hypophysectomized rats bearing hypothalamic lesions. *Am. J. Physiol.* **218**: 769, 1970.

CHAPTER 10

Amino Acids in the Brain
During Fetal Growth and the
Effects of Prenatal Hormonal
and Nutritional Imbalance

Claude Bachmann, William L. Nyhan, Stanko Kulovich, and Mary Etta Hornbeck

INTRODUCTION

The amino acids provide the substrate for protein synthesis which is fundamental to cellular growth. They may also be concerned with the regulation of protein synthesis. These compounds and their metabolites are also involved in many of the specific functions of the central nervous system. For example, several amino acids are themselves neurotransmitters; the concentration of the substrate tryptophan is thought to be a determining factor in the formation of serotonin; tyrosine is a precursor of catecholamines; and methionine and choline may serve as methyl donors for the synthesis of catecholamines.

Tissue concentrations of amino acids result from a dynamic equilibrium produced by their synthesis, degradation, incorporation into proteins, and transport in and out of the cell. The goal of this study was to determine whether or not there were changes in the concentrations of amino acids during normal fetal primate development and under experimental conditions that might be expected to alter fetal growth. Elucidation of any relevant aspects of amino acid metabolism could provide information on the mechanisms of cellular growth.

This work was supported by Research Grant HDO4588 from the National Institute of Child Health and Human Development, National Institutes of Health, Bethesda, Maryland, and by a grant from the Swiss National Foundation for Scientific Research.

169

MATERIALS AND METHODS

The animals studied were from the same series of primates investigated throughout this book. Details of their care, experimental plan, and other data pertaining to growth are documented elsewhere in this book.

Methods (Chemical)

After the animals were killed, tissue samples were weighed, homogenized in water (90–100 mg tissue/ml), and kept frozen until analysis. Aliquots of the homogenates of cerebrum and cerebellum were deproteinized with cold 0.4 N perchloric acid (1:1).[1] Ion exchange chromatography was performed in accordance with the method of Spackman and co-workers[2] using Beckman Spinco Model 120 and 120 C Automatic Amino Acid Analyzers. Norleucine was employed as an internal standard. The concentrations of tryptophan in cerebrum and cerebellum were determined separately using a fluorometric method[3] after deproteinization of the homogenate with 6% trichloracetic acid (TCA) (0.5–1.0 ml of homogenate was diluted with TCA to a total volume of 4.0 ml).

Calculations

Amino acid concentrations were calculated as micromoles per liter of blood or per kilogram of tissue, using the original wet weight of the tissue samples. Concentrations were also related to the DNA in the tissues. In addition ratios of the micromolar concentrations of individual nonessential and essential amino acids were calculated, as these have seemed useful in assessing the amino acid concomitants of abnormal human growth.[4] We also calculated the ratio of the micromolar sum of the concentrations of serine, glycine, alanine, tyrosine, and ornithine, divided by the sum of the concentrations of threonine, valine, methionine, isoleucine, leucine, phenylalanine, lysine, and histidine. This quotient is referred to as the ratio of nonessential to essential amino acids, although not all of the nonessential and essential amino acids are included. The designation of an amino acid as essential was extrapolated from studies in man and in laboratory animals other than monkeys.

Group comparisons were made statistically using a t-test for unpaired samples. Computer facilities at the University of California, San Diego, and at the National Institutes of Health were of invaluable assistance in handling the large volumes of data generated in these studies. Correlation coefficients were calculated between fetal plasma corticosteroid levels* and the concentrations of amino acids.

NORMAL GROWTH

Results

The monkeys were divided into groups for comparison as follows:

    Group 1.   Fetuses delivered between 75 and 112 days of pregnancy.
    Group 2.   Fetuses delivered between 122 and 140 days.

---

* Generously supplied by Dr. Claude Migeon, Professor of Pediatrics, The Johns Hopkins School of Medicine. We are grateful to Dr. Inez Beitins who carried out the determinations.

Group 3.   Fetuses delivered between 145 and 160 days.

Group 4.   Born naturally and killed between 12 hours and 32 days of postnatal
           age.

Group 5.   Normal, growing monkeys between the ages of 60 and 122 days.

Group 6.   Adult monkeys.

The amino acids present in highest concentration in brain tissues were taurine and
glutamic acid, whose concentrations generally exceeded 5 mM/kg. Alanine, whose
concentration usually exceeded that of glycine, was usually about 2 to 4 mM/kg.
Glycine and serine were generally 1 to 2 mM/kg. Aspartic acid, threonine, glutamine, proline, valine, leucine, lysine, and arginine generally exceeded 500 μM/kg.
γ-Aminobutyric acid concentrations were quite variable, with values observed from
500 to 5,000 μM/kg. Methionine, isoleucine, tyrosine, phenylalanine, and histidine
were usually over 100 μM/kg, and tryptophan was usually less than 100 μM/kg.
Cystathionine concentration was less than 100 μM/kg in the cerebrum of the
younger fetuses, rising with age. In the cerebellum it was generally over 500 μM/kg.

The mean concentrations of amino acids in the brain have been set out per unit
DNA in Table 10.1 and per unit tissue weight in Table 10.2. The animals represented
a wide spread from prior to birth (groups 1–3), immediately after birth (groups 4 and
5), to adult animals (group 6). The results of statistical comparisons among the
groups are shown in Table 10.3. These data are shown graphically in Figure 10.1.
Tables 10.4, 10.5, and 10.6 and Figure 10.2 provide the same treatments of the data
for cerebellum. The concentrations of most amino acids per gram of DNA were
higher in the cerebrum than in the cerebellum. An exception to this was citrulline
in group 5. The analysis of glutamine by ion exchange chromatography is not reli-

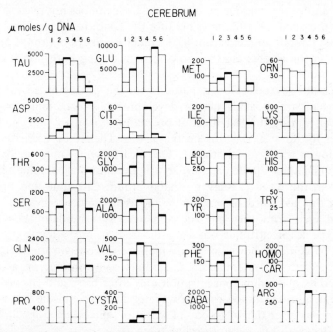

Fig. 10.1.   Concentrations of amino acids in cerebrum during development. The values are expressed
per gram of DNA. The heavy bars indicate changes that are significant when compared to the first
of the second preceding group.

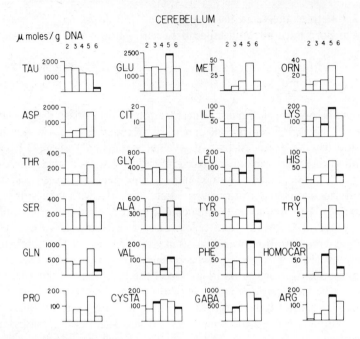

Fig. 10.2. Concentrations of amino acids in cerebellum during development. The values are expressed per gram of DNA. The heavy bars indicate changes that are significant when compared to the first or the second preceding group.

able. This amide is not separated from asparagine. There is conversion to both glutamic acid and to pyrrolidone carboxylic acid which does not react to ninhydrin. The data are provided for glutamine because the conditions were the same for all of the analyses. Cystathionine, except in the older monkeys in groups 5 and 6, was always higher in the cerebellum than in cerebrum during both prenatal and postnatal life.

In the cerebrum several different patterns can be distinguished in the cellular concentrations of amino acids during development. Most amino acids reached maximum levels during the last third of pregnancy (groups 2 and 3). These were maintained in the first 30 days of postnatal life. Then they decreased, reaching significantly lower levels in adulthood. The dicarboxylic amino acids glutamate and aspartate and their amide counterparts in glutamine/asparagine reached their maxima only in the 60-to-122-day postnatal group. Citrulline and ornithine declined during the last third of pregnancy and then suddenly peaked after birth. They declined again from then on. These changes were subtle in the case of ornithine, but the peak for citrulline was quite different from the levels at other times.

Cystathionine content showed a steady increase in concentration. Its maximum cerebral concentration was found in the adults. γ-Aminobutyric acid (GABA) clearly reached its maximum concentration only after birth and showed no significant decrease in adults. Homocarnosine was not detectable in the first two groups; it began to appear after the 145th day of gestation and reached much higher concentrations after birth but did not decline thereafter.

The ratios of glycine to the branched-chain amino acids (Figure 10.3) steadily increased, reaching maxima in adulthood. The ratio of nonessential to essential

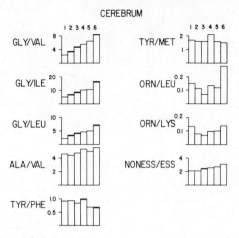

Fig. 10.3. Ratios of amino acid concentrations in cerebrum. The amino acid concentration per gram of DNA was used for calculation of the ratios.

amino acids followed the same pattern, but the changes in this ratio were so small that one might say there was very little change. The concentrations of most free amino acids computed on a weight basis (micromoles per kilogram) were higher in cerebrum and cerebellum than in plasma (micromoles per liter). Methionine and histidine were exceptions to this in the age group of 130 to 140 days prenatally but not in the group studied at 75 to 120 days.

The ratios of alanine to valine, tyrosine to phenylalanine, and ornithine to leucine or lysine also appeared to be of little benefit in detecting age-related change. The ratio of tyrosine to methionine was also without obvious developmental pattern.

In the cerebellum there were a number of changes in amino acid concentration that were statistically significant (Table 10.6) when they were related to DNA concentration or when concentrations were expressed per tissue weight. The general pattern was of a postnatal peak in group 5 (60–122 postnatal days), followed by a decline to reach low levels in adulthood. A number of amino acids such as leucine and phenylalanine did not vary much in group 1 through group 3, and then did not decline much beyond this level in adulthood. Homocarnosine was not measurable until the group immediately preceding birth and increased markedly after delivery. Its concentration was lower afterwards. The ratios of glycine to isoleucine and of glycine to leucine (Figure 10.4) reached a significant maximum in the neonatal group (group 4). The glycine:valine ratio showed a similar pattern. The alanine: valine ratio did not change much, although differences between groups 2 and 3 and between groups 4 and 5 were significant statistically. In contrast to the situation in the cerebrum the tyrosine:phenylalanine ratio appeared to decline steadily with development.

In the cerebrum there were significant positive correlations between fetal levels of corticosteroids in plasma and the concentrations of some amino acids (Table 10.7). Positive correlations were found for cystathionine, leucine, citrulline, and homocarnosine prenatally. Concentrations of glycine and valine were significantly

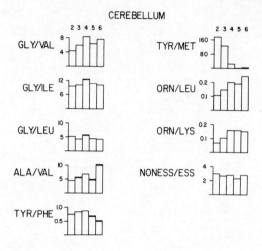

Fig. 10.4. Ratios of amino acid concentrations in cerebellum. The amino acid concentration per gram of DNA was used for calculation of the ratios.

negatively correlated with plasma corticoids before birth. In the two postnatal groups (groups 4 and 5), a negative correlation with the concentration of proline was present.

In the case of the cerebellum the concentration of corticosteroid in plasma was positively correlated with the concentration of cystathionine in group 4.

Summary of Changes during Normal Growth

Concentration of Amino Acids

1. The concentrations of most free amino acids were higher in the cerebrum than in the cerebellum and both had levels higher than in the plasma.

2. There was some variation in the concentrations of amino acids in the cerebrum and cerebellum. In general the decreasing order of concentration was as follows: taurine and glutamic acid (concentrations greater than 5 mM/kg), alanine (2–4 mM/kg), glycine and serine (1–2 mM/kg), aspartic acid, threonine, glutamine, proline, valine, leucine, lysine, and arginine (greater than 500 μM/kg), γ-aminobutyric acid (variable, 500–5,000 μM/kg), methionine, isoleucine, tyrosine, phenylalanine, and histidine (usually over 100 μM/kg), tryptophan (usually less than 100 μM/kg). Cystathionine concentration was less than 100 μM/kg in the cerebrum and over 500 μM/kg in the cerebellum.

3. In the cerebellum the general pattern that emerged was a postnatal peak, followed by a decrease with low levels in adults. There were some exceptions, for example, leucine and phenylalanine (high prenatally, no marked decrease) and homocarnosine (not measurable until birth, then a marked increase immediately after delivery, followed by a decrease).

TABLE 10.1
Concentrations of Amino Acids per Unit of DNA in Primate Cerebrum During Development*

(µmoles/g DNA)

	GROUP 1			GROUP 2			GROUP 3			GROUP 4			GROUP 5			GROUP 6		
	MEAN	S.E.M.	N	MEAN	S.E.M.	N	MEAN	S.E.M.	N	MEAN	S.E.M.	N	MEAN	S.E.M.	N	MEAN	S.E.M.	N
TAURINE	1906.0	352.2	7	3928.0	391.4	8	4403.0	623.0	11	4111.9	475.2	9	2169.7	219.1	7	907.2	201.5	6
ASPARTIC ACID	379.1	46.1	6	1186.4	162.6	9	1671.9	196.3	10	3075.0	294.5	8	5123.3	422.5	5	4758.1	721.2	6
THREONINE	271.7	37.8	6	460.5	86.2	9	501.9	58.4	10	675.2	97.1	7	481.2	89.5	3	289.5	30.8	5
SERINE	488.5	66.4	6	783.2	55.5	9	1200.4	158.2	11	1275.8	137.9	9	1191.8	84.4	7	708.4	47.7	6
GLUTAMINE	157.6	27.5	6	631.4	163.2	9	652.5	129.2	11	1174.0	196.3	8	2405.8	586.2	7	750.9	318.7	6
PROLINE	0.0	0.0	2	436.2	45.6	9	691.4	155.5	9	157.3	156.5	3	589.7	105.5	3	0.0	0.0	0
GLUTAMIC ACID	2211.1	292.2	7	4988.4	431.9	9	7528.7	1098.1	11	7591.9	443.9	9	9617.8	896.0	9	7964.2	755.5	6
CITRULLINE	21.0	8.9	7	12.7	12.4	7	3.9	3.8	9	60.5	15.4	9	9.7	9.5	6	0.5	0.1	6
GLYCINE	566.8	69.1	7	1175.2	101.5	9	2019.0	286.3	11	2109.2	171.5	9	2282.2	92.7	7	1619.0	143.9	6
ALANINE	978.1	107.2	7	1464.7	98.2	9	2023.7	281.7	11	2030.3	198.5	9	1739.1	132.1	7	1058.9	105.4	6
VALINE	226.3	33.7	7	336.9	17.4	9	447.9	67.9	11	399.0	58.1	9	360.8	41.3	7	191.2	10.2	6
CYSTATHIONINE	2.9	1.9	7	41.5	6.9	9	103.4	11.5	11	104.8	9.9	9	152.3	19.7	7	321.8	64.6	6
METHIONINE	55.6	9.7	7	87.9	9.4	9	124.1	14.7	11	105.1	15.8	9	134.7	28.3	7	55.8	12.5	6
ISOLEUCINE	114.2	16.8	7	169.2	10.9	9	238.2	31.7	11	209.7	23.6	9	221.2	23.9	7	100.9	9.3	6
LEUCINE	255.0	34.7	7	334.6	19.0	9	499.3	73.7	11	478.2	65.5	9	487.8	69.9	7	231.1	26.3	6
TYROSINE	91.7	11.8	7	138.7	9.9	9	190.6	21.8	11	201.5	29.4	9	203.0	27.2	7	74.6	5.9	6
PHENYLALANINE	99.4	11.8	7	147.8	10.8	9	234.4	32.8	11	202.2	25.4	9	296.5	38.3	7	110.0	11.5	6
GABA**	250.1	43.7	7	888.5	68.4	9	1198.0	148.1	11	2626.7	275.1	9	2288.5	444.9	7	2325.5	382.5	6
ORNITHINE	42.1	12.1	6	40.1	18.7	9	36.2	11.0	11	64.4	12.2	8	52.2	20.5	7	54.9	15.4	6
LYSINE	283.8	50.8	7	469.2	38.7	9	469.2	41.6	11	609.2	88.3	9	495.3	81.3	7	371.8	63.9	6
HISTIDINE	66.4	17.8	7	161.6	16.8	9	145.3	22.8	11	196.3	34.7	9	154.9	18.3	7	103.8	18.1	6
TRYPTOPHAN	13.3	1.6	7	15.7	3.0	7	45.2	11.2	10	36.0	4.6	8	47.9	4.5	4	0.0	0.0	0
ARGININE	129.6	39.9	7	284.7	66.6	9	233.5	41.3	11	420.2	82.8	9	362.6	82.5	7	383.9	71.6	6
HOMOCARNOSINE	0.0	0.0	7	0.0	0.0	9	43.7	43.6	11	214.7	55.8	9	201.8	57.7	7	202.4	74.1	6

* The groups were as follows: 1, 75–112 days of fetal life; 2, 122–140 days of fetal life; 3, 145–160 days of fetal life; 4, 12 hours–32 days of postnatal life; 5, 60–122 days of postnatal life; and 6, adult monkeys. The data were the means, the standard errors of the means (S.E.M.), and the number of animals (N).
** GABA: γ-Aminobutyric acid.

TABLE 10.2
Concentrations of Amino Acids Per Unit Tissue Weight in Primate Cerebrum During Development*

(μmoles/kg)

	GROUP 1			GROUP 2			GROUP 3			GROUP 4			GROUP 5			GROUP 6		
	MEAN	S.E.M.	N	MEAN	S.E.M.	N	MEAN	S.E.M.	N	MEAN	S.E.M.	N	MEAN	S.E.M.	N	MEAN	S.E.M.	N
TAURINE	5526.5	833.1	7	5866.6	333.3	8	5676.6	813.9	11	5108.2	531.8	9	3008.6	292.4	7	1131.4	243.8	6
ASPARTIC ACID	1163.1	82.3	6	1795.3	206.9	9	2161.4	265.4	10	3897.8	388.0	8	7196.6	652.7	5	6012.0	927.4	6
THREONINE	824.9	70.3	6	693.1	102.1	9	645.7	72.1	10	839.6	108.6	7	657.2	111.2	3	370.9	41.6	5
SERINE	1474.9	104.8	6	1210.9	72.2	9	1527.7	187.5	11	1588.3	152.6	9	1661.2	122.6	7	891.0	58.5	6
GLUTAMINE	498.2	78.0	6	930.4	207.8	9	830.8	160.9	11	1470.4	251.6	8	3334.7	806.8	7	969.3	435.0	6
PROLINE	0.0	0.0	2	675.1	65.8	9	881.6	188.9	9	203.0	202.0	3	814.7	130.2	3	0.0	0.0	0
GLUTAMIC ACID	6380.2	420.9	7	7739.5	712.6	9	9548.8	1307.2	11	9540.0	538.3	9	13345.2	1190.7	7	10001.8	895.7	6
CITRULLINE	53.1	22.2	7	22.6	22.2	7	5.3	5.1	9	74.1	18.1	9	13.8	13.4	7	0.6	0.2	6
GLYCINE	1633.1	93.7	7	1835.6	160.8	9	2558.6	337.4	11	2638.5	187.2	9	3172.4	110.0	7	2028.6	156.2	6
ALANINE	2859.7	174.5	7	2296.8	200.1	9	2573.9	336.0	11	2525.8	211.7	9	2423.4	191.5	7	1323.0	106.4	6
VALINE	646.1	54.2	7	523.5	27.2	9	571.5	82.7	11	494.9	66.4	9	500.6	53.6	7	240.5	12.4	6
CYSTATHIONINE	12.1	8.0	7	62.0	8.0	9	131.6	13.3	11	131.1	11.1	9	212.0	26.8	7	402.0	78.8	6
METHIONINE	157.2	18.9	7	134.2	11.1	9	158.1	17.6	11	130.8	18.4	9	185.8	37.3	7	71.5	18.0	6
ISOLEUCINE	326.2	28.2	7	262.2	15.4	9	303.4	38.0	11	260.6	26.1	9	306.5	30.2	7	127.5	13.4	6
LEUCINE	728.9	50.6	7	520.5	29.8	9	635.0	88.0	11	594.6	74.9	9	675.3	90.6	7	293.2	38.5	6
TYROSINE	262.6	16.9	7	214.5	13.7	9	242.6	25.5	11	250.6	34.2	9	280.8	35.1	7	94.7	9.5	6
PHENYLALANINE	287.3	11.7	7	227.9	13.0	9	299.2	39.7	11	251.0	28.4	9	410.9	50.1	7	139.2	16.2	6
GABA	703.4	78.2	7	1367.8	73.1	9	1524.5	183.3	11	3314.2	360.0	9	3167.3	616.2	7	2919.5	477.3	6
ORNITHINE	119.6	25.1	6	68.0	32.8	9	48.0	15.0	11	80.6	15.6	8	72.8	28.7	7	68.7	19.9	6
LYSINE	822.3	104.4	7	727.9	54.4	9	600.6	53.6	11	759.8	107.5	9	685.5	112.0	7	470.3	82.7	6
HISTIDINE	181.7	35.2	7	246.5	17.8	9	185.2	28.3	11	246.3	42.9	9	214.1	23.5	7	130.9	23.0	6
TRYPTOPHAN	38.8	2.7	7	25.0	4.1	7	57.7	13.4	10	45.5	6.6	8	67.5	6.7	4	0.0	0.0	0
ARGININE	344.8	88.7	7	459.1	125.3	9	296.8	53.8	11	525.3	99.7	9	500.3	111.4	7	484.4	91.8	6
HOMOCARNOSINE	0.0	0.0	7	0.0	0.0	9	52.9	52.8	11	276.2	71.6	9	278.6	79.1	7	258.7	95.1	6
GLY/VAL	2.5	0.1	7	3.5	0.2	9	4.8	0.4	11	5.7	0.4	9	6.6	0.5	7	8.4	0.5	6
GLY/ILE	5.1	0.2	7	7.0	0.5	9	8.7	0.6	11	10.6	0.9	9	10.7	0.6	7	16.2	1.0	6
GLY/LEU	2.2	0.08	7	3.5	0.3	9	4.3	0.4	11	4.7	0.4	9	5.0	0.4	7	7.3	0.8	6
ALA/VAL	4.6	0.4	7	4.3	0.1	9	4.7	0.3	11	5.3	0.3	9	5.0	0.4	7	5.5	0.5	6
TYR/PHE	0.9	0.06	7	0.9	0.04	9	0.8	0.03	11	0.9	0.04	9	0.6	0.05	7	0.6	0.03	6
TYR/MET	1.7	0.1	7	1.6	0.1	9	1.6	0.1	11	2.1	0.4	9	1.6	0.1	7	1.4	0.1	6
ORN/LEU	0.1	0.02	6	0.1	0.05	9	0.07	0.1	11	0.1	0.02	8	0.1	0.05	7	0.2	0.09	6
ORN/LYS	0.1	0.02	6	0.08	0.03	9	0.09	0.02	11	0.09	0.02	8	0.1	0.04	7	0.1	0.02	6
NONESS/ESS	2.1	0.1	5	2.1	0.08	9	2.5	0.1	11	2.6	0.1	8	2.7	0.2	7	3.1	0.3	6

* Abbreviations employed include GABA, γ-aminobutyric acid; GLY, glycine; VAL, valine; ILE, isoleucine; LEU, leucine; ALA, alanine; TYR, tyrosine; PHE, phenylalanine; MET, methionine; ORN, ornithine; LYS, lysine; and NONESS: ESS, the ratio of nonessential to essential amino acids. The groups were the same as those in Table 10.1.

TABLE 10.3
Statistical Comparison of the Data Shown in Tables 10.1 and 10.2 *

	μmoles 1/2		μmoles 2/3		μmoles 1/3		μmoles 3/4		μmoles 5/6		μmoles 4/6	
Groups compared	/kg 1/2	/gDNA 1/2	/kg 2/3	/gDNA 2/3	/kg 1/3	/gDNA 1/3	/kg 3/4	/gDNA 3/4	/kg 5/6	/gDNA 5/6	/kg 4/6	/gDNA 4/6
TAURINE		0.005				0.01			0.001	0.005	0.001	0.001
ASPARTIC ACID	0.05	0.005			0.02	0.001	0.005	0.001			0.05	0.05
THREONINE						0.02			0.05	0.05	0.01	0.01
SERINE		0.005		0.05		0.01	0.05	0.05	0.001	0.001	0.005	0.01
GLUTAMINE		0.05				0.02			0.05	0.05		
GLUTAMIC ACID		0.001				0.005						
CITRULLINE					0.05		0.005	0.005	0.001	0.005	0.01	0.01
GLYCINE		0.001		0.025	0.05	0.005			0.001	0.005	0.05	0.005
ALANINE		0.005				0.02			0.005	0.005	0.001	0.02
VALINE	0.05	0.01				0.05			0.05	0.005	0.005	0.005
CYSTATHIONINE	0.001	0.001	0.001	0.001		0.001			0.025	0.05	0.005	0.005
METHIONINE		0.05				0.005			0.001	0.05	0.05	0.05
ISOLEUCINE		0.02				0.01			0.005	0.005	0.005	0.005
LEUCINE	**0.005**					0.025			0.005	0.01	0.01	0.02
TYROSINE	0.05	0.01				0.005			0.001	0.005	0.005	0.005
PHENYLALANINE	0.01	0.01		0.05		0.01			0.001	0.005	0.02	0.02
GABA	0.001	0.001			0.005	0.001	0.001	0.001				
ORNITHINE					0.02							
LYSINE		0.02				0.05						
HISTIDINE		0.005				0.05			0.05			
TRYPTOPHAN	0.02			0.05		0.05	0.05	0.05				
ARGININE							0.02	0.025				
HOMOCARNOSINE												
GLY/VAL	0.02		0.05		0.005				0.05		0.005	
GLY/ILE	0.01				0.001				0.001		0.005	
GLY/LEU	0.005				0.005				0.05		0.01	
ORN/LYS												
TYR/PHE							0.02				0.001	
NONESS/ESS	0.05		0.05									

* The data shown are P values ($P < 0.05$, etc). Where no values are given the differences were not significant.

177

TABLE 10.4
Concentrations of Amino Acids per Unit of DNA in Primate Cerebellum During Development

(μmoles/gDNA)

	GROUP 2			GROUP 3			GROUP 4			GROUP 5			GROUP 6		
	MEAN	S.E.M.	N	MEAN	S.E.M.	N	MEAN	S.E.M.	N	MEAN	S.E.M.	N	MEAN	S.E.M.	N
TAURINE	1544.1	94.6	9	1542.0	128.1	9	1247.8	117.3	7	1120.2	294.8	7	269.8	39.5	6
ASPARTIC ACID	338.7	30.5	8	441.1	46.8	9	580.4	116.5	5	1658.7	544.7	5	0.0	0.0	1
THREONINE	132.2	7.7	8	123.4	8.1	8	100.1	11.4	4	239.5	84.8	4	0.0	0.0	1
SERINE	257.7	11.7	8	235.0	22.0	10	183.6	20.2	8	373.9	72.9	7	190.8	35.0	6
GLUTAMINE	463.7	96.9	8	371.6	102.7	10	494.3	96.7	8	861.8	167.8	7	202.1	60.0	6
PROLINE	20.1	20.0	4	82.3	50.2	4	76.7	20.1	6	164.9	91.7	4	34.3	13.6	5
GLUTAMIC ACID	1529.6	120.8	9	1562.5	83.5	10	1412.7	113.3	8	2421.3	453.1	7	1445.1	198.9	6
CITRULLINE	0.07	0.02	9	1.0	1.0	10	1.6	1.6	9	13.7	13.7	7	0.03	0.03	6
GLYCINE	384.3	27.5	9	409.5	43.0	10	354.2	37.6	8	699.8	137.2	7	335.9	63.1	6
ALANINE	407.0	19.9	9	424.1	37.3	10	287.6	20.0	8	555.8	158.2	7	412.4	50.8	6
VALINE	87.5	5.6	9	72.7	4.9	10	44.1	6.3	8	115.2	27.1	7	62.6	26.9	6
CYSTATHIONINE	81.0	11.5	9	126.2	10.8	10	141.1	16.2	8	130.6	12.7	7	93.0	13.2	6
METHIONINE	1.6	1.5	8	7.1	3.1	10	15.6	3.2	8	44.2	11.5	7	16.5	9.6	6
ISOLEUCINE	42.8	4.6	9	43.9	6.7	10	28.9	4.4	8	72.3	21.3	7	39.4	15.4	6
LEUCINE	77.6	5.9	9	94.0	6.2	10	65.9	10.0	8	179.5	54.1	7	92.5	33.7	6
TYROSINE	31.8	2.8	9	38.9	6.4	10	34.8	3.9	8	74.6	18.6	7	24.5	6.8	6
PHENYLALANINE	40.3	3.3	9	44.7	7.1	10	39.5	6.7	8	107.4	29.1	7	57.8	25.8	6
GABA	274.0	40.4	9	450.6	32.4	10	486.1	69.7	8	933.2	241.1	7	708.1	42.3	6
ORNITHINE	7.9	4.0	9	12.1	3.9	10	14.2	4.9	6	32.6	10.4	6	18.0	5.2	6
LYSINE	103.8	15.5	9	126.3	8.1	10	84.6	6.7	8	187.9	27.4	7	139.3	39.7	6
HISTIDINE	9.6	5.4	8	24.0	6.8	10	26.5	3.6	7	70.9	14.0	7	26.3	8.6	6
TRYPTOPHAN	0.0	0.0	0	0.0	0.0	1	5.8	0.8	3	7.6	2.4	4	5.8	0.8	5
ARGININE	11.9	8.0	9	46.4	14.6	10	63.9	8.1	8	164.1	22.5	7	127.0	45.5	6
HOMOCARNOSINE	0.0	0.0	9	10.2	10.2	9	70.3	9.7	9	87.6	26.3	7	27.5	12.8	6

178

TABLE 10.5

Concentrations of Amino Acids per Unit Tissue Weight in Primate Cerebellum During Development

(μmoles/kg)

	GROUP 2			GROUP 3			GROUP 4			GROUP 5			GROUP 6		
	MEAN	S.E.M.	N	MEAN	S.E.M.	N	MEAN	S.E.M.	N	MEAN	S.E.M.	N	MEAN	S.E.M.	N
TAURINE	9822.1	657.7	9	10138.4	835.9	9	9248.4	1272.3	7	6787.1	1800.2	7	1410.6	226.3	6
ASPARTIC ACID	2152.3	195.7	8	2950.3	301.1	9	4055.6	535.5	5	10019.2	3343.1	5	0.0	0.0	1
THREONINE	783.9	49.3	8	828.6	52.6	8	716.3	25.5	4	1421.0	527.8	4	0.0	0.0	1
SERINE	1638.8	71.1	8	1568.1	135.6	10	1320.6	147.2	8	2269.0	448.5	7	999.4	201.1	6
GLUTAMINE	2962.5	597.2	8	2426.7	640.7	10	3518.8	617.4	8	5231.6	1008.8	7	1077.1	328.7	6
PROLINE	118.4	117.8	4	553.2	337.3	4	554.4	151.4	6	1012.4	557.0	4	174.0	69.7	5
GLUTAMIC ACID	9727.0	802.6	9	10473.7	528.7	10	10145.1	779.2	8	14639.4	2756.0	7	7534.6	1106.6	6
CITRULLINE	0.4	0.1	9	8.7	8.3	10	12.2	11.9	8	83.9	83.6	7	0.1	0.1	6
GLYCINE	2436.9	179.4	9	2729.2	264.1	10	2519.2	216.0	8	4228.1	833.3	7	1765.7	361.1	6
ALANINE	2585.7	136.0	9	2838.1	234.9	10	2092.5	191.4	8	3368.5	965.9	7	2152.4	291.8	6
VALINE	554.7	33.5	9	491.4	36.3	10	320.0	48.5	8	698.9	165.5	7	334.2	150.2	6
CYSTATHIONINE	518.8	76.6	9	838.1	56.8	10	1009.8	105.9	8	793.7	82.1	7	476.4	63.4	6
METHIONINE	11.2	10.3	8	50.4	23.3	10	118.2	26.0	8	267.7	70.3	7	88.9	53.4	6
ISOLEUCINE	272.0	29.1	9	293.0	43.4	10	207.9	32.0	8	438.5	130.1	7	209.6	86.2	6
LEUCINE	491.0	34.9	9	630.8	42.0	10	475.1	73.2	8	1089.5	330.7	7	490.8	189.3	6
TYROSINE	202.3	18.0	9	260.7	42.5	10	250.2	28.7	8	453.2	113.9	7	129.0	38.5	6
PHENYLALANINE	256.3	21.8	9	299.5	46.8	10	282.1	46.3	8	651.9	177.5	7	308.7	144.4	6
GABA	1755.2	263.9	9	3040.9	243.6	10	3528.2	525.4	8	5616.7	1415.9	7	3641.4	165.5	6
ORNITHINE	48.3	24.3	9	85.7	28.0	10	104.3	34.3	6	197.0	63.4	7	95.3	28.1	6
LYSINE	665.5	100.6	9	845.7	48.9	10	611.3	53.4	8	1139.8	168.9	7	731.2	224.8	6
HISTIDINE	58.5	33.1	8	163.9	46.2	10	193.8	28.6	7	429.9	85.4	7	137.4	48.3	6
TRYPTOPHAN	0.0	0.0	0	0.0	0.0	1	45.4	3.5	3	46.3	15.1	4	29.6	3.4	5
ARGININE	72.8	49.4	9	325.0	100.8	10	454.5	48.3	8	995.1	138.3	7	669.1	255.8	6
HOMOCARNOSINE	0.0	0.0	9	81.8	81.7	9	522.0	82.1	8	533.1	159.4	7	143.2	66.1	6
GLY/VAL	4.4	0.2	9	5.9	0.9	10	8.4	0.8	8	6.4	0.5	7	7.6	1.3	6
GLY/ILE	9.6	1.0	9	9.7	0.7	10	12.9	1.0	8	10.9	1.1	7	10.7	1.3	6
GLY/LEU	5.2	0.7	9	4.3	0.3	10	5.7	0.4	8	4.5	0.5	7	4.4	0.5	6
ALA/VAL	4.7	0.2	9	5.8	0.3	10	6.9	0.5	8	4.8	0.4	7	10.2	1.8	6
TYR/PHE	0.8	0.07	9	0.8	0.04	9	0.9	0.05	8	0.7	0.01	7	0.5	0.04	6
TYR/MET	176.6	34.9	7	131.4	66.7	8	30.9	28.8	8	1.7	0.1	7	2.5	0.4	6
ORN/LEU	0.1	0.05	9	0.1	0.05	10	0.2	0.05	6	0.1	0.02	7	0.2	0.1	6
ORN/LYS	0.07	0.03	8	0.1	0.03	10	0.1	0.05	6	0.1	0.02	7	0.1	0.05	6
NONESS/ESS	3.0	0.2	7	2.7	0.1	10	2.8	0.1	6	2.3	0.2	7	2.8	0.4	6

179

TABLE 10.6
Statistical Comparison of the Data Shown in Tables 10.4 and 10.5

Groups Compared	µmoles /kg 2/3	µmoles /gDNA 2/3	µmoles /kg 3/4	µmoles /gDNA 3/4	µmoles /kg 4/5	µmoles /gDNA 4/5	µmoles /kg 5/6	µmoles /gDNA 5/6	µmoles /kg 4/6	µmoles /gDNA 4/6
TAURINE							0.02	0.025	0.001	0.001
ASPARTIC ACID	0.05									
THREONINE										
SERINE						0.025	0.05			
GLUTAMINE							0.005	0.01	0.01	0.05
PROLINE										
GLUTAMIC ACID						0.05	0.05			
CITRULLINE										
GLYCINE						0.025	0.05	0.05		
ALANINE			0.05	0.01						0.05
VALINE			0.02	0.005	0.05	0.02				
CYSTATHIONINE	0.005	0.02					0.02		0.005	0.05
METHIONINE						0.05				
ISOLEUCINE										
LEUCINE	0.025			0.05		0.05				
TYROSINE						0.05	0.05	0.05	0.025	
PHENYLALANINE						0.05				
GABA	0.005	0.005								0.05
ORNITHINE										
LYSINE			0.01	0.005	0.01	0.025				
HISTIDINE					0.025	0.02	0.02	0.05		
TRYPTOPHAN									0.025	
ARGININE	0.05				0.005	0.001				
HOMOCARNOSINE			0.005	0.001					0.01	0.02
GLY/VAL										
GLY/ILE			0.02							
GLY/LEU			0.05							
ALA/VAL	0.05				0.02		0.02			
TRY/PHE					0.005		0.005		0.001	
TYR/MET										
ORN/LEU										
ORN/LYS										
NONESS/ESS										

Ratio of Amino Acids to DNA

1. The concentrations of most amino acids per gram of DNA were generally higher in the cerebrum than in the cerebellum. Cystathionine in contrast was always higher in concentrations in the cerebellum than in the cerebrum except in the older monkeys in groups 5 and 6.

2. In the *cerebrum* most amino acid ratios reached their maxima during the last third of pregnancy; these were maintained in the first 30 days of postnatal life and then decreased. Exceptions to this general pattern were glutamine and asparagine (maxima reached 60–122 days postnatally), citrulline and ornithine (decreased during last third of pregnancy then suddenly peaked after birth), cystathionine, γ-aminobutyric acid, and homocarnosine (maxima reached only after birth).

3. In the *cerebellum* there were no significant changes with time in the ratio of amino acids to DNA.

Correlation of Amino Acid Concentrations with Plasma Corticosteroid Levels

1. In the *cerebrum*, prenatally, correlations were found for cystathionine, GABA, citrulline, and homocarnosine and negative correlations for glutamine, glycine, valine, and leucine. Postnatally a negative correlation existed for proline.

2. In the *cerebellum* prenatally, there was a positive correlation for glycine, cystathionine, and methionine. Postnatally, positive correlations appeared for cystathionine.

TABLE 10.7
Correlation Coefficients Between Corticosteroid Concentration in Fetal Plasma and Amino Acid Concentrations in Primate Cerebrum and Cerebellum During Development*

	Cerebrum				Cerebellum			
	Group	Correlation Coefficient	Degrees of Freedom	Probability	Group	Correlation Coefficient	Degrees of Freedom	Probability
THREONINE	1 /DNA	-0.95	2	0.05	10 /kg	-0.90	3	0.05
SERINE	1 /DNA	-0.99	2	0.01	10&12 /kg	-0.86	5	0.02
PROLINE	4&5 /kg	-0.95	4	0.005				
	4&5 /DNA	-0.95	4	0.005				
	11&13 /kg	0.99	1	0.05				
	4 /kg	-0.99	1	0.01				
CITRULLINE	3 /kg	0.76	6	0.05				
	3 /DNA	0.76	6	0.05				
GLYCINE	1 /DNA	-0.96	2	0.05				
	11 /kg	-0.99	1	0.05				
VALINE	1 /DNA	-0.99	2	0.01				
CYSTATHIONINE	1 /kg	0.98	2	0.02	4 /kg	0.96	3	0.01
	1 /DNA	0.98	2	0.02	4&5 /kg	0.67	10	0.02
LEUCINE	1 /DNA	0.98	2	0.02	3 /kg	0.66	7	0.05
PHENYLALANINE					2 /kg	0.76	6	0.05
GABA					4&5 /DNA	-0.61	10	0.05
LYSINE	2 /kg	-0.83	6	0.01				
HOMOCARNOSINE	3 /kg	0.65	8	0.05				
	3 /DNA	0.65	8	0.05				
ORN/LEU					4&5	-0.65	9	0.05
TYR/PHE					5	0.80	5	0.05
TYR/MET					4&5	-0.65	9	0.05
NONESS/ESS					11&13	-0.99	1	0.02

* Only those correlations that were significant statistically are shown. The designations /DNA and /kg indicate that the values were those of the amino acid concentrations in micro-moles per gram of DNA and per kilogram of tissue, respectively. Groups 1–6 are those described in Table 10.1. Group 10, fetal monkeys injected with streptozotocin at 154–160 days of gestation and delivered by cesarean section at 154–160 days; group 11, injected at the same time but born naturally; group 12, injected at 130 days of gestation and delivered by cesarean section at 157 and 158 days; and group 13, injected at 130 days and born naturally.

Discussion

It has been assumed that the DNA content of the brain is proportional to the cell number during prenatal and postnatal life, and therefore that the concentrations of amino acids relative to DNA can be thought of as the cellular concentration of amino acids. The methods were imprecise in that the tissues of the brain in which the determinations were performed consist of a mixture of white and gray matter containing different cell types; corrections were not made for the extracellular fluid space and its amino acid content, and the number of animals in each group was small. Appraisal of these factors is consistent with a considerable degree of variation of the data within each group. Nevertheless, the number of statistically significant differences found was high. Furthermore, the patterns that emerged revealed developmental changes that were parallel for a number of amino acids and to some extent tissue specific for cerebrum or cerebellum.

Very few data are available on the concentrations of amino acids in the brain in humans during development. Taurine was found to be considerably higher in fetal human brain than in the adult brain, which is consistent with our data; similarly, GABA was much lower in fetal brain, cystathionine nearly absent, and homocarnosine absent. [5, 6] The data are also consistent with those of Volpe and Laster[7] who studied the sulfur-containing amino acids and the process of transsulfuration in the brain of the developing rhesus monkey. In their studies cystathionine increased with the transition from late fetal to postnatal life. In contrast, taurine concentration decreased as the brain matured. In the adult group (group 6) our data agree closely with those of Perry et al[9] for human cortex and cerebellum, with the exception of the concentration for glutamine.

The concentrations of amino acids in the brain were higher than those in the plasma even in the youngest fetuses in this study. This could indicate that active transport mechanisms for amino acids essential for the brain are already present at this stage of development. The metabolic pathways for the synthesis of nonessential amino acids (alanine, aspartic acid, glutamine, glycine, and GABA) from glucose metabolites also seem to be operative very early. In the cerebrum the peak in the cellular concentrations of most amino acids could reflect intense protein synthesis during periods of rapid growth. Rats and guinea pigs[8] differ in the pattern of development in that the period of rapid definition of myelin occurs after birth in the rat and just before birth in the guinea pig, the concentrations of amino acids in the brain tending to conform to these two patterns. In contrast to these two species, amino acid concentrations in the fetus of the primate tended to be higher earlier in fetal life. Nevertheless, in the case of many amino acids the peak concentrations were postnatal. In the rat the developmental patterns for glycine, serine, alanine, and leucine were parallel. This was also true in the primate.

Developmental changes that are specific to an amino acid are of special interest, since they could point to biochemical functions that are specific for the tissue analyzed. The high citrulline values in the immediate neonatal period and their subsequent decrease probably represent the development of enzyme adaptation to the sudden load of extraneous protein. Prenatally the fetus can rely on maternal enzyme.

The late peak of glutamate and aspartate may reflect the synthesis of these dicarboxylic amino acids from Krebs cycle intermediates in brain. Glutamine concentrations also peaked in brain in group 5. These changes could reflect the development of mechanisms for the handling of ammonia. GABA concentration displayed its own developmental pattern. Its concentration did not parallel development of activity of glutamate decarboxylase in the human fetus.[5] Perry et al[9] indicated that glutamate decarboxylase activity may persist for some time after death. However, it appears unlikely that the changes we have observed reflect postmortem activity of the enzyme because of the developmental pattern observed. Cellular concentrations of GABA were positively correlated with the concentrations of plasma corticoids.

There was a steady increase of cystathionine content of the cerebrum. Volpe and Laster[7] also noted this developmental pattern in the rhesus monkey. They found no correlation with the activity of the enzyme cystathionine synthase[7] or the methionine activating enzyme.[10] The brain of monkey and man is richer in cystathionine that the brain of nonprimate animals.[11] The presence of cystathionine in high concentration in the brain of primates and its pattern of development suggest that it has a function that is specific to brain.

Volpe and Laster[7] have emphasized the high content of cystathionine in the cerebellum as compared with other areas of the brain. We found much higher concentrations of cystathionine earlier in development in cerebellum than in cerebrum. This may be consistent with the idea that the cerebellum develops ahead of the forebrain in the course of embryogenesis.

The virtual absence of homocarnosine up to the group immediately preceding birth is followed by a sharp rise in concentration after birth. This dipeptide is synthesized from histidine and GABA. Mardens and Van Sande[6] could not detect homocarnosine in the brain of the human fetus but found it in appreciable concentration in adult human brain. The significance of these findings is not clear. It is tempting to think of this dipeptide as a storage form of GABA, which is a known neurotransmitter.

In the age group from 75 to 112 prenatal days the concentration of glycine in the cerebrum tended to be negatively correlated with the plasma concentration of corticosteroids, whereas in cerebellum this was not the case. It may be that the mechanisms regulating glycine concentration in cerebrum and cerebellum are qualitatively different.

ABLATION OF PANCREATIC BETA CELLS IN THE FETUS BY STREPTOZOTOCIN

In this and subsequent sections of this chapter data are reviewed on the series of interventions that were undertaken to influence the course of fetal growth. In this series of monkeys, groups 10 through 13, streptozotocin was injected into the fetus *in utero* to produce a chemical ablation of the pancreatic beta cells (see Chapter 9). The effect of this procedure on amino acids in the brain is described in tabular form.

Comparisons were made with control fetuses delivered at the same age (group 3). Comparisons were also made between the naturally born monkeys and those delivered by cesarean section. Groups 12 and 13 were too small for separate statistical treatment. Therefore they were combined with group 10 or 11, respectively, to detect potential trends.

Group	Injection of Streptozotocin	Delivery
10	110 days gestation	Cesarean section 154–160 days
11	110 days gestation	Naturally born
12	130 days gestation	Cesarean section 157–158 days
(Two monkeys)		
13	130 days gestation	Naturally born
(One monkey)		

Results

The results are shown in Tables 10.8 through 10.13. Whenever a t-test was significant the P value is indicated in the table. There were few statistically significant differences; they are summarized below:

1. There was no significant difference in composition of cerebrum or cerebellum between naturally born fetuses and those delivered by cesarean section.
2. Cerebrum: In streptozotocin-injected animals there were higher levels of glutamine, taurine, aspartic acid, and GABA and raised ratios for tyrosine to methionine and glycine to isoleucine. Levels of serine, glycine, and alanine decreased.
3. Cerebellum: In streptozotocin-injected animals there were raised levels of glutamine and phenylalanine. The level of ornithine decreased as did the ratios of alanine to valine, ornithine to leucine, and nonessential to essential amino acids.

Discussion

Assessment of the role of experimental fetal diabetes on the metabolism of amino acids in the brain is complex. Primarily there is the lack of fetal insulin. However, a reactive hyperplasia in some may have occurred, as discussed in Chapter 9. The endocrine imbalance that results could represent an unmasking of the effects of other hormones.

The elevation in glutamine concentration in both cerebrum and cerebellum appears to be meaningful since the glutamic acid was not decreased. This could reflect an increased gluconeogenesis, for example, an effect of glucocorticoids not antagonized by insulin. Increased gluconeogenesis might lead to increased formation of ammonia which could be handled effectively through the formation of glutamine. Certainly alanine and pyruvate can be converted to glutamine by the cerebral cortex of the rat *in vitro*.[14] The decrease in the ratio of nonessential to essential amino acids points also to increased gluconeogenesis.

ABLATION OF THE PANCREATIC BETA CELLS OF THE MOTHER USING STREPTOZOTOCIN

These experiments were undertaken to assess the effects of maternal diabetes produced by injection of streptozotocin into the maternal circulation at midpregnancy. Fetal concentrations of amino acids in the brain in this group (group 9) were compared with the values of the age-matched control group (group 3) using the t-test.

Results

In the cerebrum the concentration of glutamine was significantly higher in the treated animals. There was a trend to higher concentrations of taurine and threonine with beta-cell ablation in the mother. No homocarnosine could be detected in these fetal brains (see Tables 10.14–10.16).

In the cerebellum the concentration of glutamic acid was significantly lower as was the ratio of alanine to valine and of nonessential to essential amino acids. There was a marked increase in the concentration of methionine.

Discussion

The changes in the concentrations of amino acids in the brain of the fetus following the treatment of the mother with streptozotocin were highly specific. In the liver, the concentration of virtually every amino acid was markedly decreased following this treatment (Chapter 20). In the brain, on the other hand, the concentrations of most amino acids changed very little. Those of glutamine, aspartic acid, threonine, serine, GABA, and arginine were increased when compared per unit of DNA. When compared per kilogram of wet tissue, only glutamine appeared to differ from the control values. The absence of homocarnosine is interesting. The greater concentration of glutamine in the cerebrum of treated animals is accompanied by an increase in the mean concentration of glutamic acid. This is consistent with the result obtained with treatment of the fetus itself with streptozotocin where, as pointed out, reactive islet cell hyperplasia was thought to occur in some fetuses.

The high concentrations of threonine and methionine, both of which are essential and not synthesized in brain, are not simply reflections of plasma changes, since in the plasma the mean concentrations of these amino acids were actually lower in the group with maternal diabetes than in the controls. This finding must imply that active transport mechanisms are operating or that binding in brain tissue is significant. Transport may be facilitated by hyperinsulinism in the fetus, a process quantitatively more important than an expected increased incorporation into proteins.

These data are consistent with an increased transport of amino acids into the central nervous system and an increase in the synthesis of proteins in the brain.

MATERNAL NUTRITIONAL RESTRICTION

Methods

The plan for this experiment is described in Chapter 6. Briefly it was a pilot study (Pilot No. 2) involving the following nutritional restrictions to pregnant rhesus monkeys with subsequent analyses of fetal brains:

Group	Calories	Protein	Weight Gain during Pregnancy
1	Normal	Normal	Normal
2	Normal	Deficient	Normal
3	Deficient	Normal	Zero
4	Deficient	Deficient	Zero

TABLE 10.8
Concentrations of Amino Acids per Unit of DNA in Primate Cerebrum of Streptozotocin-Treated Fetuses

(μmoles/gDNA)

	GROUP 10			GROUP 11			GROUP 10+12			GROUP 11+13		
	MEAN	S.E.M.	N	MEAN	S.E.M.	N	MEAN	S.E.M.	N	MEAN	S.E.M.	N
TAURINE	5034.0	456.1	3	4418.4	1189.1	4	5109.7	331.2	8	4185.2	950.2	5
ASPARTIC ACID	1795.6	98.3	6	1600.6	254.4	5	1696.6	101.8	8	1516.2	224.2	6
THREONINE	474.1	27.0	4	457.6	43.6	5	461.5	19.7	6	445.6	37.6	6
SERINE	1056.9	95.8	6	923.5	102.2	5	1050.3	70.9	8	906.6	85.1	6
GLUTAMINE	1386.8	219.8	6	1562.4	456.4	5	1752.9	316.8	8	1641.2	380.9	6
PROLINE	0.0	0.0	2	607.7	75.7	5	565.2	73.5	3	617.6	54.5	4
GLUTAMIC ACID	7524.0	615.1	6	6708.4	826.9	6	7410.4	507.0	8	6409.0	738.5	6
CITRULLINE	0.7	0.01	6	0.5	0.1	5	0.7	0.01	8	0.6	0.1	6
GLYCINE	1848.1	132.1	6	1729.4	216.5	5	1881.8	101.4	8	1669.7	186.6	6
ALANINE	1460.9	72.2	6	1450.1	79.5	5	1499.6	64.3	8	1362.7	108.8	6
VALINE	359.2	21.4	6	308.0	47.5	5	346.9	18.8	8	287.5	42.1	5
CYSTATHIONINE	119.6	11.0	6	93.9	16.4	4	119.5	8.1	8	96.6	13.7	6
METHIONINE	88.0	7.2	6	98.4	20.6	5	84.2	7.1	8	96.1	17.0	6
ISOLEUCINE	177.8	6.7	6	172.2	22.3	5	173.8	5.8	8	165.3	19.5	6
LEUCINE	365.6	25.7	6	368.0	52.6	5	350.5	23.2	8	344.6	48.9	6
TYROSINE	210.7	36.7	6	227.7	19.0	5	192.0	29.6	8	212.7	21.6	6
PHENYLALANINE	221.6	25.0	6	218.1	27.6	5	198.2	23.9	8	208.4	24.6	6
GABA	1536.1	109.0	6	1459.9	210.8	5	1496.0	100.8	8	1487.0	174.2	6
ORNITHINE	29.7	10.4	6	65.3	13.0	5	33.4	9.3	8	58.9	12.3	6
LYSINE	414.1	39.6	6	560.1	99.9	5	382.5	37.7	8	520.9	90.5	6
HISTIDINE	168.0	23.0	6	216.4	38.3	5	160.0	20.4	8	203.3	33.9	6
TRYPTOPHAN	0.0	0.0	6	0.0	0.0	5	0.0	0.0	8	0.0	0.0	6
ARGININE	215.0	66.7	5	240.8	117.7	5	195.2	57.3	7	241.7	96.1	6
HOMOCARNOSINE	39.5	26.8	6	43.1	27.3	5	29.7	20.6	8	36.0	23.4	6

TABLE 10.9

Concentrations of Amino Acid per Unit Tissue Weight in Primate Cerebrum of Streptozotocin-Treated Fetuses

(μmoles/kg)

	GROUP 10			GROUP 11			GROUP 10+12			GROUP 11+13		
	MEAN	S.E.M.	N	MEAN	S.E.M.	N	MEAN	S.E.M.	N	MEAN	S.E.M.	N
TAURINE	7072.4	447.9	3	6138.0	1894.2	4	6998.7	325.1	4	5782.0	1509.8	5
ASPARTIC ACID	2454.2	111.1	6	2126.0	371.8	5	2294.7	140.4	8	2016.1	322.9	6
THREONINE	657.6	34.7	4	608.2	76.4	5	627.0	31.0	6	592.9	64.2	6
SERINE	1438.8	111.4	6	1223.8	161.2	5	1413.0	85.1	8	1203.5	133.2	6
GLUTAMINE	1882.7	279.5	6	2022.0	536.8	5	2330.8	390.3	8	2139.6	453.8	6
PROLINE	0.0	0.0	2	856.0	131.8	3	793.4	127.8	3	858.8	93.2	4
GLUTAMIC ACID	10237.3	670.8	6	8753.7	906.9	5	9974.1	610.6	8	8391.8	824.2	6
CITRULLINE	1.0	0.0	6	0.8	0.2	5	1.0	0.0	8	0.8	0.1	6
GLYCINE	2517.6	138.4	6	2268.3	261.3	5	2530.0	103.0	8	2196.5	225.1	6
ALANINE	2002.8	100.8	6	1923.1	168.1	5	2026.0	86.1	8	1809.4	178.2	6
VALINE	492.4	30.9	6	422.5	83.5	4	469.9	28.6	8	393.1	71.0	5
CYSTATHIONINE	163.7	14.7	6	124.1	23.0	5	161.4	10.9	8	128.1	19.2	6
METHIONINE	120.0	8.2	6	133.4	33.5	5	113.8	9.2	8	130.1	27.6	6
ISOLEUCINE	243.9	10.6	6	231.3	39.6	5	235.4	9.9	8	222.0	33.7	6
LEUCINE	503.0	42.0	6	495.5	91.2	5	476.3	37.8	8	463.8	80.9	6
TYROSINE	285.7	46.7	6	304.7	38.5	5	258.3	38.8	8	284.6	37.2	6
PHENYLALANINE	303.0	32.2	6	293.3	49.7	5	268.7	32.5	8	280.1	42.6	6
GABA	2108.5	162.3	6	1927.3	281.3	5	2028.6	151.8	8	1968.4	233.3	6
ORNITHINE	41.4	14.6	6	87.0	19.1	5	45.6	12.8	8	78.6	17.7	6
LYSINE	569.6	59.6	6	757.9	163.5	5	520.7	56.8	8	704.5	143.9	6
HISTIDINE	229.0	31.2	6	290.2	58.8	5	216.2	28.1	8	272.5	51.2	6
TRYPTOPHAN	0.0	0.0	6	0.0	0.0	5	0.0	0.0	8	0.0	0.0	6
ARGININE	292.4	92.4	5	325.3	172.4	5	263.8	78.4	7	326.1	140.7	6
HOMOCARNOSINE	54.8	37.8	6	62.8	40.2	5	41.2	29.0	8	52.5	34.4	6
GLY/VAL	5.1	0.3	6	6.0	1.2	4	5.4	0.3	8	6.1	0.9	5
GLY/ILE	10.4	0.7	6	10.6	2.0	5	10.8	0.6	8	10.6	1.6	6
GLY/LEU	5.1	0.5	6	5.1	1.1	5	5.5	0.4	8	5.2	0.9	6
ALA/VAL	4.1	0.2	6	4.8	0.4	4	4.3	0.2	8	4.7	0.3	5
TYR/PHE	0.9	0.1	6	1.0	0.07	5	0.9	0.09	8	1.0	0.06	6
TYR/MET	2.4	0.4	6	2.5	0.3	5	2.3	0.3	8	2.3	0.3	6
ORN/LEU	0.08	0.03	6	0.1	0.02	5	0.09	0.02	8	0.1	0.02	6
ORN/LYS	0.06	0.02	6	0.1	0.02	5	0.08	0.02	8	0.1	0.02	6
NONESS/ESS	2.5	0.1	6	2.3	0.3	4	2.8	0.2	8	2.4	0.2	5

TABLE 10.10

Concentrations of Amino Acids per Unit DNA in Primate Cerebellum of Streptozotocin-Treated Fetuses

(μmoles/gDNA)

	GROUP 10			GROUP 11			GROUP 10+12			GROUP 11+13		
	MEAN	S.E.M.	N	MEAN	S.E.M.	N	MEAN	S.E.M.	N	MEAN	S.E.M.	N
TAURINE	1572.6	24.7	5	1695.6	257.2	3	1595.2	30.3	6	1658.0	185.7	4
ASPARTIC ACID	551.9	55.6	5	494.0	165.9	3	563.3	42.7	7	453.5	124.1	4
THREONINE	124.4	11.2	4	171.9	46.9	3	125.8	9.5	6	151.3	39.0	4
SERINE	270.9	25.8	5	282.5	83.6	3	260.5	19.0	7	242.6	71.3	4
GLUTAMINE	920.5	86.7	5	766.5	172.3	3	1052.0	147.3	7	895.6	177.5	4
PROLINE	0.0	0.0	0	0.0	0.0	2	0.0	0.0	1	135.3	48.3	3
GLUTAMIC ACID	1512.1	82.6	5	1796.7	490.5	3	1516.8	64.8	7	1568.3	415.3	4
CITRULLINE	0.02	0.02	5	0.09	0.04	3	0.03	0.02	7	0.07	0.04	4
GLYCINE	464.7	44.5	5	440.0	122.9	3	451.3	32.6	7	377.1	107.2	4
ALANINE	338.9	14.2	5	468.3	121.1	3	336.3	10.0	7	410.5	103.3	4
VALINE	77.5	6.4	5	108.0	29.4	3	76.7	4.9	7	88.7	28.3	4
CYSTATHIONINE	154.7	10.3	5	164.9	50.3	3	158.7	16.2	7	162.5	35.7	4
METHIONINE	14.5	3.2	5	17.7	8.8	3	20.1	5.8	7	14.2	7.1	4
ISOLEUCINE	46.4	3.2	5	51.3	12.8	3	45.4	2.8	6	43.6	11.9	4
LEUCINE	106.1	13.4	5	176.4	50.9	3	102.1	10.5	7	142.2	49.7	4
TYROSINE	41.7	2.7	5	67.6	25.5	3	44.1	2.4	7	55.1	21.9	4
PHENYLALANINE	59.4	5.0	5	97.1	25.0	3	58.4	3.5	7	79.2	25.1	4
GABA	447.5	46.9	5	308.1	27.3	3	415.9	62.1	7	259.6	52.1	4
ORNITHINE	0.1	0.007	5	1.8	1.6	3	0.7	0.5	7	1.7	1.1	4
LYSINE	136.9	16.1	5	116.8	37.6	3	120.8	20.3	7	92.5	36.0	4
HISTIDINE	42.4	14.9	5	29.3	21.1	3	41.4	12.0	7	24.0	15.8	4
TRYPTOPHAN	0.0	0.0	5	0.0	0.0	3	0.0	0.0	7	0.0	0.0	4
ARGININE	72.5	27.1	5	43.3	32.1	3	53.4	22.4	7	34.8	24.2	4
HOMOCARNOSINE	38.5	26.0	5	54.2	32.9	3	44.8	21.0	7	49.3	23.8	4

TABLE 10.11

Concentrations of Amino Acids per Unit Tissue Weight in Primate Cerebellum of Streptozotocin-Treated Fetuses

(μmoles/kg)

	GROUP 10			GROUP 11			GROUP 10+12			GROUP 11+13		
	MEAN	S.E.M.	N	MEAN	S.E.M.	N	MEAN	S.E.M.	N	MEAN	S.E.M.	N
TAURINE	10249.1	352.4	5	11451.6	2076.5	3	10357.6	307.5	6	11648.6	1481.4	4
ASPARTIC ACID	3646.1	462.5	5	3389.8	1220.7	3	3799.2	389.2	7	3199.4	883.9	4
THREONINE	835.5	86.0	4	1165.7	348.9	3	861.4	85.5	6	1051.4	271.9	4
SERINE	1751.2	141.2	5	1921.1	619.2	3	1719.2	105.0	7	1684.4	497.7	4
GLUTAMINE	6022.5	621.9	5	5198.0	1337.4	3	7140.4	1240.0	7	6438.9	1560.1	4
PROLINE	0.0	0.0	5	0.0	0.0	2	0.0	0.0	1	938.6	339.3	3
GLUTAMIC ACID	9912.1	781.7	5	12246.9	3680.6	3	10155.0	698.9	7	10933.9	2915.0	4
CITRULLINE	0.2	0.2	5	0.6	0.3	3	0.2	0.1	7	0.5	0.2	4
GLYCINE	3039.6	309.1	5	3012.4	924.0	3	2999.7	215.0	7	2633.0	755.6	4
ALANINE	2211.4	125.8	5	3176.8	906.5	3	2237.1	96.3	7	2852.0	718.6	4
VALINE	503.6	39.7	5	730.5	217.3	3	507.4	27.8	7	609.3	195.7	4
CYSTATHIONINE	1006.0	63.9	5	1135.2	374.8	3	1067.0	135.8	7	1158.6	266.1	4
METHIONINE	98.1	25.4	5	115.3	57.1	3	141.5	46.2	7	94.2	45.6	4
ISOLEUCINE	300.7	13.7	5	348.5	96.6	3	293.6	13.2	6	301.7	82.7	4
LEUCINE	692.4	86.1	5	1185.3	365.9	3	675.4	62.9	7	967.6	338.1	4
TYROSINE	269.4	8.1	5	464.7	185.6	3	292.7	16.9	7	383.9	154.1	4
PHENYLALANINE	383.1	17.3	5	650.8	178.2	3	385.7	14.7	7	538.5	168.8	4
GABA	2957.0	386.1	5	2050.5	117.1	3	2745.8	422.0	7	1764.3	297.9	4
ORNITHINE	1.0	0.0	5	10.9	9.9	3	5.2	4.2	7	11.5	7.0	4
LYSINE	890.8	98.0	5	761.4	212.6	3	786.4	127.0	7	610.3	213.1	4
HISTIDINE	272.3	93.3	5	182.7	125.7	3	267.8	77.9	7	153.0	93.7	4
TRYPTOPHAN	0.0	0.0	5	0.0	0.0	3	0.0	0.0	7	0.0	0.0	4
ARGININE	470.4	175.3	5	269.4	191.6	3	348.6	144.5	7	220.3	144.1	4
HOMOCARNOSINE	229.7	156.1	5	342.6	198.0	3	276.9	128.2	7	325.5	141.0	4
GLY/VAL	6.1	0.6	5	4.1	0.8	3	5.9	0.4	7	4.6	0.7	4
GLY/ILE	10.0	0.8	5	8.5	1.1	3	10.2	0.6	6	8.6	0.8	4
GLY/LEU	4.9	1.2	5	2.7	0.8	3	4.8	0.8	7	3.2	0.7	4
ALA/VAL	4.4	0.3	5	4.3	0.2	3	4.4	0.2	7	5.1	0.8	4
TYR/PHE	0.7	0.03	5	0.7	0.2	3	0.7	0.04	7	0.7	0.1	4
TYR/MET	4.1	1.4	5	273.5	271.8	3	3.5	1.1	7	206.3	203.6	4
ORN/LEU	0.002	0.0	5	0.01	0.01	3	0.009	0.008	7	0.01	0.01	4
ORN/LYS	0.001	0.0	5	0.01	0.009	3	0.03	0.03	7	0.02	0.01	4
NONESS/ESS	2.3	0.05	5	2.1	0.4	3	2.2	0.06	6	2.5	0.5	4

189

TABLE 10.13
Statistical Analysis of the Data Shown in Tables 10.10 and 10.11

Groups compared	μmoles /kg 7/8	/gDNA 7/8	μmoles /kg 10/3	/gDNA 10/3	μmoles /kg 10+11/3	/gDNA 10+11/3	μmoles /kg 10+12/3	/gDNA 10+12/3
TAURINE								
ASPARTIC ACID								
THREONINE								
SERINE	0.005	0.001						
GLUTAMINE			0.005	0.005	0.005	0.005	0.005	0.005
PROLINE								
GLUTAMIC ACID								
CITRULLINE								
GLYCINE								
ALANINE								
VALINE								
CYSTATHIONINE								
METHIONINE								
ISOLEUCINE								
LEUCINE								
TYROSINE								
PHENYLALANINE					0.05	0.05		
GABA								
ORNITHINE					0.025	0.025	0.05	0.05
LYSINE								
HISTIDINE								
TRYPTOPHAN	0.02	0.025						
ARGININE								
HOMOCARNOSINE								
GLY/VAL								
GLY/ILE								
GLY/LEU								
ALA/VAL			0.05		0.02		0.02	
TYR/PHE			0.05					
TYR/MET								
ORN/LEU					0.05			
ORN/LYS					0.05			
NONESS/ESS					0.05		0.025	

* Groups 3, 10, 11, and 12 are those described in previous tables. Groups 7 and 8 are the control and hypothyroid monkeys, respectively, described in Tables 10.22 and 10.23.

TABLE 10.12
Statistical Analysis of the Data Shown in Tables 10.8 and 10.9 '

	μmoles/kg 7/8	/gDNA 7/8	μmoles/kg 10/3	/gDNA 10/3	μmoles/kg 10+11/3	/gDNA 10+11/3	μmoles/kg 10+12/3	/gDNA 10+12/3
Groups compared								
TAURINE								
ASPARTIC ACID								
THREONINE								
SERINE								
GLUTAMINE			0.005	0.01	0.005	0.01	0.005	0.005
PROLINE								
GLUTAMIC ACID								
CITRULLINE								
GLYCINE								
ALANINE								
VALINE								
CYSTATHIONINE								
METHIONINE								0.05
ISOLEUCINE								
LEUCINE								
TYROSINE								
PHENYLALANINE								
GABA					0.05			
ORNITHINE								
LYSINE								
HISTIDINE								
TRYPTOPHAN	0.01	0.05						
ARGININE								
HOMOCARNOSINE								
GLY/VAL								
GLY/ILE							0.05	
GLY/LEU								
ALA/VAL								
TYR/PHE	0.05							
TYR/MET					0.02			
ORN/LEU								
ORN/LYS								
NONESS/ESS								

191

TABLE 10.14

Concentrations of Amino Acids in Primate Cerebrum of the Fetus
Following Maternal Beta Cell Ablation with Streptozotocin

GROUP 9	(μmoles/kg)			(μmoles/g DNA)		
	MEAN	S.E.M.	N	MEAN	S.E.M.	N
TAURINE	7718.6	1011.2	9	6688.0	878.1	9
ASPARTIC ACID	2460.0	203.2	7	2126.3	182.2	7
THREONINE	1069.7	272.3	6	951.0	253.1	6
SERINE	1703.3	148.9	8	1485.7	145.3	8
GLUTAMINE	1830.7	265.8	8	1585.0	241.5	8
PROLINE	0.0	0.0	1	0.0	0.0	1
GLUTAMIC ACID	10139.2	1239.0	9	8787.2	1078.3	9
CITRULLINE	20.4	13.2	9	17.8	11.4	9
GLYCINE	2498.6	208.9	9	2172.3	193.1	9
ALANINE	2462.3	189.7	9	2135.6	165.8	9
VALINE	640.4	70.9	9	558.8	65.8	9
CYSTATHIONINE	147.5	28.0	9	129.4	26.1	9
METHIONINE	210.2	38.2	9	182.2	33.3	9
ISOLEUCINE	307.9	29.3	9	268.6	27.9	9
LEUCINE	624.7	57.8	9	544.7	54.6	9
TYROSINE	263.9	17.4	9	228.6	16.1	9
PHENYLALANINE	279.6	23.0	9	243.0	21.5	9
GABA	1983.8	279.2	9	1717.7	246.7	9
ORNITHINE	76.2	18.4	9	65.8	15.9	9
LYSINE	752.8	120.2	9	654.1	107.7	9
HISTIDINE	211.1	32.5	9	183.1	28.8	9
TRYPTOPHAN	35.7	2.4	9	30.9	2.2	9
ARGININE	396.5	77.3	9	346.0	69.5	9
HOMOCARNOSINE	0.0	0.0	9	0.0	0.0	9
GLYCINE/VALINE	4.0	0.2	9			
GLYCINE/ISOLEUCINE	8.3	0.4	9			
GLYCINE/LEUCINE	4.0	0.1	9			
ALANINE/VALINE	3.9	0.2	9			
TYROSINE/PHENYLALANINE	0.9	0.04	9			
TYROSINE/METHIONINE	1.4	0.1	9			
ORNITHINE/LEUCINE	0.1	0.02	9			
ORNITHINE/LYSINE	0.1	0.02	8			
NONESSENTIAL/ESSENTIAL	2.4	0.2	8			

TABLE 10.15

Concentrations of Amino Acids in Primate Cerebellum of the Fetus
Following Maternal Beta Cell Ablation with Streptozotocin

GROUP 9	(μmoles/kg.)			(μmoles/gDNA)		
	MEAN	S.E.M.	N	MEAN	S.E.M.	N
TAURINE	7718.2	885.6	7	1054.9	134.6	7
ASPARTIC ACID	2839.2	210.0	9	381.4	32.1	9
THREONINE	867.3	54.3	8	114.1	7.9	8
SERINE	1676.8	86.6	9	226.1	16.3	9
GLUTAMINE	3483.3	133.8	9	467.9	25.4	9
PROLINE	0.0	0.0	1	0.0	0.0	1
GLUTAMIC ACID	8192.3	467.5	9	1091.9	55.4	9
CITRULLINE	19.5	18.8	9	2.4	2.3	9
GLYCINE	2419.9	132.2	9	324.4	20.4	9
ALANINE	2304.4	128.7	9	308.0	17.2	9
VALINE	512.1	32.0	9	68.8	5.2	9
CYSTATHIONINE	884.7	92.8	9	119.7	14.2	9
METHIONINE	161.5	17.2	9	21.8	2.6	9
ISOLEUCINE	264.1	22.4	9	35.6	3.6	9
LEUCINE	525.9	40.9	9	70.7	6.5	9
TYROSINE	254.8	14.4	9	34.0	1.9	9
PHENYLALANINE	265.7	13.7	9	35.5	2.0	9
GABA	2737.1	312.8	9	361.7	36.6	9
ORNITHINE	218.6	83.5	9	29.6	11.4	9
LYSINE	1017.7	95.2	9	135.5	12.9	9
HISTIDINE	272.1	25.8	9	36.2	3.5	9
TRYPTOPHAN	32.4	3.6	5	4.4	0.4	5
ARGININE	487.4	91.5	9	64.9	12.4	9
HOMOCARNOSINE	179.4	94.9	9	23.6	12.3	9
GLYCINE/VALINE	4.8	0.2	9			
GLYCINE/ISOLEUCINE	9.5	0.6	9			
GLYCINE/LEUCINE	4.7	0.2	9			
ALANINE/VALINE	4.5	0.2	9			
TYROSINE/PHENYLALANINE	0.9	0.03	9			
TYROSINE/METHIONINE	1.6	0.1	9			
ORNITHINE/LEUCINE	0.3	0.1	9			
ORNITHINE/LYSINE	0.2	0.08	9			
NONESSENTIAL/ESSENTIAL	2.3	0.1	9			

TABLE 10.16
Statistical Analysis of the Data Shown in Tables 10.14 and 10.15

Groups compared	Cerebrum μmoles /kg 9/3	/gDNA 9/3	Cerebellum μmoles /kg 9/3	/gDNA 9/3
TAURINE		0.05		0.025
ASPARTIC ACID				
THREONINE		0.05		
SERINE				
GLUTAMINE	0.005	0.005		
PROLINE				
GLUTAMIC ACID			0.01	0.001
CITRULLINE				
GLYCINE				
ALANINE				0.02
VALINE				
CYSTATHIONINE				
METHIONINE			0.005	0.005
ISOLEUCINE				
LEUCINE				0.025
TYROSINE				
PHENYLALANINE				
GABA				
ORNITHINE				
LYSINE				
HISTIDINE				
TRYPTOPHAN				
ARGININE				
HOMOCARNOSINE				
GLY/VAL				
GLY/ILE				
GLY/LEU				
ALA/VAL			0.02	
TYR/PHE	0.05			
TYR/MET				
ORN/LEU				
ORN/LYS				
NONESS/ESS			0.05	

Results

The results are shown in Tables 10.17 to 10.20. It must be remembered that this was a pilot study. However, the data on amino acid concentrations were analyzed by a 2 × 2 factorial analysis of variance (with the generous help of Dr. Jonas Ellenberg of the N.I.N.D.S.).

Group 2 (protein deficient):
Cerebrum.   Concentration of most amino acids decreased, especially arginine.
Cerebellum.   Decreased concentrations (especially GABA, lysine, and taurine).

Group 3 (calorie deficient):
Cerebrum.   Elevation of most amino acid concentrations, especially for GABA and alanine.
Cerebellum.   Definite decreases (aspartate, glycine, cystathionine, methionine, tyrosine, phenylalanine, and histidine).

Group 4 (calorie and protein deficient):
Cerebrum.   Concentration of most amino acids increased, especially aspartate, threonine, and glycine.
Cerebellum.   Decreased concentrations—general.

Discussion

When considering changes in tissue amino acid concentrations, one also considers transport, *de novo* synthesis of nonessential amino acids, breakdown of proteins, incorporation into proteins, as well as amino acid metabolism per se.

In calorie restriction, for example, the increased alanine in the cerebrum might arise from increased protein breakdown or decreased protein synthesis. In the cerebellum most amino acids were reduced in concentration. Cerebellar tyrosine, phenylalanine, and histidine were notably reduced on this diet. Taurine, which is known to have a high concentration in the fetal cerebellum,[7] was also reduced in the presence of a reduction in methionine or cystathionine.

The enzyme activating methionine is operative in early fetal life [10] in the cerebellum and S-adenosylmethionine is involved in methylation of important catecholamines.

In protein restriction one might expect a decreased concentration of arginine and ornithine since these are intermediaries in the urea cycle. Moreover, essential amino acids in the cerebellum were decreased (groups 1 and 4) while those of the nonessential amino acids tended to increase. Since the growth of the cerebellum is faster than the cerebrum from midgestation, changes in cerebellar growth might be expected to be more significant in that organ.

In the cerebrum in protein deficiency (group 2) or calorie deficiency (group 3) there was an increase in glycine and threonine. One could speculate that in protein deficiency there is increased transamination of glucose metabolites leading to increased glycine synthesis. In calorie restriction more protein is broken down for gluconeogenesis which also elevates the level of glycine. When protein plus calorie deficiency presents, there would be a lack of glucose metabolites as well as minimal protein synthesis, and thus the increment in glycine would be minimal.

Clearly further work is necessary to clarify these results.

TABLE 10.17

Concentrations of Amino Acids Per Unit DNA in the Cerebrum of Fetuses of Nutritionally Deprived Maternal Monkeys*

(μmoles/gDNA)

| | GROUP 1 | | | GROUP 2 | | | GROUP 3 | | | GROUP 4 | | | SIGNIFICANCE P ← | | |
	MEAN	S.D.	N	MEAN	S.D.	N	MEAN	S.D.	N	MEAN	S.D.	N	RESTRICTION OF PROTEIN	WEIGHT GAIN	INTERACTION
TAURINE	7063.0	3271.0	4	7145.0	3006.0	3	8709.0	3161.0	4	7927.0	3133.0	6			
ASPARTIC ACID	891.0	263.0	4	1406.0	557.0	3	1364.0	271.0	4	1105.0	353.0	6			0.05
THREONINE	378.0	102.0	4	505.0	210.0	3	629.0	113.0	4	447.0	135.0	6			0.05
SERINE	901.0	308.0	4	1047.0	347.0	3	1235.0	118.0	4	992.0	352.0	6			
GLUTAMINE	2585.0	514.0	4	3045.0	765.0	3	3349.0	1046.0	4	2621.0	719.0	6			
GLUTAMIC ACID	5473.0	1445.0	4	6979.0	2262.0	3	7447.0	650.0	4	6114.0	994.0	6			0.025
GLYCINE	1341.0	297.0	4	1816.0	611.0	3	1854.0	132.0	4	1426.0	302.0	6			
ALANINE	1072.0	293.0	4	705.0	598.0	3	1428.0	253.0	4	1102.0	288.0	6		0.05	
VALINE	393.0	191.0	4	349.0	96.0	3	350.0	127.0	4	323.0	125.0	6			
CYSTATHIONINE	107.0	24.0	4	84.0	39.0	3	64.0	46.0	4	79.0	31.0	6			
METHIONINE	43.0	41.0	4	53.0	25.0	3	45.0	21.0	4	43.0	26.0	6			
ISOLEUCINE	188.0	52.0	4	183.0	62.0	3	195.0	69.0	4	180.0	51.0	6			
LEUCINE	371.0	114.0	4	335.0	122.0	3	358.0	116.0	4	318.0	97.0	6			
TYROSINE	182.0	65.0	4	166.0	70.0	3	144.0	63.0	4	143.0	49.0	6			
PHENYLALANINE	183.0	94.0	4	165.0	70.0	3	142.0	49.0	4	144.0	47.0	6			
GABA	1474.0	360.0	4	1377.0	243.0	3	2007.0	454.0	4	1962.0	521.0	6		0.025	
ORNITHINE	50.0	35.0	4	45.0	18.0	3	66.0	25.0	4	61.0	23.0	6			
LYSINE	427.0	204.0	4	290.0	95.0	3	559.0	208.0	4	424.0	118.0	6			
HISTIDINE	234.0	144.0	4	144.0	53.0	3	247.0	97.0	4	218.0	81.0	6			
ARGININE	352.0	192.0	2	176.0	77.0	3	312.0	86.0	4	252.0	68.0	6	0.05		
TRYPTOPHAN	29.6	3.4		19.4	10.1	3	25.0	6.5	4	22.1	2.7	6			

* Groups are as follows: 1, controls; 2, protein restriction; 3, calorie restriction; and 4, calorie and protein restriction. Significant differences from the control group are indicated by the *P* values at the right. S.D.: Standard deviation.

196

TABLE 10.19

Concentrations of Amino Acids per Unit Tissue Weight in the Cerebrum of Fetuses of Nutritionally Deprived Maternal Monkeys

(μmoles/kg)

| | GROUP 1 | | | GROUP 2 | | | GROUP 3 | | | GROUP 4 | | | SIGNIFICANCE P< | | |
	MEAN	S.D.	N	MEAN	S.D.	N	MEAN	S.D.	N	MEAN	S.D.	N	RESTRICTION OF PROTEIN	WEIGHT GAIN	INTERACTION
TAURINE	9112.0	3963.0	4	10391.0	4600.0	3	11294.0	3731.0	4	10333.0	4050.0	6			
ASPARTIC ACID	1162.0	352.0	4	2017.0	705.0	3	1772.0	240.0	4	1452.0	509.0	6			0.05
THREONINE	490.0	123.0	4	731.0	306.0	3	819.0	103.0	4	585.0	182.0	6			0.025
SERINE	1158.0	334.0	4	1515.0	496.0	3	1616.0	127.0	4	1295.0	462.0	6			
GLUTAMINE	3351.0	723.0	4	4383.0	889.0	3	4332.0	1116.0	4	3439.0	1081.0	6			
GLUTAMIC ACID	6999.0	1218.0	4	10026.0	2878.0	3	9785.0	1255.0	4	7986.0	1476.0	6			0.025
GLYCINE	1724.0	262.0	4	2617.0	817.0	3	2424.0	109.0	4	1867.0	441.0	6			0.01
ALANINE	1382.0	319.0	4	1665.0	669.0	3	1857.0	225.0	4	1439.0	388.0	6			
VALINE	505.0	220.0	4	505.0	133.0	3	453.0	146.0	4	422.0	164.0	6			
CYSTATHIONINE	430.0	572.0	4	122.0	57.8	3	82.1	53.6	4	104.0	41.5	6			
METHIONINE	57.6	57.6	4	76.3	35.1	3	58.8	24.6	4	57.5	35.4	6			
ISOLEUCINE	246.0	71.3	4	265.0	89.3	3	253.0	81.0	4	236.0	70.6	6			
LEUCINE	484.0	164.0	4	484.0	169.0	3	465.0	13.4	4	417.0	134.0	6			
TYROSINE	236.0	89.6	4	241.0	99.6	3	186.0	72.6	4	187.0	65.9	6			
PHENYLALANINE	239.0	135.0	4	240.0	99.6	3	185.0	54.4	4	189.0	62.9	6			
GABA	1952.0	644.0	4	1997.0	372.0	3	2617.0	527.0	4	2535.0	598.0	6			
ORNITHINE	67.3	48.5	4	66.4	26.6	3	87.5	32.7	4	80.1	31.2	6			
LYSINE	560.0	272.0	4	423.0	147.0	3	728.0	258.0	4	551.0	149.0	6			
HISTIDINE	305.0	189.0	4	210.0	81.8	3	324.0	130.0	4	282.0	108.0	6			
TRYPTOPHAN	38.3	1.4	4	27.8	13.2	3	33.0	9.5	4	29.0	4.8	6			
ARGININE	466.0	301.0	2	256.0	116.0	3	409.0	114.0	4	328.0	85.0	6			
GLY/VAL	3.8	1.2	4	5.1	0.4	3	5.8	1.9	4	4.7	0.9	6			
GLY/ILE	7.3	1.7	4	9.9	1.1	3	10.4	3.5	4	8.0	0.8	6			0.05
GLY/LEU	3.7	0.9	4	5.4	0.4	3	5.5	1.5	4	4.6	0.5	6			0.025
ALA/VAL	3.0	1.1	4	3.2	0.5	3	4.3	1.0	4	3.5	0.6	6			
TYR/PHE	1.0	0.1	4	1.0	0.1	3	0.9	0.1	4	0.9	0.09	6			
TYR/MET	3.7	1.0	3	3.0	0.7	3	3.2	0.8	4	3.5	1.4	6			
ORN/LEU	0.1	0.03	3	0.1	0.03	3	0.1	0.07	4	0.2	0.08	6			
ORN/LYS	9.1	0.03	3	0.1	0.01	3	0.1	0.05	4	0.1	0.04	6			
NONESS/ESS	1.7	0.5	4	2.2	0.3	3	1.9	0.4	4	1.7	0.1	6			

TABLE 10.19
Concentrations of Amino Acids per Unit DNA in the Cerebellum of Fetuses of Nutritionally Deprived Maternal Monkeys

(μmoles/gDNA)

	GROUP 1			GROUP 2			GROUP 3			GROUP 4			SIGNIFICANCE $P \leqslant$		
	MEAN	S.D.	N	MEAN	S.D.	N	MEAN	S.D.	N	MEAN	S.D.	N	RESTRICTION OF PROTEIN	WEIGHT GAIN	INTERACTION
TAURINE	2339.0	74.0	2	1361.0	476.0	2	1956.0	99.0	2	1619.0	526.0	3			
ASPARTIC ACID	423.0	78.0	4	485.0	268.0	3	282.0	74.0	4	283.0	119.0	6		0.05	
THREONINE	125.0	21.0	4	162.0	102.0	3	115.0	48.0	4	103.0	21.0	6			
SERINE	246.0	53.0	4	287.0	187.0	3	172.0	50.0	4	186.0	60.0	6			
GLUTAMINE	1438.0	203.0	4	1055.0	230.0	3	1171.0	389.0	4	1130.0	225.0	6			
GLUTAMIC ACID	1477.0	78.0	4	2704.0	2613.0	3	1039.0	520.0	4	1209.0	234.0	6			
GLYCINE	345.0	60.0	4	413.0	243.0	3	235.0	46.0	4	237.0	65.0	6		0.025	
ALANINE	283.0	66.0	4	286.0	168.0	3	228.0	70.0	4	195.0	31.0	6			
VALINE	64.0	9.0	4	81.0	56.0	3	58.0	21.0	4	43.0	8.0	6		0.05	
CYSTATHIONINE	133.0	17.0	4	131.0	100.0	3	66.0	28.0	4	78.0	52.0	6		0.05	
METHIONINE	13.0	5.0	3	13.0	10.0	3	6.0	2.0	3	5.0	2.0	6			
ISOLEUCINE	36.0	9.0	4	33.0	17.0	3	32.0	5.0	4	27.0	5.0	6			
LEUCINE	72.0	16.0	4	69.0	36.0	3	58.0	9.0	4	49.0	8.0	6			
TYROSINE	39.0	5.0	4	36.0	17.0	3	29.0	8.0	4	22.0	5.0	6		0.025	
PHENYLALANINE	39.0	6.0	4	39.0	21.0	3	29.0	5.0	4	22.0	5.0	6		0.025	
GABA	458.0	99.0	4	385.0	113.0	3	432.0	130.0	4	349.0	78.0	6			
ORNITHINE	18.0	9.0	3	9.0	2.0	3	15.0	8.0	4	17.0	11.0	6			
LYSINE	77.0	21.0	4	63.0	5.0	3	75.0	9.0	4	57.0	5.0	6			
HISTIDINE	45.0	11.0	4	32.0	4.0	3	26.0	3.0	4	27.0	9.0	6	0.025		
ARGININE	53.0	22.0	4	43.0	10.0	3	49.0	12.0	4	39.0	8.0	6		0.025	
TRYPTOPHAN	7.0	2.4	4	5.4	1.0	3	6.3	0.5	4	5.8	1.2	6			

198

TABLE 10.20
Concentrations of Amino Acids Per Unit Tissue Weight in the Cerebellum of Fetuses of Nutritionally Deprived Maternal Monkeys

(μmoles/kg)

	GROUP 1			GROUP 2			GROUP 3			GROUP 4			SIGNIFICANCE P<		
	MEAN	S.D.	N	MEAN	S.D.	N	MEAN	S.D.	N	MEAN	S.D.	N	RESTRICTION OF PROTEIN	WEIGHT GAIN	INTERACTION
TAURINE	16481.0	2094.0		9053.0	1986.0	2	14218.0	2520.0	2	12082.0	1918.0	3	0.025		
ASPARTIC ACID	2835.0	556.0	4	3380.0	1987.0	3	2016.0	440.0	4	2092.0	762.0	6		0.05	
THREONINE	843.0	186.0	4	1121.0	741.0	3	812.0	287.0	4	778.0	106.0	6			
SERINE	1629.0	237.0	4	1993.0	1366.0	3	1227.0	301.0	4	1368.0	236.0	6			
GLUTAMINE	9669.0	1769.0	4	7309.0	1747.0	3	8314.0	2163.0	4	8443.0	656.0	6			
GLUTAMIC ACID	9922.0	1311.0	4	18933.0	18991.0	3	7321.0	3465.0	4	9049.0	871.0	6			
GLYCINE	2322.0	474.0	4	2869.0	1781.0	3	1685.0	215.0	4	1782.0	447.0	6		0.05	
ALANINE	1881.0	370.0	4	1985.0	1226.0	3	1627.0	393.0	4	1473.0	116.0	6			
VALINE	430.0	55.3	4	4563.0	406.0	3	413.0	123.0	4	330.0	67.0	3			
CYSTATHIONINE	895.0	149.0	4	918.0	729.0	3	473.0	172.0	4	623.0	484.0	6			
METHIONINE	94.5	22.8	3	92.0	71.0	3	46.8	9.8	3	46.4	17.8	3			
ISOLEUCINE	241.0	59.4	4	234.0	120.0	3	273.0	30.5	4	209.0	43.6	6			
LEUCINE	478.0	95.3	4	478.0	262.0	3	419.0	40.3	4	373.0	66.8	6			
TYROSINE	267.0	50.0	4	252.0	128.0	3	212.0	65.3	4	171.0	23.0	6			
PHENYLALANINE	264.0	54.6	4	278.0	151.0	3	212.0	33.6	4	172.0	32.7	6		0.05	
GABA	3031.0	387.0	4	2618.0	493.0	3	3142.0	1036.0	4	2615.0	426.0	6			
ORNITHINE	120.0	49.3	3	67.5	19.9	3	115.0	68.8	4	123.0	63.3	6			
LYSINE	511.0	104.0	4	435.0	44.7	3	547.0	78.9	4	435.0	70.3	6	0.05		
HISTIDINE	298.0	52.8	4	228.0	39.4	3	193.0	25.6	4	214.0	89.2	6			
TRYPTOPHAN	46.7	14.5	4	37.6	5.4	3	45.9	4.2	4	45.2	12.5	6			
GLY/VAL	3.9	2.1	4	5.5	0.7	3	4.2	0.8	4	5.6	1.7	6		0.05	
GLY/ILE	9.9	2.8	4	12.0	1.9	3	7.3	1.4	4	8.8	2.6	6		0.05	
GLY/LEU	4.9	1.3	4	5.9	0.6	3	4.0	0.4	4	4.8	0.9	6			
ALA/VAL	4.4	0.8	4	3.7	0.3	3	4.0	0.4	4	4.5	0.8	6			
TYR/PHE	1.0	0.03	4	0.9	0.03	3	0.9	0.1	4	1.0	0.09	6			
TYR/MET	3.1	1.1	3	3.1	0.8	3	3.9	0.7	3	3.9	0.9	3			
ORN/LEU	0.2	0.08	3	0.1	0.1	3	0.2	0.1	4	0.3	0.2	6			
ORN/LYS	0.2	0.07	4	0.1	0.05	3	0.2	0.09	4	0.2	0.1	6			
NONESS/ESS	1.9	0.09	4	1.8	0.5	3	1.7	0.1	4	2.1	0.4	6			

INDUCED PLACENTAL INSUFFICIENCY

Method

The general design of the experiment has been described[15] (Chapter 7). Briefly, it was designed to study the effects on the fetus of the *in utero* reduction of placental mass during gestation.

Results

This reduction of functioning placental mass led to clear-cut intrauterine growth retardation. The weight of the brain was less affected than any other tissue in these growth-retarded fetuses.

The mean concentration of virtually every amino acid was lower in the placental insufficiency group than in controls (Table 10.21). The effect was seen in both essential and nonessential amino acids, while the overall ratio of nonessential to essential amino acids did not change. The concentrations of many amino acids in the plasma were significantly higher than those of the controls.

Discussion

The number of animals studied appeared to be too small and the variation about the means too great to permit statistically significant differences. However, the uniform nature of the changes and their magnitude, as well as the size of the *t* values observed, indicated that the differences might have biologic significance.

The data suggest that the decreased concentrations of amino acids in the brain, together with the increased concentrations in the plasma, are a consequence of altered transport in the face of a diminished supply. It is of interest that the pattern of uniform reduction of amino acid content in the brain in these animals was quite different from that observed in the fetus of the nutritionally deprived mother.

A limitation of energy for the active transport from blood to the extracellular compartment and then into the brain cells could explain these data. The consequence of a depleted amino acid pool could be a diminished intracellular protein synthesis with instability of polysomes.[16] The role of tryptophan depletion in experimental hyperphenylalaninemia on the disaggregation of brain polyribosomes has been shown.[17] A depleted protein synthesis in the brain might lead to irreversible damage, especially if it occurred during a vulnerable phase of brain development. Proteolipids are an essential part of myelin, and delayed or defective myelination could lead to irreversible functional defects. It is not known if changes in amino acids levels affect synaptogenesis.

PRENATAL HYPOTHYROIDISM

The design of this experiment is described by Holt, Cheek, and Kerr.[18] Groups compared were control and prenatally hypothyroid monkeys. Control and experimental animals were from the Wisconsin Regional Primate Center.

TABLE 10.21
Concentrations of Amino Acids in the Fetal Primate Cerebrum Following Placental Insufficiency*

| | (μmoles/kg) | | | | | | (μmoles/g DNA) | | | | | |
| | GROUP 14 | | | GROUP 15 | | | GROUP 14 | | | GROUP 15 | | |
	MEAN	S.E.M.	N	MEAN	S.E.M.	N	MEAN	S.E.M.	N	MEAN	S.E.M.	N
TAURINE	6439.1	356.2	5	5957.7	517.7	5	4749.7	370.8	5	4098.3	260.3	5
ASPARTIC ACID	2897.4	349.2	5	2985.5	608.1	5	2155.4	330.4	5	2061.5	408.6	5
THREONINE	1079.2	149.4	5	920.8	251.6	5	806.5	136.6	5	633.8	170.5	5
SERINE	1914.5	198.4	5	1563.6	366.2	5	1425.0	197.4	5	1075.1	245.5	5
GLUTAMINE	458.5	42.4	5	441.3	69.3	5	338.8	39.4	5	305.7	46.6	5
PROLINE	1233.5	131.7	5	967.0	316.5	5	920.2	137.3	5	663.7	214.5	5
GLUTAMIC ACID	10792.8	427.5	5	9353.5	1099.5	5	7969.7	612.0	5	6472.4	745.7	5
CITRULLINE	69.6	22.0	5	68.6	68.6	5	52.4	17.2	5	47.0	47.0	5
GLYCINE	2864.0	144.3	5	2605.1	394.5	5	2118.0	185.1	5	1794.7	257.3	5
ALANINE	3491.6	320.6	5	2625.3	402.0	5	2597.7	339.1	5	1797.7	248.5	5
VALINE	796.3	110.9	5	597.4	235.9	5	596.0	106.8	5	411.4	160.6	5
CYSTATHIONINE	121.3	21.8	5	91.1	18.0	5	91.4	20.5	5	63.0	12.1	5
METHIONINE	159.1	24.2	5	147.3	61.8	4	119.0	22.6	5	100.6	42.7	4
ISOLEUCINE	410.9	57.3	5	336.1	114.1	5	307.0	54.0	5	230.4	77.4	5
LEUCINE	838.6	127.3	5	645.0	234.0	5	627.9	119.1	5	442.9	158.9	5
TYROSINE	284.4	46.7	5	251.8	97.5	5	213.6	43.9	5	172.9	66.3	5
PHENYLALANINE	349.8	44.3	5	294.2	111.4	5	261.5	43.9	5	202.9	75.7	5
GABA	2011.3	194.5	5	1640.7	130.2	5	1497.0	199.7	5	1146.3	112.9	5
ORNITHINE	82.5	14.5	5	86.4	18.5	5	62.1	13.7	5	60.0	12.2	5
LYSINE	782.0	92.4	5	715.0	106.1	5	582.4	86.4	5	502.5	82.4	5
HISTIDINE	166.7	18.5	5	180.1	35.9	5	124.2	18.1	5	126.5	26.4	5
ARGININE	326.0	37.6	5	306.1	68.1	5	243.3	37.0	5	216.5	51.1	5
HOMOCARNOSINE	32.5	32.0	5	0.0	0.0	5	23.6	23.2	5	0.0	0.0	5
GLY/VAL	3.7	0.3	5	5.5	0.8	5						
GLY/ILE	7.3	0.7	5	9.2	1.1	5						
GLY/LEU	3.6	0.3	5	4.9	0.6	5						
ALA/VAL	4.4	0.2	5	5.6	1.1	5						
TYR/PHE	0.7	0.03	5	0.8	0.1	5						
TYR/MET	1.7	0.1	5	2.1	0.3	4						
ORN/LEU	0.09	0.006	5	0.1	0.05	5						
ORN/LYS	0.1	0.01	5	0.1	0.02	5						
NONESS/ESS	2.5	0.1	5	2.7	0.3	4						

* Group 14, controls; group 15, monkeys with intrauterine growth retardation.

201

Results

In the cerebrum most of the amino acids remained unchanged in the cretinoid monkeys (Table 10.22). However, the levels per unit tissue of GABA, ornithine, lysine, histidine, and cystathionine showed a trend toward an increase in the experimental group. There was a trend toward a reduction of nonessential amino acids. Both aspartic and glutamic acid showed some reduction in cerebrum and cerebellum (per unit DNA). In both the cerebrum and cerebellum there was a slight but significant increase in tryptophan and in the cerebellum there was in addition an increase in serine (Table 10.23).

Discussion

The significance of the change in tryptophan is not known but the synthesis of serotonin in the brain may well be substrate dependent. It is known that tyrosine concentration is reduced in hypothyroidism and since both amino acids have a similar carrier system into the central nervous system it is possible that the activity of this carrier system is increased in this situation.[19]

The change in serine leaves open the question of whether this substrate is under hormonal control.

The production of fetal hypothyroidism was the only experimental condition in this series of experiments that appeared to affect the cerebellum much less than the cerebrum. It was also unique insofar as the major effect appeared to be to lower the concentrations of nonessential amino acids, thus decreasing the calculated ratios, while under virtually all of the other conditions studied, the ratios were increased.

CONCLUDING COMMENTS

These data help to define the chemical anatomy of the central nervous system during development. The experiments performed examined the effects of a number of conditions that interfere with the normal processes of fetal growth.

The most impressive changes in amino acid concentrations observed were those that took place at different stages of normal fetal and postnatal development. A number of highly specific patterns was observed, and there was a number of highly significant differences when groups at different stages of development were compared. The patterns in cerebellum and cerebrum were quite different. Certain amino acids, like homocarnosine, appear in fetal brain only after a certain period of development. A somewhat similar pattern was observed for cystathionine and γ-aminobutyric acid. All three amino acids appear to be especially important to the central nervous system.

Interventions that altered the rates of fetal growth generally had a much greater effect on the amino acid concentrations of the cerebellum than on those of the cerebrum. This is consistent with the hypothesis that this tissue develops from mid-gestation at a greater rate than does the cerebrum.

TABLE 10.22

Concentrations of Amino Acids in the Cerebrum of Control and Hypothyroid Primate Fetuses*

(μmoles/kg)

	GROUP 7 MEAN	GROUP 7 S.E.M.	GROUP 7 N	GROUP 8 MEAN	GROUP 8 S.E.M.	GROUP 8 N
TAURINE	3852.0	677.9	6	3443.4	573.8	6
ASPARTIC ACID	1323.4	223.4	6	1138.8	206.7	6
THREONINE	507.9	73.8	6	554.6	92.1	6
SERINE	1003.0	127.1	6	1031.9	171.9	6
GLUTAMINE	844.7	114.8	6	815.9	185.7	6
PROLINE	608.2	89.9	6	505.6	95.5	5
GLUTAMIC ACID	6007.0	968.7	6	5414.6	921.2	6
CITRULLINE	16.5	15.7	6	40.1	28.6	6
GLYCINE	1574.6	243.2	6	1450.8	253.5	6
ALANINE	1537.1	202.0	6	1475.7	192.5	6
VALINE	381.3	58.8	6	359.9	58.0	6
CYSTATHIONINE	63.6	8.0	6	100.1	42.3	6
METHIONINE	98.2	13.5	6	118.3	23.4	6
ISOLEUCINE	233.9	30.7	6	219.9	33.4	6
LEUCINE	419.6	58.3	6	419.2	65.9	6
TYROSINE	186.9	28.6	6	199.5	34.8	6
PHENYLALANINE	167.0	43.7	6	202.1	37.6	6
GABA	1079.1	179.2	6	1101.0	136.9	6
ORNITHINE	58.0	18.8	5	86.2	8.6	5
LYSINE	582.0	95.4	6	788.9	60.6	6
HISTIDINE	180.7	23.8	6	234.6	30.0	6
TRYPTOPHAN	6.8	0.3	6	9.4	0.7	6
ARGININE	349.7	91.4	6	383.2	108.6	5
HOMOCARNOSINE	0.1	0.1	6	0.0	0.0	6
GLY/VAL	4.1	0.2	6	3.9	0.1	6
GLY/ILE	7.0	0.2	6	6.4	0.2	6
GLY/LEU	3.7	0.1	6	3.4	0.1	6
ALA/VAL	4.1	0.1	6	4.2	0.3	6
TYR/PHE	0.8	0.01	5	0.9	0.03	5
TYR/MET	1.9	0.1	6	1.7	0.08	6
ORN/LEU	0.1	0.06	5	0.2	0.06	5
ORN/LYS	0.09	0.02	5	0.1	0.009	6
NONESS/ESS	2.0	0.1	5	1.7	0.1	5

(μmoles/g DNA)

	GROUP 7 MEAN	GROUP 7 S.E.M.	GROUP 7 N	GROUP 8 MEAN	GROUP 8 S.E.M.	GROUP 8 N
TAURINE	3068.7	641.5	6	2544.0	384.7	6
ASPARTIC ACID	1053.2	211.7	6	837.4	135.2	6
THREONINE	402.9	70.1	6	409.2	60.6	6
SERINE	793.7	121.4	6	761.6	114.1	6
GLUTAMINE	669.4	110.1	6	598.1	124.8	6
PROLINE	483.0	85.2	6	378.4	64.4	5
GLUTAMIC ACID	4782.9	934.0	6	3996.9	615.1	6
CITRULLINE	12.7	12.1	6	28.2	20.0	6
GLYCINE	1251.9	232.9	6	1070.8	169.5	6
ALANINE	1219.3	197.4	6	1099.3	136.1	6
VALINE	302.7	55.3	6	266.7	39.6	6
CYSTATHIONINE	50.4	7.9	6	72.3	29.1	6
METHIONINE	77.6	12.1	6	87.4	16.0	6
ISOLEUCINE	177.2	28.7	6	163.1	22.6	6
LEUCINE	331.8	53.9	6	310.8	44.9	6
TYROSINE	148.1	26.7	6	147.7	23.8	6
PHENYLALANINE	131.1	37.8	6	149.1	25.2	6
GABA	860.6	162.7	6	837.8	123.8	6
ORNITHINE	44.5	14.3	6	65.2	7.9	6
LYSINE	464.7	88.1	6	597.2	60.4	6
HISTIDINE	143.4	21.8	6	178.2	26.0	6
TRYPTOPHAN	5.3	0.2	6	7.1	0.6	6
ARGININE	280.6	78.8	6	287.4	83.6	5
HOMOCARNOSINE	0.1	0.1	6	0.0	0.0	6

* Groups 7 and 8, control and hypothyroid monkeys, respectively, are described and compared statistically in Tables 10.12 and 10.13.

TABLE 10.23

Concentrations of Amino Acids in the Cerebellum of Control and Hypothyroid Primate Fetuses*

	(μmoles/kg) GROUP 7			GROUP 8			(μmoles/g DNA) GROUP 7			GROUP 8		
	MEAN	S.E.M.	N	MEAN	S.E.M.	N	MEAN	S.E.M.	N	MEAN	S.E.M.	N
TAURINE	0.0	0.0	2	0.0	0.0	1	0.0	0.0	2	0.0	0.0	1
ASPARTIC ACID	3581.6	315.8	6	2968.5	145.7	6	414.3	39.5	6	345.6	15.6	6
THREONINE	1095.3	31.8	6	1216.6	60.7	6	126.3	4.5	6	141.9	7.4	6
SERINE	1954.2	96.6	6	2507.7	80.1	6	225.0	10.6	6	292.2	9.4	6
GLUTAMINE	2653.1	358.5	6	3827.0	521.3	6	305.2	41.3	6	442.6	54.7	6
PROLINE	0.0	0.0	2	1308.2	40.1	3	0.0	0.0	2	150.6	8.1	3
GLUTAMIC ACID	15674.8	2031.8	6	13946.9	1247.1	6	1815.1	245.1	6	1619.1	123.4	5
CITRULLINE	150.6	56.6	5	205.8	38.3	5	18.0	7.1	5	23.8	4.6	5
GLYCINE	3250.0	227.0	6	3409.9	180.4	6	375.9	30.6	6	397.0	19.1	6
ALANINE	2379.8	141.3	6	2714.7	115.9	6	274.7	17.5	6	316.1	12.0	6
VALINE	668.0	39.9	6	658.5	32.4	6	76.7	3.6	6	76.9	4.5	6
CYSTATHIONINE	771.3	139.7	6	743.1	120.9	6	88.7	16.2	6	86.1	13.1	6
METHIONINE	234.1	16.9	6	253.8	25.2	6	27.2	2.4	6	29.6	2.9	6
ISOLEUCINE	366.7	12.1	6	382.8	19.6	6	42.3	1.8	6	44.6	2.5	6
LEUCINE	779.7	33.3	6	849.3	36.9	6	90.1	5.0	6	99.0	4.7	6
TYROSINE	270.0	57.0	6	368.9	47.6	6	31.1	6.6	6	43.1	5.7	6
PHENYLALANINE	331.9	71.2	6	467.3	15.8	6	38.2	8.2	6	54.5	2.3	6
GABA	2211.8	208.5	6	1769.0	196.3	6	255.0	24.3	6	204.7	19.8	6
ORNITHINE	128.6	29.8	6	163.4	14.1	6	14.8	3.3	6	19.0	1.7	6
LYSINE	1461.6	126.2	6	1379.1	93.4	6	168.8	15.5	6	161.5	13.0	6
HISTIDINE	352.8	19.4	6	404.9	22.9	6	40.7	2.7	6	47.3	2.9	6
TRYPTOPHAN	9.2	0.7	6	11.6	0.4	6	1.0	0.08	6	1.3	0.1	6
ARGININE	798.7	41.7	6	573.9	124.4	6	92.1	5.5	6	66.5	14.7	6
HOMOCARNOSINE	447.4	77.4	6	400.1	143.4	6	51.6	8.9	6	45.3	16.3	6
GLY/VAL	4.9	0.4	6	5.2	0.3	6						
GLY/ILE	8.9	0.4	6	8.9	0.3	6						
GLY/LEU	4.1	0.1	6	4.0	0.1	6						
ALA/VAL	3.6	0.2	6	4.1	0.1	6						
TYR/PHE	0.8	0.02	5	0.7	0.09	6						
TYR/MET	1.2	0.2	6	1.4	0.1	6						
ORN/LEU	0.1	0.03	6	0.1	0.02	6						
ORN/LYS	0.09	0.03	6	0.1	0.01	6						
NONESS/ESS	1.9	0.1	6	2.0	0.1	6						

REFERENCES

1. Nyhan, W. L., Yujnovsky, A. O., and Wehr, R. F.: Amino acids and cell growth, In: Cheek, D. B. (Ed.): *Human Growth: Body Composition, Cell Growth, Energy, and Intelligence.* Lea & Febiger, Philadelphia, 1968, p. 396.

2. Spackman, D. H., Stein, W. H., and Moore, S.: Automated recording apparatus for use in the chromatography of amino acids. *Anal. Chem.* **30:** 1190, 1958.

3. Udenfriend, S.: *Fluorescence Assay in Biology and Medicine.* Academic Press, New York, 1968, p. 396.

4. Bejar, R. L., Smith, G. F., Park, S., Spellacy, W. N., Wolfson, S. L., and Nyhan, W. L.: Cerebral gigantism: Concentrations of amino acids in plasma and muscle. *J. Pediatr.* **76:** 105, 1970.

5. Colombo, J. P.: Congenital disorders of the urea cycle and ammonia detoxication. *Monogr. Paediatr.* **1:** 1, 1971.

6. Mardens, Y., and Van Sande, M.: Identification and quantitation of ninhydrin positive substances in the human central nervous system. *Technicon Symp.* **2:** 239, 1967.

7. Volpe, J. J., and Laster, L.: Transsulphuration in primate brain: Regional distribution of cystathionine synthase, cystathionine, and taurine in the brain of the rhesus monkey at various stages of development. *J. Neurochem.* **17:** 425, 1970.

8. Oja, S. S., Uusitalo, A. J., Vahvelainen, M. L., and Piha, R. S.: Changes in cerebral and hepatic amino acids in the rat and guinea pig during development. *Brain Res.* **11:** 655, 1968.

9. Perry, T. L., Hansen, S., Berry, K., Mok, C., and Lesk, D.: Free amino acids and related compounds in biopsies of human brain. *J. Neurochem.* **18:** 521, 1971.

10. Volpe, J. J., and Laster, L.: Transsulphuration in primate brain: Regional distribution of methionine-activating enzyme in the brain of the rhesus monkey at various stages of development. *J. Neurochem.* **17:** 413, 1970.

11. Tallan, H. H., Moore, S., and Stein, W. H.: L-Cystathionine in human brain. *J. Biol. Chem.* **230:** 707, 1968.

12a. Zachmann, M., Tocci, P., and Nyhan, W. L.: The occurrence of γ-aminobutyric acid in human tissues other than brain. *J. Biol. Chem.* **241:** 1355, 1966.

12b. Davison, A. N., and Kaczmarek, L. K.: Taurine, a possible neurotransmitter. *Nature* **234:** 107, 1971.

13. Cheek, D. B., Brayton, J. B., and Scott, R. E.: Overnutrition, overgrowth and hormones (with special reference to the infant born of the diabetic mother). In *Nutrition and Malnutrition.* Eds. Roche, A. F. and Falkner, F. *Adv. Exp. Med. Biol.* **49:** 47, 1974.

14. Cory, H. T., and Rose, S. P. R.: Alanine metabolism in rat cortex *in vitro. J. Neurochem.* **17:** 1477, 1970.

15. Myers, R. E., Hill, D. E., Holt, A. B., Scott, R. E., Mellits, E. D., and Cheek, D. B.: Fetal growth retardation produced by experimental placental insufficiency in the rhesus monkey. *Biol. Neonate* **18:** 379, 1971.

16. Miller, S. A.: Nutrition in the neonatal development of protein metabolism. *Fed. Proc.* **29:** 1497, 1970.

17. Aoki, K., and Siegel, F. L.: Hyperphenylalaninemia: Disaggregation of brain polyribosomes in young rats. *Science* **168:** 129, 1970.

18. Holt, A. B., Cheek, D. B., and Kerr, G. R.: Prenatal hypothyroidism and brain composition in a primate. *Nature* **243:** 413, 1973.

19. Yuwiler, A.: Conversion of D- and L-tryptophan to brain serotonin and 5-hydroxyindoleacetic acid and to blood serotonin. *J. Neurochem.* **20:** 1099, 1973.

PART II

THE GROWTH OF THE SOMA

CHAPTER 11

Growth of Visceral Organs
in the Fetus

E. David Mellits, Donald E. Hill, and Clayton H. Kallman

In this chapter the change in weight of various fetal organs is compared for the human and other mammals. The literature is extensive and all available data have not been used, the prime concern being to compare data from the macaque with those from the human fetus. An allometric approach to the growth of kidney, spleen, heart, pituitary, adrenal, thyroid, and thymus in relation to body weight increments was used. (Aspects of liver and placental growth are discussed in the following chapters.) The resulting relationships (Table 11.1) indicate that there are differences in the mode of growth of fetal organs between primate and nonprimate orders. It is apparent that a more detailed study documenting these differences could be attempted to extend the information that we present in this chapter.

The offspring of *Macaca mulatta* were delivered either by cesarean section at specified times during gestation or spontaneously at term. Anthropometric data and the weights of individual organs were obtained either immediately on delivery or at various times to 120 days of postnatal life.

Mathematical analyses of the measurements obtained throughout the gestational and perinatal period indicated complex relationships between the growth of individual organs and various other parameters. A discussion of the relationships that evolved from treatment of the anthropometric data illustrates the approach taken in the presentation of the data. For example, the overall relationship between body weight and conception age can be described by a straight line from 80 days through to 300 days, as measured from date of conception ± 2 days (Figure 11.1, Equation 1). This relationship, however, may be subdivided into a fetal growth curve (Equation 2) and an infant or postnatal growth curve (Equation 3), a very slight discontinuity being apparent between the two lines. For our purposes, the discontinuity is insufficient to improve the fit materially. Therefore, the use of the single linear

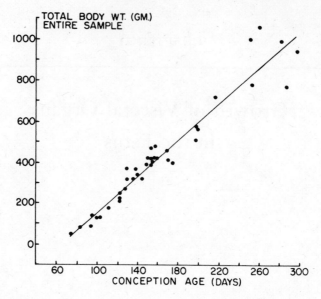

Fig. 11.1.   Total body weight (g) as a function of conception age (days) (Equation 1).

KEY TO TABLE 11.1

The headings on the table are described from left to right.

1.   *Time span* is the time in days over which the data are described. *CA* indicates the age from conception while *PN* (postnatal age) indicates the age from birth. Birth is considered to occur in the macaque at 165 ± 5 days from conception. The estimated time in days from conception is accurate to ± 2 days.

2.   *n* indicates the number of subjects in each age bracket used to derive the equation.

3.   *Y* is the value to be predicted from the equation for a dependent variable *X*. *X* will relate to either age (*CA* or *PN*), body length, or body weight.

4.   *Equation* describes the mathematical relationship of *X* to *Y*. Predictions of *Y* are valid only when applied to data obtained within the designated *time span* for the equation. It is emphasized that where applicable the equations are based on *conceptual age* (*CA*). Relationships that refer to the postnatal period are, of course, expressed in terms of *postnatal days* (*PN*). (In the corresponding figures, fetal monkeys are plotted on conception age, which is scaled to 160 days. A second scale for postnatal monkeys, postnatal age, utilizes age from birth and is plotted on the same abscissa. The abscissa point 160 days for conception age corresponds to 0 days, age from birth.)

5.   *SD* Standard deviation around the fitted line.

6.   *Fit*. The decimalized figure for each equation represents the probability value *P*. When *linear* equations are documented, the *P* value indicating the significance level of an "F test" was used to test the existence of regression. In the case of linear equations the correlation coefficient *r* is also given. In the case when *quadratic* expressions are used, the *P* value indicates the significance level of an F test used to test the improvement (ie, reduction in variance) from fitting the listed equation over the linear equation.

TABLE 11.1   Equations describing organ and body size in Macaca mulatta.

	TIME SPAN	n	Y units	X units	Equation Y =	SD	Fit
1.	80 days CA to 120 days PN	39	Total body weight (g)	CA (days)	$-\,287.49 + 4.4235\,(X)$	67.8	0.001 linear r = 0.97
2.	80 days CA to Birth	26	Total body weight (g)	CA (days)	$-\,365.31 + 5.0708\,(X)$	31.8	0.001 linear r = 0.97
3.	Birth to 120 days PN	13	Total body weight (g)	PN (days)	$414.68 + 4.7303\,(X)$	112	0.001 linear r = 0.89
4.	80 days CA to 120 days PN	39	Total body weight (g)	Body length (cm)	$108.65 - 16.045\,(X) + 0.88698\,(X)^2$	48.0	0.001 quadratic
5.	80 days CA to 120 days PN	39	Log Total Body weight (g)	Log Body length (cm)	$-\,2.8529 + 2.6147\,(X)$	0.094	0.001 linear r = 0.99

CA=Days from Conception   PN=Postnatal days   SD=Standard deviation   n=Number of subjects

Table 11.1   (Cont.)

	TIME SPAN	n	Y units	X units	Equation Y =	SD	Fit
6.	80 days CA to 120 days PN	39	Total body weight$^{1/3}$ (g)	CA (days)	$- 0.80212 + 0.071754(X) - 0.00012245 (X)^2$	0.341	0.001 quadratic
7.	80 days CA to 120 days PN	39	Body length (cm)	CA (days)	$- 6.5017 + 0.31355 (X) - 0.00052929 (X)^2$	1.57	0.001 quadratic
8.	80 days CA to 120 days PN	39	Carcass weight (g)	CA (days)	$- 187.80 + 2.6277 (X)$	39.7	0.001 linear r = 0.97
9.	80 days CA to 120 days PN	39	Carcass weight (g)	Body length (cm)	$106.94 - 13.762 + 0.59792 (X)^2$	26.6	0.001 quadratic
10.	80 days CA to 120 days PN	33	Total visceral weight (g)	CA (days)	$- 46.214 + 0.90329$	13.6	0.001 linear r = 0.97
11.	80 days CA to 120 days PN	33	Total visceral weight (g)	Body length (cm)	$- 20.796 + 0.78662 (X) + 0.11208 (X)^2$	10.7	0.001 quadratic
12.	80 days CA to 120 days PN	18	Skin wet weight (g)	CA (days)	$- 59.157 + 0.74742 (X)$	20.7	0.001 linear r = 0.95

No.	Time period	n	Variable (y)	Variable (x)	Equation		Sig.	Type	r
13.	80 days CA to 120 days PN	18	Skin wet weight (g)	Body length (cm)	$28.198 - 4.0713\,(X) + 0.17235\,(X)^2$	15.2	0.01	quadratic	
14.	80 days CA to Birth	20	Lung weight (g)	CA (days)	$-7.6674 + 0.10804\,(X)$	0.944	0.001	linear	$r = 0.94$
15.	Birth to 120 days PN	13	Lung weight (g)	PN (days)	$4.9763 + 0.01592\,(X)$	0.727	0.01	linear	$r = 0.72$
16.	80 days CA to birth	20	Lung weight (g)	Body weight (g)	$0.01867 + 0.02184\,(X)$	0.600	0.001	linear	$r = 0.98$
17.	Birth to 120 days PN	13	Lung weight (g)	Body weight (g)	$3.2367 + 0.00385\,(X)$	0.411	0.001	linear	$r = 0.92$
18.	80 days CA to Birth	20	Lung weight (g)	Body length (cm)	$6.1968 - 0.69803\,(X) + 0.026735\,(X)^2$	0.849	0.01	quadratic	
19.	Birth to 120 days PN	13	Lung weight (g)	Body length (cm)	$-0.53813 + 0.17941\,(X)$	0.569	0.01	linear	$r = 0.84$
20.	80 days CA to 120 days PN	39	Heart weight (g)	CA (days)	$-2.5753 + 0.039592\,(X) - 0.000055180\,(X)^2$	0.437	0.01	quadratic	

Table 11.1   (Cont.)

TIME SPAN	n	Y units	X units	Equation Y =	SD	Fit
21. 80 days CA to Birth	26	Heart weight (g)	Total Body weight (g)	$-$ 0.35942 + 0.01009 (X) $-$ 0.000096929 (X)^2	0.171	0.001 quadratic
22. Birth to 120 days PN	13	Heart weight (g)	Total Body weight (g)	0.72447 + 0.00387 (X)	0.377	0.001 linear r = 0.93
23. 80 days CA to Birth	26	Log heart weight (g)	Log Total Body weight (g)	$-$ 5.1079 + 0.98321 (X)	0.125	0.001 linear r = 0.98
24. 80 days CA to 120 days PN	33	Kidney weight (g)	CA (days)	$-$ 1.2676 + 0.02221 (X)	0.576	0.001 linear r = 0.92
25. 80 days CA to 120 days PN	33	Kidney weight (g)	Total Body weight (g)	0.21365 + 0.00499 (X)	0.464	0.001 linear r = 0.95
26. 80 days CA to Birth	20	Kidney weight (g)	Body length (cm)	$-$ 1.2202 + 0.11463 (X)	0.201	0.001 linear r = 0.95

No.	Period	n	Dependent variable	Independent variable	Equation		Significance
27.	Birth to 120 days PN	13	Kidney weight (g)	Body length (cm)	$-6.2692 + 0.27365\,(X)$	0.927	0.001 linear r = 0.82
28.	80 days CA to 120 days PN	37	Pituitary weight (mg)	CA (days)	$-18.508 + 0.29205\,(X) - 0.00050441\,(X)^2$	2.97	0.01 quadratic
29.	80 days CA to 120 days PN	37	Pituitary weight (mg)	Body length (cm)	$-11.092 + 0.86788\,(X)$	2.91	0.001 linear r = 0.92
30.	80 days CA to Birth	26	Adrenal weight (mg)	CA (days)	$-223.20 + 3.3804\,(X)$	50.8	0.001 linear r = 0.86
31.	80 days CA to Birth	26	Adrenal weight (mg)	Total Body weight (g)	$20.169 + 0.66720\,(X)$	46.0	0.001 linear r = 0.89
32.	80 days CA to Birth	26	Thyroid weight (mg)	CA (days)	$-175.17 + 2.2400\,(X)$	32.9	0.001 linear r = 0.86
33.	80 days CA to Birth	26	Thyroid weight (mg)	Total body weight (g)	$-16.426 + 0.45074\,(X)$	27.3	0.001 linear r = 0.91
34.	80 days CA to 120 days PN	39	Pancreas weight (mg)	CA (days)	$200.80 - 3.5973\,(X) + 0.024386\,(X)^2$	131	0.001 quadratic

215

Table 11.1 (Cont.)

TIME SPAN	n	Y units	X units	Equation Y =	SD	Fit
35. 80 days CA to 120 days PN	39	Pancreas weight (mg)	Total body weight (g)	$81.298 - 0.14658 (X) + 0.0012652 (X)^2$	97.5	0.001 quadratic
36. 80 days CA to Birth	22	Spleen weight (g)	CA (days)	$- 0.41267 + 0.00694 (X)$	0.108	0.001 linear $r = 0.84$
37. 80 days CA to Birth	22	Spleen weight (g)	Body length (cm)	$- 0.41737 + 0.03570 (X)$	0.0844	0.001 linear $r = 0.91$
38. 80 days CA to Birth	20	Thymus weight (g)	CA (days)	$- 1.3986 + 0.01776 (X)$	0.298	0.001 linear $r = 0.81$
39. 80 days CA to Birth	20	Thymus weight (g)	Total body weight (g)	$- 0.16894 + 0.00372 (X)$	0.246	0.001 linear $r = 0.88$

CA=Days from Conception   PN=Postnatal days   SD=Standard deviation   n=Number of subjects relationship using the entire sample is recommended. For subsequent analyses of the data, it is recommended that the two lines be fitted separately only where there is marked discontinuity or change in growth pattern when comparing the fetal line to the postnatal line.

A linear relationship indicates pure additive growth and can be applied to the examination of data over a small range of time within which additive growth is assumed to occur. Usually nonlinear relationships best represent exponential, multiplicative, or other types of growth that occur over longer periods of time. Often these nonlinear variables are transformed in order to be analyzed by linear models. The transformation using logarithms may yield other growth models representing true exponential or multiplicative growth. Whether to use polynomial equations, a log-log approach, the cube root of body weight, or some other transformation, depends on the theoretical biological model the investigator chooses to assume in describing the growth process. We have used what we consider to be the simplest model in order to present growth phenomena in a readily usable and understandable manner.

The relationship illustrated by Figure 11.2 between total body weight and body length for the entire sample is an example of nonlinear growth (Equation 4). It probably represents a portion of a pure multiplicative or log-log growth model. Following transformation to a log-log scale, the logarithm of total body weight is a linear function of the logarithm of body length (Equation 5). This linear, or arithmetic, relationship appears to hold throughout the range of our data and indicates that body weight increases at a constant rate (or power) with body length. The relationship between the cube root of body weight and gestational age (Figure 11.3) is nonlinear and continues through the postnatal period, being similar in form to the plot of body length as a function of gestational age for the entire data (Figure 11.4, Equation 7).

In describing visceral organ growth, the various components have been examined as functions of time and other parts of the body as a whole. In most instances the

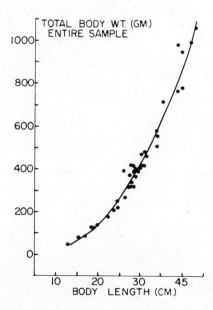

Fig. 11.2. Total body weight (g) as a function of body length (cm) (Equation 4).

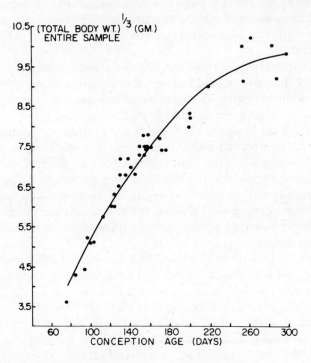

Fig. 11.3. (Total body weight)$^{1/3}$ (g) as a function of conception age (days). Fetal line, Equation 6.

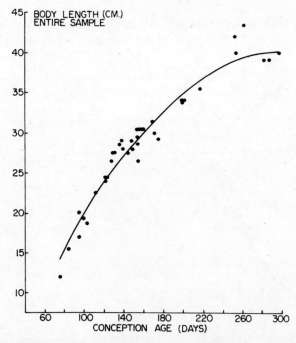

Fig. 11.4. Body length (cm) as a function of conception age (days) (Equation 7).

growth of an organ is related to time from conception. However, when the relationship with length describes the growth pattern more precisely, this relationship is illustrated. For example, when the carcass weight (Equation 9), visceral weight (Equation 11), and skin weight (Figure 11.5, Equation 13) are expressed as functions of body length, the scatter that is apparent in the relationship with age (Equations 8, 10, and 12) is diminished. The points fitting a quadratic relationship with body length, for example, yield precise equations that can be used in comparing normal and abnormal growth in the fetal and perinatal periods of the macaque.

In Figures 11.6 and 11.7, the lung weight is related to age (Equations 14 and 15) and body length (Equations 18 and 19), respectively; it is readily apparent that postnatal growth of the lung is discontinuous with that of the fetus. Lung weight as a function of body weight is best described by a linear fit during fetal life (Equation 16). In some respects the increase in weight of the lung near term indicates the extent to which water contributes to the total lung weight. There is a dramatic change in weight at birth that is obviously due to the replacement of fluid with air. At no time during the postnatal period does the weight of the lung exceed its weight at the end of gestation. Examining the postnatal lines, it is evident that the best fits are related to total body weight and body length, there being considerable scatter when lung weight is related to postnatal age.

The relationship of heart weight to conception age for the entire sample is best described by a quadratic line (Figure 11.8, Equation 20). In contrast to this, when heart weight is related to total body weight two separate lines yield the best description, the points for the fetal line (Equation 21) fitting a quadratic curve and the points for the postnatal period being best described by a linear fit (Equation 22).

It is of particular interest to note the growth of individual organs in relation to total body weight. If the fetal period only is examined, the growth of the heart may be viewed as a multiplicative function of total body weight. When the heart weight is plotted against total body weight on a log-log grid for the fetal period, the slope of this relationship (Equation 23) corresponds to the power of total body weight to which the fetal heart is growing. The slope of this line is approximately unity,

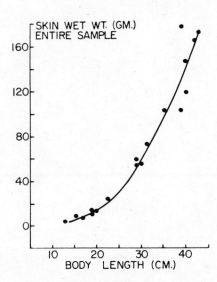

Fig. 11.5. Skin wet weight (g) as a function of body length (cm) (Equation 13).

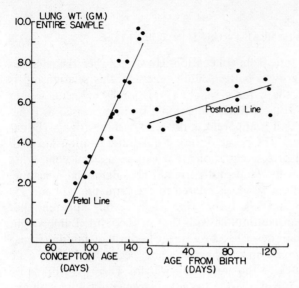

Fig. 11.6. Lung weight (g) as a function of conception age during fetal life and age from birth (days). Fetal line, Equation 14; postnatal line, Equation 15.

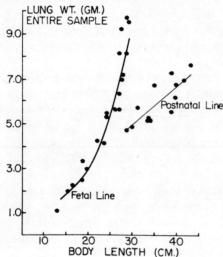

Fig. 11.7. Lung weight (g) as a function of body length (cm) during fetal life and after birth. Fetal line, Equation 18; postnatal line, Equation 19.

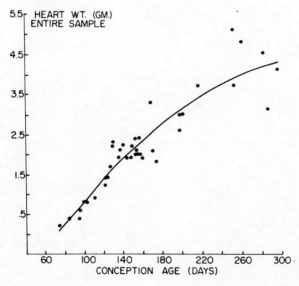

Fig. 11.8. Heart weight (g) as a function of conception age (days) (Equation 20).

indicating that the heart is growing as a constant proportion of total body weight during the fetal period.

The pattern of growth in the kidney is almost identical to that of the liver (Chapter 12) in that there is a slightly better fit for kidney weight in relation to body weight (Equation 25) than for age (Equation 24, Figure 11.9). When kidney weight is expressed against body length (Figure 11.10) unlike the liver there is no indication of nonlinearity in the fetal group. The growth pattern, therefore, is best expressed as two separate straight lines (Equations 26 and 27), the lines holding no special biologic significance but indicating that linear functions express the data best.

In sharp contrast to previous organs examined, the pituitary weight is best described by a quadratic relationship with age (Figure 11.11, Equation 28). However, when expressed as a function of body length there is a strong linear fit (Figure 11.12, Equation 29). The relationship of pituitary weight to body weight was similar to that expressed against conception age.

Figure 11.13 represents the total adrenal weight (both adrenals) expressed as a function of conception age for the fetal period only (Equation 30). Equation 31 represents the relationship with body weight. There is obviously a great deal of scatter in the data for postnatal animals. Data from other experiments in our own laboratory and those of Kerr et al[1, 2] indicate that there is a rather sharp increase in adrenal weight very near term, and a subsequent decrease to the lower weight values shown on the graphs. The curves for total adrenal weight expressed as functions of height and weight have not been plotted as they are very similar to the figure shown.

When thyroid weight during the fetal period is expressed as a function of conception age (Figure 11.14, Equation 32) or total body weight (Equation 33), the best description of the data is obtained by using a linear fit. The correlation co-

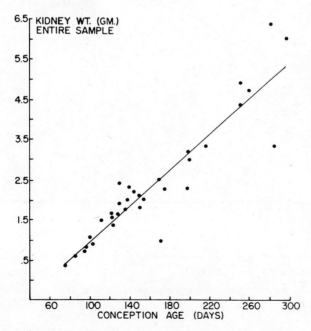

Fig. 11.9.   Kidney weight (g) as a function of conception age (days) (Equation 24).

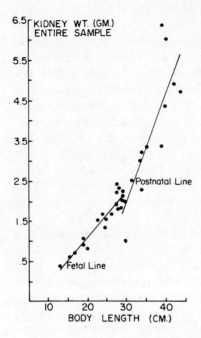

Fig. 11.10. Kidney weight (g) as a function of body length (cm). Fetal line, Equation 26; postnatal line, Equation 27.

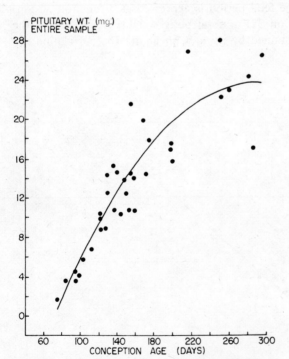

Fig. 11.11. Pituitary weight (mg) as a function of conception age (days) (Equation 28).

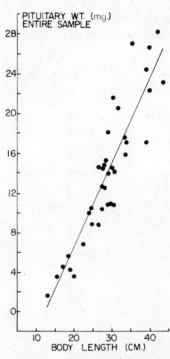

Fig. 11.12. Pituitary weight (mg) as a function of body length (cm) (Equation 29).

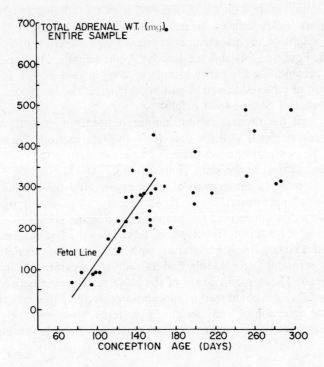

Fig. 11.13. Total adrenal weight (mg) as a function of conception age (days). Fetal line, Equation 30.

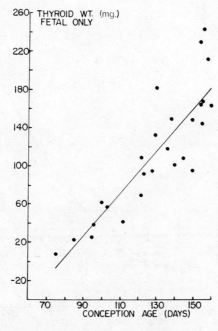

Fig. 11.14. Thyroid weight (mg) as a function of conception age (days). Fetal line, Equation 32.

223

efficients are comparable with those obtained with the adrenal weights. A similar postnatal pattern exists with considerable spread in the points.

When the weight of the pancreas is expressed as a function of conception age (Figure 11.15, Equation 34) and total body weight (Figure 11.16, Equation 35) a quadratic fit presents for the entire sample in both instances. The same holds for the relationship of pancreatic weight and body length. The quadratic fit for weight is better than that of either age or height.

The spleen and the thymus exhibit similar patterns of growth. Mathematical relationships can be fitted well for data from the fetal period (Equations 36–39). However, in the postnatal period there is too much scatter to enable any mathematical representation of the data (Figures 11.17–11.19). In this respect, some similarity exists between the growth of these organs and that of the adrenal and thyroid mentioned previously.

These relationships concerning the growth of endocrine glands may have certain implications for mechanisms involved in fetal growth. Increments in pituitary weight showed a strong linear correlation with increasing body length throughout the fetal and perinatal periods, this finding differing significantly from the other organs examined. The demonstration of the close relationship between pancreatic weight and body weight could lead to speculation that the pancreas exerts a regulatory role in the accretion of body weight in the fetus. However, the growth of the pituitary differs from the growth of the pancreas when the relationship with gesta-

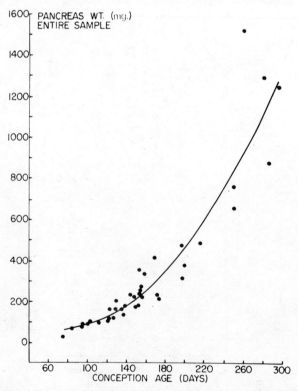

Fig. 11.15. Pancreas weight (mg) as a function of conception age (days) (Equation 34).

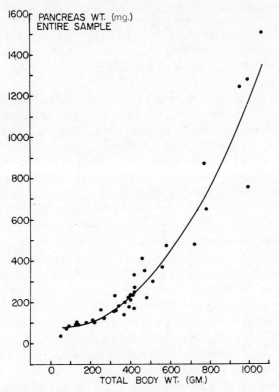

Fig. 11.16. Pancreas weight (mg) as a function of total body weight (g) (Equation 35).

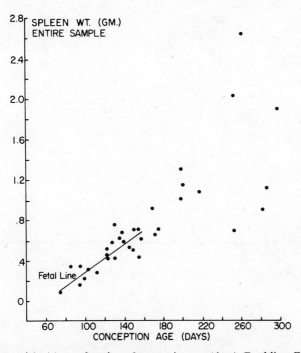

Fig. 11.17. Spleen weight (g) as a function of conception age (days). Fetal line, Equation 36.

tional age is considered (Figures 11.11 and 11.15). The curve for the data relating to the pituitary is convex, indicating a more rapid growth spurt earlier in fetal life followed by deceleration. The pancreas, however, is growing at an accelerated rate with increasing time.

The rapid increase in adrenal weight at term is possibly due to the appearance of the fetal zone of the cortex which is known to atrophy some time near birth. The data of Lanman[3] suggest that the fetal cortex of the macaque disappears prior to birth. However, his study was based on five animals with a wide range in age. If this finding is verified by more extensive studies, it would explain the involution to a total adrenal weight of 400 mg in the postnatal animal. Variation in the rate of atrophy could account for the large individual variation in weight found in this study.

Of importance is the inspection of the growth of organs from one mammal to the next and the relative growth of an organ to the body as a whole (eg, the weight of the kidney relative to the total body weight). The allometric formula (discussed in Chapter 2) can be expressed as $y = bx^k$ or $\log y = k \log x + \log b$, where y is the weight of the organ, x is the total body weight, and k is the gradient or slope of the line. By comparing the slopes for different mammals information is obtained with respect to the similarity or dissimilarity of growth of the particular organ. The use of such an approach is discussed in detail elsewhere.[7,8] The usual approach has been a comparison of organ growth between mature mammals, while here organ growth during fetal development is being examined.

It will be recalled that the growth of the brain relative to the total body weight yielded a slope of unity for the primate during fetal life, which indicated that the brain and the body were growing at the same rate.

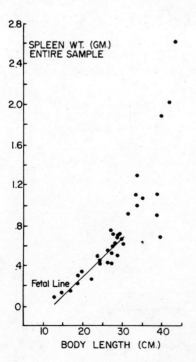

Fig. 11.18.   Spleen weight (g) as a function of body length (cm). Fetal line, Equation 37.

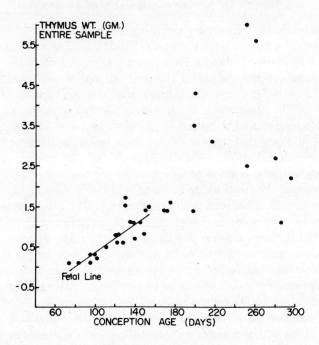

Fig. 11.19. Thymus weight (g) as a function of conception age (days). Fetal line, Equation 38.

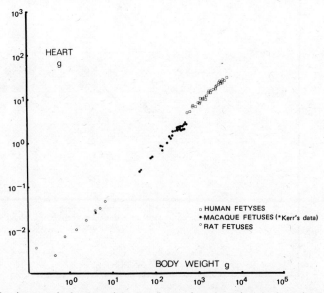

Fig. 11.20. The increase in heart weight has been plotted against body weight for the human, monkey, and rat fetus. A log-log scale has been used. (For references, see text.)

Data available in the literature concerning the human fetus[9-12] and the rat[13] have been plotted on log grids (Figures 11.20–11.25). The rate of growth of the heart (Figure 11.20) is similar for human, monkey, and rat fetus. The gradient approximates unity, again indicating the proportional growth. The figures depicting relative growth for the lung, kidney, and spleen (Figures 11.21–11.23) all show similarity. The gradients of the lines (not shown) representing the points are similar for the human and the monkey. By contrast, data for the adrenal glands (Figure 11.24) indicate that while a similar slope holds for the monkey and for the human fetus, the interception on the y axis would differ by a factor of 10, when, for example, body weight is equivalent to 1 g.

A comparison of the relationship between body weight and body length emphasizes the close similarity between primates (Figure 11.25). When the anthropometric data are considered, it becomes clear that the growth curves derived from measurements of the fetal rhesus monkey are comparable to those of human fetal growth curves.[4] This is particularly true when relating total body weight to the one-third power as a function of conception age, the lines for the human fetus and macaque fetus being almost identical.[5] The slope of the line describing this relationship was 0.059 from the data of Dawes[5] and 0.042 from Spencer et al.[6] When a linear relationship was utilized to describe points for the fetal period a slope of 0.046 evolved, which is in agreement with these earlier investigations (Figure 11.3). This similarity is of importance when normal and abnormal growth are compared using the macaque as the experimental model. In many smaller mammals, such as rabbits, guinea pigs, sheep, and rats, the expression of the fetal growth curve as a function of age yields an entirely different slope, indicating a more rapid accumulation of all body constituents.[6]

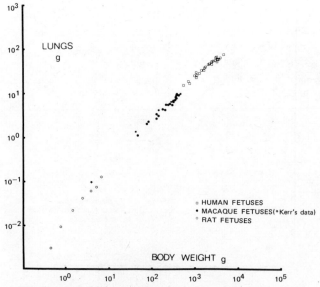

Fig. 11.21. The increase in lung weight has been plotted against body weight for the human, monkey, and rat fetus. A log-log scale has been used. (For references, see text.)

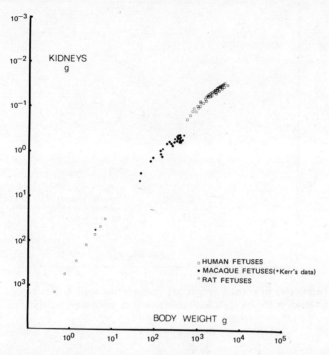

Fig. 11.22. The increase in kidney weight has been plotted against body weight for the human, monkey, and rat fetus. A log-log scale has been used. (For references, see text.)

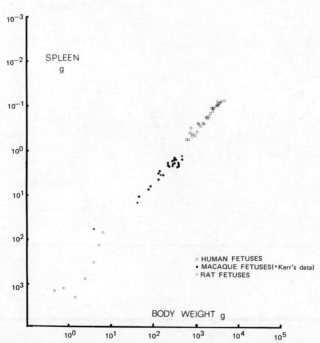

Fig. 11.23. The increase in spleen weight has been plotted against body weight for the human, monkey, and rat fetus. A log-log scale has been used. (For references, see text.)

229

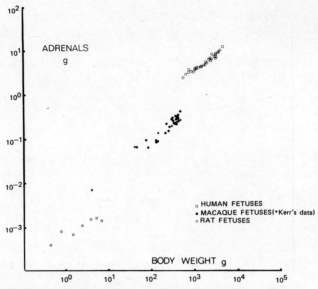

Fig. 11.24. The increase in adrenal weight has been plotted against body weight for the human, monkey, and rat fetus. A log-log scale has been used. (For references, see text.)

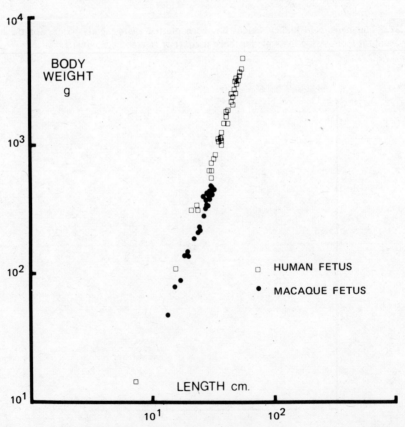

Fig. 11.25. The relationship between body weight and body length for the fetal macaque and human. A log-log scale has been used. (For references, see text.)

In summary, this chapter describes the growth pattern of fetal and postnatal rhesus monkeys with respect to total body weight and major components of the body. In most instances the growth curves are related to time although a number of organs are better related to height or weight. The data, in some cases, have been transformed to express mathematical relationships. This is illustrated well in transformation to a log-log scale of organ growth data allowing the computation of relative growth rates. Comparisons have been made with human growth and that of other mammals indicating that the intrauterine growth slope during late gestation is similar. These relationships may be of considerable help in the interpretation of experiments in which growth has been altered and in the extrapolation of such experiments to human disorders.

REFERENCES

1. Kerr, G. R., Kennan, A. L., Waisman, H. A., and Allen, J. R.: Growth and development of the fetal rhesus monkey. 1. Physical growth. *Growth* **33**: 201, 1969.

2. Kerr, G. R., and Waisman, H. A.: Fetal biology of the rhesus monkey. *Medical Primatology, 1970. Proc. 2nd Conf. Exp. Med. Surg. Primates, New York, 1969.* Karger, Basel, 1971, p. 590.

3. Lanman, J. T.: The adrenal fetal zone: Its occurrence in primates and a possible relationship to chorionic gonadotropin. *Endocrinology* **61**: 684, 1957.

4. Roberts, R. C.: On the lineal growth of the human foetus. *Lancet* **1**: 295, 1906.

5. Dawes, G. S.: *Foetal and Neonatal Physiology.* Yearbook, Chicago, 1969, p. 52.

6. Spencer, R. P., Coulombe, M. J., and van Wagenen, G.: Intraspecies comparison of fetal growth. *Growth* **30**: 1, 1966.

7. Naroll, R. S., and von Bertalanffy, L.: The principle of allometry in biology and the social sciences. *Gen. Systems* **1**: 76, 1956.

8. von Bertalanffy, L., and Priozynski, W. J.: Ontogenetic and evolutionary allometry. *Evolution* **6**: 387, 1952.

9. Potter, E. H., and Adair, F. L.: *Fetal and Neonatal Death.* University of Chicago Press, Chicago, 1949.

10. Schulz, D. M., Giordano, D. A., and Schulz, D. H.: Weights of organs of fetuses and infants. *Arch. Pathol.* **74**: 244, 1962.

11. Gruenwald, P., and Minh, H. N.: Evaluation of body and organ weights in perinatal pathology. 1. Normal standards derived from autopsies. *Am. J. Obstet. Gynecol.* **34**: 247, 1960.

12. Emery, J. L., and Methal, A.: The weights of kidneys in late intra-uterine life and childhood. *J. Clin. Pathol.* **13**: 490, 1960.

13. Sikov, M. R., and Thomas, J. M.: Prenatal growth of the rat. *Growth* **34**: 1, 1970.

CHAPTER 12

Growth of the Liver

Donald E. Hill

Doljanski[1] has reviewed the processes of normal liver growth in mammalian and avian species. Morphologically the adult liver is unique in that varied metabolic functions, which in other organs are carried out by different types of cells, are performed by one cell type. Therefore, a study of liver growth in the fetus is concerned not only with the overall increase in size but also with a changing population of cell types. Differences appear in the rate of change in the cell population when comparisons are made between species. The relative liver weight, that is, the weight of the liver per 100 g body weight, decreases during the embryonic growth of mammals,[1] this being partly due to the involution of hemopoietic islands in the liver during the embryonic phase. A fall in the relative number of hepatic cells per 100 g body weight which correlates with the decreasing rate of growth of the fetus has been demonstrated by Dick[2] in the fetal sheep. On the basis of this observation he hypothesized that the relative number of hepatic cells in the fetus is determined by the functional requirements of body growth and metabolism. The relative liver weight of the human fetus in late pregnancy is about 5.2 per 100 g body weight compared with the rhesus monkey at term, which is approximately 2.8 per 100 g body weight.[1, 3, 4]

In this chapter the somatic and cellular growth of the liver in the fetal and postnatal rhesus monkey is reported and compared with human liver growth. The mathematical relationships derived from the data and cited in the following paragraphs are presented in Table 12.1.

Figures 12.1 and 12.2 outline the growth of the macaque liver in relation to conception age (Equation 1) and body length (Equation 2), respectively. The relationship with total body weight (Equation 3) is similar to that of conception age but is more precise. There is no apparent discontinuity at birth; therefore the overall sample is shown and the line represents continuous growth through the postnatal period. As was previously seen, in relating organ growth to length, a quadratic fit

Table 12.1 Equations describing liver composition in Macaca mulatta.

	TIME SPAN	n	Y units	X units	Equation Y =	SD	Fit
1.	80 days CA to 120 days PN	38	Liver weight (g)	CA (days)	$-6.7278 + 0.12063 (X)$	2.52	0.001 linear r=0.93
2.	80 days CA to 120 days PN	38	Liver weight (g)	Body length (cm)	$4.7234 - 0.48934 (X) + 0.025038 (X)^2$	1.30	0.001 quadratic
3.	80 days CA to 120 days PN	38	Liver weight (g)	Total Body weight (g)	$1.0956 + 0.02719 (X)$	1.22	0.001 linear r=0.98
4.	80 days CA to 160 days CA	26	DNA mg/g	CA (days)	$14.87797 - 0.07169 (X)$	1.23	0.001 linear r=-0.83
5.	80 days CA to 160 days CA	26	DNA mg/g	CA (days)	$-487.87906 + 13.239 (X) - 0.10954 (X)^2 + 0.0003026 (X)^3$	5.98	0.01 cubic
6.	Birth to 120 days PN	12	DNA mg/g	PN (days)	$46.26133 + 0.59912 (X)$	15.39	0.001 linear r=0.87
7.	80 days CA to 160 days CA	26	Protein mg/g	CA (days)	$188.70692 - 0.34348 (X)$	11.14	0.001 linear r=-0.63
8.	Birth to 120 days PN	12	Protein mg/g	PN (days)	$156.50220 + 0.45933 (X)$	13.68	0.01 linear r=0.83

No.	Period	Variable	Units	Equation		Significance
9.	80 days CA to 160 days CA	Protein g	CA (days)	$-0.98040 + 0.01743\,(X)$	0.176	0.001 linear $r=0.93$
10.	Birth to 120 days PN	Protein g	PN (days)	$1.90024 + 0.03118\,(X)$	0.815	0.001 linear $r=0.86$
11.	80 days CA to 120 days PN	Prot: DNA	CA (days)	$-17.92734 + 0.47968\,(X) -0.00087504\,(X)^2$	4.86	0.01 quadratic
12.	80 days CA to 120 days PN	RNA: DNA	CA (days)	$-0.06674 + 0.017565\,(X) -0.000038784\,(X)^2$	0.244	0.01 quadratic
13.	80 days CA to 120 days PN	$\%H_2O$	CA (days)	$84.57803 - 0.099536\,(X) +0.00017942\,(X)^2$	1.164	0.01 quadratic
14.	80 days CA to 120 days PN	Plasma Proteins g%	CA (days)	$-2.33768 + 0.059176\,(X) -0.00010087\,(X)^2$	0.508	0.001 quadratic

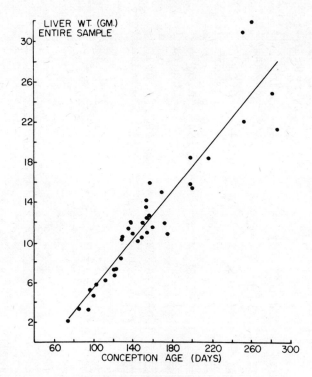

Fig. 12.1. Liver weight (g) as a function of conception age (days) (Equation 1).

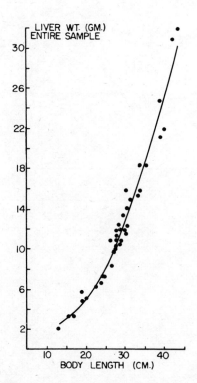

Fig. 12.2. Liver weight (g) as a function of body length length (cm) (Equation 2).

adequately expresses the data. The precision of this line is comparable to that for body weight.

The growth of the liver relative to the increase in body weight during the gestational period of the human,[5-7] macaque, and rat [8] is depicted in Figure 12.3. (Additional information on normal rat liver growth is available from a number of sources).[3, 9-12] The slopes of the growth curves are very similar, indicating a close parallel between the three mammals in growth rate relative to body weight during fetal life. Although the liver appears to be growing at a constant rate relative to body weight, when log-log conversions of the liver weight and body weight are made for the fetal period, the coefficient is 0.84, compared to a value of 1 for organs such as heart and cerebrum. This indicates that the fetal rate of growth of the liver is slower than that of the heart and cerebrum or that of the body as a whole. In a comparison of postnatal liver growth between human and subhuman primates, the reported slopes of the growth curves were 0.87 for the human and 0.93 for the subhuman primate, indicating that the similarity persists after birth.[13]

The chemical composition of the fetal liver has been reported for both human[14] and rhesus monkey.[15, 16] Although other organs have been studied extensively with respect to their cellular growth it, was not until 1972 that Widdowson et al[17] systematically documented the cellular development of the human liver prior to birth.

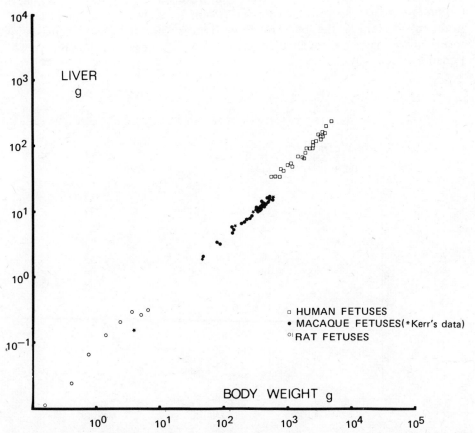

Fig. 12.3. The growth of the liver relative to the body as a whole for man, macaque, and the rat during fetal life.

In Figure 12.4 the DNA concentration in fresh liver is shown plotted against gestational days and postnatal days. There is a sharp decline in liver concentration of DNA from 80 days to 160 days (Equation 4), at which time the DNA concentration appears to reach a constant value (mean concentration of DNA = 4.1 mg/g) and remains so through postnatal life. A similar pattern is seen in developing chicks, [18] rats,[19-21] and humans.[17] This decline in DNA concentration could possibly be explained by the involution of some of the hematopoietic elements in the liver, as well as a relative greater increase in protein and lipid as the liver matures. There is, however, an increase in the total DNA (Figure 12.5) when the values are plotted against gestational age (Equations 5 and 6). The pattern of increase in total DNA is similar to that described by Widdowson et al[17] for human fetuses. The increase is not as rapid when plotted on comparable logarthmic scales. The macaque data were collected after midgestation and the growth rate was obviously slower than that for human liver.

In most species the amount of ploidy present in liver at birth is small, and in man it is estimated that up to the age of 6 years most liver cells are diploid.[22] The information is not known for the rhesus monkey. It is possible that the majority of cells in the liver of fetal monkeys, as in the human, are diploid in type.

In contrast, the protein concentration decreases slightly in fetal life (Equation 7) and increases slowly in postnatal life to adult values (Equation 8, Figure 12.6). These data are similar to those of Kerr and Waisman.[15] In humans, the concentration of nitrogen (protein) increases 11% from 13 weeks of gestation to term.[14] In the rhesus monkey, the total protein in liver, as with total DNA, increases in a steady linear manner throughout prenatal and early postnatal life (Figure 12.7, Equations 9 and 10).

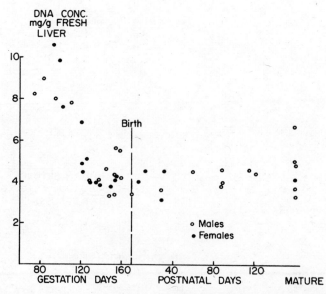

Fig. 12.4. Changes in DNA concentration for the fetal liver of the macaque against time.

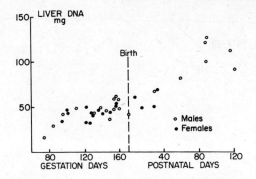

Fig. 12.5. Total DNA within the liver is shown relative to time in the fetal macaque.

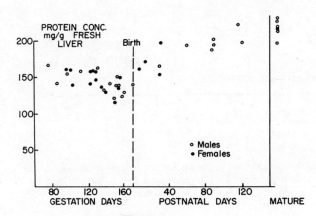

Fig. 12.6. Protein concentration in the liver is plotted against time in the fetal macaque. Note the decrease prior to birth, a finding that agrees with the work of Kerr and Waisman.[15]

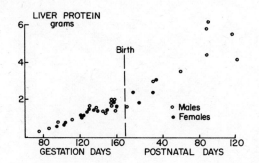

Fig. 12.7. The change in protein content with time in the fetal macaque liver.

The protein:DNA ratio, as defined earlier, can be used as an index of cell size at some specific point of study, provided that the amount of polyploidy is not significant or provided the increase in cytoplasm is commensurate. Polyploidy in fetal life is minimal; therefore Figure 12.8 documents the rapid increase in cell size at 120 days of gestation (Equation 11). In postnatal life it is likely that the incidence of polyploidy increases up to 50% of the total cell population. Therefore the protein: DNA ratio may be a less valid index of cell size. In humans, the increase in the protein:DNA ratio occurs during the last 10 weeks of gestation[17] and the pattern of growth is very similar to that of the rhesus monkey (Figure 12.8). The changes in RNA concentration parallel those in protein concentration. In the rhesus monkey, the increase in the RNA:DNA ratio after 120 days of gestation is similar to that of the protein:DNA ratio (Figure 12.9, Equation 12).

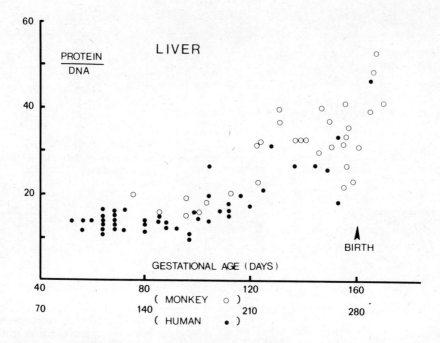

Fig. 12.8. The protein:DNA ratio (index of cell size) is shown for the human fetus and for the macaque. Note that the protein:DNA ratio increases for the macaque after 120 days of gestation and the increase for the human fetus are similar (last trimester). The human data are from the work of Widdowson et al.[17]

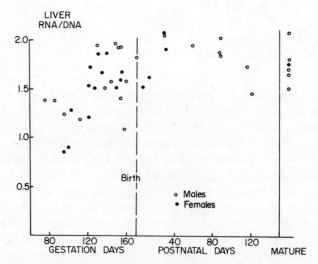

Fig. 12.9. The relationship of RNA to DNA is shown for the fetal macaque liver.

The percentage of water in fresh liver follows the pattern of other body organs in that a reduction occurs with increasing gestational age and postnatal life, the adult values leveling off at 68 to 71% (Figure 12.10, Equation 13). This is consistent with the data of Kerr and Waisman.[15] We do not have data on the glycogen content of liver throughout prenatal life; however, the level in control animals at term was 60 mg/g of fresh liver and was reduced within 10 to 20 hours to very low levels, 5 mg/g.[24] In monkeys, overnight fasting will decrease the glycogen level in the liver to less than 4 mg/g (unpublished data).

Finally, in view of the important role the liver plays in protein synthesis and in the regulation of protein degradation, the increase in plasma protein concentration relative to conception age is presented (Figure 12.11, Equation 14).

In summary the pattern of liver growth in the rhesus monkey and man is similar. The monkey provides the investigator with a satisfactory model for further research into the nature of cellular growth in the liver.

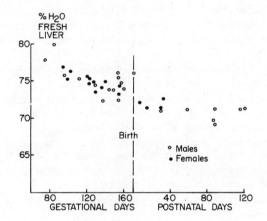

Fig. 12.10. The percentage of water in the liver is shown for the fetus and during early postnatal life.

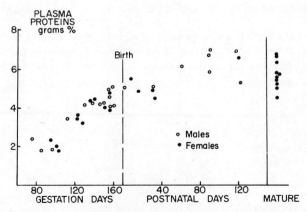

Fig. 12.11. The plasma protein concentrations prior to birth and in the early postnatal period are shown for the macaque.

REFERENCES

1. Doljanski, F.: The growth of the liver with special reference to mammals. *Int. Rev. Cytol.* **10:** 217, 1960.

2. Dick, A. T.: Growth and function in the fetal liver. *J. Embryol. Exp. Morphol.* **4:** 97, 1956.

3. Brody, S.: *Bioenergetics and Growth.* Van Nostrand-Reinhold, Princeton, New Jersey, 1945, p. 641.

4. Dawes, G. S.: *Fetal Physiology.* Yearbook, Chicago, 1968, Chapter 1.

5. Gruenwald, P., and Minh, H. N.: Evaluation of body and organ weights in perinatal pathology. I. Normal standards derived from autopsies. *Am. J. Obstet. Gynecol.* **34:** 247, 1960.

6. Schulz, D. M., Giordano, D. A., and Schulz, D. H.: Weights of organs of fetuses and infants. *Arch. Pathol.* **74:** 244, 1962.

7. Potter, E. L., and Adair, F. L.: *Fetal and Neonatal Death*, 2nd ed. University of Chicago Press, Chicago, 1949.

8. Sikov, M. R., and Thomas, J. M.: Prenatal growth of the rat. *Growth* **34:** 1, 1970.

9. Williamson, M. B.: Growth of the liver in fetal rats. *Growth* **12:** 145, 1948.

10. Givol, D. M.: Sci. Thesis, Department of Zoology, Hebrew University, Jerusalem, 1957.

11. Leblond, C. P., and Walker, B. E.: Renewal of cell populations. *Physiol. Rev.* **36:** 255, 1956.

12. Cheek, D. B.: *Human Growth.* Lea & Febiger, Philadelphia, 1968, Chapter 21.

13. Stahl, W. R., and Gummerson, J. Y.: Systematic allometry in five species of adult primates. *Growth* **31:** 24, 1967.

14. Widdowson, E. M.: Growth and composition of the fetus and newborn. In *Biology of Gestation*, Ed. Assali, N. S. Vol. 2. Academic Press, New York, 1968.

15. Kerr, G. R., and Waisman, H. A.: Fetal biology of the rhesus monkey. *Medical Primatology, 1970. Proc. Conf. Exp. Med. Surg. Primates, New York*, 1969. Karger, Basel, 1971, p. 590.

16. Hill, D. E., Myers, R. E., Holt, A. B., Scott, R. E., and Cheek, D. B.: Fetal growth retardation produced by experimental placental insufficiency in the rhesus monkey. II. Biochemical constituents of the carcass, brain, liver and muscle. *Biol. Neonate* **19:** 68, 1971.

17. Widdowson, E. M., Crabb, D. E., and Milner, R. D. G.: Cellular development of some human organs before birth. *Arch. Dis. Child.* **47:** 652, 1972.

18. Weston, J. C.: The effect of cortisone on some chemical constituents of developing chick liver. *Growth* **20:** 75, 1956.

19. Geschwind, I., and Li, C. H.: Nucleic acid content of fetal rat liver. *J. Bio. Chem.* **180:** 467, 1949.

20. Fukuda, M., and Sibatani, A.: Biochemical studies on number and composition of liver cells in postnatal growth of the rat. *J. Biochem.* **40:** 95, 1953.

21. Cheek, D. B., and Graystone, J. E.: Changes in enzymes (GOT and GDH) and metals (Zn, Mn, and Mg) in liver of rats during endocrine imbalance and caloric restriction. *Pediatr. Res.* **3:** 433, 1969.

22. Swartz, F. J.: The development in the human liver of multiple deoxyribose nucleic acid (DNA) classes and their relationship to the age of the individual. *Chromosoma* **8:** 53, 1956.

23. Shelley, H. J.: Glycogen reserves and their changes at birth. *Br. Med. Bull.* **17:** 137, 1961.

24. Shelley, H. J., and Neligan, G. A.: Neonatal hypoglycaemia. *Br. Med. Bull.* **22:** 34, 1966.

CHAPTER 13

Muscle Development in the Fetus

Donald B. Cheek, Clarissa H. Beatty, Rachel E. Scott, and Rose Mary Bocek

GROWTH OF SKELETAL AND CARDIAC MUSCLE

Donald B. Cheek and Rachel E. Scott

Introduction

Embryonic muscle begins its development when myoblasts differentiate from the primitive mesodermal cells, replicate, and eventually fuse to form the embryonic myotube. The work of Yaffe and Fuchs[1] and Marchok and Herrman[2] shows that the synthetic processes in the myoblast are primarily concerned with the formation of nucleic acids necessary for protein synthesis and for nuclear replication. With the fusion of myoblasts to form myotubes, there is probably a major shift from DNA replication to protein synthesis within the myotube. The available data suggest that the endocrine system may control the time at which these two processes or stages occur, as discussed in this chapter. With fusion of single myogenic cells to form multinucleated myotubes,[3,4] there are changes in metabolic patterns of the participating cells which affect enzymes and structural proteins.[5] For example, there is a decrease in the rate of total RNA synthesis in fused as compared with unfused cells [1] and also an abrupt inhibition of DNA synthesis in the fused cells with a concomitant rapid decline in DNA polymerase which is not accompanied by an increase in DNAase.[6,7]

Some Observations on Chick Embryo Muscle

Love and his co-workers[8] have studied the endocrine regulation of embryonic muscle development in the chick. In early work in 1958 Love and Konigsberg produced hypophysectomy in the chick embryo by partial decapitation[9] and thyroid ablation by the injection of thiourea.[10] The work suggested that the endocrine system played a role in regulating the pattern of growth in embryonic muscle. In the normal embryo a sharp decrease in DNA accumulation occurs after the 16th day (term is 20 days) which is accompanied by an increase in total protein accretion. These changes did not occur in experimental embryos with partial decapitation; at term there was a 20% increase in the DNA content of the muscle over that of the control animals.

At the 16th day the morphology of normal embryonic muscle in the chick embryo is similar to that of adult muscle. The myotubes are similar; the nuclei are located peripherally; and the myofibrils are in compact units in the center of the fiber. Very few extrasarcolemmal nuclei (either myoblast or fibroblast) are present. However, in the hypophysectomized chick, the usual decrease in myoblasts with a corresponding increase in myotubes does not occur. Even with a transplanted pituitary, the ratio of myoblasts to myotubes tends to remain the same. In the normal embryo it is difficult to identify myoblasts by day 18 since they are incorporated with the myotube. In pituitary insufficiency, however, the myoblasts are still replicating and have not formed myotubes, hence the increase in DNA. The myotubes that have been formed are larger than normal. These results are supported by the work of De la Haba et al[11] who showed *in vitro* that growth hormone and insulin produce enhanced fusion of myoblasts. However, it is possible that hormones control only the rate at which the two major events occur and not the actual fusion of myoblasts or DNA replication.

Of further interest from the work of Love et al was the demonstration that in term embryos that have been subjected to hypophysectomy, the nuclei within the myoblasts were not diploid but tetraploid, indicating that division was still taking place but was not complete. Hypophysectomized embryos receiving pituitary transplants remained in an intermediate position with some tetraploid and some diploid nuclei. With cessation of DNA replication a decrease in RNA synthesis occurred in the chick embryo, a twofold decrease in RNA content of chick muscle being shown from day 9 to 18 by Marchok and Wolff.[12]

The DNA Unit and Muscle Growth

At the turn of the last century it was shown that in the human, the mean cross-sectional area of muscle fibers at birth increased ninefold during subsequent growth.[15,16] A tenfold increase in fiber diameter has been shown for other mammals.[17–22] The measurement of fiber diameter or cross-sectional area, however, throws little light on the actual increase in fiber mass, which is three dimensional. Studies on mice have indicated that fiber length correlates with the growth of lean body mass;[23,24] this parameter may indicate total muscle growth more accurately.

Whether or not fiber numbers increase after birth is a contentious subject since apparent increments could arise from myotubes present at birth.[25–27] Tello[28] and Montgomery[29] believe fiber numbers increase in the human postnatally.

The nuclei within the myofibers move to the periphery of the cell, being displaced by the myofibrils; this is apparent in the human during the last trimester as shown by MacCallum in 1898.[16] Surrounding the muscle bundles discrete connective tissue sheaths exist but collagen per se does not make up more than 1% of the fresh weight of a sample taken from muscle.[30] Histiocytes, fibroblasts, neuronal cells, adipocytes, or endothelial cells (from capillaries) may be present in muscle so that the DNA content of the sample is not entirely within the myofiber. Dr. Charles Freidman working in our laboratory and using the method of Dunnill[31] found that 25% of nuclei were outside the myofiber.

This realization led to the concept of "the DNA unit."[32] It was suggested that each nucleus within the myofiber has jurisdiction over a certain volume or mass of cytoplasm to form the DNA unit, and that the protein:DNA ratio comprises a functional measure of muscle cell size.

Cytoplasmic mass may be measured by the distribution of chloride outside the myotubes. Chloride accounts for the extracellular space including the connective tissue phase of muscle[33] and, unlike nitrate or sulfate, penetrates the transverse and longitudinal canals within the myofiber[34] which are important for muscle contraction. The continuity of these canals with the extracellular phase has not been recognized when, for example, the distribution of chloride is compared with the distribution of nitrate or sulfate.[35] Muscle weight minus the chloride space is therefore a measure of cytoplasmic mass and together with a knowledge of the number of nuclei per gram, one can measure the DNA unit. In other words, one gram of muscle minus the extracellular fluid in that gram, divided by the number of nuclei per gram equals one unit. More simply the protein per gram divided by the number of nuclei per gram (from the DNA content) also equals one unit.

Within human muscle the DNA increases up to 20-fold postnatally as shown by Cheek et al.[32] Thus the old thesis that all muscle growth involved only increments in fiber size is no longer tenable. Muscle contains only diploid nuclei, and mitotic division within the myofiber is almost never observed.[32] If nuclei within the myofiber do not undergo mitosis, how is it that DNA increases within the myofiber? In 1961 Mauro[36] described the satellite cell which is a mononucleated cell that is wedged between the basal or plasma membrane of the muscle fiber and the myotube. These cells are abundant during embryonic life and it is not clear how they participate in myogenesis. However, during muscle repair, these cells incorporate tritiated thymidine; thus it is clear that they participate in muscle repair [37, 38] and it would appear that they could be the progenitors of the myoblast. Moreover, each new nucleus donated from the satellite cell to the myofiber is possibly responsible for the synthesis of a given number of myofibrils.[39]

Thus the satellite cell is the most likely candidate for the cell that undergoes DNA replication and the cell that is influenced by hormonal and nutritional factors during normal and abnormal growth.[32, 40] According to Lee [41] and Klinkerfuss[42] the plasma membrane surrounding satellite cells penetrates into the sarcoplasm and additional nuclei are added to the myofiber. Shafiq et al[43] noted that satellite cells are so close to the myofibers that the nuclei appear by microscopy to be within the myotube. Kelly and Zacks[44] and Wirsen and Larsson[45] have discussed the role of the satellite cell during embryological development.

Observations on Skeletal Muscle Growth in Macaca Mulatta

The work of Beatty and Bocek (see the latter part of this chapter) has shown that the muscle mass makes up 20 to 25% of the body weight from midgestation until term. Our own work has shown that of the carcass (muscle mass plus skeletal mass) approximately 50% is muscle by weight. Since in neonatal monkeys and in older primates the values for DNA and protein content in various muscle groups show agreement[32] it is valid to assume that a sample of muscle taken from the gastrocnemius muscle is representative of the total muscle mass.

The nuclear number in muscle rises from 5×10^9 to about 40×10^9 from midgestation to term, an eightfold increase (Figure 13.1; see Table 13.1, Equation 1). The concentration of DNA falls from a value of 3 mg/g muscle in midgestation, to a value of 2 at birth (Figure 13.2, Equation 3), and to a value of 1 at maturation. As cytoplasmic growth increases the nuclei become more sparsely separated.

Protein:DNA ratio (milligram per milligram) increases from a value of 30 units at midgestation to 80 units at birth, a 2.6-fold increase. Following birth cytoplasmic growth continues and at 100 days postnatally the ratio is 140 units. This is well below the value of 240 units for the mature rhesus monkey (Figure 13.3, Equation 2). The concentration of protein (Figure 13.4) increases steadily from midgestation until birth, then a stable value is reached (Equations 4–6).

The percent water content of muscle falls steeply shortly after midgestation until birth but reaches a steady state after birth (Figure 13.5, Equations 7 and 8).

In figure 13.6 the chloride space per 100 grams of muscle is shown (Cl content divided by the concentration of Cl in a plasma ultrafiltrate) together with the nonchloride space (total water minus the chloride space in 100 grams of muscle). From midgestation the amount of cell water per 100 grams of muscle (nonchloride space) increases significantly while the extracellular volume decreases (Equations 9 and 10). At birth a reasonably stable or mature value is reached for cell water. Thus there is a growth of the cellular phase relative to the extracellular.

The values obtained for the concentration of chloride (as a plasma ultrafiltrate) are shown in Figure 13.7. There is an indication that the values rise from a mean of 115 prenatally to about 125 meq/l postnatally (Equation 11).

The RNA concentration falls with time from midgestation until birth. In view of the previous discussion this finding is not unexpected if myoblastic or satellite cell activity diminishes as birth approaches. A further decrease in RNA concentration would appear to occur after birth (Figure 13.8, Equation 12). The RNA:DNA ratio remained constant from 80 days prenatally to 120 days postnatally (Figure 13.9).

Very little information of this nature is available for the human fetus. Widdowson et al[46] studied muscle and myocardial growth in 28 fetuses delivered by hysterotomy for therapeutic abortion and also 28 fresh stillborn or live-born infants who died within the first week of life. All fetuses were normal on clinical judgment. The amount of DNA in the two gastrocnemius muscles doubled each week between the 14th and 25th week of gestation. Thereafter the rate of increase declined. By contrast the increment in protein:DNA ratio was not very remarkable from the middle of the first trimester until the beginning of the third. From 30 weeks of gestation until birth (or shortly after) there was a steep rise from 40 units to 120. A comparison between these data and those in *Macaca mulatta* has been made (Figure 13.10).

Observations on Myocardial Growth in Macaca Mulatta

Observations by Miller[47] on rats during the suckling period show that initially the heart grows at a rate similar to the body but eventually the body growth outstrips

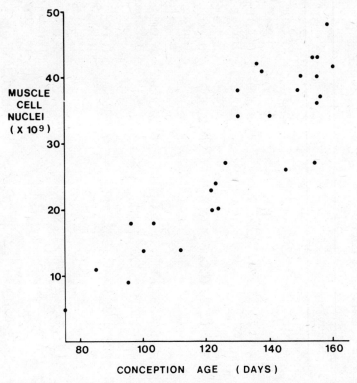

Fig. 13.1. The increment in number of nuclei with time in the skeletal muscle of the fetal macaque.

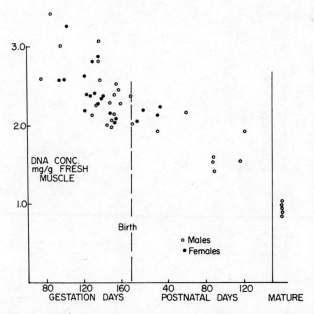

Fig. 13.2. The relationship between DNA concentration and time in the skeletal muscle of the fetal and postnatal macaque.

Table 13.1   The mathematical relationship describing biochemical changes in skeletal muscle during the development of the macaque in the fetal and perinatal period

	Time span	n	Y units	X units	Equation Y =	SD	Fit
1.	80 days CA to birth	26	MCP* x 10^9	CA (days)	$-30.271 + 0.456\,(X)$	4.490	0.001 linear
2.	80 days CA to 120 days PN	38	Prot/DNA	CA (days)	$-9.57445 + 0.53577\,(X)$	10.6309	0.001 linear r = 0.94
3.	80 days CA to 120 days PN	39	DNA FFFM mg/g	CA (days)	$3.31743 - 0.00664\,(X)$	0.283037	0.001 linear r = -0.80
4.	80 days CA to 120 days PN	39	Prot FFFM mg/g	CA (days)	$-69.23325 + 2.1858\,(X) - 0.0041925\,(X)^2$	8.97566	0.001 quadratic
5.	80 days CA to 160 days CA	26	Prot FFFM mg/g	CA (days)	$-9.22393 + 1.15373\,(X)$	7.75662	0.001 linear r = 0.97
6.	Birth to 120 days PN	13	Prot FFFM mg/g	PN (days)	$193.52564 + 0.17936\,(X)$	6.50773	0.01 linear r = 0.79
7.	80 days CA to 120 days PN	39	% H$_2$O	(CA days)	$114.96209 - 0.44322\,(X) + 0.0017103\,(X)^2 - 0.0000022240\,(X)^3$	0.916187	0.01 cubic

No.		N				
8.	80 days CA to 160 days CA	26	% H_2O	CA (days)	$28.89810 + 1.8360 (X) - 0.017763 (X)^2 + 0.000051685 (X)^3$	0.688026	0.001 cubic
9.	80 days CA to 120 days PN	35	Cl space mg/g	CA (days)	$1.74912 - 0.020716 (X) + 0.00009089 (X)^2 - 0.00000013439 (X)^3$	0.058821	0.05 cubic
10.	80 days CA to 120 days PN	35	Non-Cl space mg/g	CA (days)	$-0.58413 + 0.015875 (X) - 0.000070457 (X)^2 + 0.0000001051 (X)^3$	0.052725	0.05 cubic
11.	80 days CA to 120 days PN	39	Cl^- plasma ultrafiltrate (mEq/L plasma H_2O)	CA (days)	$108.01890 + 0.07352 (X)$	5.2358	0.001 linear r = 0.63
12.	80 days CA to 120 days PN	39	RNA FFFM mg/g	CA (days)	$3.85364 - 0.00906 (X)$	0.345629	0.001 linear r = -0.83

Key: CA = Days from conception; PN = Postnatal days; SD = Standard deviation; N = Number of subjects

FFFM = Fresh fat free muscle

* MCP = Muscle cell population i.e. cell No. per gram x $\dfrac{\text{lean carcass mass}}{2}$

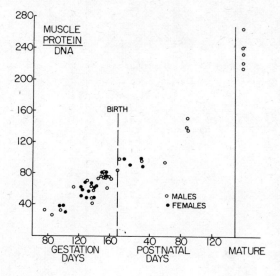

Fig. 13.3. The relationship of the protein:DNA ratio with time in skeletal muscle in the macaque.

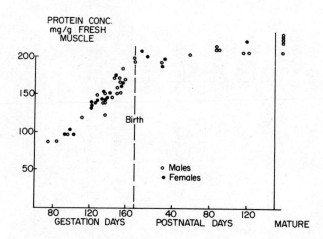

Fig. 13.4. The change in protein concentration with time in skeletal muscle in the macaque.

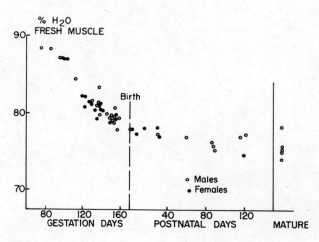

Fig. 13.5. The change with time in the percentage of water in skeletal muscle in the macaque.

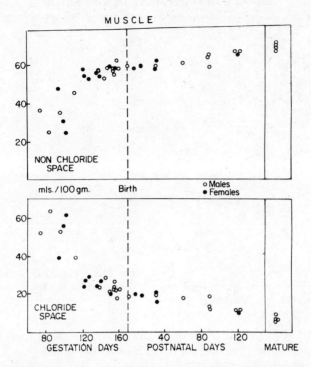

Fig. 13.6. The change with time of the values for chloride and nonchloride space per 100 grams of skeletal muscle in the macaque.

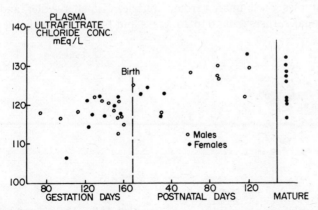

Fig. 13.7. The change with time of the chloride concentration (plasma ultrafiltrate) in the fetal macaque.

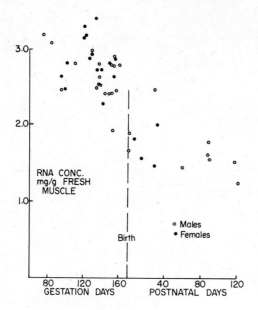

Fig. 13.8. The change with time of the RNA concentration in skeletal muscle in the macaque.

that of the heart. For the rat the protein content of the heart increases until just after sexual maturation. The work of Rakuson and Poupal (cited by Miller[47]) indicates that cytoplasmic protein and contractile protein concentrations reach maxima at the time of sexual maturation (40 days). These concentrations then fall until day 120. Stromal proteins increase only slightly postnatally (birth to 40 days). Enesco and Leblond[48] showed that for the rat embryo the total DNA content increased from day 7 until day 48 postnatally.

Widdowson et al[46] have reported some values for the human fetal heart. The total DNA in the whole heart increased from the first trimester to term (14–40 weeks) from 0.5 to 32 mg, the amount of DNA in heart doubling each week from the 14th to 25th week of gestation, with a subsequent decline in the rate of increase. At term the total DNA was 20% of the adult value. The protein:DNA ratio increased in the last 10 weeks of gestation. Before 30 weeks of gestation the increase was only gradual.

In other studies on human cardiac muscle, Kapeller-Adler and Hammad[49] studied 14 human fetuses from 6 to 20 weeks and found for the heart that the RNA

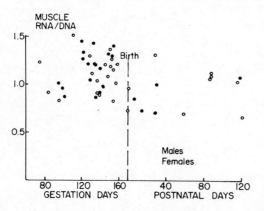

Fig. 13.9. The change with time of the RNA:DNA ratio in skeletal muscle of the macaque.

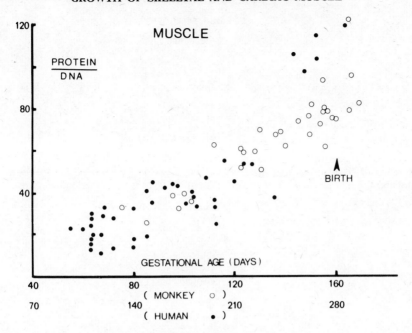

Fig. 13.10. The ratio of protein to DNA in skeletal muscle of the macaque and human. The human data are taken from Widdowson et al;[46] the gestational period for the monkey has been scaled to make it equivalent to that of the human.

and DNA concentrations were highest early in pregnancy, both falling thereafter. The RNA:DNA ratio remained relatively stable during the period of study. The protein:DNA ratio increased steeply during the first half of gestation.

We have studied the ventricular muscle of the rhesus monkey with respect to the concentration of certain components. Total ventricular weight was not measured but in a previous chapter it was shown that the heart (like the brain) grew commensurately with the soma (total body weight) and a tenfold increase in weight occurred from midgestation to birth.

The concentration of DNA appeared to remain constant (Figure 13.11) both prenatally and postnatally, hence presumably the DNA content increased commensurately with cardiac weight (tenfold). The weight increase appeared to slow at 120 days postnatally (Chapter 11).

Protein concentration in the macaque showed a definite but small increase prior to birth and constancy was reached early in the postnatal period (Figure 13.12; see Table 13.2, Equation 1). The reverse changes occurred when the percent water was inspected; a decrease from midgestation and a more constant value for the first 120 days postnatally were observed (Figure 13.13, Equation 2). The concentration of RNA showed an overall but gradual decrease prenatally and postnatally (Figure 13.14, Equation 3). The ratio of protein to DNA showed a gradual increase (Figure 13.15, Equation 4).

It would appear that the patterns of growth are somewhat different for the rodent and primate. Work with rats suggests that the accretion of protein is greater after fetal life,[48] while for the mouse the concentration of DNA per 100 g decreases rapidly following birth and attains adult values after weaning as shown by Peterson

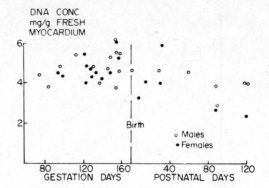

Fig. 13.11. The change with time of the concentration of DNA in the macaque myocardium.

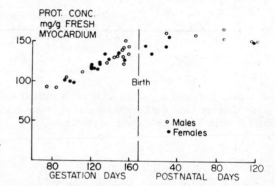

Fig. 13.12. The change with time of protein concentration in macaque myocardium.

and Baserga[50] and Walker and Adrian.[51] Moreover, the concentration of RNA decreases with time in the primate whereas RNA concentration increases for the rodent; peaks of RNA synthesis have been described for the rat by Peterson and Baserga[50] at 12 days postpartum. Our own observations on the RNA:DNA ratio (Figure 13.16, Equation 5) would indicate a gradual decline in the ratio from 80 to 160 days of gestation.

Myocardial growth patterns in primates show similarities. From our own work on *Macaca mulatta* and the work of others in the human, the cellular number in the heart (or myocardium) increases remarkably even though the cell density (DNA concentration) remains much the same in fetal and postnatal life for the monkey, and shows an actual decrease in humans.[49] Protein concentration increases slightly from midgestation in the monkey (100 mg/g to 150 at birth). In the human[46] the accretion of protein within the myocardial fibers is significant also and the accumulation of DNA at birth is 20% of the adult value. In Figure 13.17 our own data for protein:DNA ratio in myocardium are plotted on an extended time scale to coincide with the human data of Widdowson et al.[46] Although the increase prior to birth is greater in the human the similarity between the two species is striking.

Thus it would appear that during the last half of gestation, growth of the myocardium of the primate is mainly by cell number increase with a slightly greater cytoplasmic enlargement of each cell. The information available would suggest that the growth of cell number in the monkey is faster than that in the human.

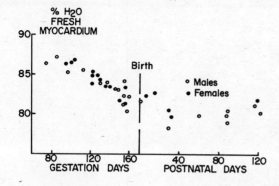

Fig. 13.13. The change with time in percent water in macaque myocardium.

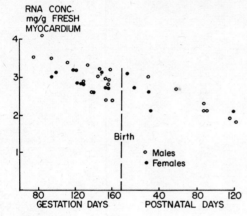

Fig. 13.14. The change with time of RNA concentration in the macaque myocardium.

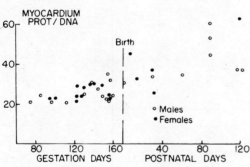

Fig. 13.15. The change with time of the ratio of protein to DNA in the macaque myocardium.

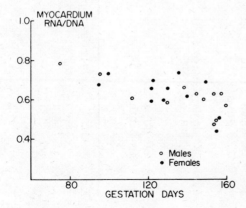

Fig. 13.16. The change with time of the ratio of RNA to DNA in the macaque myocardium.

Table 13.2 The mathematical relationships describing the biochemical changes in cardiac muscle in the macaque in the fetal and perinatal periods

	Time span	n	Y units	X units	Equation Y =	SD	Fit
1.	80 days CA to 120 days PN	38	Prot mg/g	CA (days)	$-31.44225 + 1.5934\,(X) - 0.0033028\,(X)^2$	15.4122	0.001 quadratic
2.	80 days CA to 120 days PN	38	% H_2O	CA (days)	$85.77538 + 0.082729\,(X) - 0.0010529\,(X)^2 + 0.0000024777\,(X)^3$	0.845943	0.01 cubic
3.	80 days CA to 120 days PN	38	RNA mg/g	CA (days)	$31.99068 - 0.00725\,(X)$	0.274881	0.001 linear $r = -0.84$
4.	80 days CA to 120 days PN	38	Prot/DNA	CA (days)	$7.11620 + 0.14662\,(X)$	6.40966	0.001 linear $r = 0.80$
5.	80 days CA to birth	25	RNA/DNA	CA (days)	$1.10387 - 0.00352\,(X)$	0.089498	0.001 linear $r = -0.71$

Key: CA = Days from conception; PN = Postnatal days; SD = Standard deviation; n = Number of subjects

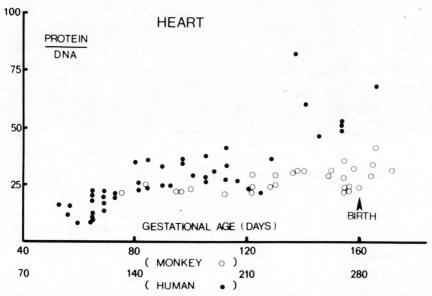

Fig. 13.17. The ratio of protein to DNA in myocardium of the macaque and human. The human data are taken from Widdowson et al;[46] the gestational period for the monkey has been scaled to make it equivalent to that of the human.

METABOLIC ASPECTS OF FETAL SKELETAL MUSCLE

Clarissa H. Beatty and Rose Mary Bocek

The percentage of body weight represented by skeletal muscle was determined by careful dissection of the total muscle mass. From 90 days fetal age to 4 days post-natally, voluntary skeletal muscle accounted for about 20 to 25% of the body weight; in the adult rhesus, this value increased to 40%. Similar values have been found in another series of monkeys by Dr. Theodore I. Grand of the Oregon Regional Primate Research Center (personal communication). In six adult macaques the percentage of body weight represented by skeletal muscle was as follows: *Macaca nigra* male, 37%; *Macaca nemestrina* male, 49%; *Macaca mulatta* male, 43%; and *Macaca mulatta* female, 40 and 41%. In a 13-month-old female *Macaca mulatta*, this value was similar to that of the adult, 39%; in three *Macaca mulatta* fetuses close to term, the value was much lower, 21 to 27%. By virtue of its mass, the metabolism of this tissue is of major importance in the total body economy and may have a greater effect on homeostasis in the adult than in the fetus or neonate.

Myotubes, present in the voluntary skeletal muscle of the rhesus fetus by 55 to 59 days of gestation, increase in number by 65 days (Figures 13.18*a* and *b*). The total number of fibers per unit area of muscle increases still more by 90 days, but depending on the area only 2 to 10% of the fibers are still at the myotube stage (Figure 13.18*c*). At 109 days, muscle contains only an occasional myotube with a central nucleus (Figure 13.18*d*), and the pattern of fiber differentiation determined by the histochemical reaction for succinic dehydrogenase resembles that of 120-day fetal and adult muscle (Figure 13.18*e*). Before 109 days, it is not possible to distinguish histochemically between red and white fibers; but by 90 days of gestation,

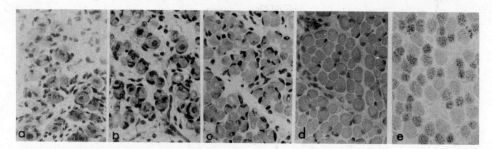

Fig. 13.18. Histological changes in rhesus fetal muscle with development: (*a*) 59 days, leg muscle. All fibers are in the myotube stage and the number of fibers per unit area is low; (*b*) 65 days, leg muscle. Fibers are in the myotube stage; (*c*) 90 days, leg muscle; the number of fibers has increased; a few myotubes are still evident; (*d*) 109 days, brachioradialis; (*e*) 109 days, brachioradialis stained for succinic dehydrogenase activity. Differentiation into the adult checkerboard pattern of small, intermediate and large sized fibers is apparent. (Sections labeled *a-d* were stained with hematoxylin-eosin; magnification ×210 in all photographs.)

quantitative differences in enzyme activity and hydroxyproline levels can be demonstrated. Red muscle has a higher succinic dehydrogenase enzyme activity and a lower hydroxyproline content than white muscle (Tables 13.3 and 13.4).[52] Although red and white muscle can be differentiated quantitatively on the basis of succinic dehydrogenase activity as early as 90 days of fetal age, the succinic dehydrogenase activity remains low throughout gestation and the first 6 weeks postpartum. By 2 years of age, adult values are reached.[52]

The nitrogen content and percent wet weight are similar in red and white muscle at each age studied (Table 13.4). Although the newborn rhesus monkey is somewhat more advanced physically than the human neonate, rhesus skeletal muscle shows histochemical differentiation into red and white fiber types at about the same time (67% of term) as human muscle (50% of term).[53]

Table 13.3 Succinic dehydrogenase activity in homogenates of soleus (Sol) and brachioradialis (BR) muscles of rhesus monkeys as measured by formazon production

Series	μg formazon/10 mg wet weight			μg formazon/mg N[o]		
	Sol	BR*	P<	Sol	BR	P <
Fetal						
90-day	1.6 ± 0.1	1.3 ± 0.1	0.02	11.9 ± 0.4	9.8 ± 0.8	0.02
120-day	3.3 ± 0.2	1.8 ± 0.2	0.005	14.2 ± 0.6	8.1 ± 1.0	0.005
150-day	3.4 ± 0.4	1.8 ± 0.2	0.005	13.5 ± 0.9	6.6 ± 1.0	0.005
Infant						
1-4 day	3.3, 3.2	1.6, 1.8		11.5, 11.4	5.3, 7.0	
2-6 week	3.5, 4.7	1.9, 2.4		11.5, 15.3	6.4, 7.6	
2-year	10.6, 11.1	2.7, 2.5		32.0, 34.0	8.1, 7.9	
Adult	10.8 ± 0.6	2.3 ± 0.3	0.005	33.1 ± 2.8	6.3 ± 0.6	0.005

Values are means $\pm$ SE. Statistical analysis on basis of paired observations.
*Samples of BR obtained from superficial portion.
[o]Kjeldahl digestion.

(Reprinted from Beatty et al: J. Histochem. Cytochem. 15: 93, 1967, with the permission of Williams & Wilkins Co.)

Table 13.4 Hydroxyproline, total nitrogen, and percent dry weight in predominantly red and white muscle of the rhesus monkey.

Series	Hydroxyproline (mg/100 g wet wt)	Hydroxyproline (mg/g N)	Nitrogen (wet wt) (g/100g)	Dry wt (%)
Fetal				
90-day red[+]	127 ± 5	99 ± 4	1.29 ± 0.03	11.9 ± 0.4
white*	169 ± 14°	132 ± 11°	1.27 ± 0.03	11.8 ± 0.4
120-day red	240 ± 11	107 ± 5	2.27 ± 0.07	18.2 ± 0.2
white	322 ± 36°°	146 ± 16°°	2.21 ± 0.08	
150-day red	245 ± 22	93 ± 8	2.63 ± 0.07	20.2 ± 0.4
white	418 ± 17**	159 ± 10**	2.62 ± 0.08	
Infant				
1-5 day red	292 ± 28	101 ± 10	2.88 ± 0.06	20.6 ± 0.4
white	386 ± 15°°	134 ± 5°°		
2-6 week red	305 ± 9	98 ± 3	3.17 ± 0.07	21.9 ± 0.3
white				
Adult red[++]	182 ± 15	56 ± 5	3.24 ± 0.05	24.3 ± 0.2
white*	353 ± 29**	108 ± 9**	3.27 ± 0.06	24.8 ± 0.2

Values are means ± SE. P values calculated on the basis of paired observations.
* Brachioradialis. + Mixed thigh muscle, predominantly red.
° P for red vs. white muscle < 0.02. °° P for red vs. white muscle < 0.05.
** P for red vs. white muscle < 0.01. ++ Sartorius.
(Reprinted from Beatty et al: J. Histochem. Cytochem. 15: 93, 1967, with the permission of Williams & Wilkins Co.)

Glycogen Metabolism

On the basis of nitrogen content, glycogen levels in rhesus fetal muscle are higher in the 50- and 65-day series than in the 100-day series but similar to those near term. Values in the neonate are low (Figure 13.19). Shelley[54] has reported similar levels for total carbohydrate in muscle from rhesus fetuses (recalculated on the basis of nitrogen). Both glycogen synthetase and phosphorylase activities can be demonstrated histochemically as early as 55 days of gestation, and synthetase I and D and phosphorylase a and b activities can be quantified as early as 78 days of gestation (Figure 13.19). Determinations on younger fetal tissues were impossible because of insufficient amounts of muscle for analysis.[55, 56] Apparently glycogen concentrations in fetal muscle cannot be attributed solely to changes in the activity of the synthetase and phosphorylase enzymes since correlation between the glycogen level and the amount of synthetase I and phosphorylase a were not always demonstrable. Glycogen levels were highest at 65 days of gestation, when synthetase I activities were low; however, between 100 and 120 days both glycogen levels and synthetase I activities rose abruptly. Phosphorylase a levels did not change much from 78 days through parturition. On the basis of total enzyme activity, the balance between synthetic and catabolic processes seems to favor glycogen deposition by about 2 to 1 at 78 days of fetal age and glycogenolysis by a similar factor near term.

The significant amount of phosphorylase and synthetase activities as early as 78 days fetal age (50% of term) suggests that glycogen stores in rhesus fetal muscle

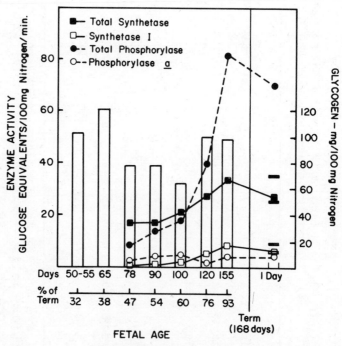

Fig. 13.19. Relationship between glycogen content, indicated by bars, and glycogen synthetase and phosphorylase. Glycogen content, in 1-day neonates, is indicated by horizontal bars. (Reprinted from Bocek et al: *Pediatic. Res.* **3**:525, 1969, with the permission of the Editor.)

are potentially available as an energy source early in gestation. Such thinking agrees with our results on muscle fiber groups incubated *in vitro*.

Glycogenolysis can be studied by incubating muscle in a medium containing glucose labeled with ^{14}C. A minimum value for glycogenolysis can be estimated by determining the dilution of the specific activity of [^{14}C]lactate formed from substrate [^{14}C]glucose by unlabeled lactate from glycogen.[57] Midway through gestation almost half of the lactate originates from glycogen. Incubation under hypoxic conditions significantly increases the lactate production and such is particularly the case close to term.

During the latter half of gestation the percent lactate formed from glycogen remains about the same but rises to 60% at term and continues at this level until 6 weeks postnatally when only 32% of lactate is formed from glycogen.

The fact that muscle glycogen can be mobilized by the fetus may be of significance. Even though muscle glycogen does not have a direct effect on circulating blood glucose levels, the principal end product of glycogenolysis, lactate, can be utilized by peripheral tissues, such as the heart, and converted to glucose in the liver. Results obtained in *in vitro* experiments may not reflect the *in vivo* situation; the data do, however, represent the potential ability of the tissues to perform specific metabolic tasks.

Respiration Rate and Glucose Utilization

For many years it was believed that the mammalian fetus develops in a hypoxic environment with a low rate of cellular metabolism.[58] However, it is difficult to reconcile this belief with the fact that the growing fetus can perform synthetic processes at a rapid rate. Synthetic processes are relatively expensive in terms of the high-energy compounds such as adenosine triphosphate. Adequate oxygenation is necessary for the efficient production of these energy stores. Recently Brinkman,[59] who studied this problem with *in vivo* preparations of mammals, including nonhuman primates, concluded that despite the low fetal blood oxygen tension, fetal oxygen consumption is maintained within the normal adult range by mechanisms such as increased hemoglobin concentration, a favorable relationship of the oxyhemoglobin dissociation curve, and increased rates of blood flow.

To explore further the respiration rate of individual fetal tissues during development, muscle fiber groups from monkeys were incubated in a medium containing 5.6 mM glucose and [^{14}C]glucose.[60] The oxygen consumption and CO_2 production of this muscle preparation from fetuses of various ages and from infants and adults were determined. The QO_2 values and the CO_2 productions were higher at 90 days, similar at 125 days, and lower at 155 days gestational age than those of adult muscle; no difference was observed between the infant and adult series (Table 13.5). These data were calculated on the basis of noncollagenous protein nitrogen (NCN) to correct for variations in the content of water and collagenous protein. The glucose uptake of this preparation of fetal muscle was higher at 90 and 125 days gestational age than that of adult muscle and similar in the 150-day fetal, neonatal, infant, and adult series (Table 13.5).

Variations in the values just given demonstrate that results on fetal metabolism must be reported for specific gestational periods. Lactate and [^{14}C]lactate produc-

Table 13.5   Oxygen consumption, CO_2 production, and glucose uptake of muscle fiber groups from the rhesus monkey

	Fetal days			Infant		Adult
	89-90	120-129	150-160	1-5 days	2-6 wk	
QO_2 μmoles/mg NCN/hr	1.11 ± 0.03*	0.69 ± 0.04	0.58 ± 0.02*		0.65 ± 0.04	0.72 ± 0.04
CO_2 μmoles/mg NCN/hr	0.84 ± 0.07*	0.52 ± 0.03	0.46 ± 0.03+			0.55 ± 0.02
Glucose uptake μg/mg NCN/hr	78 ± 6*	57 ± 2*	47 ± 1	44 ± 4	48 ± 3	42 ± 2

Muscle incubated for 2 hours in Krebs medium plus 1 mg glucose per ml medium, 1.2 uc glucose-^{14}C per ml. Values are means ± SE.   NCN = noncollagenous protein nitrogen.
* P for fetal vs. adult series <0.01.   + P for fetal vs. adult series <0.05.
(Reprinted from Beatty et al: Pediatrics 42: 5, 1968, with the permission of the Editor.)

tions were higher in the earlier fetal series than in those of the adult (Figure 13.20). These data suggest that aerobic glycolysis is more active in fetal and neonatal than in adult muscle. Birth did not cause a significant change in any metabolic parameter. Under hypoxic conditions, the relative increases in glucose uptake and lactate and [^{14}C]lactate productions in fetal and adult muscle suggest that the glycolytic pathway of fetal muscle does not respond more effectively to hypoxia. The percentage of total CO_2 derived from glucose rose during gestation from 2% at 90 days to 4.4% at 155 days; in the adult series, 9% of the total CO_2 originated from glucose. Villee[61] has also demonstrated that the pathways of oxidative metabolism are present in human fetal muscle during the first half of gestation, but comparisons with older fetal and adult tissues were not possible. The sum of ^{14}C activities appearing in lactate, pyruvate, and CO_2 was higher in fetal and neonatal than in adult muscle.[60]

Respiration and glucose utilization were also studied in skeletal muscle homogenates prepared with a Bronwill CO_2 cooled homogenizer (Table 13.6.).[62] The highest values for QO_2 and CO_2 production were observed in the 155-day fetal series; the QO_2 appeared to drop in the 3-day postnatal series. However, there were only two monkeys (eight flasks) in this series and no statistical comparisons were made. The percentage of total CO_2 and the micromoles of CO_2 arising from glucose plus glycogen (carbohydrate) were similar in homogenates of fetal, neonatal, and adult muscle.

In all age groups, about 70% of the total CO_2 produced originated from a source or sources other than glucose and glycogen; thus homogenates of fetal, neonatal, and adult muscle are potentially able to obtain a large part of their energy from the oxidation of substrates other than carbohydrates.

Pentose Cycle

One might expect that the pentose cycle would be quantitatively more important in fetal muscle than in adult muscle. In fetal muscle a maximum rate of protein synthesis should be associated with an increasing RNA content. To test this hypothesis, muscle fiber groups from fetal, infant, and adult rhesus monkeys were incubated in media containing [1-^{14}C]glucose and [6-^{14}C]glucose, and the pentose cycle activity was estimated by the equations of Katz and Wood.[63] The results indicated that pentose cycle activity is more important in fetal than in neonatal and adult

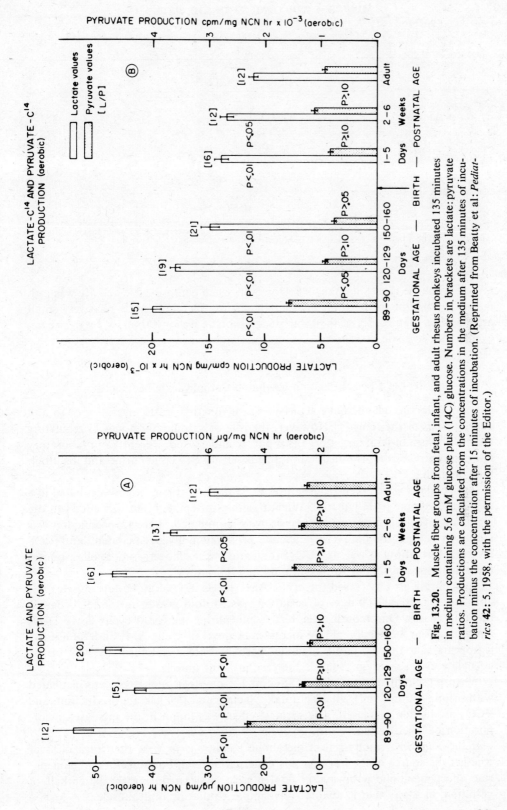

Fig. 13.20. Muscle fiber groups from fetal, infant, and adult rhesus monkeys incubated 135 minutes in medium containing 5.6 mM glucose plus (14C) glucose. Numbers in brackets are lactate:pyruvate ratios. Productions are calculated from the concentrations in the medium after 135 minutes of incubation minus the concentration after 15 minutes of incubation. (Reprinted from Beatty et al: *Pediatrics* **42**: 5, 1958, with the permission of the Editor.)

Table 13.6   Metabolism of homogenates of skeletal muscle from fetal, neonatal, and adult rhesus monkeys

	Fetal		Neonatal	Adult
	113 days	155 days	3 days	
umoles/g protein/30 min				
O_2 consumption	170 ± 27	232 ± 27*	162 ± 17	157 ± 9
CO_2 production	149 ± 18	230 ± 20*	204 ± 25	159 ± 10
% total CO_2 from glucose-^{14}C	23 ± 2*	21 ± 3*	25 ± 3	31 ± 4
% total CO_2 from glucose-^{14}C + glycogen	30 ± 4	27 ± 4	27 ± 3	34 ± 3
umoles CO_2 from carbohydrate/g protein/30 min	45 ± 4	62 ± 5	55 ± 5	54 ± 4

Values are means ± SEM, duplicate flasks on each observation. Homogenates were incubated for 30 min at 37° in TES buffered medium, pH 7.4, plus 0.21 uCi glucose-U-^{14}C per ml.
* P Fetal vs. adult < 0.005.
(Reprinted from Beatty et al: Pediatr. Res. 6: 813, 1972, with the permission of the Editor.)

muscle from the rhesus monkey.[64] However, when pentose cycle activity was estimated in relation to the total amount of glucose metabolized, a relatively small amount, less than 0.4%, of the total glucose uptake was metabolized by this route, even under hypoxic conditions.

Effect of Epinephrine and Insulin on Carbohydrate Metabolism

Fetal endocrine glands have a physiological function in the overall growth and development of the fetus.[65] However, the role of specific hormones in regulating the metabolism of fetal target organs is poorly understood. Recently our laboratory has demonstrated that rhesus fetal muscle is sensitive to epinephrine and insulin in midgestation.[5,15]

Muscle fibers were taken from fetuses at 95 days of gestation and incubated in a medium containing [^{14}C]glucose. When 6 μmoles of epinephrine was added to the medium, glycolysis and glycogenolysis were stimulated. Lactate production was increased but glucose uptake, [^{14}C]lactate production, glycogen content, and [^{14}C]-glycogen formation, as well as $^{14}CO_2$ production, were all decreased. Such responses to epinephrine are similar to those found in adult muscle.

Epinephrine also increased the cyclic AMP levels in fetal and adult muscle. The absolute increase at 100 days of gestation was twofold greater in the fetal than in the adult series. One month after birth, epinephrine increased cyclic AMP levels almost tenfold. Since epinephrine increases the level of cyclic AMP in fetal muscle, it appears that this hormone regulates carbohydrate metabolism by way of the adenylate cyclase system. Such is the case in adult muscle.

When muscle fiber groups from 85- and 125-day fetal monkeys were incubated with insulin (10 mU/ml), glucose uptake, lactate and [^{14}C]lactate production, and $^{14}CO_2$ production increased. The greatest effect was found in the increased incorporation of labeled glucose into glycogen.[56,66]

If these in vitro results reflect metabolic conditions in vivo, then regardless of whether the source of the hormones is maternal or fetal, both insulin and epinephrine affect metabolic pathways in fetal muscle, at least during the latter half of gestation, in a way that is qualitatively similar to that in adult muscle.

Palmitate Metabolism

The current assumption is that glucose derived transplacentally is the major source of energy throughout fetal life; but the relationship between the various potential fuels has not been quantified.[67] Fifteen years ago carbohydrate was also generally assumed to be the fuel for adult muscle. It has since been established that lipids are also an important energy source for this tissue in the adult. Since brain, lung, and liver of human fetuses can oxidize [14C]palmitate to $^{14}CO_2$,[68] one may then assume that some oxidation of lipid occurs in fetal muscle. To determine whether it does, a preparation of muscle fiber groups from rhesus monkeys of various ages was incubated in medium containing 0.5 mM palmitate plus [14C]palmitate with a molar ratio of free fatty acid to albumin of 3.[69] When calculated on the basis of NCN, the oxygen consumption and palmitate uptakes were higher in the fetal and neonatal series than in the adult (Table 13.7). The amount of palmitate converted to lipid was also higher in the two fetal series than in the adult (Table 13.7), and the *in situ* lipid levels per gram of NCN were higher in fetal than in adult muscle (Table 13.8). The micromoles of palmitate converted to CO_2 were similar in fetal, neonatal, and adult muscle and accounted for 11% of the total respiration in the neonate and adult, and 4 to 7% in the fetal series (Table 13.7).

Amino Acid Oxidation

Amino acid transferases have recently been found in high concentration in skeletal muscle. Several groups of workers have reported that a number of 14C-labeled amino acids are oxidized to $^{14}CO_2$ by skeletal muscle of the adult rat.[70] However, these workers did not measure oxygen consumption or total CO_2 production and were unable to calculate amino acid oxidation in terms of the overall rate of respiration. Therefore, we incubated muscle fiber groups, from fetal (155 day) and adult rhesus monkeys, in media plus 14C-labeled amino acids at concentrations approximating plasma levels. The uptake and conversion of leucine, valine, alanine, and

Table 13.7 Muscle fiber groups from the rhesus monkey incubated in medium containing palmitate-1-14C

	Fetal age, days 99-101	Fetal age, days 150-160	Neonatal, days 1-4	Adult
Palmitate uptake, μmoles/g wet wt/hr	0.54 ± 0.03	0.44 ± 0.03	0.46 ± 0.03	0.46 ± 0.02
μmoles/g NCN/hr	50 ± 3*	27 ± 2*	26 ± 1*	20 ± 1
Palmitate to lipid, μmoles/g NCN/hr	36 ± 4*	21 ± 1*	18 ± 2	14 ± 1
Palmitate to CO_2, μmoles/g NCN/hr	2.0 ± 0.4	2.1 ± 0.2	3.1 ± 0.5	2.9 ± 0.2
% CO_2 from palmitate	4.3 ± 0.8*	7.3 ± 0.7*	10.6 ± 0.9	10.6 ± 0.9
QO_2, μmoles/mg NCN/2 hr	1.74 ± 0.04*	1.27 ± 0.05+	1.32 ± 0.04+	1.16 ± 0.06
CO_2, μmoles/mg NCN/2 hr	1.44 ± 0.14*	0.95 ± 0.09	0.94 ± 0.06	0.95 ± 0.04

Values are means ± SE. Muscle fiber groups were incubated in Krebs medium plus 5.6 umoles glucose, 0.5 umoles palmitate (FFA/albumen = 3) and 0.13 uc palmitate-1-14C per ml. NCN = non collagenous protein nitrogen.
* P for rapidly growing vs. adult muscle <0.025. + P for rapidly growing vs. adult muscle <0.05. (Beatty and Bocek: Am. J. Physiol. 219 : 1311, 1970)
Reprinted from Beatty and Bocek, Am. J. Physiol., 219: 1311, 1970, with permission of the Editor.

Table 13.8   Total lipid content of rhesus muscle during development.

	mg/100 mg NCN	n
Fetal*-days		
60	116	1
82	122 ± 5	10
120	88 ± 2	9
155	81 ± 2	10
Infant**		
4-5 days	68, 69	2
2-6 weeks	76 ± 4	4
Adult**	65 ± 2	20

Values are means ± SE, duplicate analyses on each monkey. NCN = non-collagenous protein nitrogen. * Predominantly red thigh muscle. ** Sartorius. (Beatty et al.: Am. J. Physiol. 219: 1311, 1970) Reprinted from Beatty and Bocek, Am. J. Physiol., 219: 1311, 1970, with permission of the Editor.

glutamic acid to $^{14}CO_2$ as well as the QO_2 and total CO_2 production were measured. It appeared that in both the fetal and adult series the oxidation of these four amino acids could account for about 10% of the total oxygen consumption.

3′,5′-Cyclic Adenosine Monophosphate (Cyclic AMP)

Recent evidence has suggested that cyclic AMP functions to regulate growth of mammalian cells in culture,[71] and therefore its relationship to cell proliferation in the mammalian system *in vivo* is of interest. Robison [72] has recently commented that cyclic AMP probably has one or more important roles to play during growth and development, even before the receptors for most hormones are present. The highest levels of cyclic AMP found in the voluntary skeletal muscle of the rhesus monkey occurred at about midgestation, calculated either in terms of wet weight or nitrogen (Figure 13.21). Insufficient amounts of muscle precluded any determination on muscle from younger fetuses. There was no change in the level of cyclic AMP from 150 days fetal age (91% of term) to 1 month after birth. Theoretically, the period of greatest cell proliferation is the presumptive myoblast stage and should precede the fall in cyclic AMP and the appearance of myotubes. Histological evidence indicates that the period of maximum cell proliferation occurred before 80 days (Figure 13.18). Therefore, the data on rhesus muscle agree with the hypothesis that a decrease in cyclic AMP is correlated with a decrease in cell proliferation, not only in cell culture but also in mammalian tissues such as rhesus muscle. Prostaglandin E_2 increased cyclic AMP accumulation in all the fetal series as well as in the infant and adult muscle.

SUMMARY

We make the proposal that a certain amount of cytoplasm is under the jurisdiction of each diploid nucleus within the myofiber and can be defined as a "DNA unit."

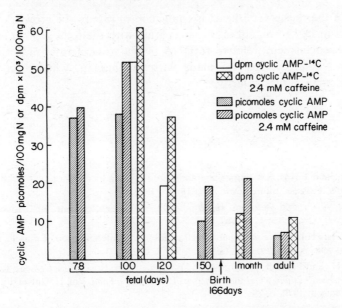

Fig. 13.21. Developmental changes in control levels of cyclic AMP in fetal, infant, and adult voluntary skeletal muscle fibers of the rhesus monkey. Cyclic AMP was determined (a) by a protein kinase binding assay and (b) by the amount of cylic AMP-¹⁴C formed from ATP-¹⁴C prelabeled by incubation with (8-¹⁴C) adenosine.

Fiber diameter probably has little significance in terms of growth and, while fiber length does relate to body size, it is reasonable to believe that the DNA unit is the more meaningful as a measure of growth. The amount of DNA in fetal muscle shows an eightfold increase from midgestation to term while the protein:DNA ratio increases 2.5-fold in the rhesus monkey.

The satellite cell is considered to be responsible not only for muscle repair but probably also for the large increase in DNA units through fetal and postnatal life. The satellite cell may be the progenitor of the myoblast.

From midgestation muscle tissue represents a large fraction of weight (25%); red and white fibers can be identified and glycogen synthetase and phosphorylase appear at low levels. *In vitro* tests show that glycogen turnover occurs and that respiratory rates are higher than for adult muscle.

Glucose uptake *in vitro* reaches a high level at 90 and 125 gestational days (by comparison with adult muscle) and glycolysis is active in fetal and neonatal muscle.

As early as 100 days of gestation, significant amounts of palmitate can be oxidized to CO_2, suggesting that fats might be metabolized by the fetus.

During the latter half of gestation fetal muscle is sensitive *in vitro* to epinephrine, insulin, and prostaglandin E_2. The cyclic AMP level reaches a maximum value at midgestation when cell or nuclear division also reaches a maximum—and apparently both decline together subsequently.

Finally, the role of hormones, particularly growth hormone, thyroxin, and insulin, in the coordination of embryonic growth of muscle, has not yet been clarified. It is possible that myoblast replication, fusion, and protein synthesis are coordinated or directed by hormones.

Growth of the rhesus fetal heart is equivalent in rate to the growth of the soma. The increase in DNA content is commensurate with the total growth of the heart. The accretion of protein, relative to DNA increase, accelerates only slightly from midgestation. Comparisons are made with the human, while data concerning rodents demonstrate dissimilarities.

REFERENCES

1. Yaffe, D., and Fuchs, S.: Autoradiographic study of the incorporation of uridine-H³ during myogenesis in tissue culture. *Dev. Biol.* **15**: 33, 1967.

2. Marchok, A. C., and Herrman, H.: Studies of muscle development. 1. Changes in cell proliferation. *Dev. Biol.* **15**: 129, 1967.

3. Holtzer, H.: Proliferative and quantal cell cycles in the differentiation of muscle, cartilage, and red blood cells. *Symp. Int. Soc. Cell Biol.* **9**: 69, 1970.

4. Holtzer, H., and Bischoff, R.: Mitosis and myogenesis. In: Briskey, E., Casseus, R., and March, B. (Eds.): *The Physiology and Biochemistry of Muscle as a Food*, Vol. II. University of Wisconsin Press, Madison, 1970, p. 29.

5. O'Neill, M. C., and Stockdale, F. E.: Differentiation without cell division in cultured skeletal muscle. *Dev. Biol.* **29**: 410, 1972.

6. Stockdale, F. E., and Holtzer, H.: DNA synthesis and myogenesis. *Exp. Cell Res.* **24**: 508, 1961.

7. O'Neill, M., and Strohman, R. C.: Studies of the decline of deoxyribonucleic acid polymerase activity during embryonic muscle cell fusion *in vitro*. *Biochemistry* **9**: 2832, 1970.

8. Love, D. S., Stoddard, F. J., and Grasso, J. A.: Endocrine regulation of embryonic muscle development: Hormonal control of DNA accumulation, pentose cycle activity and myoblast proliferation. *Dev. Biol.* **20**: 563, 1969.

9. Love, D. S., and Konigsberg, I. R.: Enhanced DNA and retarded protein accumulation in skeletal muscle of "hypophysectomized" chick embryos. *Endocrinology* **62**: 378, 1958.

10. Konigsberg, I. R.: Thyroid regulation of protein and nucleic acid accumulation in developing skeletal muscle of the chick embryo. *J. Cell. Comp. Physiol.* **52**: 13, 1958.

11. De la Haba, G., Cooper, G. W., and Elting, V.: Hormonal requirements for myogenesis of striated muscle *in vitro*: Insulin and somatotropin. *Proc. Natl. Acad. Sci. U.S.A.* **56**: 1719, 1966.

12. Marchok, A., and Wolff, J. A.: Studies of muscle development. IV. Some characteristics of RNA polymerase activity in isolated nuclei from developing chick muscle. *Biochim. Biophys. Acta* **155**: 378, 1968.

13. Beatty, C. H., Basinger, G. M., and Bocek, R. M.: Pentose cycle activity in muscle from fetal, neonatal and infant rhesus monkeys. *Arch. Biochem. Biophys.* **117**: 275, 1966.

14. Giacanelli, M., Reniers, J., and Martin, L.: Morphology and histology of foetal muscles. *Biol. Neonate* **13**: 281, 1968.

15. Godlewski, E. Jr.: Die Entwicklung des Skelet-und-Hertzmuskelgewebes der Saugethiere. *Arch. Mikrobiol. Anat.* **60**: 111, 1902.

16. MacCallum, J. B.: On the histogenesis of the striated muscle fibres, and the growth of the human sartorius muscle. *Bull. Johns Hopkins Hosp.* **90-91**: 208, 1898.

17. Chiakulas, J. J., and Pauly, J. E.: A study of postnatal growth of skeletal muscle in the rat. *Anat. Rec.* **152**: 55, 1965.

18. Goldspink, G.: Studies on postembryonic growth and development of skeletal muscles. *Roy. Irish Acad. Proc.* **61**: 135, 1962.

19. Hammond, J., and Appleton, A. P.: *Growth and Development of Mutton Qualities in Sheep.* Oliver & Boyd, Edinburgh, 1932.

20. Heidenrich, C. H.: Der Einfluss der histologischen Bestandeile des Muskels auf die Qualitat des Fleisches. *Wiss. Arch. Landwirtsch.* **6**: 366, 1931.

21. Joubert, D. M.: An analysis of factors influencing postnatal growth and development of the muscle fibre. *J. Agric. Sci.* **47**: 59, 1956.

22. Staun, H.: Various factors affecting number and size of muscle fibres in the pig. *Acta Agric. Scand.* **13**: 293, 1963.

23. Goldspink, G.: Increase in length of skeletal muscle during normal growth. *Nature* **204**: 1095, 1964.

24. Cheek, D. B., and Holt, A. B.: Growth and body composition in the mouse. *Am. J. Physiol.* **205**: 913, 1963.

25. Chiakulas, J. J., and Pauly, S. E.: A study of postnatal growth of skeletal muscle in the rat. *Anat. Rec.* **152**: 55, 1965.

26. Rowe, R. W., and Goldspink, G.: Surgically induced hypertrophy in skeletal muscles of the laboratory mouse. *Anat. Rec.* **161**: 69, 1968.

27. Goldspink, G.: The proliferation of myofibrils during muscle fibre growth. *J. Cell Sci.* **6**: 593, 1970.

28. Tello, J. F.: Die Enstehung der motorischen und lsensiblen nervendigungen. I. In dem loko-motorischen System der hoheren Wirbeltiere. Muskulare Histogenese. *Z. Anat. Entwicklungs-gesch.* **64**: 384, 1922.

29. Montgomery, R. D.: Growth of human striated muscle. *Nature* **195**: 194, 1962.

30. Cheek, D. B., Graystone, J., and Mehrizi, A.: The importance of muscle cell number in children with congenital heart disease. *Bull. Johns Hopkins Hosp.* **118**: 140, 1966.

31. Dunnill, M. S.: In: Dyke, S. C. (Ed.): *Quantitative Methods in Histology, Recent Advances in Clinical Pathology*, Series V. Little, Brown, Boston, 1968, p. 401.

32. Cheek, D. B., Holt, A. B., Hill, D. E., and Talbert, J. L.: Skeletal muscle cell mass and growth: The concept of the deoxyribonucleic acid unit. *Pediatr. Res.* **5**: 312, 1971.

33. Cheek, D. B., West, C. D., and Golden, C. C.: The distribution of Na and Cl and the extra-cellular fluid volume in the rat. *J. Clin. Invest.* **36**: 340, 1957.

34. Huxley, H. E.: Evidence for continuity between the central elements of the triads and extra-cellular space in frog sartorius muscle. *Nature* **202**: 1067, 1964.

35. Barrett, T. M., and Walser, McK.: Extracellular fluid in individual tissue and in whole animals: The distribution of radio sulphate and radio bromide. *J. Clin. Invest.* **48**: 56, 1969.

36. Mauro, A.: Satellite cell of skeletal muscle fibres. *J. Biophys. Biochem. Cytol.* **9**: 493, 1961.

37. Reznik, M.: Possible origin of myoblasts during muscle regeneration. *J. Cell Biol.* **39**: 110, 1968.

38. Reznik, M.: Thymidine-^{3}H uptake by satellite cells of regenerating skeletal muscle. *J. Cell Biol.* **40**: 568, 1969.

39. Moss, F. P.: The relationship between the dimensions of the fibres and the number of nuclei during normal growth of skeletal muscle in the domestic fowl. *Am. J. Anat.* **122**: 555, 1968.

40. Stockdale, F. E.: Changing levels of DNA polymerase activity during the development of skel-etal muscle tissue *in vivo*. *Dev. Biol.* **21**: 462, 1970.

41. Lee, J. C.: Electron microscope observations on myogenic free cells of denervated skeletal muscle. *Exp. Neurol.* **12**: 123, 1965.

42. Klinkerfuss, G. H.: An electron microscopic study of myotonic dystrophy. *Arch. Neurol.* **16**: 181, 1967.

43. Shafiq, S. A., Gorycki, M. A., and Mauro, A.: Mitosis during postnatal growth in skeletal and cardiac muscle of the rat. *J. Anat.* **103**: 135, 1968.

44. Kelly, A. M., and Zacks, S. I.: The histogenesis of rat intercostal muscle. *J. Cell Biol.* **42**: 135, 1969.

45. Wirsen, C., and Larsson, K. S.: Histochemical differentiation of skeletal muscle in foetal new-born mice. *J. Embryol. Exp. Morphol.* **12**: 759, 1964.

46. Widdowson, E. M., Crabb, D. E., and Milner, R. D. G.: Cellular development of some human organs before birth. *Arch. Dis. Child.* **47**: 652, 1972.

47. Miller, S. A.: Protein metabolism during growth and development. In: Munro, H. N. (Ed.): *Mammalian Protein Metabolism*, Vol. II, Academic Press, New York, 1969, p. 213.

48. Enesco, M., and Leblond, C. P.: Increase in cell number as a factor in the growth of organs and tissue of the young male rat. *J. Embryol. Exp. Morphol.* **10**: 530, 1962.

49. Kapeller-Adler, R., and Hammad, W. A.: A biochemical study on nucleic acids and protein synthesis in the human fetus and its correlation with relevant embryological data. *J. Obstet. Gynaecol. Br. Commonw.* **79**: 924, 1972.

50. Peterson, R. O., and Baserga, R.: Nucleic acid and protein synthesis in cardiac muscle of growing and adult mice. *Exp. Cell Res.* **40**: 340, 1965.

51. Walker, B. E., and Adrian, E. K. Jr.: DNA synthesis in the myocardium of growing, mature, senescent and dystrophic mice. *Cardiologia* **49**: 319, 1966.

52. Beatty, C. H., Basinger, G. M., and Bocek, R. M.: Differentiation of red and white fibers in muscle from fetal, neonatal, and infant rhesus monkeys. *J. Histochem.* **15**: 93, 1967.

53. Dubowitz, V.: Enzyme histochemistry of skeletal muscle. II. Developing human muscle. *J. Neurol. Neurosurg. Psychiatr.* **28**: 519, 1965.

54. Shelley, H. J.: Glycogen reserves and their changes at birth and in anoxia. *Br. Med. Bull.* **17**: 137, 1961.

55. Bocek, R. M., Basinger, G. M., and Beatty, C. H.: Glycogen synthetase, phosphorylase, and glycogen content of developing rhesus muscle. *Pediatr. Res.* **3**: 525, 1969.

56. Bocek, R. M., Young, M. K., and Beatty, C. H.: Effect of insulin and epinephrine on the carbohydrate metabolism and adenylate cyclase of rhesus fetal muscle. *Pediatr. Res.* **7**: 787, 1973.

57. Bocek, R. M., and Beatty, C. H.: Glycogen metabolism in fetal, neonatal and infant muscle of the rhesus monkey. *Pediatrics* **40**: 412, 1967.

58. Villee, C. A., Hagerman, D. D., Holmberg, N., Lind, J., and Villee, D. B.: Effects of anoxia on the metabolism of human fetal tissues. *Pediatrics* **22**: 953, 1958.

59. Brinkman, C. R.: Umbilical blood flow and fetal oxygen consumption. In: Mann, L. I. (Ed.): *Clinical Obstetrics and Gynecology*. Harper & Row, New York, 1970, Chapter 13, p. 565.

60. Beatty, C. H., Basinger, G. M., and Bocek, R. M.: Oxygen consumption and glycolysis in fetal, neonatal, and infant muscle of the rhesus monkey. *Pediatrics* **42**: 5, 1968.

61. Villee, C. A.: The intermediary metabolism of human fetal tissues. *Cold Spring Harbor Symp. Quant. Biol.* **19**: 186, 1954.

62. Beatty, C. H., Young, M. K., Dwyer, D., and Bocek, R. M.: Glucose utilization of cardiac and skeletal muscle homogenates from fetal and adult rhesus monkeys. *Pediatr. Res.* **6**: 813, 1972.

63. Katz, J., and Wood, H. G.: The use of $C^{14}O_2$ yields from glucose-1- and glucose-6-C^{14} for the evaluation of the pathways of glucose metabolism. *J. Biol. Chem.* **238**: 517, 1963.

64. Beatty, C. H., Basinger, G. M., and Bocek, R. M.: Pentose cycle activity in muscle from fetal, neonatal, and infant rhesus monkeys. *Arch. Biochem. Biophys.* **117**: 275, 1966.

65. Jost, A.: The extent of foetal endocrine autonomy. In: *Foetal Autonomy*, a CBA Foundation Symposium. Churchill, London, 1969, p. 79.

66. Bocek, R. M., and Beatty, C. H.: Effect of insulin on the carbohydrate metabolism of fetal rhesus monkey muscle. *Endocrinology* **85**: 615, 1969.

67. Adams, P. A. J.: Control of glucose metabolism in the human fetus and newborn infant. In: Levine, R., and Luft, R. (Eds.): *Advances in Metabolic Disorders*, Vol. 5. Academic Press, New York, 1971, p. 183.

68. Roux, J. F., and Yoshioko, T.: Lipid metabolism in the fetus during development. In: Mann, L. I. (Ed.): *Clinical Obstetrics and Gynecology*. Harper & Row, New York, 1970, Chapter 13, p. 595.

69. Beatty, C. H., and Bocek, R. M.: Metabolism of palmitate by fetal, neonatal, and adult muscle of the rhesus monkey. *Am. J. Physiol.* **219**: 1311, 1970.

70. Goldberg, A. L., and Odessey, R.: Oxidation of amino acids by diaphragms from fed and fasted rats. *Am. J. Physiol.* **223**: 1384, 1972.

71. Otten, J., Johnson, G. S., and Pastan, I.: Regulation of cell growth by cyclic adenosine 3′,5′-monophosphate. *J. Biol. Chem.* **247**: 7082, 1972.

72. Robison, G. A.: The biological role of cyclic AMP: An updated overview. In: Kahn, R. H., and Lands, W. E. M. (Eds.): *Prostaglandins and Cyclic AMP.* Academic Press, New York, 1973, p. 229.

CHAPTER 14

Fetal Lung Development

Louis Gluck and Marie V. Kulovich

INTRODUCTION

An outstanding example of the complexities of differentiation in the embryo and fetus is the development and maturation of the lung, where ability to function is basic to survival of the organism in the extrauterine environment. This complex organ goes from its anlage through numerous branchings and subdivisions[1-4] to achieve an exchange surface for respiratory gases, the alveolus. This is capable of supporting life when it matures biochemically to form a specialized surfactant lining that maintains alveolar stability.

EARLY EMBRYOLOGICAL DEVELOPMENT[1,4,5]

An endodermal and mesodermal derivative, the embryonic lung begins as a ventral groove in the cervical endodermal tube at 24 days of development in the human. Growth and evagination of the groove form the primitive lung buds which grow and develop in the median mass of mesenchyme.

A series of asymmetric branchings begins on both the developing right and left lung buds, three lobes forming on the right and two on the left. Contributions from the mesenchyme include muscle, cartilage, and connective tissue for the airways and the elastic and collagen tissues of pleura and septum.

Between weeks 10 and 14, the growth and subdivisions result in about 75% of the total number of branchings.[1,6] By the 16th week of gestation, the bronchial tree, the "structural lung," is complete through the terminal bronchioles. The

Supported by National Institutes of Health Grants HDO4143, HDO4380, HDO3015, SCOR HL-14169, Maternal and Child Health Funds of the California State Department of Health, and the Gerber Products Company.

respiratory bronchioles begin developing by the 16th week and expand into alveolar structures. The development of the respiratory part of the lung occurs principally after birth.

PHASES OF LUNG DEVELOPMENT

Investigators describe three phases of lung development: [1, 7–9] a *glandular* phase, a *canalicular* phase, and an *alveolar* phase. In the *glandular* phase there is no respiration although the bronchial divisions are established. From the 16th week the *canalicular* phase begins with vascularization and delineation of the respiratory portion of the lungs. The *alveolar* phase begins at about 24 to 26 weeks and extends well into postnatal life. With the alveolar phase, surfactant appears in the tracheal fluid.

Alveolar Development

Although information about the general morphologic aspects is necessary to understand lung development, the focus of this discussion is almost completely on alveolar development and specifically on the development of the surfactant that maintains alveolar stability. In alveolar development, the lung bud initially is lined by columnar epithelium, which by about week 13 of gestation has developed cilia. The epithelium changes in character at the bronchiolar level from columnar to cuboidal. [1, 8] In the canalicular phase there is marked proliferation of blood vessels around terminal bronchioles. The respiratory bronchiole then begins to differentiate from the terminal bronchiole, whose distal parts develop into areas of gas exchange (respiratory elements). The lining epithelium changes from cuboidal [1, 8] and the cellular continuity is lost as the cells become attenuated and flattened, presumably due to the growth of underlying vascular tissue. In the respiratory tissue, by about 24 weeks, saccules appear, which differentiate from respiratory bronchiolar endoderm. [1, 6] An alveolar membrane covers the capillaries and from 20 to 24 weeks there is the very important differentiation of the alveolar epithelium into two cell types: type I cells with a small perinuclear body and cytoplasmic extensions which line a very large part of the alveolar surface; and type II cells with a larger perinuclear body which contain no extensions but instead contain characteristic, unusual lamellar structures, the osmiophilic inclusion bodies. [10]

Balis et al [11] described fetal and early postnatal lungs as having respiratory areas with thick intra-alveolar septa, few capillaries in contact with air spaces, many type II alveolar cells, and fewer type I cells. Between 32 and 40 weeks of gestation there is about a sixfold increase in the number of alveoli per terminal lung unit. [12]

SURFACE TENSION FORCES IN LUNG

The major biochemical event in the development of alveoli is the formation of surfactant which appears in lung fluid and amniotic fluid. The significance of the surfactant system was suggested in 1929[13] with the experiments of the Swiss physiologist von Neergaard, who showed with pressure/volume curves of extirpated lungs distended with air or with liquid that the lungs were much more easily distensible with liquid than with air. He postulated that most of the force acting to deflate the air-distended lung came from surface tension forces at the air-tissue interface. He also noted that the pressure/volume (P/V) curve derived from saline filling and emptying was an almost equivalent curve, 1 ml of saline producing 1 g of pressure. The P/V curve with air required much more pressure to produce the same volume distension. When the lung was emptied of saline, the deflation curve coincided exactly with the inflation curve while deflation from air filling described a different curve from that of inflation; this wandering is called *hysteresis*. These effects can all be ascribed to surface tension forces.[14-16]

SURFACTANT

The phenomenon of surface tension at the air-liquid interface of the alveolar lining is the key to the understanding of these aspects of lung function since alveoli act like bubbles. According to the Laplace equation, as a bubble becomes smaller in radius, its wall (surface) tension rises in inverse proportion. Since alveoli become smaller on expiration, their surface tension would become very high and they would collapse if it were not for the detergent lining, *surfactant*, that imparts alveolar stability. In fact, lack of surfactant is the problem in infants who develop the respiratory distress syndrome (RDS).

Surfactant is a generic name for a complex group of molecules consisting largely of phospholipids, which bind water in the outer layers of the alveolar surface, at the interface with air, lowering the surface tension which otherwise would rise upon expiration when the alveolus reaches its minimum size. This important physiological phenomenon is the basis of what variously is termed alveolar stability, functional residual capacity, prevention of atelectasis, and so on.

SURFACTANT LECITHIN AND ITS SYNTHESIS

The major surfactant molecule is *surface active lecithin*, basically a three-carbon glycerol molecule, with phosphocholine on one terminal carbon and with two saturated fatty acid esters on the α- and β-carbons. The α-carbon fatty acid ester is palmitic (16:0) and the β-carbon ester either palmitic or myristic (14:0).[17]

The synthesis of surface active lecithin occurs by more than one pathway. The major pathway is

(1) CDP choline $+$ D-α,β-diglyceride $\rightarrow$ lecithin.[18,19]

There appear to be three other routes for the biosynthesis of surface active lecithin in lung, including:

(2) phosphatidylethanolamine $+$ 3CH$_3$ (from methionine) $\rightarrow$ lecithin.[18,19]
(3) lecithin $\rightarrow$ (lysolecithin $+$ β-carbon fatty acid) $+$ palmitic acid $\rightarrow$ dipalmitoyl lecithin.[20]
(4) incompletely defined as of this writing.[21]

In the human the timing of these different synthetic pathways is such that the fetal lung begins making surface active lecithin at about 22 to 24 weeks.[19, 22] Pathway (1) becomes active at about 35 weeks in the human[19, 22] with a sudden burst in enzymatic activity and the synthesis of dipalmitoyl lecithin; at this time the lung may be considered to be mature biochemically.

PHOSPHOLIPIDS IN AMNIOTIC FLUIDS

The development of the fetal lung is reflected by the phospholipids in amniotic fluid in the human and other primates. The lung maturity of the fetus can be evaluated from the ratio between the concentrations of surfactant lecithin and the sphingomyelin (L:S) in amniotic fluid.[22-24] There is little of either compound, but sphingomyelin predominates until about the 32nd week of gestation, when the concentrations become approximately equal. By the 35th week there is a sudden rise in concentration of lecithin. The sphingomyelin concentration levels off and then falls. When these findings are translated into ratios, an L:S ratio of 2 (by densitometry or planimetry) indicates maturity of lung.

ESTABLISHING AN ANIMAL MODEL

Studies in part from our laboratory[25] on the rhesus monkey (*Macaca mulatta*) established that the rhesus monkey is very similar biochemically to the human with respect to lung development. It was of particular interest to compare this bio-chemical development with that of the baboon (*Papio papio*). As Table 14.1 shows, during the sequence of biochemical development of surfactant in the fetus, the structure of lecithin changes in the β-carbon fatty acid esters from a predominance of palmitoyl-myristoyl lecithin to a significant percentage of dipalmitoyl lecithin at term. In this respect the rhesus and the human resemble each other closely.[22, 25, 26] The baboon, by contrast, undergoes no similar changes. With maturation there is the characteristic increase in L:S ratio. However, there is surprising constancy of the β-carbon fatty acids on the lecithin. Palmitoyl-myristoyl lecithin is the major surface active compound throughout the gestation of the baboon fetus.

The time sequence of maturation of the L:S ratios themselves shows an abrupt maturation time in the rhesus at about 154 to 158 days, while in the baboon it is about 172 to 174 days.

The biochemical difference thus indicates that the rhesus is a closer model of the human than is the baboon. These findings are similar whether one examines the amniotic fluid or the fetal lung.

Continuity of the fetal lung with amniotic fluid has been established by a series of recent observations.[25-30] Older observations dealt with the impressive volume of tracheal fluid that issued from fetal sheep;[31, 32] with similarities between tracheal fluid phospholipids in sheep and those in amniotic fluid;[33] and with "laryngeal sphincter" mechanisms whereby the flow of tracheal fluid into amniotic fluid could possibly be controlled.[34] More definitive studies include those by Reynolds et al[27] using radioactive precursors of phospholipids; a study of lamellar bodies

Table 14.1 Composition by mean percent of fatty acids esterified on the β-carbons of surface active lecithin from amniotic fluid of normal humans, rhesus monkeys and baboons (22, 25)

Fatty acid	Human		Rhesus days		Baboon days	
	31 wk	term	108-154	155-171	110-171	172-184
14.0	71.6	48.1	80.3	35.9	67.2	66.9
16.0	12.9	29.2	9.2	21.0	16.5	17.8
16.1	4.6	5.9	1.5	3.5	3.6	1.3
18.0	2.9	3.0	3.3	6.9	3.9	4.2
18.1	5.0	8.7	3.2	24.8	5.9	13.6
18.2	3.0	5.8	1.1	6.2	2.1	3.0
18.3	Tr	-	0.7	1.6	1.0	-
20.0	Tr	Tr	1.3	-	3.3	-
Saturated	87.4	80.3	93.8	63.8	88.8	81.8
Unsaturated	12.6	20.4	6.7	36.1	11.2	18.2

from lung in amniotic fluid;[28] studies showing profound differences in amniotic fluid lecithin following ligation of the fetal lung;[25] a specific lung surfactant protein found also in amniotic fluid;[29] and a report by Biggs et al measuring directly the outpouring of surfactant into amniotic fluid.[30]

MATERNAL DIET AND FETAL SURFACTANT LECITHIN IN MONKEYS

Preliminary studies reported here on the maturation and development of fetuses with different maternal dietary regimens have particular significance in the lung. Table 14.2 shows the four categories of diet into which pregnant monkeys were grouped and the findings on the β-carbon fatty acid esterified on surface active lecithin from amniotic fluid and lung. All determinations were done on unknown samples, which were coded by Cheek's laboratory.

The controls in this group have acyl esters that are very similar to the group of normal control monkeys previously studied[25] in relation to their L:S ratios in amniotic fluid and to the composition of β-carbon fatty acid esters on the surface active lecithin. Two groups with aberrations of development were found. The group whose protein and calorie intakes were lowered symmetrically did not vary significantly from normal controls. However, the group whose intakes included either adequate calories and low protein or low calories with normal protein showed deviations from normal on both regimens, with the fatty acid esters on the β-carbons of lecithins different from those of normal controls.

What effect starvation may have on development of fetal lung, perhaps by limiting adequate substrates, is not clear from these preliminary studies. They suggest, however, that the lung may be an especially good target organ to study for measurable effects of dietary deprivations.

VARIATIONS IN FETAL LUNG DEVELOPMENT IN HUMANS

Studies previously published showed that in the human a number of diseases of mothers, placenta, and fetus may result in deviations from normal in maturation of the fetal lung.[24]

These studies on biochemical maturation of human fetal lung disclosed that the population of pregnant patients may be broken down into three groups. Fetal lungs in the normal population mature between 33 and 37 weeks, clustering relatively tightly around a mean of 35 weeks. A second group of patients shows acceleration of maturation with normal L:S ratios prior to 33 weeks (26–32 weeks). In the third group there is a definite delay in maturation at 37 or more weeks of gestation.

The two abnormal groups are of particular interest vis-à-vis the monkeys in the present study on nutrition. Human fetuses showing acceleration of maturation of lung almost always have been subjected to some sort of chronic intrauterine stress, most often with a placental insufficiency.[24] The most potent stimulus appears to be a chronic retroplacental bleeding (chronic abruptio placentae), with placental infarction, where maturation of lung and mature L:S ratios as early as 26 weeks of gestation have been seen. Other conditions of mother and placenta associated with accelerated maturation of fetal lung include severe ("chronic") toxemia,

Table 14.2 Composition by mean percent of fatty acids
esterified on the β-carbon of surface active
lecithin from amniotic fluid of rhesus monkeys
on four dietary regimens as indicated

Fatty acid	100 Cal/kg 4.2 gm Prot/kg	100 Cal/kg 2.1 g Prot/kg	50 Cal/kg 4.2 g Prot/kg	50 Cal/kg 2.1 g Prot/kg
8.0		1.48		
10.0	24.3	4.10		14.31
12.0		1.89		
14.0	39.60	6.54	11.85	32.08
14.1	1.61	1.02	2.78	3.97
16.0	17.53	21.36	23.38	20.97
16.1	3.98	8.04	5.13	5.88
18.0	4.44	14.71	12.07	8.98
18.1	4.81	16.74	10.05	6.9
18.2	8.12	14.95	9.81	2.02
18.3	12.87	4.71	6.02	8.36
20.0		1.49	17.95	
L/S ratio at term	2.34	1.49	1.49	2.73
% Sat.	74.03	62.65	66.06	72.51
% Unsat.	25.97	47.36	33.94	27.49

chronic (degenerative) diabetes mellitus (D, E, F types), heroin/morphine addiction, sickle-C hemoglobinopathy, maternal infections (some urinary tract infections and amnionitis), premature rupture of membranes, and placental infarctions. The group with delayed maturation of fetal lung development is best exemplified by gestational or mild maternal diabetes mellitus (types A, B, C) and by hydrops fetalis.[24]

Acceleration of maturation of fetal lung also may be induced experimentally in the rhesus monkey.[25] Stress in the form of fetal surgery and maternal glucose intolerance with streptozotocin caused marked acceleration of maturation of monkey fetal lung, from the normal 154 to 158 days to 130 days, with changes similar to those seen in the human.[25]

POSSIBLE HORMONAL EFFECTS

The exact mechanisms in acceleration of maturation of lung are unknown, although it is tempting to suggest that the effects may be mediated by hormones. Studies by Liggins and Howie[35] on sheep and on humans treated with betamethasone suggest a possible role by glucocorticosteroids. Acceleration of maturation of fetal lung with steroids was found by others on rabbits.[35a] Farrell and Zachman[36] reported *in vitro* enhancement of pathway (1) (CDP-choline + D-α,β-diglyceride → lecithin) with cortisone. Cortisone levels were reported to be elevated in cord bloods as

compared to normals in babies born after premature rupture of membranes.[37]
Also in babies with RDS, serum estriol levels were lower than in normal controls.[37] Interpretations of these studies include possibilities that corticosteroids in
primates (humans) do affect the synthesis of lecithins, but that the effects possibly
are mediated by the fetal adrenal which processes the precursor DHA (dehydro-
epiandrosterone).[38, 39] The hormonal effects possibly relate to specific receptor
binding protein in cells and certainly the concept in the lung of the sequence of "hormone-receptor-DNA-RNA-new enzyme synthesis" postulated by
Giannopoulos is one of the exciting areas for the future.[40] It has particular
relevance for investigation since studies have now shown convincingly that the
Macaca mulatta is an excellent model for human lung development.[25] This is true
both during normal fetal lung development and in its response to stress by accelerated maturation.

SPECULATION

The preliminary findings here that surfactant metabolism is affected where normal
calorie/protein proportions are altered suggest that this is a particular area for
future fruitful research, since possible effects of starvation and/or malnutrition on
organ development can be followed using surfactant as a model. This would permit
also the effects of steroids to be followed and established.

In the long view, conceivably, this could be a model system to study "fetal
engineering" and particularly to try to establish and correct any possible adverse
effects on brain development produced by malnutrition. Studies on infants with
accelerated lung maturation due to chronic stress, especially those born after
chronic abruptio placentae, showed also that there is a parallelism between development of the central nervous system and surfactant development, in that some
infants whose lung development was significantly accelerated also showed marked
acceleration of neurological age.[24] The surfactant system may be a relevant
model here too, since the phospholipids in the central nervous system and lung
are almost identical and are synthesized similarly and may therefore be influenced
by similar conditions. Perhaps the most useful feature of the model is the accessibility
of amniotic fluid whose phospholipid changes reflect the changes occurring in the
fetal lung.

REFERENCES

1. Charnock, E. L., and Doershuk, C. F.: Developmental aspects of the human lung *Pediatr. Clin. North Am.* **20**: 275, 1973.
2. Weibel, E.: *Morphometry of the Human Lung.* Academic Press, New York, 1963.
3. Horsfield, K., and Cumming, G.: Morphology of the bronchial tree in man. *J. Appl. Physiol.* **24**: 373, 1968.
4. Avery, L. B.: *Developmental Anatomy.* Saunders, Philadelphia, 1965.
5. Avery, M. E.: *Lung Development: The Lung and Its Disorders in the Newborn Infant*, 2nd ed. Saunders, Philadelphia, 1968.
6. Bucher, U., and Reid, L.: Development of the intrasegmental bronchial tree: The pattern of branching and development of cartilage at varying stages of intrauterine life. *Thorax* **16**: 207, 1961.

7. Boyden, E. A.: Observation on the anatomy and development of the lungs. *Lancet* **73:** 509, 1953.

8. Emery, J.: Embryogenesis. In: *The Anatomy of the Developing Lung*. Heinemann, London, 1969.

9. Reid, L.: The embryology of the lung. In: *Development of the Lung*, a Ciba Foundation Symposium. Little, Brown, Boston, 1967.

10. Campiche, M. A., Gautier, A., Hernandez, E., et al: An electron microscopic study of the development of human lung. *Pediatrics* **32:** 976, 1963.

11. Balis, J. U., Delivoria, M., and Conen, D. E.: Maturation of postnatal human lung and the idiopathic respiratory distress syndrome. *Lab. Invest.* **15:** 530, 1966.

12. Emery, J. L., and Mithal, A.: The number of alveoli in the terminal respiratory unit of man during late intrauterine life and childhood. *Arch. Dis. Child.* **35:** 544, 1960.

13. von Neergaard, K.: Neue Auffassungen uber Einen Gundbegriff der Alemmechanik Die Retiaktionskraft der lunge abhangig von der Oberflackenspannung in der Alveolen. *Z. Ges. Exp. Med.* **66:** 373, 1929.

14. Pattle, R. E.: Surface lining of lung alveoli. *Physiol. Rev.* **45:** 48, 1965.

15. Clements, J. A., Hustead, R. F., Johnson, R. P., and Gibetz, I.: Pulmonary surface tension and alveolar stability. *J. Appl. Physiol.* **16:** 444, 1961.

16. Avery, M. E., and Mead, J.: Surface properties in relation to atelectasis and hyaline membrane disease. *Am. J. Dis. Child.* **97:** 517, 1959.

17. Gluck, L., Landowne, R. A., and Kulovich, M. V.: Biochemical development of surface activity in mammalian lung. III. Structural changes in lung lecithin during development of the rabbit fetus and newborn. *Pediatr. Res.* **4:** 352, 1970.

18. Gluck, L., Sribney, M., and Kulovich, M. V.: Biochemical development of surface activity in mammalian lung. II. The biosynthesis of phospholipids in the lung of the developing rabbit fetus and newborn. *Pediatr. Res.* **1:** 247, 1967.

19. Gluck, L., Kulovich, M. V., Eidelman, A. I., Cordero, L., and Khazin, A. F.: Biochemical development of surface activity in mammalian lung. IV. Pulmonary lecithin synthesis in the human fetus and newborn and etiology of the respiratory distress syndrome. *Pediatr. Res.* **6:** 81, 1972.

20. Hallman, M., and Raivio, K.: Studies on the biosynthesis of disaturated lecithin of the lung: Importance of the lysolecithin pathway. Submitted for publication.

21. Hallman, M., Kulovich, M. V. and Gluck, L.: Unpublished observations.

22. Gluck, L., Kulovich, M. V., Borer, R. C., Jr., Brenner, P., Anderson, G. G., and Spellacy, W. N.: Diagnosis of the respiratory distress syndrome by amniocentesis. *Am. J. Obstet. Gynecol.* **109:** 440, 1971.

23. Borer, R. C., Gluck, L., Freeman, R. K., and Kulovich, M. V.: Prenatal prediction of the respiratory distress syndrome. *Pediatr. Res.* **5:** 655, 1971.

24. Gluck, L., and Kulovich, M. V.: Lecithin/sphingomyelin ratios in amniotic fluid in normal and abnormal pregnancy. *Am. J. Obstet. Gynecol.* **115:** 539, 1973.

25. Gluck, L., Chez, R. A., Kulovich, M. V., Hutchinson, D. L., and Nieman, W. H.: Comparison of phospholipid indicators of fetal lung maturity in amniotic fluid of monkey (*Macaca mulatta*) and baboon (*Papio papio*). *Am. J. Obstet. Gynecol.*, in press.

26. Gluck, L., Kulovich, M. V., Borer, R. C., Jr., and Keidel, W. N.: The interpretation and significance of the lecithin/sphingomyelin ratio in amniotic fluid. *Am. J. Obstet. Gynecol.*, in press.

27. Reynolds, W. A., Pitkin, R. M., and Filer, L. J., Jr.: *Proceedings, Medical Perintology, 1972. Proc. 3rd Conf. Exp. Med. Surg. Primates, Lyon 1972*, Part III. Karger, Basel, 1972, pp. 368–375.

28. Novy, M. J., Portman, O. W., and Bell, M.: Evidence for pulmonary and other sources of amniotic fluid phospholipids in the rhesus monkey. In: Villee, C. A., Villee, D. B., and Zuckerman, J. (Eds.): *Respiratory Distress Syndrome*. Academic Press, New York, 1973, pp. 205–218.

29. Clements, J. A.: Composition and properties of pulmonary surfactant. In: Villee, C. A., Villee, D. B., and Zuckerman, J. (Eds.): *Respiratory Distress Syndrome*. Academic Press, New York, 1973, pp. 77–98.

30. Biggs, J. J. G., Gaffney, T. J., and McGeary, H.: Evidence that fetal lung fluid and phospho-lipids pass into amniotic fluid in human pregnancy. *J. Obstet. Gynaecol. Br. Commonw.* **80:** 125, 1973.

31. Setnikar, I., Agostoni, E., and Taglietti, A.: The fetal lung, a source of amniotic fluid. *Proc. Soc. Exp. Biol. Med.* **101:** 842, 1949.

32. Boston, R. W., Humphreys, P. W., Normand, I. C. S., Reynolds, E. O. R., and Strang, L. B.: Formation of liquid in the lungs of foetal lambs. *Biol. Neonate* **12:** 306, 1968.

33. Scarpelli, E. M.: The lung, tracheal fluid and lipid metabolism of the fetus. *Pediatrics* **40:** 951, 1967.

34. Adams, F. H., Desilets, D. J., and Towers, B.: Control of flow of fetal lung fluid at the laryngeal outlet. *Resp. Physiol.* **2:** 302, 1967.

35. Liggins, G. C., and Howie, R. N.: A controlled trial of antepartum glucocorticoid treatment for prevention of the respiratory distress syndrome in premature infants. *Pediatrics* **50:** 515, 1972.

35a. Kotas, R. V., and Avery, M. E.: Accelerated appearance of pulmonary surfactant in the fetal rabbit. *J. Appl. Physiol.* **30:** 358, 1971. Also Motoyama, E. K., Orzalesi, M. M., Kikkawn, Y., et al: Effects of cortisol on the development of fetal rabbit lungs. *Pediatrics* **48:** 547, 1971.

36. Farrell, P. M., and Zachman, R. D.: Induction of choline phosphotransferase and lecithin syn-thesis in the fetal lung. *Science* **179:** 297, 1973.

37. Bauer, C. R., Stern, L., and Colle, E.: Prolonged rupture of membranes associated with a de-creased incidence of respiratory distress syndrome. *Pediatrics* **53:** 7, 1974.

38. Conly, P. W., LeMaire, W. J., Monkus, E. F., and Cleveland, W. W.: Plasma estriol concen-tration in infants with the respiratory distress syndrome. *J. Pediatr.* **83:** 851, 1973.

39. Pakravan, P., Kenny, F. M., Depp, R., and Allen, A. C.: Familial congenital absence of adrenal glands; evaluation of glucocorticoid, mineralocorticoid, and estrogen metabolism in the peri-natal period. *J. Pediatr.* **84:** 74–78, 1974.

40. Giannopoulos, G., Mulay, S., and Solomon, S.: Cortisol receptors in rabbit fetal lung. *Bio-chem. Biophys. Res. Commun.* **47:** 411, 1972. Also see Giannopoulos, G.: *Fed. Proc.* **32:** 651, 1973.

CHAPTER 15

Cellular Growth of the Rhesus Monkey Placenta

Donald E. Hill

Systematic study of the cellular growth of the placenta has received increasing attention in the past 10 years. Winick and Noble[1] documented that weight, protein, and RNA content increase linearly until day 20 in rat placenta, whereas DNA fails to increase after day 17. They interpret this to indicate a cessation of DNA synthesis prior to term. Similarly, the data of Winick et al[2] in humans indicate that DNA content does not increase after 34 to 36 weeks of gestation while RNA and protein increase linearly until term. This has been supported by the data of Weinberg et al[3] in which autoradiography of placental tissue slices indicated less ^{3}H-thymidine uptake in trophoblasts or fibroblasts with advancing gestation. On the other hand, the data of Dayton et al[4] indicate that DNA content of the placenta increases linearly until term. Although the data of Laga et al[5] show a positive correlation between DNA content and gestational age, they have insufficient numbers in late gestation to support or negate either thesis.

Since the placenta has a mixture of cell types in variable amounts throughout pregnancy, the use of DNA content as an index of cell number is less valid than in other tissues. However, it can be used to relate to other cell constituents and as a total amount probably reflects the overall growth of the placenta. Determination of the relative trophoblast mass has recently been accomplished[6] and gives a better estimate of the cell type and cell population present at any given time in the placenta. Other considerations such as the presence of metabolic DNA[7, 8] and abnormalities in DNA synthesis such as those occurring in chromosome disorders[9, 10] or in intrauterine viral infections[11] make the use of DNA as an index of placental cell number subject to greater error than is morphometry.

In this chapter biochemical data are reported for normal rhesus monkey placentas from 80 to 160 days of gestation. The *Macaca mulatta* placenta is composed of two discs in the majority (80%) of pregnancies and is hemochorial in type. All fetuses were delivered by cesarean section, and the placentas were processed:

The excess blood and amniotic fluid was drained off and the total weight was obtained. The placentas were then trimmed of membranes, cord, and surface blood vessels, as well as the decidua on the maternal side. The trimmed, wet weight was the value used in determining total amounts of constituents. One-half of the primary and one-half of the secondary placenta were frozen at —20°C and later homogenized for DNA and RNA determinations. The remaining portions were dried and ether extracted to obtain the water, protein, collagen, and lipid content according to previously described methods.

In Figures 15.1 and 15.2, the placenta weight is shown plotted against gestational age and body weight, respectively. The best fit of the data for both graphs in the last third of pregnancy is linear with highly significant correlation coefficients ($P < 0.001$).

Figure 15.3 depicts the total placental DNA as a function of gestational age, and it also increases linearly until term. There is no indication of a plateau in late pregnancy. When compared with placental weight the correlation is greater.

Similarly, the placental RNA increases linearly until term although the slope is not as steep as with DNA (Figure 15.4). This increase in total RNA occurs while the concentration of RNA (milligrams per gram of fresh placenta) is gradually declining (Figure 15.5). The concentration of collagen is also declining (Figure 15.6) toward term. Total noncollagen protein increased linearly to term with a highly significant ($P < 0.001$) positive correlation (Figure 15.7). The equations describing these relationships are shown in Table 15.1.

The linear increase in DNA content to term in normal monkey placenta agrees with the data of Dayton et al[4] for well-nourished human populations. The reason for the discrepancy between these findings and those of Winick et al[2] is not clear. One possible explanation is that the data of the latter authors are plotted versus placental weight (which is used in computing total DNA content) and the variability is large nearer term. When the placental DNA is plotted against fetal weight, the apparent cessation of DNA synthesis is less striking. If the data were plotted against gestational age, there may in fact be a quadratic relationship overall and a linear relationship in late gestation.

Our data in the monkey for RNA values agree with the data of Winick and Noble[1] in rats, and Winick et al[2] in humans. Laga et al[5] found a negative correlation between gestational age and placental RNA while the correlation was positive to term with birth weight and placental weight. This finding is as yet unexplained. It is unlikely that where strongly positive correlations exist between birth weight and gestational age there would be a negative correlation between RNA content and the variable. The same comments apply to the negative correlation found with protein content in their study. Our data on protein content are in agreement with the findings of Winick et al[2] for human placenta.

The strongly positive linear correlations between placental weight and fetal weight in the latter one-third of pregnancy are in agreement with data in humans[12, 15] and rhesus monkeys.[16, 17] Similarly, the relationships between placental weight and gestational age follow the pattern seen in humans. Although the numbers in this series are small, the variation is also small and the correlations are highly significant.

The growing placenta in normal rhesus monkeys continues to increase in DNA, RNA, and protein content until term. This would suggest that although the growth velocity is slowing near term, the placenta is still actively accreting cells and protein.

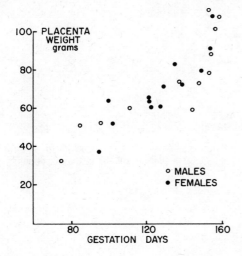

Fig. 15.1. The change during gestation in placental weight in the macaque.

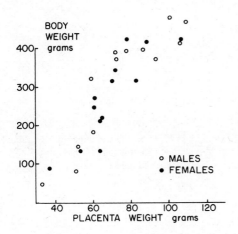

Fig. 15.2. The change during gestation in placental weight with body weight in the macaque.

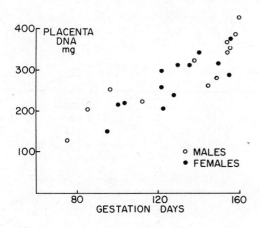

Fig. 15.3. The change during gestation in the total placental DNA in the macaque.

285

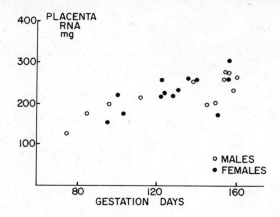

Fig. 15.4. The change during gestation in placental RNA in the macaque.

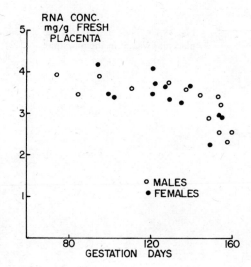

Fig. 15.5. The change during gestation in concentration of placental RNA in the macaque.

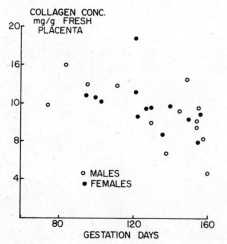

Fig. 15.6. The change during gestation in collagen concentration in the placenta in the macaque.

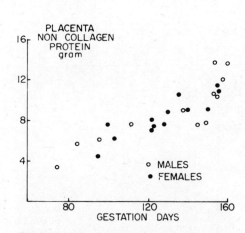

Fig. 15.7. The change during gestation in placental noncollagen protein in the macaque.

286

Table 15.1 Equations describing placental size in Macaca mulatta.

	TIME SPAN	n	Y units	X units	Equation Y =	SD	Fit
1.	80 days CA to 160 days CA	25	Placenta weight g	CA (days)	$-18.97955 + 0.69856 \, (X)$	10.56	0.001 linear r = 0.86
2.	80 days CA to 160 days CA	25	Placenta weight g	Body weight g	$31.49052 + 0.13875 \, (X)$	9.59	0.001 linear r = 0.89
3.	80 days CA to 160 days CA	25	DNA mg	CA (days)	$-52.53063 + 2.61381 \, (X)$	37.57	0.001 linear r = 0.87
4.	80 days CA to 160 days CA	25	RNA mg	CA (days)	$66.31873 + 1.25296 \, (X)$	30.71	0.001 linear r = 0.73
5.	80 days CA to 160 days CA	25	RNA mg/g	CA (days)	$0.91415 + 0.059058 \, (X) - 0.00030175 \, (X)^2$	0.34	0.5 quadratic
6.	80 days CA to 160 days CA	25	Collagen mg/g	CA (days)	$19.88806 - 0.06563 \, (X)$	2.48	0.01 linear r = -0.57
7.	80 days CA to 160 days CA	25	Non Collagen Protein g	CA (days)	$-2.75952 + 0.08827 \, (X)$	1.30	0.001 linear r = 0.87

REFERENCES

1. Winick, M., and Noble, A.: Quantitative changes in DNA, RNA, and protein during normal growth of rat placenta. *Nature* **212**: 5057, 1966.

2. Winick, M., Coscia, A., and Noble, A.: Cellular growth of human placenta. I. Normal placental growth. *Pediatrics* **39**: 248, 1967.

3. Weinberg, P. C., Camerson, I. L., Parnley, T., Jetter, J. R., and Pauerstein, C. J.: Gestational age and placental cellular replication. *Obstet. Gynecol.* **36**: 692, 1970.

4. Dayton, D. H , Filer, L. J., and Canosa, C.: Cellular changes in the placentas of undernourished mothers in Guatemala. *Fed. Proc.* **28**: 488, 1969.

5. Laga, E. M., Driscoll, S. G., and Munro, H. N.: Quantitative studies of human placenta. II. Biochemical characteristics. *Biol. Neonate* **23**: 260, 1973.

6. Laga, E. M., Driscoll, S. G., and Munro, H. N.: Quantitative studies of human placenta. I. Morphometry. *Biol. Neonate* **23**: 231, 1973.

7. Stroun, M., Charles, P., Anker, P., and Pele, R. C.: Metabolic DNA in heart and skeletal muscle and in the intestine of mice. *Nature (London)* **216**: 716, 1967.

8. Ficqo, A., Pavan, C., and Brachet, J.: Metabolic processes in chromosomes. *Exp. Cell Res. Suppl.* **6**, 105–114, 1958.

9. Kaback, M. M., and Bernstein, L. H.: Biologic studies of trisonic cells growing *in vitro*. *Ann. N.Y. Acad. Sci.* **171**: 526, 1970.

10. German, J.: Bloom's syndrome. I. Genetical and clinical observations in the first twenty-seven patients. *Am. J. Human Genet.* **21**: 196, 1969.

11. Plotkin, S. A., Bove, L. A., and Bove, J. G.: The *in vitro* growth of rubella virus in human embryo cells. *Am. J. Epidemiol.* **81**: 71, 1965.

12. Adair, F. L., and Thelander, H.: A study of the weight and dimensions of the human placenta in its relation to the weight of the newborn infant. *Am. J. Obstet. Gynecol.* **10**: 172, 1925.

13. McKeown, T., and Record, R. G.: The influence of placental size on foetal growth in man, with special reference to multiple pregnancy. *J. Endocrinol.* **9**: 418, 1953.

14. Hendricks, C. H.: Patterns of fetal and placental growth: The second half of normal pregnancy. *Obstet. Gynecol.* **24**: 357, 1964.

15. Aherne, W.: A weight relationship between the human foetus and placenta. *Biol. Neonate* **10**: 113, 1966.

16. Dawes, G. S.: The placenta and foetal growth. In: *Foetal and Neonatal Physiology*. Yearbook, Chicago, 1969.

17. Kerr, G. R., Campbell, J. A., Helmuth, A. C., and Waisman, H. A.: Growth and development of the fetal rhesus monkey (*Macaca mulatta*). II. Total nitrogen, protein, lipid, glycogen, and water composition of major organs. *Pediatr. Res.* **5**: 151, 1971.

CHAPTER 16

Skeletal Growth
in the Fetal Macaque

George R. Kerr

INTRODUCTION

The progess of growth culminates in the achievement of "maturity," with maturation of each process occurring at a different chronologic age. [1] A variety of environmental and hereditary agents are capable of influencing both the velocity of developmental changes and the chronologic ages at which maturity occurs. [2, 3] Linear
growth of the body ceases after puberty, but many of the agents that interfere with
linear growth also delay the onset of puberty, allowing growth to continue for a
period of time that is longer than would be anticipated on the basis of chronologic
age. The amount of this prepubertal delay, and the potential for "catchup" growth,
is most easily quantified by evaluating the processes of skeletal maturation. [4-13]
    The rate of growth is fastest during fetal life but a variety of agents cause growth
failure in the human fetus. [14, 15] Unfortunately the stage of maturation of the newborn skeleton is of little clinical value in predicting the growth potential since
radiologically it is difficult to establish reference points, the majority of which ossify
only after birth. [16]
    Major differences have been found between species with respect to placental
structures, [17] rates of fetal growth, [18] and timing of important maturational
processes. [19] The macaque placenta resembles that of the human and other subhuman primates. This similarity extends to fetal skeletal growth, [20, 21] from which
arises our interest in the study of skeletal tissues from normal fetuses (*Macaca
mulatta*) of exact gestational age. [22, 23]

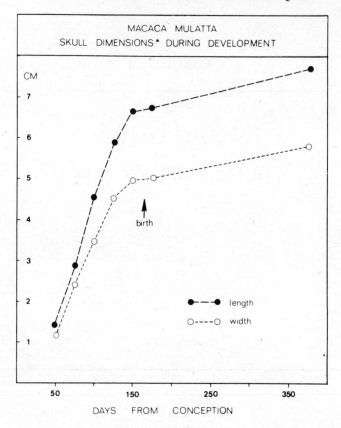

Fig. 16.1. Development of the fetal skeleton in *M. mulatta:* Linear dimensions of the skull. (*Length of ossified bone in centimeters.)

OBSERVATIONS ON SKELETAL GROWTH

The amount of mineral present in the 50-day fetal skeleton was small and ossification could be visualized and measured in only the humerus, radius, ulna, femur, tibia, and fibula. After 75 days of gestation, no difficulty was encountered in measuring the length of each tubular bone, or in identifying the presence of ossification in the epiphyseal centers and round bones of the appendicular skeleton. The linear dimensions of the skull and the long bones of the extremities are presented in Figures 16.1 and 16.2. These illustrations are constructed from previously published data.[23] The sequences and timing of ossification of round bones and epiphyses are presented in Tables 16.1 and 16.2. A graphical representation of the data shown in these tables is presented in Figure 16.3.

The tarsal calcaneus was the first epiphyseal center in which ossification could be detected in fetal life. This appeared by 75 days of gestation. The tarsal talus was apparent in fetuses of 100 gestational days, and by 125 days, ossification centers were visible at the distal radial epiphysis and in the epiphyses of the second, third, and fourth metacarpals. A few of the fetuses showed ossification of the proximal epiphysis of the humerus, the carpal capitate, hamate, triangular and scaphoid, the proximal and distal epiphyses of the tibia, the tarsal cuboid, and the third cuneiform bone.

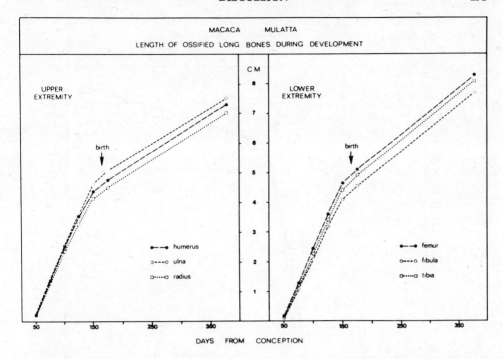

Fig. 16.2. Development of the fetal skeleton in *M. mulatta*: Linear dimensions of the long bones of the upper extremity (humerus, radius, ulna) and lower extremity (femur, tibia, fibula).

By 150 days of gestation all centers of epiphyseal ossification in the lower extremities were present in some of the fetuses, but about half of them did not show visible ossification in the tarsal navicular and second cuneiform bones and the second and fifth middle phalanges; only a few showed ossification at the first metatarsal and the distal phalanges. In the upper extremity, a few animals showed ossification at the distal epiphyses of the ulna, the first metacarpal, and the third and fourth distal phalanges. Ossification could not be identified in any animal at the proximal epiphyses of the radius and ulna, the carpal centrale and trapezium, and the epiphyses of the first proximal phalanx and the first, second, and fifth distal phalanges. The remaining epiphyses and round bones were ossified in almost all of the animals.

By 175 days of gestational age it was possible to identify ossification centers in the proximal epiphyses of the radius and ulna, the carpal centrale and trapezium, the epiphyses of the first proximal phalanx, and the second and fifth distal phalanges in about half of the fetuses. All epiphyses and round bones were ossified in the lower extremity in most animals, with only a few showing lack of ossification at the epiphyses of the first proximal phalanx and the second and fifth distal phalanges. By 7 months postnatal age, all epiphyseal centers and round bones were well ossified.

DISCUSSION

The maximal rates of development occur during early gestation, which is a period of vulnerability.[1, 24] A wide variety of infectious,[25] socioeconomic,[26, 27] ge-

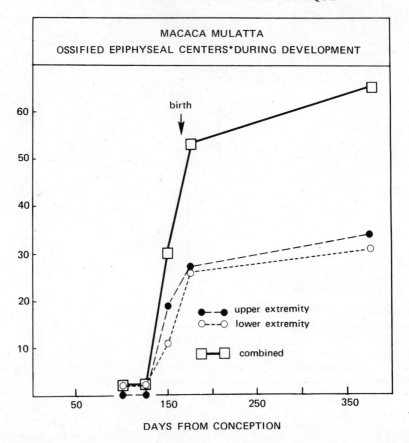

Fig. 16.3. Development of the fetal skeleton in *M. mulatta*: Epiphyseal ossification in the upper and lower extremity. (*A total of 67 sites of ossification was examined. The number on the ordinate represents that number *of* sites which were ossified in *all* animals examined. For complete assessment of these data consult Tables 16.1 and 16.2).

netic,[28] pharmacological,[29,30] nutritional,[31,32] and other factors are associated with developmental abnormalities and growth failure of the human fetus. Over 90% of the fatalities between conception and the end of the first year of postnatal life occur prior to full-term gestation.[33] Insults that interfere with normal fetal development produce disabilities.[34-41]

Measurement of growth retardation in terms of organ size and composition is difficult.[42,43] Such terms as "placental insufficiency" or "fetal malnutrition" disguise our ignorance of causative mechanisms.

The ability to evaluate skeletal development by radiologic means has been of clinical value in *postnatal* life. Many factors that alter the rate of linear growth delay the processes of skeletal maturation. As linear growth continues until skeletal maturation is complete, the growth failure from certain disorders may be reversed by a period of "catchup" growth during which the velocity of linear growth is greater than that appropriate for the chronologic age, or by a period of growth of normal velocity but which is longer in duration than that of the age peers.

Table 16.1   Development of the fetal skeleton in M. mulatta: epiphyseal ossification in the upper extremity*

Upper extremity	\	Conceptual age (days)				
	75	100	125	150	175	378
Humerus - proximal			1/11	*	*	*
- distal				*	*	*
Radius - proximal					7/13	*
- distal			11/12	*		*
Ulna - proximal					5/13	*
- distal				1/10	*	*
Carpal - capitate			2/12	*	*	*
- hamate			2/12	*	*	*
- triangular			1/12	*	*	*
- scaphoid			1/12	*	*	*
- centrale					6/13	*
- pisiform				8/10	*	*
- trapezoid				8/10	*	*
- trapezium					10/13	*
- lunate				9/10	*	*
Metacarpal - 1				1/10	*	*
- 2			5/12	*	*	*
- 3			7/12	*	*	*
- 4			7/12	*	*	*
- 5				*	*	*
Proximal phalanges - 1					5/13	*
- 2				*	*	*
- 3				*	*	*
- 4				*	*	*
- 5				*	*	*
Middle phalanges - 2				*	*	*
- 3				*	*	*
- 4				*	*	*
- 5				*	*	*
Distal phalanges - 1					*	*
- 2					12/13	*
- 3				3/10	*	*
- 4				1/10	*	*
- 5					7/11	*

* Indicates epiphyseal ossification in all animals; numbers represent number of epiphyses showing ossification/total number of epiphyses. Reprinted from Kerr et al: Growth 36:59, 1972, with the permission of the Editor.

Development of the appendicular skeleton in humans occurs through three sequential stages superimposed upon the continuing processes of linear skeletal growth: (1) ossification of the tubular bones, largely established during fetal life; (2) ossification of the round bones (carpals and tarsals) and the epiphyses of the tubular bones, commencing during late fetal life and continuing until the onset of puberty; and (3) unification of the epiphyses with the diaphyses of the tubular bones which commences with the onset of puberty and within a few years terminates the processes of linear skeletal growth.

A variety of studies of different areas of the skeleton have been utilized to determine the state of skeletal maturation, with ease of technique and the number of reference skeletal structures determining the relative value of each area.[44-46, 55]

Table 16.2　　　　　Development of the fetal skeleton in
M. mulatta: epiphyseal ossification
in the lower extremity*

Lower extremity	Conceptual age (days)					
	75	100	125	150	175	378
Femur - proximal				8/9	*	*
- distal				*	*	*
Tibia - proximal			4/11	*	*	*
- distal			1/12	*.	*	*
Fibula - distal				8/10	*	*
Tarsal						
Calcaneus	6/10	*	*	*	*	*
Talus		*	*	*	*	*
Cuboid			1/12	*	*	*
Navicular				5/10	*	*
1st Cuneiform				*	*	*
2nd Cuneiform				5/10	*	*
3rd Cuneiform			1/12	*	*	*
Metatarsal - 1				1/10	*	*
- 2				*	*	*
- 3				*	*	*
- 4				*	*	*
- 5				9/10	*	*
Proximal - 1					10/13	*
phalanges - 2				8/10	*	*
- 3				9/10	*	*
- 4				9/10	*	*
- 5				8/10	*	*
Middle - 2				5/10	*	*
phalanges - 3				9/10	*	*
- 4				9/10	*	*'
- 5				5/10	*	*
Distal - 1				4/10	*	*
phalanges - 2				2/10	2/13	*
- 3				2/10	11/13	*
- 4				2/10	11/13	*
- 5				1/10	3/13	*

* Indicates epiphyseal ossification in all animals; numbers
represent number of epiphyses showing ossification/total
number of epiphyses. Reprinted from Kerr et al: Growth
36:59, 1972 with the permission of the Editor.

It has not been appreciated, however, that there is a range of normal values for each skeletal structure at each developmental age, and that agents which interfere with skeletal growth may affect the development of one structure more than another. This is so, for example, in fetal dysmorphogenesis.[28]

The fact that most of the reference points in the skeleton appear only after full-term gestation hampers the use of such points to assess retarded growth or catchup growth.[56]

Most investigators of fetal biology utilize experimental animals as "models" in which hypotheses related to human fetal growth and development may be explored. Subhuman primates, while showing some differences from those of man, also show many similarities. Moreover, it is possible to design studies that would not be possible during human pregnancies.[57-66] During the last 10 years studies have shown that placental structures and the rates of linear growth of the fetal rhesus monkey are generally similar to those of man.[67-74] Moreover, the normal patterns of post-natal growth,[75] learning,[76] and social behavior[77] have also been quantified, and it is possible to determine the ultimate developmental consequences of agents applied to the mother or fetus during gestation. The rhesus monkey is of value for investigating problems of pregnancy.[78-82]

Definition of the sequences of skeletal development and the availability of norms for skeletal maturation and linear growth are of value in the study of a wide variety of factors influencing the growth of the human fetus.

Fetal skeletal maturation in the rhesus monkey has been studied by Schultz[20] and van Wagenen and Asling[21] and by our group.[23] Details of the skeletal system of adult monkeys are available in the dissection manual of Berringer et al[83] and in Hill's series, *Primates: Comparative Anatomy and Taxonomy*.[84] However, each of these studies utilized different methodology in describing the growth of the fetal skeleton. Schultz dealt primarily with the external dimensions of the fetus[20] and van Wagenen and Asling's study was more concerned with the timing of epiphyseal ossification than with the details of linear growth.[21] Our study, by defining exact linear dimensions in fetuses of known gestational ages and born to females of known health and reproductive experience, provides more precise data for the quantitation of skeletal maturation. Moreover, as the rates of linear growth have also been defined, such data may be of value in identifying the gestational ages at which postulated teratogenic agents could most logically be evaluated.

The radiographic procedures utilized in our study proved to be highly precise. The relative lack of variability between animals at each fetal age attested to the potential value of this species as a model. The sequences of ossification that we found are almost identical with those reported by van Wagenen and Asling.[21] The main exceptions occurred with the carpal centrale and the proximal epiphysis of the ulna which were ossified in about half of our 175-day fetuses whereas they did not report it prior to 177 days. The reason for these minor differences is not apparent. Epiphyseal ossification occurs in a predictable sequence but the exact gestational ages obscure the small differences in the sequence of skeletal maturation that should be expected in all primate species.

REFERENCES

1. Falkner, F. (Ed.): *Human Development*. Saunders, Philadelphia, 1966.
2. Cheek, D. B. (Ed.): *Human Growth. Body Composition, Cell Growth, Energy and Intelligence*. Lea & Febiger, Philadelphia, 1968.
3. Wolanski, N.: Genetic and ecological factors in human growth. *Human Biol*. **42**: 349, 1970.
4. Tanner, J. M. *Growth at Adolescence*. Thomas, Springfield, Illinois, 1962.
5. Hansman, C. F., and Maresh, M. M.: A longitudinal study of skeletal maturation. *Am. J. Dis. Child*. **101**: 305, 1961.
6. Moss, M., and Noback, C. R.: Longitudinal study of digital epiphyseal fusion in adolescence. *Anat. Rec*. **131**: 19, 1958.
7. Dreizen, S., Spirakis, C. N., and Stone, R. E.: A comparison of skeletal growth and maturation in undernourished and well-nourished girls before and after menarche. *J. Pediatr*. **70**: 256–263, 1967.
8. Hansen, J. D. L., Freesemann, C., Moodie, A. D., and Evans, D. E.: What does nutritional growth retardation imply? *Pediatrics* **47**: 299, 1971.
9. Dreizen, S., Snodgrass, R. M., Webbpeploe, H., and Spies, T. D.: The retarding effect of protracted undernutrition on the appearance of the postnatal ossification centers in the hand and wrist. *Human Biol*. **30**: 253, 1958.

10. Raisy, L. G., and Bengham, P. J.: Effect of hormones on bone development. *Ann. Rev. Pharmacol.* **12**: 335, 1972.

11. Sontag, L. W., and Lipford, J.: The effect of illness and other factors on appearance patterns of skeletal epiphyses. *J. Pediatr.* **23**: 391, 1943.

12. Acheson, R. M.: Effects of nutrition and disease on human growth. In: Tanner, J. M. (Ed.): *Human Growth, Sympos. Soc. Study Human Biol.* **3**: 73–92, 1960.

13. Roche, A. F. (Ed.): Assessment of skeletal maturation. *Am. J. Phys. Anthropol.* **35**: 315–470, 1972.

14. Andrews, B. F. (Ed.): The small-for-date infant. *Pediatr. Clin. North Am.*, Vol. 17. Saunders Philadelphia, 1970.

15. Editorial: Fetal growth retardation. *Aust. N. Z. J. Obstet. Gynecol.* **9**: 75, 1969.

16. Stuart, H. C., Pyle, S. I., Cornoni, J., and Reed, R. B.: Onsets, completions and spans of ossification in the 29 bone-growth centers of the hand and wrist. *Pediatrics* **29**: 237–249, 1962.

17. Wynn, R. M.: Morphology of the placenta. In: Assali, N. S. (Ed.): *Biology of Gestation*, Vol. 1. Academic Press, New York, 1968, pp. 94–184.

18. Widdowson, E. M.: Growth and composition of the fetus and newborn. In: Assali, N. S. (Ed.): *Biology of Gestation*, Vol. II. Academic Press, New York, 1968, pp. 1–49.

19. Dobbing, J.: Vulnerable periods in developing brain. In: Davison, A. M., and Dobbing, J. (Eds.): *Applied Neurochemistry*. Blackwell, Oxford, 1968, pp. 287–315.

20. Schultz, A. H.: Fetal growth and development of the rhesus monkey. *Cont. Embryol. # 155*, Carnegie Institute of Washington, 1937.

21. van Wagenen, G., and Asling, C. W.: Ossification in the fetal monkey (*Macaca mulatta*). Estimation of age and progress of gestation by roentgenography. *Am. J. Anat.* **114**: 107, 1964.

22. Kerr, G. R., Scheffler, G., and Waisman, H. A.: Growth and development of infant *M. mulatta* fed a standardized diet. *Growth* **33**: 185, 1969.

23. Kerr, G. R., Wallace, J. H., Chesney, C. F., and Waisman, H. A.: Growth and development of the fetal rhesus monkey. III. Maturation and linear growth of the skull and appendicular skeleton. *Growth* **36**: 59, 1972.

24. Brown, D. M.: Determination of cell development, differentiation, and growth. *Pediatr. Res.* **1**: 395–408, 1967.

25. Ross, C. A. C., Bell, E. J., Kerr, M. M., and Williams, K. A. B.: Infective agents and embryopathy in the west of Scotland, 1966–1970. *Scot. Med. J.* **17**: 252–258, 1972.

26. Gruenwald, P., Funakawa, H., Mitani, S., Nishimura, T., and Takeuchi, S.: Influence of environmental factors on fetal growth in man. *Lancet* **1**: 1026–1029, 1967.

27. Naeye, R. E., Diener, M. M., Harcke, H. T., Jr., and Blanc, W. A.: Relation of poverty and race to birth weight and organ and cell structure in the newborn. *Pediatr. Res.* **5**: 17–22, 1971.

28. Smith, D. W.: *Recognizable Patterns of Human Malformation. Genetic, Embryologic and Clinical Aspects.* No. 7 in series, *Major Problems in Clinical Pediatrics*, Schaffer, A. J. (Ed.). Saunders, Philadelphia, 1970.

29. Haworth, J. C., and Ford, J. D.: Comparison of the effects of maternal undernutrition and exposure to cigarette smoke on the cellular growth of the rat fetus. *Am. J. Obstet. Gynecol.* **112**: 653–656, 1972.

30. Friedler, G., and Cochin, J.: Growth retardation in offspring of female rats treated with morphine prior to conception. *Science* **175**: 654–656, 1972.

31. Bergner, L., and Susser, M. W.: Low birth weight and prenatal nutrition: An interpretive review. *Pediatrics* **46**: 946–966, 1970.

32. Neligan, G. A.: The effect of intrauterine malnutrition upon later development of humans. *Psychiatr. Neurol. Neurochir.* **74**: 453–461, 463–479, 1971.

33. Stickle, G.: Defective development and reproductive wastage in the United States. *Am. J. Obstet. Gynecol.* **100**: 442–447, 1968.

34. Editorial: Low birth weight infants. *Obstet. Gynecol.* **31**: 283–287, 1968.

35. North, A. F., Jr.: Small-for-dates neonates. II. Maternal, gestation and neonatal characteristics. *Pediatrics* **38**: 1013–1019, 1966.

36. Sinclair, J. C., and Coldiron, J. S.: Low birth weight and postnatal physical development. *Dev. Med. Child. Neurol.* **11**: 314–329, 1969.

37. Babson, S. G.: Growth of low-birth-weight infants. *J. Pediatr.* **77**: 11–18, 1970.

38. van den Berg, B. J., and Yerushalmy, J.: The relationship of the rate of intrauterine growth of infants of low birth weight to mortality, morbidity, and congenital anomalies. *J. Pediatr.* **69**: 531–545, 1966.

39. McDonald, A. D.: Intelligence in children of very low birth weight. *Br. J. Prev. Soc. Med.* **18**: 59–74, 1964.

40. Weiner, G., Rider, R. V., Oppel, W. C., Fischer, L. K., and Harper, P. A.: Correlates of low birth weight: Psychological status at six to seven years of age. *Pediatrics* **35**: 434–444, 1965.

41. Andrews, B. F. (Ed.): The small-for-date infant. *Pediatr. Clin. North Am.*, Vol. 17. Saunders, Philadelphia, 1970.

42. Gruenwald, P., and Minh, H. N.: Evaluation of body and organ weights in perinatal pathology. I. Normal standards derived from autopsies. *Am. J. Clin. Pathol.* **34**: 247–253, 1960.

43. Schultz, D. M., Giordano, D. A., and Schultz, D. H.: Weights of organs of fetuses and infants. *Arch. Pathol.* **74**: 80–86, 1962.

44. Acheson, R. M.: Maturation of the skeleton. In: Falkner, F. (Ed.): *Human Development*. Saunders, Philadelphia, 1966, pp. 465–501.

45. Rodahl, K.: Bone development. In: Falkner, F. (Ed.): *Human Development*. Saunders, Philadelphia, 1966, pp. 503–509.

46. Rotch, T. M.: A study of the development of the bones in childhood by the roentgen method, with a view of establishing a developmental index for the grading of and the protection of early life. *Trans. Assoc. Am. Physicians* **24**: 603–630, 1909.

47. Pyle, S. I., and Hoerr, N. L.: *Radiographic Atlas of Skeletal Development of the Knee*. Thomas, Springfield, Illinois, 1955.

48. Greulich, W. W., and Pyle, S. I.: *Radiographic Atlas of Skeletal Development of the Hand and Wrist*. Stanford University Press, Palo Alto, California, 1959.

49. Hansman, C. F., and Maresh, M. M.: A longitudinal study of skeletal maturation. *Am. J. Dis. Child.* **101**: 305–321, 1961.

50. Hoerr, N. L., Pyle, S. I., and Francis, C. C.: *Radiographic Atlas of Skeletal Development of the Foot and Ankle*. Thomas, Springfield, Illinois, 1962.

51. Tanner, J. M., and Whitehouse, R. H.: *Standards of Skeletal Maturity*. International Childrens Center, Paris, 1959.

52. Tanner, J. M., Whitehouse, R. H., and Healy, M. J. R.: A new system for estimating skeletal maturity from the hand and wrist, with standards derived from a study of 2600 healthy British children. International Childrens Center, Paris, 1962.

53. Bardeen, C. R.: The relationship of ossification to physiological development. *J. Radiol.* **2**: 1–8, 1921.

54. Flory, C. D.: Osseous development in the hand as an index of skeletal development. *Monogr. Soc. Res. Child Dev.* **1**: 1936.

55. Todd, T. W.: *Atlas of Skeletal Maturation*. Mosby, St. Louis, Missouri, 1937.

56. Emery, J. L.: Evidence from bone growth that most of the infants dying in the neonatal period had been ill before birth. *Acta Pediatr. Scand. Suppl.* **172**: 55–59, 1967.

57. Kerr, G. R., and Waisman, H. A.: Phenylalanine: Transplacental concentrations in rhesus monkeys. *Science* **151**: 824–825, 1966.

58. Reynolds, S. R. M., Paul, W. M., and Huggett, A. St. G.: Physiological study of the monkey fetus *in utero*: A procedure for blood pressure recording, blood sampling and injection of the fetus under normal conditions. *Bull. Johns Hopkins Hosp.* **95**: 256–268, 1954.

59. Behrman, R. E., and Lees, M. H.: Organ blood flows of the fetal, newborn and adult rhesus monkey. *Biol. Neonate* **18**: 330–340, 1971.

60. Myers, R. E.: Two patterns of perinatal brain damage and their conditions of occurrence. *Am. J. Obstet. Gynecol.* **112**: 246–270, 1972.

61. Delahunt, G. S., and Rieser, N.: Rubella-induced embryopathies in monkeys. *Am. J. Obstet. Gynecol.* **99**: 580–588, 1967.

62. Speert, H.: Swallowing and gastrointestinal activity in the fetal monkey. *Am. J. Obstet. Gynecol.* **45:** 69–82, 1943.

63. de Gallardo, F. O. E., Fleischman, R. W., and de Arellano, M. I. R. R.: Electroencephalogram of the monkey fetus *in utero*, and changes in it at birth. *Exp. Neurol.* **9:** 73–84, 1964.

64. Parer, J. T., de Lannoy, C. W., Hoverland, A. S., and Metcalfe, J.: Effect of decreased uterine blood flow on uterine oxygen consumption in pregnant macaques. *Am. J. Obstet. Gynecol.* **100:** 813–820, 1968.

65. Hill, D. E., Myers, R. E., Holt, A. B., Scott, R. E., and Cheek, D. B.: Fetal growth retardation produced by placental insufficiency in the rhesus monkey. *Biol. Neonate* **19:** 68–82, 1971.

66. Adamsons, K., James, L. S., Lucey, J. F., and Towell, M. E.: The effect of anemia upon cardiovascular performances and acid-base state of the fetal rhesus monkey. *Ann. N.Y. Acad. Sci.* **162:** 225–239, 1969.

67. Martin, C. B., and Ramsey, E. M.: Gross anatomy of the placenta of rhesus monkeys. *Obstet. Gynecol.* **36:** 167–177, 1970.

68. Allen, J. R., and Ahlgren, S. A.: A comparative study of the hematologic changes in pregnancy in the *Macaca mulatta* monkey and the human female. *Am. J. Obstet. Gynecol.* **100:** 894–903, 1968.

69. Kerr, G. R.: The free amino acids of serum during development of *Macaca mulatta*. II. During pregnancy and fetal life. *Pediatr. Res.* **2:** 493–500, 1968.

70. Kerr, G. R., and Kennan, A. L.: The free amino acids of amniotic fluid during pregnancy of the rhesus monkey. *Am. J. Obstet. Gynecol.* **105:** 363–368, 1969.

71. Kerr, G. R., Kennan, A. L., Waisman, H. A., and Allen, J. R.: Growth and development of the fetal rhesus monkey. I. Physical growth. *Growth* **33:** 201–213, 1969.

72. Campbell, J. A.: DNA, RNA and protein in developing organs of the fetal rhesus monkey. M.S. Thesis, University of Wisconsin, 1973.

73. Kerr, G. R., Helmuth, A., Campbell, J., and Waisman, H. A.: Growth and development of the fetal rhesus monkey. II. Total protein, lipid, glycogen and water composition of major organs. *Pediatr. Res.* **5:** 151–158, 1971.

74. Kerr, G. R., Helmuth, A. C., and Waisman, H. A.: Growth and development of the fetal rhesus monkey. IV. Fractional lipid analysis of the developing brain. *Growth*, 1973 (in press).

75. Kerr, G. R., Scheffler, G., and Waisman, H. A.: Growth and development of infant *M. mulatta* fed a standardized diet. *Growth* **33:** 185–199, 1969.

76. Harlow, H. F.: The development of learning in the rhesus monkey. *Am. Sci.* **47:** 459–479, 1959.

77. Harlow, M. K., and Harlow, H. F.: Affection in primates. *Discovery* **27:** 11–17, 1966.

78. Kerr, G. R., Chamove, A. S., Harlow, H. F., and Waisman, H. A.: "Fetal PKU"—The effect of maternal hyperphenylalaninemia during pregnancy in the rhesus monkey (*M. mulatta*). *Pediatrics* **42:** 27–36, 1968.

79. Kerr, G. R., Allen, J. R., Scheffler, G., and Waisman, H. A.: Malnutrition studies in the rhesus monkey (*M. mulatta*). I. The effect on physical growth. *Am. J. Clin. Nutr.* **23:** 739–748, 1970.

80. Kerr, G. R., Waisman, H. A., Allen, J. R., Wallace, J. H., and Scheffler, G.: Malnutrition studies in *M. mulatta*: 2. Effect on organ size and growth of the skull and appendicular skeleton. *Am. J. Clin. Nutr.*, 1973 (in press).

81. Kerr, G. R., and Helmuth, A. C.: Malnutrition studies in *M. mulatta*. III. Effect on cerebral lipids. *Am. J. Clin. Nutr.*, 1973 (in press).

82. Kerr, G. R., Tyson, I. B., Allen, J. R., Wallace, J. H., and Scheffler, G.: Deficiency of thyroid hormone and development of the fetal rhesus monkey. *Biol. Neonate* **21:** 282, 1972.

83. Berringer, O. M., Browning, F. M., and Schroeder, C. R.: *An Atlas and Dissection Manual of Rhesus Monkey Anatomy.* Anatomy Lab. Aids, Tallahassee, Florida, 1968.

84. Hill, W. C. O.: *Primates: Comparative Anatomy and Taxonomy*, Vols. 1–8. University of Edinburgh Press, Edinburgh, Scotland, 1953–1970.

85. Poznanski, A. K., Garn, S. M., Kuhns, L. R., and Sandusky, S. T.: Dysharmonic maturation of the hand in the congenital malformation syndromes. *Am. J. Phys. Anthropol.* **35:** 417, 1972.

CHAPTER 17

Changes in Somatic Growth
After Placental Insufficiency
and Maternal Protein Deprivation

Donald B. Cheek and Donald E. Hill

PLACENTAL INSUFFICIENCY

In Chapter 7 the effects of placental insufficiency on brain growth of the rhesus monkey fetus were described and contrasted with those data available from other animal experiments and human data. In this chapter the changes in cell and somatic growth of the other visceral organs and the carcass are summarized.

Significant growth retardation in fetal rhesus monkeys has been achieved by the ligation of interplacental blood vessels in previously reported studies. [1–3] In the first study, ligation of interplacental vessels at 100 to 110 days of gestation was achieved by briefly removing the fetus through a hysterotomy and directly identifying and ligating the vessels. In more recent work, a total extraamniotic approach has been used. This procedure has effectively reduced the mortality from 60% to 30% and produces significant growth retardation in 70% of experimental animals. The animals that have minimal effects on growth at term usually have a primary placenta that is sufficiently large to compensate for any loss in placental mass secondary to the ligation procedure. The most severely affected animals are those in which the secondary placenta accounts for nearly 50% of the total placental mass. We have had a limited number of placentas available for examination. However, it has become clear that below 110 g of total placental weight significant growth retardation occurs (Figure 17.1).

The typical appearance of the experimental small-for-gestational-age monkeys is similar to that of severe marasmus. The head appears disproportionately large, and total body length is frequently not as severely affected as weight (Figure 17.2).

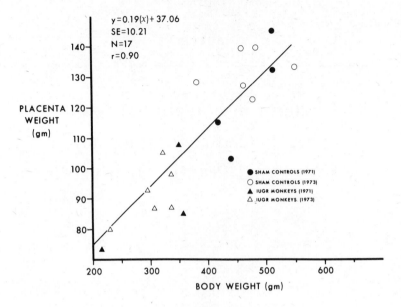

Fig. 17.1. The relationship between placental weight and body weight is shown for control macaques and for those with placental insufficiency. Note that if the placental tissue weight is below 100 g significant growth retardation occurs.

In Figure 17.3, the relative organ involvement in these animals is compared with the human data of Gruenwald[4] and Naeye.[5] There is close agreement with the human data with the exception of the adrenal gland, which is much more reduced in size in the human. This may be related to the fact that most of the human data were obtained from infants who were a few days old and had been severely stressed. Since the liver is severely affected and the brain is relatively spared there is a significant increase in the brain:liver ratio. A similar situation pertains for the human. The total amount of glycogen available for fuel is reduced and hence there is a tendency to spontaneous hypoglycemia.[6] We have observed hypoglycemia in three newborn monkeys with growth retardation. In spite of the severe growth retardation produced, the chemical composition in most of the organs was maintained proportionately, the exception to this being lipid content which was significantly reduced on a percentage basis in most of the organs examined.

The chemical composition of the liver is shown in Figure 17.4, and it can be seen that there is little or no change in the relative composition except for the fat content. Similarly, the nucleic acid and the protein contents were not altered on a concentration basis as outlined in Table 17.1. However, total amounts of constituents were obviously reduced and this is particularly true for nucleic acids. The total DNA content was significantly reduced in the liver for both gestational age and body weight. Similarly, there was a reduction in both total RNA and total protein of a significant degree. The protein:DNA ratios were unchanged in the growth-retarded group compared with age mates, indicating that the deficits in DNA and protein were proportional. The small amount of data from human low-birth-weight infants[7] indicates that there is no change in the protein:DNA ratio in the liver and that the total DNA is on the lower limits of normal. The relatively small deficit in DNA in the human material may indicate that the growth-retarding

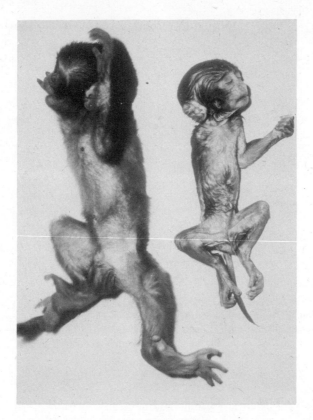

Fig. 17.2. A full-term fetal macaque is shown (left side) and compared with a fetus of the same gestational age but with intrauterine growth retardation due to ligation of placental vessels at 100 days of gestation. Note that the head appears disproportionately large in the growth-retarded fetus. (Reprinted from Richardson (Ed.): "Brain and Intelligence." Copyright 1973 by National Educational Press, 5604 Rhode Island Ave., Hyattsville, Md., 20781.)

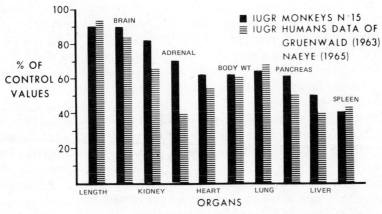

Fig. 17.3. If the normal growth of different organs of the human and macaque is placed at 100% for full growth, then the percentage of normal reached by human and macaque fetuses when placental insufficiency is present can be defined. Note the close agreement (except for the adrenal gland) between the human and monkey. (Data are from Gruenwald[4] and Naeye.[5])

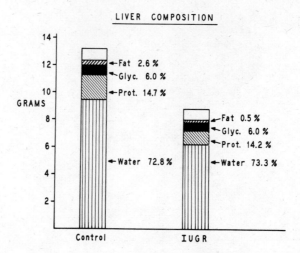

Fig. 17.4. The chemical composition is shown for the liver of the macaque fetus with intrauterine growth retardation. By comparison with the control, the percent reduction of various constituents is proportional except for fat which is more reduced in the liver of the growth-retarded fetus. (Reprinted from Hill et al., *Biol. Neon.* 19: 68, 1974, with permission of S. Karger A. G. Basel.)

influence develops late in gestation. Uterine artery ligation in rats[8] produced a small liver with reduced DNA and protein content. It would appear therefore that the deficit in liver growth is primarily related to an arrest in cell replication or at least in DNA content and has a secondary effect on protein synthesis.

Muscle mass, as obtained by direct weighing of dissected muscle, was reduced to 65% of control values and this tissue, like the liver, was not appreciably altered in composition. The nucleic acid concentrations and protein concentrations were also normal, as indicated in Table 17.2. The deficit in total DNA was less than that of the liver, while the total protein deficit was highly significant. However, when the protein:DNA ratio in the muscle was calculated, it was low. In experiments with runted pigs and newborn guinea pigs who were born of undernourished mothers, Widdowson[9] reported a reduction in total DNA as well as in the protein:DNA ratio in the quadriceps muscle of these animals. In the human data, also from Widdowson et al,[7] the DNA in the gastrocnemius muscle of five small-for-dates infants was in the lower range of normal, while the protein:DNA ratio for two of these infants was below the normal range. Again, it is not known at what point these infants suffered growth failure so it is difficult to make absolute comparisons with the data from monkeys. The data on the rhesus monkeys would suggest that protein synthesis is arrested or slowed out of proportion to the slowing in DNA replication.

The changes in the carcass (muscle mass plus skeletal mass) were again confined to a relative reduction in fat content and a total reduction in other constituents. Since the reduction in body length was minimal, the carcass mass relative to the muscle mass maintained the same ratio.

In Table 17.3, the experimental models that have been used for studying intrauterine growth retardation are summarized and contrasted.[10-15] In each of these

Table 17.1   The effect of intra-uterine growth retardation
(IUGR) produced by placental insufficiency on
the composition of the liver in the fetal
macaque

		Controls (N = 8)	IUGR (N = 7)
Weight	g	13.1 ± 2.4	** 8.4 ± 2.0
DNA	mg/g	4.21 ± 0.76	4.16 ± 0.63
RNA	mg/g	7.85 ± 0.21	8.18 ± 1.37
Protein	mg/g	147 ± 14	144 ± 27
Prot/DNA		37 ± 3	35 ± 8
Total DNA	mg	56 ± 15	* 34 ± 9
Total RNA	mg	100 ± 20	*** 70 ± 12
Total protein	g	1.95 ± 0.6	***1.2 ± 0.3

Difference from controls: * P = less than 0.02
** P = less than 0.005   *** P = less than 0.001

experiments the circulation has been compromised either at the uterine level or
placental level. There appears to be a fairly uniform pattern produced in each of
these experiments; however, the degree of involvement of various organs would
appear to be related to the timing of the insult. Each organ has its own specific
growth pattern and its own stage of hyperplasia or hypertrophy, which would
influence the growth of these organs and their chemical composition at the time of
study.

It is also evident that, in primates (man and monkeys), severe somatic growth
arrest can occur with less growth arrest of the brain. The reasons for this are not yet
clear and may be related in part to regional differences in blood flow. The growth

Table 17.2   The effect of intra-uterine growth retardation
(IUGR) produced by placental insufficiency on
the composition of the muscle in the fetal
macaque

		Controls (N = 8)	IUGR (N = 7)
Carcass weight	g	251 ± 36	*** 161 ± 34
Muscle mass	g	124 ± 20	*** 83 ± 18
DNA (FFFM)	mg/g	2.11 ± 0.27	2.57 ± 0.71
RNA (FFFM)	mg/g	2.09 ± 0.51	1.95 ± 0.32
Protein	mg/g	176 ± 10.0	172 ± 7.0
Protein/DNA ratio		77 ± 3.7	*** 59 ± 6
Total DNA	mg	359 ± 70	299 ± 90
Total RNA	mg	377 ± 107	* 229 ± 55
Total protein	g	30 ± 4.2	** 20 ± 4.6

FFFM = Fat free fresh muscle
Difference from controls: * P = less than 0.02
** P = less than 0.005   *** P = less than 0.001

Table 17.3　　　A comparison of intravascular
insufficiency experiments.

	Rat (Uterine artery ligation)	Sheep (Emboliz-ation)	Monkey (Intraplacental blood vessel ligation)
Body weight	50-70*	70	25
Brain weight	90-100	90	90 (cerebrum) 82 (cerebellum)
Brain: liver weight ratio	135-150	120	130
Total brain DNA	100	ND	100 (cerebrum) 80 (cerebellum)
Total liver DNA	60	ND	45

* Each figure is the value expressed as a
percentage of the control　　ND = Not determined
For references see text.

arrest may be due primarily to a reduction in overall substrate supply, that is, amino acids, glucose, and fatty acids, or may be due to severe fetal hypoxia and/or reduced blood volume. Dynamic studies of the transfer of nutrients following vascular ligations of various types will be required to determine the exact nature of the insult. Further work on the mechanisms that arrest protein and DNA synthesis is also required in order that mechanisms to stimulate catchup growth can be defined. Although this model of intrauterine growth retardation is similar to that of the human in biochemical and morphologic features, this form of reduced blood supply (vascular insufficiency) is not a common cause of the syndrome in humans.

MATERNAL PROTEIN DEPRIVATION

The effects of maternal protein-calorie restriction on the brain of the offspring have been discussed (Chapter 7) and the present discussion is on the somatic effects produced by reduction in maternal diet. Factors influencing fetal circulation, viral infections, or other deleterious factors that have been classed as factors causing "fetal malnutrition" are not discussed.

The effects of maternal nutrition on the course of pregnancy and on the offspring were discussed by a special committee in Washington, D.C., in 1970.[16] It was pointed out at the conference that a departure from the time-honored anthropometric assessment of growth was needed. Further information should come from the study of factors influencing cell multiplication and cytoplasmic growth.

It is recognized that liver glycogen is reduced and hypoglycemia and hypothermia occur in the full-term fetus that is reduced in weight. Moreover, the milk production of the mother is liable to be reduced, and even if satisfactory food intake is offered from weaning, catchup growth does not occur and the animal may never reach expected weight. There is a higher mortality in neonatal life when a low birth weight is recorded.

The rate of growth of the fetus is related to the weight of the fetus at term and to the length of gestation, and the size of the fetus is related to maternal size. The supply of food to the growing fetus depends on the maternal blood perfusing the placenta in which the concentrations of nutrients are the same in all species. As discussed by Widdowson[17] the mouse fetus normally grows at a rate of 0.09 g/day, the human at 12.5 g/day, and the blue whale at 9,000 g/day. Further, for guinea pigs the usual litter contains four offspring which together comprises 50% of maternal body weight, which may explain the finding that undernutrition in pregnant guinea pigs results in a marked growth retardation of the fetus.[18]

The early work of Wallace[19–21] demonstrated that nutritional deprivation in pregnant sheep decreased the size of the offspring.

The rat has received close attention by Chow and his co-workers[22, 23] who showed that rats subjected to restriction during their period in utero gained less weight per gram of food eaten than did the controls. Zamenhof et al[24] reduced maternal intake to one-third in pregnant rats and found that the litter showed reduced body weight. Thaler[25] made similar observations by subjecting the pregnant rats to periods of starvation. Maternal protein deprivation led to a decrease in cell number in the offspring, the deficit continuing during the postnatal period even if the litters were reduced to four.[26] Of interest is the fact that the protein: DNA ratio in tissues was usually normal, especially if adequate nutrition was given postnatally.

Zeman and Stanbrough reviewed 12 papers showing that the offspring of rats fed a protein-deficient diet during pregnancy have a reduced weight at term.[27] They also investigated the effects of maternal protein deficiency on cellular growth of the rat fetus. At term, organ weights and carcass weight were all reduced and all organs showed a reduction in cell number (liver, kidney, heart, thymus, brain, and carcass). However, there were no reductions in RNA:DNA or protein:DNA ratios, indicating that a reduction in the rate of cell division is an important feature. Some slight decrease in cell size was detected in the brain. In a later study it was shown that under controlled conditions such deprived newborn rats did not make good the loss in cell number.[26] This work is in agreement with early work of Winick and Noble,[29] who also emphasized that the time of insult was important since periods of hyperplasia, for example, were halted by nutritional deprivation.[30] Fisher and Leathem[31] demonstrated the ability of the rat fetus to store electrolyte, protein, and vitamins prior to parturition and at the expense of the maternal organism.

In studies in the dog, Platt and Stewart[32] subjected bitches to protein-calorie malnutrition during pregnancy and lactation. The newborn offspring showed reduction in weight and developed bone abnormalities and ataxia if restriction continued. Similar studies in the pig[33, 34] revealed reduced cytoplasmic growth in muscle even when the newborn was fed to adulthood. Restricted nutrition in pigs 1 month to 1 year lowered the humoral and cellular immunity.[35]

Little work has been done on the role of hormones in animals that are stunted due to gestational deprivation. Evidence available suggests that growth hormone and the cell multiplying factor (somatomedin) is reduced in restricted nutrition while a possible role for adrenocortical activity has been mentioned. Lee[38] injected insulin and growth hormone into neonatal mice, either gestationally deprived or subjected to a neonatal enterovirus, and reversed many of the defects in protein biosynthesis that follow such insults. Lee and Dubos[39] subsequently showed that growth hormone per se would correct the derangement of catechol metabolism present in the central nervous system. It is known that 1 mg of cortisone given to rats on the second day of life will cause growth retardation[36] while Howard[37] reported growth retardation in mice receiving corticosterone. Such retardation was comparable with that produced by restricted nutrition.

As we turn to the primate there is a paucity of information. Maternal protein or calorie restriction as a separate entity is only now receiving attention while, as stated earlier, the term "fetal malnutrition" has included many different circumstances. Naeye,[40] with histologic and histometric observations on human material, has emphasized that organ growth differs according to circumstances of fetal malnutrition. Cell size and cell number are also influenced differently.

Another complicating factor, as pointed out by Gruenwald,[41] is that birth weight will vary according to socioeconomic conditions, the mother's own development influencing the situation. Term weight may not reach optimal conditions for several generations after the reversal of poor socioeconomic conditions. Subhuman primates are also sensitive to environmental conditions. The variability of birth weights in the rhesus monkey in captivity is exactly similar to that of the human, as shown by Battaglia.[42] The macaque studied in its natural surroundings gives rise to fetuses of greater birth weight than those from the first pregnancies of monkeys recently taken into captivity. Otherwise, birth weight is generally higher in established breeding colonies than in the wild.[51]

In the ongoing experiments discussed in Chapter 6 and relating to the deprivation of protein or calories or both during pregnancy in the rhesus monkey, some information is available from pilot experiments.

Muscle growth is reduced and protein synthesis is affected more than DNA replication (see Tables 17.4 and 17.5). Renal growth is affected significantly, being disproportionately reduced for body weight.

Our own experimental work on maternal protein deprivation and the effects on the fetus is still in progress, but the question arises as to why the kidney should be singled out. The work of Nuzum and Snodgrass[43] draws attention to the activation of enzymes involved in the urea cycle when protein intake is varied in the primate. The previous work of Schimke[44] demonstrated that amino nitrogen resulting from the utilization of amino acids for energy is excreted largely as urea and such enzyme activity is dependent on differences in dietary protein consumption.

It is possible that pregnant primates may, as a result of protein restriction, alter their urea cycle so that reduced amounts of amino nitrogen are delivered to the fetus and that this results in the presentation to the fetal kidney of a smaller load of urea. Battaglia's group, and in particular Tsoulos and associates[45] and James et al,[46] have shown that glucose utilization accounts for only 50% of the oxygen consumption of the sheep fetus and that more than 40% of the oxygen consumption is probably related to the catabolism of amino acids. If the availability of amino acids is reduced, it is possible that consumption of glucose or of fatty acids is increased.

Battaglia,[47] on the basis of primate studies, considers the transplacental urea clearance to be of the order of 540 mg/kg/day. Gresham et al[48] have shown that the human fetus has a higher plasma urea than the mother (the same holds true for

Table 17.4   The effect of maternal food restriction on
fetal muscle composition in the macaque

		Normal diet	Calorie and protein restricted diet
H_2O	%	78.8	* 79.9
DNA	mg/g	2.07	* 2.32
Protein	mg/g	178	** 163
Protein:DNA		86	** 71

*P = not less than 0.025   ** P = not less than 0.01

amino acids) which may suggest a diffusion of urea from fetus to mother. In the situation under discussion this may not be the case since the fetal urea may be utilized much more for protein synthesis.

In summary it is possible that the delivery of amino acids to the fetus and the activation of the urea cycle within the fetus may have an effect on the development of the kidney or on renal growth.

Whether or not these changes in kidney and other tissues such as muscle are reversed by adequate postnatal nutrition is not known. Adequate nutrition post-natally may well reverse the changes since the growth process of the soma has a remarkable distance to travel, especially with respect to muscle. The early work of Chow showed clearly that for rats irreversible changes were produced in the soma with gestational deprivation even if adequate food was offered during postnatal life. Growth hormone, if injected at an early time postnatally, did reverse the situation.[22, 49]

For the human the situation is difficult to appraise since gestational deprivation is usually associated with postnatal deprivation. The reduction in somatic growth in Jamaican children with early kwashiorkor was no different at 8 years of age

Table 17.5   The effect of maternal food restriction on
fetal kidney composition in the macaque
(pilot study)

		Kidney weight (g) (pilot experiment)
1.	Control diet	2.17 ± 0.21
2.	Calorie sufficient Protein deficient	1.61 ± 0.19
3.	Protein sufficient Calorie deficient	2.13 ± 0.15
4.	Calorie and protein deficiency	1.81 ± 0.35

By analysis of variance fetuses of groups 2 and 4 had a significantly reduced kidney weight for age.

from that found in siblings with similar genetic and economic background and no gestational deprivation.[50] However, with respect to Caucasian standards such children were reduced in growth and there is clearly a range of normal sizes for ages which must be differentiated from overnutrition, excess somatic growth, and obesity. Maximum growth versus optimal growth is discussed in Chapter 26.

SUMMARY

Ligation of the bridging vessels between the two placental discs in the pregnant rhesus monkey can successfully produce a model for the study of intrauterine growth retardation of the fetus. In this chapter the soma is discussed. The growth of organs is retarded and resembles the situation in the human except that the adrenal of the human appears to be affected more. The brain is involved the least. In general the growth in size and number of cells is compromised to a comparable degree. The changes have been compared with those found in subprimates when the blood supplied to the fetus is reduced.

Experiments concerning the restriction of calories and protein (or both) in the pregnant primate are in progress and a study is being made concerning organ growth. For most mammals a reduction in fetal weight can be demonstrated, the variability depending on the mammal. For the macaque, as pointed out by Riopelle (personal communication), the time of gestation may be prolonged with the result that the infant is of normal weight.

In rats an interruption of cell multiplication in most organs of the fetus can be shown. By contrast in the monkey an effect on protein synthesis is more apparent in muscle. In dogs evidence presents for changes in endocrine function, and the development of ataxia implies involvement of the cerebellum in the offspring.

It is pointed out that little work has been done in the experimental animal to show the therapeutic use of hormones to counter changes in tissue growth and protein synthesis except for the work of Lee and Dubos.[38][39]

A reduction in the weight of the kidney relative to body weight is found when protein is restricted in the diet of the macaque. It is suggested that the restriction of protein influences urea metabolism and the urea cycle such that the stimulus for renal growth is lacking in the fetus.

Whether or not children with intrauterine growth retardation or gestational protein deprivation subsequently reach expected growth remains to be determined.

REFERENCES

1. Myers, R. E., Hill, D. E., Holt, A. B., Scott, R. E., Mellits, E. D., and Cheek, D. B.: Fetal growth retardation produced by experimental placental insufficiency in the rhesus monkey. I. Body weight, organ size. *Biol. Neonate* **18**: 379, 1971.

2. Hill, D. E., Myers, R. E., Holt, A. B., Scott, R. E., and Cheek, D. B.: Fetal growth retardation produced by experimental placental insufficiency in the rhesus monkey. II. Chemical composition of the brain, liver, muscle and carcass. *Biol. Neonate* **19**: 68, 1971.

3. Hill, D. E.: Experimental growth retardation in rhesus monkeys. Accepted by the Ciba Foundation Symposium on *Size at Birth*, for publication, 1974.

4. Gruenwald, P.: Chronic fetal distress and placental insufficiency. *Biol. Neonate* **5**: 215, 1963.

5. Naeye, R. L.: Malnutrition, probable cause of fetal growth retardation. *Arch. Pathol.* **79:** 284, 1965.

6. Dawkins, M. J. R.: Discussion. *Proc. Roy. Soc. Med.* **57:** 1063, 1964b.

7. Widdowson, E. M., Crabb, D. E., and Milner, R. D. G.: Cellular development of some human organs before birth. *Arch. Dis. Child.* **47:** 652, 1972.

8. Roux, J. M., Tordet-Caridroit, C., and Chanez, C.: Studies on experimental hypotrophy in the rat. I. Chemical composition of the total body and some organs in the rat foetus. *Biol. Neonate* **15:** 342, 1970.

9. Widdowson, E. M.: Harmony of growth. *Lancet* **1:** 901, 1970.

10. Wigglesworth, J. S.: Experimental growth retardation in the foetal rat. *J. Pathol. Bacteriol.* **88:** 1, 1964.

11. Oh, W., and Guy, J. A.: Cellular growth in experimental intrauterine growth retardation in rats. *J. Nutr.* **101:** 1631, 1971.

12. Winick, M.: Cellular growth of the placenta as an indicator of abnormal fetal growth. In: K. Adamsons (Ed.): *Diagnosis and Treatment of Fetal Disorders.* Springer-Verlag, Berlin and New York, 1968, p. 83.

13. Harding, P., and Shelley, H. J.: Some effects of intrauterine growth retardation in the foetal rabbit. In: Horskey and Stembera, (Eds.): *Intrauterine Dangers to the Foetus.* Excerpta Medica, The Netherlands, 1967.

14. Alexander, G.: Studies on the placenta of the sheep (Ovis Aries L.). Effect of surgical reduction in the number of caruncles. *J. Reprod. Fertil.* **7:** 307, 1964.

15. Creasy, R. K., Barrett, C. T., de Swiet, M., Kahanpaa, K. V., and Rudolph, A. M.: Experimental intrauterine growth retardation in the sheep. *Am. J. Obstet. Gynecol.* **112:** 566, 1972.

16. *Maternal Nutrition and the Course of Pregnancy.* National Academy of Sciences, Washington, 1970.

17. Widdowson, E. M.: Growth and composition of the fetus and newborn. In: *Biology of Gestation,* Vol. II. Academic Press, New York, 1968.

18. Eckstein, P., and McKeown, T.: Effect of transection of one horn of guinea pig's uterus on foetal growth in other horn. *J. Endocrinol.* **12:** 97, 1955.

19. Wallace, L. R.: The growth of lambs before and after birth in relation to the level of nutrition, Part 1. *J. Agric. Sci.* **38:** 93, 1948.

20. Wallace, L. R.: The growth of lambs before and after birth in relation to the level of nutrition, Part 2. *J. Agric. Sci.* **38:** 243, 1948.

21. Wallace, L. R.: The growth of lambs before and after birth in relation to the level of nutrition, Part 3. *J. Agric. Sci.* **38:** 367, 1948.

22. Chow, B. F., and Lee, C. J.: Effect of dietary restriction of pregnant rats on body weight gain of the offspring. *J. Nutr.* **82:** 10, 1964.

23. Lee, C.-J., and Chow, B. F.: Metabolism of proteins by progeny of underfed mother rats. *J. Nutr.* **94:** 20, 1968.

24. Zamenhof, S., van Marthens, E., and Grauel, L.: Prenatal cerebral development: Effect of restricted diet, reversal by growth hormone. *Science* **174:** 954, 1971.

25. Thaler, M. M.: Effects of starvation on normal development of beta–hydroxybutyrate dehydrogenase activity in foetal and newborn rat brain. *Nature* **236:** 140, 1972.

26. Zeman, F. J.: Effect of protein deficiency during gestation on postnatal cellular development in the young rat. *J. Nutr.* **100:** 530, 1970.

27. Zeman, F. J., and Stanbrough, E. C.: Effect of maternal protein deficiency on cellular development in the fetal rat. *J. Nutr.* **99:** 274, 1969.

28. Hall, S. M., and Zeman, F. J.: Kidney function of the progeny of rats fed a low protein diet. *J. Nutr.* **95:** 49, 1968.

29. Winick, M., and Noble, A.: Quantitative changes in DNA, RNA and protein during prenatal and postnatal growth in the rat. *Dev. Biol.* **12:** 451, 1965.

30. Winick, M., and Noble, A.: Cellular response in rats during malnutrition at various ages. *J. Nutr.* **89:** 300, 1966.

31. Fisher, C. J., and Leathem, J. H.: Effect of a protein-free diet on protein metabolism in the pregnant rat. *Endocrinology* **76**: 454, 1965.

32. Platt, B. S., and Stewart, R. J. C.: Effects of protein-calorie deficiency on dogs. 1. Reproduction, growth and behaviour. *Dev. Med. Child Neurol.* **10**: 3, 1968.

33. Pond, W. G., Strachan, D. N., Sinha, Y. N., Walker, E. F., Jr., Dunn, J. A., and Barnes, R. H.: Effect of protein deprivation of swine during all or part of gestation on birth weight, postnatal growth rate and nucleic acid content of brain and muscle of progeny. *J. Nutr.* **99**: 61, 1970.

34. Pond, W. G., Wagner, W. C., Dunn, J. A., and Walker, E. F., Jr.: Reproduction and early postnatal growth of progeny in swine fed a protein-free diet during gestation. *J. Nutr.* **94**: 309, 1968.

35. Lopez, V., Davis, S. D., and Smith, N. J.: Studies in infantile marasmus. IV. Impairment of immunologic responses in the marasmic pig. *Pediatr. Res.* **6**: 779, 1972.

36. Winick, M., and Coscia, A.: Cortisone-induced growth failure in neonatal rats. *Pediatr. Res.* **2**: 451, 1968.

37. Howard, E.: Effects of corticosterone and food restriction on growth and on DNA, RNA and cholesterol contents of the brain and liver in infant mice. *J. Neurochem.* **12**: 181, 1965.

38. Lee, C.-J.: Biosynthesis and characteristics of brain protein and ribonucleic acid in mice subjected to neonatal infection or undernutrition. *J. Biol. Chem.* **245**: 1998, 1970.

39. Lee, C.-J., and Dubos, R.: Lasting biological effects of early environmental influences. VIII. Effects of neonatal infection, perinatal malnutrition, and crowding on catecholamine metabolism of brain. *J. Exp. Med.* **136**: 1031, 1972.

40. Naeye, R. L.: Structural correlates of fetal undernutrition. In: Waisman, H. A., and Kerr, G. (Eds.): *Fetal Growth and Development*. McGraw-Hill, New York, 1970.

41. Gruenwald, P.: Fetal malnutrition. In: Waisman, H. A., and Kerr, G. (Eds.): *Fetal Growth and Development*. McGraw-Hill, New York, 1970.

42. Battaglia, F. C.: Intrauterine growth retardation. *J. Obstet. Gynecol.* **106**: 1103, 1970.

43. Nuzum, C. T., and Snodgrass, P. J.: Urea cycle enzyme adaptation to dietary protein in primates. *Science* **172**: 1042, 1971.

44. Schimke, R. T.: Adaptive characteristics of urea cycle enzymes in the rat. *J. Biol. Chem.* **237**: 459, 1962.

45. Tsoulos, N. G., Colwill, J. R., Battaglia, F. C., Makowski, E. L., and Meschia, G.: Comparison of glucose, fructose and O_2 uptakes by the fetuses of fed and starved ewes. *Am. J. Physiol.* **221**: 234, 1971.

46. James, E. J., Meschia, G., and Battaglia, F. C.: A-V differences of free fatty acids and glycerol in the ovine umbilical circulation. *Proc. Soc. Exp. Biol. Med.*, **138**: 823 (1971).

47. Battaglia, F. C., Behrman, R. E., Meschia, G., Seeds, A. E., and Bruns, P. D.: Clearance of inert molecules Na and Cl ions across the primate placenta. *Am. J. Obstet. Gynecol.* **102**: 1135, 1968.

48. Gresham, E. L., Simons, P. S., and Battaglia, F. C.: Maternal-fetal urea concentration difference in man. Metabolic significance. *J. Pediatr.* **79**: 809, 1971.

49. Chow, B. F.: Effect of maternal dietary protein on anthropometric and behavioral development of the offspring. In: Roche, A. F. and Falkner, F. (Eds.), *Nutrition and Malnutrition*. Advances in Experimental Medicine and Biology, Volume 49, p. 183, 1974.

50. Garrow, J. S., and Pike, M. C.: The long-term prognosis of severe infantile malnutrition. *Lancet* **I**: 1, 1967.

51. Valerio, D. A., et al: In: *Macaca mulatta; management of a Laboratory Breeding Colony*. Academic Press, New York, 1969.

CHAPTER 18

Changes in Somatic Growth
After Ablation of Maternal
or Fetal Pancreatic Beta Cells

Donald B. Cheek and Donald E. Hill

INTRODUCTION

Our interest in this work and its relevance to the human infant born of the diabetic mother (IBDM) has been explained (Chapter 9). The methods used were described also: briefly, two approaches were made. In the first, streptozotocin, an agent that ablates pancreatic beta cells, was injected into the maternal circulation in midgestation, and in the second approach streptozotocin was injected directly into the fetal circulation at the beginning of the third trimester or shortly thereafter.

MATERNAL BETA-CELL ABLATION

Earlier in the book it was pointed out that the injection of streptozotocin (50 mg/kg) into the pregnant monkey in midgestation produces a moderate diabetes mellitus,[1] an enlargement of the pituitary and adrenal gland in the fetus, and specific changes in the brain. It was suggested that the increase in protein and zinc relative to DNA indicated an increase in cytoplasmic growth while the reduction in cerebral cell number and in cerebral phospholipid suggested growth arrest. The fact that carbonic anhydrase was increased in activity focused attention on neuroglial cells.[2]

When the monkeys born of streptozotocin-treated mothers were compared with control animals, several differences were apparent with respect to somatic growth. The weight of five out of nine of the fetal macaques was greater than that of the controls and fell more than one standard deviation above the control line, four of these being two standard deviations above (Figure 18.1). (The equation used to define body weight for age differs from earlier equations given, since here only controls are used of 140–160 days of gestation.) In five fetuses there was a disproportionate increase in length. The carcass (muscle plus skeleton) and visceral mass were higher than the controls in seven out of nine fetuses (Figure 18.2). There was visceromegaly, some organs being affected more than others (Table 18.1). There was an increased amount of fat in the carcass ($P < 0.002$), the skin ($P < 0.005$), and in the muscle ($P < 0.001$).

The DNA content per gram of muscle was reduced ($P < 0.001$), this reduction being so great that in spite of the increased muscle mass the total number of muscle nuclei was less than in control animals. The remarkable change in muscle tissue, however, was the increase in the protein:DNA ratio (Figure 18.3). A loss of water from muscle was also documented (Figure 18.4). (It is interesting to note that these were the changes that occurred in the cerebrum in these infants.) The ratio of protein to DNA in the myocardium also showed a trend toward an increment (Figure 18.5) while the concentration of RNA in the myocardium was decreased (Figure 18.6).

The visceromegaly that occurred affected the spleen, heart, pituitary, and adrenals. These findings are of interest in view of the adrenal enlargement in the human infant born of the diabetic mother,[3] spenic enlargement and increased hemopoietic tissue with cardiomegaly being also common. The occurrence of an enlarged pituitary in the human situation has been debated.[4]

Hoet[5] has considered the possible role of the hypothalamus and adrenal in fetal growth. As stated earlier in the book, the hyperplasia of the pancreas and the enlargement of the adrenal might be related to hypothalamic stimulation. The finding by Driscoll et al[6] of testicular interstitial cell hyperplasia or the formation of luteinized ovarian cysts in infants born of diabetic mothers may suggest overactivity of the pituitary-hypothalamic area. Gaunt et al[4] reviewed the literature up to 1962 concerning the status of acidophil cells in the pituitary and also the evidence concerning pancreatic beta-cell hyperplasia. While some workers have reported excess numbers of acidophil cells with, in some cases, evidence for an increased weight of the pituitary gland, Gaunt et al established that the size of acidophil cells was increased. Westphal[7] did not find a higher level of plasma growth hormone in the infant of the diabetic mothers after the infusion of glucose. However, it is possible that growth hormone release may be excessive.

Elsewhere in this book the ability of insulin to increase cytoplasmic growth in muscle without causing an increase in cell number has been emphasized. The present findings in skeletal muscle, the suggestive changes in myocardial muscle, and the changes in brain cell cytoplasm are consistent with this theory of action of insulin on cell growth. The fact that the number of cells per gram of muscle is reduced (the cerebral population was also reduced) suggests that factors involved in cell multiplication may also be compromised.

An important cause of death in infants of diabetic mothers is related to the development of the respiratory distress syndrome. In this study there was a decreased weight in the lungs in five out of nine instances. Work by Gluck's group in San Diego[8] suggests that there could be some correlation between the development of phospholipids in the brain and in the lung. As already noted, the development of phospholipid in the brain was retarded. Future studies on the chemistry of phospholipids in the lungs of infants of diabetic mothers may prove rewarding.

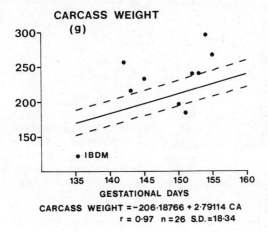

CARCASS WEIGHT =−206·18766 + 2·79114 CA
r = 0·97   n = 26   S.D. =18·34

Fig. 18.1. The weights of nine fetuses born of diabetic mothers (IBDM) are shown compared with a normal population of fetal rhesus monkeys, 140 to 160 days of gestation. The equation and plotted lines shown describe the relationship for the normal animals. Note that the weights of four of the IBDM fetuses are more than two standard deviations above the normal weight for age.

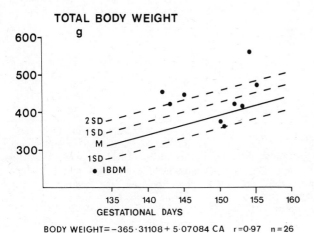

BODY WEIGHT=−365·31108 + 5·07084 CA   r=0·97   n=26
SD= 31·7548 g

Fig. 18.2. Carcass weight is plotted on gestational age for fetal monkeys born of diabetic mothers (IBDM). The plotted line and equation described the relationship for normal animals of similar gestation age. Note that seven out of the nine IBDM animals tended to have an increased carcass mass for age when compared with normal animals.

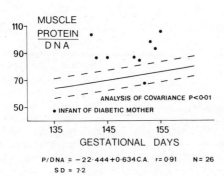

P/DNA = − 22·444+0·634 C.A.   r=0·91   N = 26
SD = 7·2

Fig. 18.3. The protein: DNA ratio (cell size) in muscle of fetal monkeys born of diabetic mothers (IBDM) is contrasted with the predicted relationship of normal animals of similar age. The plotted line and equation describe the relationship for normal animals of similar gestational age. Note that eight out of the nine IBDM animals show an increased cell size. Similar changes have been described for the brain in these animals (Chapter 9).

313

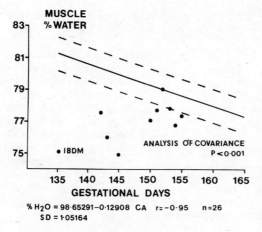

Fig. 18.4. The percentage of water in the muscle of fetal monkeys born of diabetic mothers (IBDM) is plotted on gestational age. The plotted lines and equation describe the relationship for normal animals of similar age. Note the lower concentration of muscle water in the IBDM subjects. Similar changes also occurred in the cerebrum of these animals (Chapter 9).

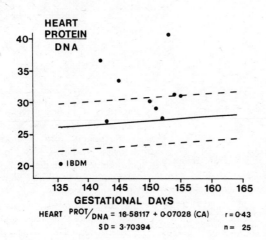

Fig. 18.5. Heart protein : DNA ratio (cell size) is plotted on gestational age for the fetal monkeys born of diabetic mothers. The plotted lines and equation describe the relationship for normal animals of similar age. Note the trend toward increased cell size in this tissue.

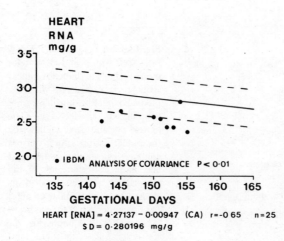

Fig. 18.6. The concentration of RNA in the heart of fetal monkeys born of diabetic mothers (IBDM) is shown in this figure. The plotted lines and equation describe the normal relationship. Note the significant decrease in concentration when IBDM are compared to normal animals of similar age.

314

Table 18.1   The effect of injection of
              streptozotocin into the maternal
              circulation at mid-gestation on the
              organ weights and percent fat in the
              fetus.

	CONTROL M±S.D.	N	I.B.D.M.* M±S.D.	N	t	p
Pituitary (mg)	13.3±2.1	19	16.0±1.2	9	4.31	<0.001
Heart (g)	2.09±0.22	22	2.34±0.32	9	2.13	<0.05
Spleen (g)	0.57±0.17	18	0.79±0.18	9	2.95	<0.01
Adrenals (mg)	240±81	22	330±96	9	2.46	=0.02
Carcass fat (g)	5.39±1.95	22	10.12±5.42	9	2.55	<0.02
Muscle (% fat)	1.03±0.42	22	2.85±1.30	9	4.10	<0.001
Skin (% fat)	5.59±2.48	11	12.80±5.99	9	3.38	<0.005

* Monkey born of diabetic mother

The question arises as to whether the effects on the infant are of any lasting nature. No information is available, for example, on subsequent pulmonary disease. On the other hand, such infants may carry a gene for diabetes: According to White,[10] 9 out of every 100 children born of a diabetic mother are already diabetic by the age of adolescence. Farquhar[9] has shown that when childhood is reached such subjects have an increased weight for height, suggesting excessive growth of lean and adipose tissue.

FETAL BETA-CELL ABLATION

The mortality in both the experimental and sham-operated group was 50% overall (Table 18.2). The deaths were designated early if the animals aborted within 10 days of the procedure, and late if they occurred some time thereafter or if the fetus was delivered stillborn. It is not uncommon for these animals to carry a stillborn macerated fetus to term. It is possible that the dosage of streptozotocin was lethal to the fetus; however, since the death rate in the sham-operated animals was of the same magnitude, and the majority of them occurred early, death was more likely to have been a consequence of the operative procedure. There was no correlation between the length of the procedure and mortality, nor did there appear to be any specific postoperative complications associated with fetal death.

In Figure 18.7 the birth weights of 12 surviving experimental animals are compared with the normal birth weight-gestational age relationship for fetal monkeys for 120 to 160 days of gestation. Three of the experimental animals had significantly

Table 18.2   Mortality following injection of streptozotocin directly into the fetal circulation at the beginning of the third trimester.

	Total	Deaths	
		Early	Late
Streptozotocin Injection	24	6	6
Sham Injection	10	5	0
Control	9	0	0

low birth weights for gestational age, while the remaining experimental animals fell within the expected range of normal. Of the latter group seven animals had a body weight greater than the mean and all had disproportionately large adrenals for their body size. This finding was of interest in that it allowed us to examine the body composition and chemistry in the experimental group in relation to the size of the adrenals. The extent of this adrenal enlargement is illustrated in Figure 18.8, where the normal adrenal weight for gestational age is shown in a shaded diagram. The seven animals with large adrenals are clearly outside the normal range.

Table 18.3 summarizes the pertinent findings with respect to muscle and carcass. The comparison here is between the controls and the seven animals that had an elevated adrenal-weight:body-weight ratio. In these animals there was a significant increase in carcass mass (skeletal mass plus muscle mass) when compared with controls. However, there was a significant decrease in the concentration of DNA in muscle and a significant increase in the protein:DNA ratio, suggesting that the increase in muscle mass for age was due mainly to an increase in the size of the muscle cells. The three low-birth-weight animals had reduced muscle mass (by inspection or dissection) and therefore less total DNA (cell number). Total RNA and percent water were reduced in the muscle of these three fetuses.

The composition of the liver in the group with the large adrenals is shown contrasted with control animals in Table 18.4. There were no changes in the concentration of constituents such as water, DNA, and protein. However, when the total amounts were compared with the control animals, there was a significant increase in total weight, DNA, protein, and RNA. There was no significant change in the protein:DNA ratio (cell size), indicating that both the DNA and protein were growing in a proportionate manner. In the small animals the total DNA was normal while the total RNA and protein were significantly reduced.

Changes in cerebral and cerebellar composition occurred in fetuses with large adrenal glands for body weight (Chapter 9). There was a reduction in water content and a trend toward an increase in protein accretion in the brain. In the cerebellum there was a definite increase in protein concentration and in the protein:DNA ratio.

The fetal plasma insulin values were similar in the control group and the seven fetuses with the large adrenals for body weight. A two- to threefold gradient existed between the maternal plasma levels and the fetal plasma levels. Of particular interest was the very low total fetal pancreatic insulin in the large adrenal weight group. In many of the large adrenal group who received streptozotocin, histological examina-

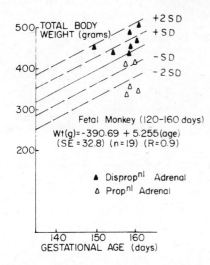

Fig. 18.7. The body weight of 12 surviving fetal monkeys that had been injected *in utero* with strepto-zotocin is shown compared with the normal population of rhesus monkeys. Those with adrenal weights that were large for body weight are depicted with closed triangles (▲) and those with normal adrenal weight are depicted with open triangles (△).

tion has shown that the pancreatic beta cells have been at least partially degranulated, and the islets have undergone definite hyperplasia. Secretion rates in these animals were not measured. However, it can be seen from Figure 18.9 that the plasma insulin values for fetal rhesus monkeys can reach "term values" as soon as 120 days. There is a slight tendency toward increased plasma insulin values as term approaches. These values were obtained essentially from animals that had not received any feeding nor had they received an infusion of any kind. Some of the scatter may be attributed to the fact that all of them had been stressed by either natural delivery or cesarean section.

The injection of streptozotocin into the fetus (75 mg/kg) at the beginning of the latter third of pregnancy thus produced a variable response. Mortality was high for the fetus. In three animals that delivered at term there was striking growth retardation that was similar in many respects to the growth retardation produced by placental insufficiency. These animals had a normal adrenal size for their body weight and there was some evidence of functioning islet tissue. The fetal plasma

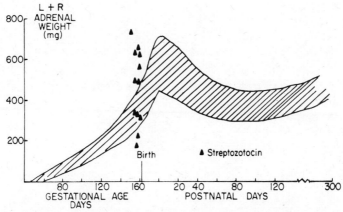

Fig. 18.8. The total adrenal weight of fetal monkeys that had been injected *in utero* with strepto-zotocin is shown contrasted with the range of normal for our primate colony.

Table 18.3   The effect on muscle and carcass of the injection of streptozotocin directly into primate fetal circulation at the beginning of the third trimester.

	CONTROLS (N=9) M±S.D.	SZ* (N=7) M±S.D.	t Test p <	Analysis of Covariance p <
Carcass Mass (g)	228.6±16.4	255.5±19.6	.02	
MUSCLE				
Water % fresh	79.21±0.81	78.14±1.09	.05	.1
DNA mg/g	2.27±0.18	1.95±0.23	.01	.025
Protein: DNA	75.1±6.44	90.8±15.2	.02	.025
RNA mg/g	2.60±0.0	2.09±0.23	.005	.01

* Streptozotocin (Increased adrenal:body weight ratio)

insulin values were in the low range of normal and there was some evidence of beta-cell granulation in the pancreas. We gained the impression that insulin secretion was poor. Although the effects on muscle and liver cell growth were of a pattern similar to that seen in fetal growth retardation produced by placental insufficiency or malnutrition, they were not as severe. This was probably related to the fact that there was still sufficient circulating insulin for at least some protein synthesis.

Table 18.4   The effect of the injection of streptozotocin into primate fetal circulation on liver composition.

	CONTROLS (N=9) M±S.D.	SZ* (N=7) M±S.D.	t test p
Weight (g)	12.5±1.7	16.4±1.7	< .005
Total DNA (mg)	50±8.0	63±8.4	< .01
Total Protein (g)	1.7±0.3	2.1±0.1	< .05
Protein:DNA	32±5.5	31±4.0	N.S.
Total RNA (mg)	84±14	105±14	< .02

* Streptozotocin (Increased adrenal:body weight ratio)

Another growth pattern emerged when the fetuses were examined on the basis of their relationship to the adrenal size. The finding of these very large adrenals was of particular interest since adrenal enlargement is known to accompany beta-cell hyperplasia and hyperinsulinemia in the infant of the diabetic mother.[11, 3] The changes in body composition including the mild changes in the cerebrum and cerebellum suggested, but not conclusively, that the pancreas had been stimulated by the injection of streptozotocin.

Since it is known that this drug can act both as an oncogenic agent[12] and oncolytic agent[13] it is not too surprising that these two patterns have emerged. The hyperplastic appearance of some of the islets in the large adrenal group was, in fact, close to a nodular hyperplasia. The dose was estimated from body weight, and therefore may have been less than that necessary for total destruction of the pancreas. The pancreas at this stage still had considerable regenerative capacity, and evidence of the formation of new islets was seen in some of the animals that had received streptozotocin.

The work of Van Assche[14] has demonstrated that the presence of an intact hypo-thalamohypophyseal tract is required for the islet cell hyperplasia in the infant of the diabetic mother. Although we have no evidence from our experiments that the stimulus for islet cell hyperplasia was due to change in glucose or amino acids, it is likely that such was the case.

In man[15] and in the rhesus monkey[16] it is evident that insulin secretion is present early in gestation. It is not known, however, at what point insulin becomes an important anabolic hormone, and further experiments of this type and others designed to ablate the fetal beta cell need to be completed in order to define the role of insulin.

Some information about the role of insulin in fetal growth has been provided by a recent case report from the Hospital for Sick Children, in Toronto, by Sherwood et al.[17] This baby was born at 40 weeks of gestation, weighed 1,200 g, and had extremely little subcutaneous tissue, virtually no muscle, and a significantly small liver. The initial glucose homeostasis was difficult to control, and after some investigation it was learned that a sibling had died 3 years prior to this birth and the autopsy record indicated that only a small portion of probably nonfunctioning pancreas

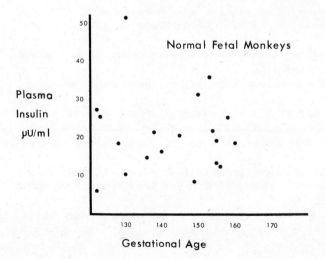

Fig. 18.9. Plasma insulin values are shown for normal fetal rhesus monkeys from 120 to 160 days of gestation. There is a wide scatter and only a moderate trend toward increase with age.

was present. This information led to a fuller investigation of the status of the pancreas in the index case. It was first demonstrated that there was a total absence of circulating insulin and glucagon, and later established at postmortem that the index case indeed did not have a pancreas. Preliminary results on some of the tissue indicated that the DNA content in both muscle and liver was reduced in total amount, and the protein:DNA ratio in muscle was extremely low and was similar to that seen in severe marasmus. It is not known at what point in time the pancreas failed to produce insulin. However, it is fairly obvious that a severe growth deficit followed, and whether this was part of the child's total problem cannot be answered at present. We feel, however, that insulin is an important anabolic hormone, and there is likely a point in late gestation when it becomes extremely important in terms of growth of muscle mass as well as fat mass in the fetus.

Milner[18] by the study of decapitated fetal rabbits concludes that the central nervous system plays a role in the development of the pancreatic beta cell. He has also indicated that a delay in beta-cell maturation can cause a transient state of diabetes mellitus in the newborn.[19] On the other hand, the levels of plasma glucagon in the maternal circulation (venous blood), umbilical artery, and fetal venous blood all remain about the same in the human at birth.[20] However, glucagon is capable of counteracting the hypersecretion of insulin in the newborn as seen in erythroblastosis.[21] The role of the brain and the balance between insulin and glucagon are discussed in Chapter 27.

REFERENCES

1. Mintz, J. H., Chez, R. A., and Hutchinson, D. L.: Subhuman primate pregnancy complicated by streptozotocin-induced diabetes mellitus. *J. Clin. Invest.* **51**: 837, 1972.

2. Millichap, J. G.: Development of seizure patterns in newborn animals: Significance of brain carbonic anhydrase. *Proc. Soc. Exp. Biol. Med.* **96**: 125, 1957.

3. Naeye, R. L.: Infants of diabetic mothers. A quantitative morphologic study. *Pediatrics* **35**: 980, 1965.

4. Gaunt, W. D., Bahn, R. C., and Hayles, A. B.: A quantitative cytological study of the anterior hypophysis of infants born of diabetic mothers. *Mayo Clin. Proc.* **37**: 345, 1962.

5. Hoet, J. J.: Normal and abnormal foetal weight gain. In: Wolstenholme, G. E. W., and O'Connor, M. (Eds.): *Foetal Autonomy*, a Ciba Foundation Symposium. Churchill, London, 1969, p. 186.

6. Driscoll, S. G., Benirschke, M., and Curtis, C. W.: Neonatal deaths among infants of diabetic mothers. *Am. J. Dis. Child.* **100**: 818, 1960.

7. Westphal, O.: Human growth hormone, a methodological and clinical study. *Acta Paediatr. Scand.* (*Suppl.* **182**), 8, 1968.

8. Gould, J. B., Gluck, L., and Kulovich, M. V.: The acceleration of neurological maturation in high stress pregnancy and its relation to fetal lung maturity. *Pediatr. Res.* **6**: 335, 1972.

9. Farquhar, J. W.: Prognosis for babies born to diabetic mothers in Edinburgh. *Arch. Dis. Child.* **44**: 36, 1969.

10. White, P.: Pregnancy complicating diabetes. In: Joslin, E. P., Root, H. F., White, P., and Marble, A. (Eds.): *The Treatment of Diabetes Mellitus*, 10th ed. Lea & Febiger, Philadelphia, and Kimpton, London, 1959, p. 690.

11. Pedersen, J.: In: Scand. Univ. Books (Eds.): *The Pregnant Diabetic and Her Newborn*. Munksgaard, Copenhagen, 1967, pp. 92–94.

12. Stolinsky, D. C., Sadoff, L., Braunwald, J., and Bateman, J. R.: Streptozotocin in the treatment of cancer: Phase II study. *Cancer* **30:** 61, 1972.

13. Volk, B. W., and Wellmann, K. F.: Pancreatic islet cell tumors induced by streptozotocin and nicotinamide (Abstr.). VIII Congress of the International Diabetes Federation Brussels, Belgium. **280:** 158, 1973.

14. Van Assche, F. A.: *The Fetal Endocrine Pancreas*. Katholieke Universiteit Leuven Press, Belgium, 1970.

15. Adam, P. A. J., Teramo, K., Raiha, N., Gitlin, D., and Schwartz, R.: Human fetal insulin metabolism early in gestation. Response to acute elevation of the fetal blood glucose concentration and placental transfer of human insulin-I-131. *Diabetes* **18:** 409, 1969.

16. Mintz, D. H., Chez, R. A., and Horger, E. O.: Fetal insulin and growth hormone metabolism in the subhuman primate. *J. Clin. Invest.* **48:** 176, 1969.

17. Sherwood, W. G., Chance, G. W., and Hill, D. E.: A new syndrome of pancreatic agenesis. The role of insulin and glucagon in cell and cell growth. *Pediatr. Res.* **8:** 360, 1974.

18. Jack, P. M. B., and Milner, R. D. G.: Effect of foetal decapitation on the development of insulin secretion in the rabbit. *J. Endocr.* **55, xxvi,** 1973.

19. Milner, R. D. G.: Brain factors in islet maturation. In: Camerini-Davalos, R. A., and Cole, H. S. (Eds.): *Early Diabetes in Early Life*, to be published, 1975.

20. Milner, R. D. G., Chouksey, S. K., Mickleson, K. N. P., and Assan, R.: Plasma pancreatic glucagon and insulin: glucagon ratio at birth. *Arch. Dis. Child.* **48:** 241, 1973.

21. Milner, R. D. G., Chouksey, S. K., and Assan, R.: Metabolic and hormonal effects of glucagon infusion in ethythroblastotic-infants. *Arch Dis. Child.* **48:** 885, 1973.

CHAPTER 19

Observations on the Tissue Lipids of Infants Born of Diabetic Monkeys

LIPID COMPOSITION OF TISSUE

W. Ann Reynolds and Ronald A. Chez

STUDIES OF LIPID METABOLISM IN VITRO

Jacques F. Roux, Ronald A. Chez, and Tapio Yoshioka

INTRODUCTION

Pregnancy in the diabetic woman may have severe consequences for the fetus and newborn. A sixfold higher perinatal mortality and a threefold increase in birth defects are encountered in infants born to diabetic women. Further, the defects that are encountered are six times more likely to be lethal ones than those found in infants born to normal women.[1]

A large percentage of all macrosomic infants are born to diabetic or prediabetic women. Infants with birthweights of 10 pounds or more exhibit a more than doubled perinatal mortality and the survivors suffer a high incidence (11%) of neurological deficit.[2]

Special gratitude goes to Mrs. Susan Beesley for expert technical assistance. "Lipid Composition of Tissue" was supported in part by grant CRBS-243 from the National Foundation.
"Studies of Lipid Metabolism *in vitro*" was supported by NICHD Grant No. HD-03261, USPHS Grant No. RR00210 from the General Clinical Research Centers Branch of the Division of Research Resources, NIH, and National Foundation Grant No. CRBS-235. It is a pleasure to acknowledge the assistance and advice of Professor D. L. Hutchinson, M.D., Department of Obstetrics and Gynecology, University of Pittsburgh School of Medicine, Pittsburgh, Pennsylvania and Ronald E. Myers, M.D., Chief, Laboratory of Perinatal Physiology, National Institute of Neurological Diseases and Stroke, Bethesda, Maryland. The technical assistance of Mrs. Z. Perry is also acknowledged.

In the infant born to a diabetic mother there is an elevated insulin level in cord blood[3] and/or failure to exhibit an early rise in plasma free fatty acids.[4,5] Osler[6,7] examined living human infants of diabetic mothers and found increased total lipid and lower water contents than in normal infants. Biochemical analyses on stillborn infants or infants suffering neonatal deaths confirmed these findings with respect to fat content.[8] Lastly, hyperplasia of the islets of Langerhans has long been recognized as a finding at autopsy of stillbirths born to diabetic women.

Only recently are studies emerging which show that careful management of the diabetic patient can result in a lower perinatal mortality. Regulation of maternal glucose metabolism *before* conception and during pregnancy has been found to reduce the rate of congenital malformations to the levels found in a normal obstetrics population.[9,10]

It can be speculated that the morphological and biochemical abnormalities observed in the infant of a diabetic mother result from abnormal maternal glucose metabolism, but which aspect of this abnormal metabolism is responsible? Based on the fundamental finding that glucose freely traverses the placenta, Pedersen[3] has proposed an attractive hypothesis to explain many of the growth abnormalities just described. He has suggested that the fetus of the poorly controlled diabetic mother is subjected to chronic hyperglycemia which results in stimulation of the fetal pancreas, eventually causing fetal hyperinsulinemia. The combination of high insulin and glucose levels in the fetus is then thought to result in overgrowth and excess fat deposition.

Beta-cell differentiation has occurred at 13 weeks of gestation in the human pancreas,[11] approximately the time that extractable insulin is first present.[12] The fetal rat pancreas does not release insulin when cultured *in vitro* in response to a glucose challenge;[13] only a glucagon stimulus can cause insulin release in such a preparation.[14] A high glucose content in the culture medium inhibits synthesis and/or storage of insulin by islet cell tissue from fetal rats of diabetic mothers.[15] Similarly, the results of all *in vivo* studies suggest that in a normal pregnancy, the fetal pancreas is incapable of releasing insulin in response to a glucose challenge. This finding, with few exceptions, holds true for early[16] and late[17-19] human pregnancy, in the sheep,[20] and in monkeys.[21,22] When tried, other agents such as tolbutamide or glucagon produced an increase in fetal plasma insulin concentration. Fetal insulin release occurred only when maternal hyperglycemia was maintained for several hours.[23]

To study the effects of prolonged hyperglycemia on the primate fetus, an accessible model of the human diabetic pregnancy characterized by chronic hyperglycemia was needed. The antibiotic streptozotocin (SZ) has been shown to cause a permanent diabetic-like state in rhesus monkeys due to its cytotoxic action specific for beta cells of the pancreas.[24] Recently, Mintz et al[25] have contrasted the responses to infused glucose or mixed amino acids in fetuses of SZ-treated glucose-intolerant monkeys. The exogenously induced fetal hyperglycemia resulted in an immediate two- to fivefold increase in fetal or neonatal plasma insulin levels in direct contrast to the unresponsive fetal pancreatic tissue characteristic of a normal macaque pregnancy. The administration of low levels of mixed amino acids was also associated with elevated plasma insulin levels; a tenfold greater concentration was necessary for similar results in the control series. It seems clear that some aspect of maternal glucose intolerance leads to precocious functional maturation and sensitivity of the primate fetal beta cells, much in line with the original Pedersen hypothesis. However, it remains to be established what causative agent(s) is responsible for the fetal biochemical and morphological abnormalities so often present in the diabetic pregnancy. As an initial step in determining the fetal responses to the diabetic pregnancy that may lead to deformity and death, we compared various biochemical parameters in fetuses born to normal monkeys and to those made glucose intolerant with streptozotocin. These studies are reported here. In the following section a report is made of *in vitro* studies on tissue from fetal macaques born to streptozotocin-treated mothers.

LIPID COMPOSITION OF TISSUES IN INFANTS BORN TO DIABETIC MONKEYS

A diabetic-like state was induced in *macaca mulatta* monkeys between 54 and 65 days of gestation or prior to conception. Streptozotocin will cross the placenta but reaches concentrations in fetal plasma of only one-twelfth or less of maternal levels, perhaps because of the rapidity of maternal degradation and placental impedance.[26] Further, direct injection of streptozotocin into the fetal circulation in monkeys during the second trimester has no observable effects on either pancreatic histology or circulating insulin levels at birth.[27, 28] In the rat, no alteration in fetal pancreatic insulin content follows the induction of maternal diabetes with streptozotocin[29] nor does the fetal pancreas respond *in vitro* to the cytotoxicity of streptozotocin. No apparent physiological or biochemical differences were found between fetuses delivered from mothers given streptozotocin prior to conception, or during the first trimester of gestation. Therefore, we have elected to induce a diabetic-like state in early gestation, which is advantageous economically due to the high cost of purchasing, maintaining, and breeding monkeys.

At the time of delivery by cesarean section, the fetuses were killed with pentobarbital, frozen rapidly in a Dry Ice and acetone slurry, and maintained at $-30°C$ until biochemical analyses could be performed. Previous studies on diabetic human infants[6, 8] generally involved determinations of the total body components. In this study separate tissue samples from four different organs (brain, liver, muscle, and placenta) were analyzed for two reasons. First, with the increasing use of the primate as a research animal for developmental studies, base-line determinations of tissue contents could prove useful to other investigators. Second, it is reasonable to expect some differences in organ responses to hyperglycemia and fetal hyperinsulinemia which might be masked in analyzing homogenized carcasses. In most instances, each tissue sample was analyzed in triplicate and an average value determined.

Analyses were carried out by the following methods:

1. Free fatty acids—Chloroform extraction, colorimetric ultramicromethod.[30]
2. Triglycerides—Extraction and saponification, colorimetric method.[31]
3. Total lipids—Colorimetric method based on sulfophosphovanillin reaction.[32]
4. Total phospholipids—Colorimetric method with perchloric acid.[33]
5. Total cholesterol—Libermann-Burchardt reaction.
6. Nitrogen—Semimicro Kjeldahl method.

Nine fetuses born to streptozotocin diabetic mothers (SZ fetuses) and six control fetuses were examined. The SZ fetuses were delivered between days 137 and 142 of gestation, while the control fetuses were delivered later in gestation, between day 144 and 150. Although the SZ fetuses were delivered at an average age that was 8.2 days less than that of the control fetuses, their average weight was 8.6% greater than that of the controls.

This apparent increase in body weight is shown to be significant if the individual body weights of the SZ and control fetuses are plotted on age and compared with data of Cheek (Figure 19.1). Macrosomia in infants born to monkeys made diabetic with streptozotocin had previously been reported[25] for this same breeding group of diabetic animals and such a finding gives further confirmation to the streptozotocin-induced monkey model of the diabetic pregnancy since macrosomia so often accompanies the diabetic human pregnancy.

The macrosomia of the fetal monkeys in this investigation is again most likely due to maternal carbohydrate intolerance. Fetal hyperinsulinemia would account for increased growth *in utero*. Hyperinsulinemia and hyperglycemia have been reported in the fetuses of SZ-diabetic monkeys during life *in utero*.[25] Direct administration of insulin to fetal rats induced macrosomia,[34] the newborn rats being characterized by high total lipid and increased lipid:nitrogen ratios, a situation not unlike that found in the infants of diabetic women.[6, 8] Similarly, fetuses born to rats made diabetic with streptozotocin were macrosomic in mild diabetes but smaller than normal in severe diabetes.[35] These newborn rats also possess higher carcass levels of fat and lower water contents than normal rat pups. Table 19.1 contains the mean

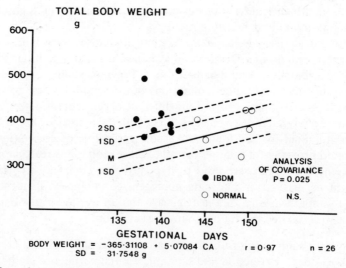

Fig. 19.1. Shown here are the weights of nine fetuses born to diabetic mothers at 137 to 142 days of gestation (IBDM) and six control fetuses born at 144 to 150 days of gestation. The equation and plotted lines shown describe the relationship for normal animals (Chapter 11). Note that IBDM fetuses as a group are significantly heavier than normal and that five of the IBDM fetuses are more than two standard deviations above the normal weight for age. The normal fetuses in this study are similar in weight for age to the normal animals in Cheek's study.

Table 19.1   Lipid Analyses of tissues from fetal monkeys born to mothers treated with streptozotocin and control fetuses.

		Brain	Liver	Muscle	Placenta
Free Fatty Acids mg/g	C	1.58 (0.18)	1.53 (0.29)	0.64 (0.16)	1.17 (0.14)
	SZ	1.47 (0.14)	1.54 (0.19)	0.22 (0.03)*	0.99 (0.10)
Triglycerides mg/g	C	14.85 (0.89)	14.33 (1.43)	8.37 (1.47)	14.87 (2.31)
	SZ	15.53 (1.67)	16.37 (1.65)	6.66 (0.81)	10.04 (1.20)
Total Lipids mg/g	C	53.83 (2.34)	41.33 (3.36)	15.17 (1.33)	29.00 (3.61)
	SZ	43.11 (2.30)*	36.67 (2.66)	13.67 (1.27)	25.22 (1.71)
Phospholipids mg/g	C	27.33 (1.14)	15.88 (1.56)	4.12 (0.87)	10.67 (0.81)
	SZ	18.59 (1.23)*	15.71 (1.00)	3.80 (0.34)	11.99 (1.09)
Cholesterol mg/g	C	5.78 (0.27)	2.68 (0.31)	0.45 (0.08)	1.97 (0.18)
	SZ	5.12 (0.20)	2.71 (0.17)	0.70 (0.06)*	2.17 (0.18)
Lipid/Nitrogen ratio	C	4.23 (0.67)	1.65 (0.28)	0.70 (0.08)	1.40 (0.00)
	SZ	4.17 (0.41)	1.95 (0.29)	0.69 (0.09)	1.38 (0.09)

C = Control Fetuses (n = 6)   SZ = Streptozotocin Diabetic Fetuses (n = 9)
Values are means with S.E.M. in parenthesis. * Values significant at 0.05 level or less.

lipid values determined from brain, liver, muscle, and placenta. With some exceptions, the SZ fetuses yielded values similar to those of the control fetuses. *Brain* analyses revealed a low concentration of total lipids ($P < 0.01$) and of phospholipids ($P < 0.02$) for the SZ fetuses as reported also by Cheek's group (Chapter 9). Thus brain was noticeably less mature in the SZ fetuses in respect to these indices. *Muscle* of the SZ fetuses was more mature than control values with respect to cholesterol concentration ($P < 0.04$). Significantly low values of free fatty acids ($P < 0.02$) were also observed. *Liver* of the SZ fetuses exhibited a trend in a more mature direction as shown by the relatively large but not significant increase in the lipid:nitrogen ratio.

The lipid:nitrogen ratio, a good indication of growth,[34] was essentially unchanged for placenta, muscle, and brain. Since there was a difference of 8.2 days in average age between the more mature control fetuses and those born to diabetic mothers, this finding implied that the tissues of the SZ fetuses were advanced for their gestational age.

The literature contains little data on fetal human or monkey tissue lipid components. Roux and Yoshioka[36] noted large increases in phospholipid and triglyceride content of the maturing human placenta. Total phospholipids increased in brain while triglycerides accumulated in liver from human fetuses studied up to 32 weeks of development.[36]

In the experiments described here, values for phospholipid composition in brain, liver, and placental samples suggest that the tissues from the control group were more mature with respect to phospholipid content (Table 19.2). The two exceptions were the concentration of phosphatidylethanolamine in brain and liver of the SZ fetuses and the concentration of monopalmitin in the brains of the same fetuses.

In the liver of the SZ group all of the lipid moieties including free fatty acids, triglycerides, lipid:nitrogen ratios, total phospholipids, and cholesterol were either increased in concentration or essentially equivalent to control values (Table 19.1). In the placenta, phospholipids and cholesterol also showed a trend toward an increased concentration in the SZ group. Except for cholesterol, the various lipids in muscle of the SZ fetuses were present in lesser amounts than in control tissues.

Table 19.2   Phospholipid composition (μg/mg) of fresh fetal tissues derived from 6 control (Co) and 9 diabetic (Sz) macaque pregnancies.

	Brain		Liver		Placenta	
	Sz	Co	Sz	Co	Sz	Co
Sphingomyelin	2.5	5.0	3.6	3.7	2.8	3.2
Lysolecithin	0.8	1.1	0.8	1.5	0.9	1.9
Dipalmitin	2.8	3.4	3.3	2.6	1.9	2.0
Monolein	1.1	1.0	4.3	---	2.2	2.5
Monopalmitin	4.9	2.9	---	---	1.1	---
Lecithin	2.5	3.5	2.8	4.2	2.2	2.2
Phosphatidyl ethanolamine	3.2	2.5	5.1	2.7	1.2	1.8

In the brain the total lipid and phospholipid concentrations were reduced, suggesting retarded growth. Only two phospholipids in the experimental group showed an increase in concentration (phosphatidylethanolamine and monopalmitin) (Table 19.2). The major proportion of total phospholipids is comprised of lecithin and phosphatidylethanolamine in the human placenta.[37] This is not so for the macaque.

The 8.2-day difference in average age between the experimental and control groups has probably accounted for the fact that the lipid determinations have revealed trends rather than significant changes. With respect to the lipid indices reported, brain tissue appeared to be behind in development while muscle and liver were as mature or more mature than in control tissues. Thus maternal carbohydrate intolerance would appear to enhance growth and hasten maturation in certain fetal tissues.

STUDIES OF LIPID METABOLISM IN VITRO

The morphologic and biochemical changes in the human newborn of mothers with diabetes mellitus have been described.[38, 39] These include an increase in body fat content of the conceptus[8] which might be related to the hyperlipidemia measured in diabetes. The heparin-treated pregnant animal demonstrates an increased fatty acid level and the fetal body fat content also shows an increase.[40] However, the fetus from a diabetic rat demonstrates a diminished fat synthesis.[41] These observations indicate that experimental alterations in carbohydrates and fatty acid levels influence fetal metabolism. It is possible that these fetal responses are mediated by an increased supply of substrate from a diabetic mother to the fetus, this substrate being metabolized by the fetus, which is hyperinsulinemic.[25]

If this assumption is correct, the metabolism *in vitro* of fetal tissue of diabetic monkey may demonstrate alterations in carbohydrate and lipid metabolism. This question was examined by measuring *in vitro* the synthesis of lipids and the production of $^{14}CO_2$ from glucose-U-^{14}C and palmitate-1-^{14}C in tissues from fetuses of normal and SZ-treated monkeys.

Timed gestations from the breeding colony of the Department of Obstetrics and Gynecology of the University of Pittsburgh School of Medicine, were used. Details of the streptozotocin-treated pregnancies have been published.[25] A total of six pregnancies were interrupted by cesarean section, four at 140 ± 1 day in the SZ-treated group and two at 147 ± 1 day in the control. The gestation period for this monkey colony is 164 ± 5 days.

The mother was premedicated with phencyclidine and anesthetized with halothane for operative delivery. The newborn was immediately killed with 30 mg intravenous pentobarbital. Placenta, lung, heart, brain, liver, and adipose tissue pooled from the omental, scapular, and buttock areas were prepared for *in vitro* incubation with 10 mM glucose-U-^{14}C (SA 0.03 μCi/mg) or 2 meq/l of albumin-palmitic-1-^{14}C (SA 0.02 μCi/mg) under an atmosphere of 95% oxygen and 5% carbon dioxide as previously described.[7] The total volume of each incubating flask was 3 ml and the incubation lasted 2 hours at 37.5°C. Each tissue (600 mg) was incubated in duplicate.

In one set of experiments, simian insulin (provided by Dr. A. M. Fisher), 3 mU/ml, was added to the incubating medium. At the end of the incubation period, total lipids, phospholipids, sterols, sterol esters, triglycerides, and free fatty acids (FFA) were isolated from each tissue and the respiratory carbon dioxide ($^{14}CO_2$) produced in each incubation flask was determined as previously described.[42]

The data are expressed as disintegrations per minute per gram of tissue wet weight. The counter efficiency was 82%. The water content was determined by dry weight measurements of the tissues.[43] Since there were no significant differences in the dry weight of both groups, the data were expressed per gram wet weight.

In one normal and one fetus born of a diabetic mother, phospholipids and triglycerides were isolated from each tissue, methylated with boron-trifluoride methanol, and their fatty acid composition determined by gas-liquid chromatography.[43]

Since small numbers of observations do not permit statistical evaluation of the data, the variability from the mean of similar tissue was determined. Tissue of nine normal fetal monkeys near term, obtained from the monkey colony in San Juan, Puerto Rico, was prepared and incubated in duplicate following the present experimental program with glucose-U-^{14}C or palmitate-1-^{14}C as substrate. The same metabolic parameters were measured and the mean and standard error of the duplicate determinations were calculated.

The plasma glucose disappearance rates observed during intravenous glucose tolerance tests were 1.6 to 3.1 times slower and the fasting venous plasma glucose concentrations 35% higher in the SZ-treated mothers than in the control group. Maternal weight gain during pregnancy, and fetal and placental weight at the time of delivery, were similar for both groups in spite of the average difference of 1 week. However, mean fetal plasma glucose concentration prior to birth was 42 ± 7 mg% in the SZ group and 38 ± 5 mg% in the control groups. The base-line fetal plasma immunoassayable insulin level of the SZ-treated groups was 1.8 ± 0.20 ng/ml, that in the control group was 0.5 ± 0.07 ng/ml ($P < 0.01$).

The percent SE (ie, standard error divided by the mean $\times$ 100) for the fetal tissue of the nine normal monkeys incubated with palmitate-1-^{14}C or glucose-U-^{14}C was 14%. However, marked variations were observed among tissues and substrates (Table 19.3).

In brain, liver, and lung of the SZ fetus, the concentration of triglycerides was about double that of the normal (Table 19.4). Placenta and fetal liver C_{14}, C_{16}, and C_{20} were in higher percentages in the SZ group than in the normal group as were fetal liver $C_{18}1$, $C_{16}1$, and fetal lung C_{20} (Table 19.5).

The incubation of placental and fetal adipose tissue, lung, and brain from streptozotocin-treated pregnancies resulted in an increase of the net conversion of palmitate-1-^{14}C to triglycerides when compared to that found in normal tissue (Table 19.6).

In liver, heart, lung, and adipose tissue, only one fetus demonstrated an increased conversion to triglycerides and there is no indication in the clinical data relative to the glucose intolerance of the mother during pregnancy to explain this difference. Compared to the normal, the production of $^{14}CO_2$ from palmitate increased consistently 1.5 to 5.1 times in each fetal tissue of the SA group.

In experiments with glucose-U-^{14}C (Table 19.7) the placenta of the SZ fetus showed two to three times more conversion of glucose to lipid than that of the normal. The production of $^{14}CO_2$ from glucose-U-^{14}C is increased 10 to 13 times in the brain and 1.4 to 4.3 times in the heart of the SZ-treated monkeys.

In the last series of experiments, the effect of insulin added to the incubation medium was examined for CO_2 production. Table 19.8 is a repeat of the data obtained in Tables 19.6 and 19.7 but the incubation with insulin has been entered. As shown in Tables 19.6 and 19.7 the SZ fetus incorporated more palmitate-1-^{14}C into lipids, triglycerides, and carbon dioxide than the normal. When glucose-U-^{14}C was used as substrate, the SZ fetal brain showed a 1.7 times increase in glucose incor-

Table 19.3   Calculated percent standard error of
the mean incorporation of palmitate-
1-14C (Palm.) and glucose-U-14C (Glu.)
in the fetal tissues of nine near term
rhesus monkeys.

Substrate	14C Lipids		14C-Tri-glycerides	$^{14}CO_2$	
	Glu	Palm	Palm	Glu	Palm
Brain	6.3%	6.3%	12%	10%	14%
Lung	3.5%	6.1%	27%	12%	11%
Liver	7.7%	5.1%	16%	31%	19%
Placenta	27.0%	11.2%	15%	12%	22%
Average	11.1%	7.2%	17.5%	16.3%	16.5%

poration into lipids as compared to the control fetus. When insulin was added to the incubation medium, palmitate-1-^{14}C incorporation into lipids was markedly increased in the placenta and heart of the SZ fetus but it remained the same in the control fetus. Similar observations apply to $^{14}CO_2$ measured in brain, lung, and liver, using palmitate-1-^{14}C as substrate. When glucose-U-^{14}C was used, insulin stimulated lipid synthesis markedly in adipose tissue and brain of the SZ fetus.

The relative scarcity of data requires a qualitative rather than a quantitative review. It has to be noted that fetal hyperinsulinemia without hyperglycemia is present in this diabetic-like model. It can be explained by an increased glucose metabolism by the fetus in this preparation that would maintain the blood glucose level at subnormal concentration.

Although statistical comparisons are not appropriate, some general comments can be made based on the known percent variations from the mean of similar prepa-

Table 19.4 Triglyceride content of fetal tissue
obtained from normal and SZ-treated
pregnant monkeys.

	Normal	SZ-Treated	Ratio
Brain	0.6	1.4 ± 0.04	2.3
Liver	2.3	4.1 ± 1.3	1.7
Lung	1.6	3.0 ± 1.1	1.9
Placenta	4.3	5.8 ± 1.4	1.3

The numbers represent the percentage of triglycerides measured in the tissue of one normal and two SZ-treated fetal monkeys. In the SZ-treated monkeys the standard error is given because two experiments were performed in duplicate.
Ratio = The percentage of triglycerides in the tissue of SZ-treated monkeys divided by that measured in the normal monkey.

Table 19.5   Percentage fatty acid composition in phospholipids in fetal organs of normal and diabetic pregnancies.

	Placenta			Liver			Brain			Lung		
	N	SZ	R	N	SZ	R	N	SZ	R	N	SZ	R
C_{14}	0.6	1.5	2.5	0.3	1.2	4.0	1.4	1.7	1.2	1.3	1.7	1.3
C_{16}	33.0	52.1	1.6	27.7	45.0	1.6	28.0	38.5	1.4	40.2	44.5	1.1
$C_{16}1$	2.5	3.4	1.4	3.5	6.1	1.7	5.1	5.6	1.1	7.3	5.4	0.7
C_{18}	29.5	21.9	0.7	23.8	14.2	0.6	25.7	24.4	0.9	13.8	16.5	1.2
$C_{18}1$	18.1	13.4	0.7	14.6	22.9	1.6	ND	19.9	ND	20.8	21.8	1.0
C_{20}	1.3	2.3	1.8	0	3.1	3.1	22.9	–	0.9	0	2.1	2.1
C_{22}	4.4	0	0	10.8	0	0	7.5	0	0	7.2	0	0
$C_{22}1$	0	0	0	0	0	0	0	7.5	ND	0	0	0
TOTALS	89.4	94.6		80.7	92.5		90.6	97.6		93.3	92.0	

The numbers are the average of duplicate determinations in the tissues of the fetuses from one normal (N) and one diabetic (D) pregnancy. R = Ratio of the percentage fatty acid composition in the diabetic fetus to that of the normal fetus (SZ/N). ND = Not detectable. N = Normal fetus.

332

Table 19.6 Conversion of palmitate-1-^{14}C to triglycerides and $^{14}CO_2$ by tissue of one normal monkey and two fetal monkeys treated with streptozotocin.

	Normal	SZ	Average	$\frac{SZ}{Normal}$
Triglyceride				
Placenta	3758	6109, 5938	6022	1.6
Adipose Tissue	18886	22897, 32271	27584	1.4
Lung	3415	4512, 8202	7042	2.1
Brain	669	929, 1812	1370	2.0
Liver	5794	5124, 10275	7699	1.3
Heart	1481	1465, 4222	2843	1.9
Carbon Dioxide				
Placenta	270	683, 1392	1038	3.8
Adipose Tissue	462	1088, –	1088	2.4
Lung	218	560, 718	639	2.9
Brain	95	119, 161	140	1.5
Liver	125	540, 540	540	4.3
Heart	207	501, 1631	1066	5.1

The results are expressed in DPM/g, wet weight of tissue/2 hours of incubation at 37.5°C. The determinations were carried out in duplicate.

rations as indicated in Tables 19.6 and 19.7. Furthermore, duplicate measurements of slices of fetal tissue did not vary more than 5%. In general, fetal tissue from SZ-treated mothers incorporates more palmitate-1-^{14}C into triglycerides than the tissue of normal fetuses but when glucose-U-^{14}C was utilized as substrate, only the placenta demonstrated an enhanced lipid synthesis. The reasons for the apparent differences in metabolism of the two substrates may be accounted for by the fact that the intracellular pool of glucose is greater than that of palmitate. This will lower the specific

Table 19.7 Conversion of Glucose-U-^{14}C to ^{14}C lipids and $^{14}CO_2$ by tissue of one normal monkey and two fetal monkeys treated with streptozotocin (SZ)

	Normal	SZ	Average	$\frac{Normal}{SZ}$
Lipids				
Brain	14399	12631, 19783	16207	1.1
Lung	8579	6574, 16104	11339	1.3
Liver	9174	13482, 14576	14029	1.5
Heart	19089	10545, 61584	36064	1.9
Adipose Tissue	59213	78622, –	78622	1.3
Placenta	18972	60679, 47294	59986	3.2
Carbon Dioxide				
Brain	7201	69840, 118276	94058	13.0
Lung	10487	9501, 17700	13600	1.3
Liver	9754	3563, 13318	8440	0.9
Heart	10365	14860, 44649	29754	2.9
Adipose Tissue	21203	21609, 52179	36894	1.7
Placenta	7169	10128, 73728	41928	5.8

The results are expressed in DPM/g, wet weight of tissue/2 hours of incubation at 37.5°C. The determinations were carried out in duplicate.

Table 19.8   Conversion of glucose-U-14C or palmitate-1-14C to lipids, triglycerides, and carbon dioxide by tissue of normal (N) and streptozotocin-treated (SZ) monkeys with and without added insulin.

	Normal	N+ Insulin	SZ-treated	SZ+ Insulin
Conversion of palmitate-1-14C to:				
Lipids				
Heart	3280	2386	9408	16506
Triglycerides				
Placenta	3758	4766	5938	9134
Heart	1481	951	4222	9180
CO_2				
Brain	7201	5931	118276	217284
Lung	10487	13066	17700	24626
Liver	5794	12119	13318	20702
Conversion of glucose-U-14C to:				
Lipids				
Brain	14399	17249	19783	26730
Adipose Tissue	59213	72117	78622	119992
CO_2				
Brain	95	604	161	ND

The results (DPM/g wet weight/hour of incubation at 37.5°C) are the means of duplicate determinations on one normal and one SZ-treated monkey. Each tissue served as its own control when insulin was added to the incubation medium. ND= Not determined.

activity of the glucose incorporated into tissue to a greater extent than that of palmitate. Furthermore, glucose is metabolized to different compounds such as glycogen, proteins, and lipids, whereas palmitate is mainly converted to lipids or carbon dioxide. The metabolic differences will be easier to detect when palmitate is utilized as a substrate because of a greater availability of radioactive palmitate for lipid studies.

Increased triglyceride synthesis from palmitate indicates that the activity of the metabolic pathways incorporating palmitate into triglyceride is greater in tissue of the SZ fetus or that the catabolism of palmitate to CO_2 is diminished in the SZ fetus. This last statement is not supported by the present data which show an increased $^{14}CO_2$ production in the SZ fetus. This increased $^{14}CO_2$ production in the tissue of the diabetic-like fetus suggests an increased activity of the enzymes of beta oxidation and of the Krebs cycle, coupled to a greater availability of L-glycerol-3-phosphate and fatty acyl-CoA. That the Krebs cycle is more active in the SZ fetus is shown by the increased conversion of glucose-U-^{14}C to $^{14}CO_2$ in adipose tissue, brain, heart, and placenta. This could be an adaptive response to the maternal glucose and fatty acid levels occurring in diabetes.

These observations may explain the increased triglyceride concentration and ^{16}C fatty acid composition of phospholipids measured in fetal tissue of the SZ-treated monkeys. It has to be noted that the fetuses from glucose-intolerant monkeys were significantly heavier than average for their gestational age. This is true of human fetuses in pregnancies complicated by poorly controlled diabetes mellitus. Direct analysis of the body composition of these fetuses indicates that their oversize is secondary to an increase in total body fat deposition.[8]

The tissue insulin response in the tissues studied was enhanced in the diabetic-like model. That this may be a reality *in utero* is suggested by the presence of fetal hyperinsulinemia and the enhanced fetal pancreatic beta-cell responsiveness to glucose or amino acid.[25]

The stimulating effect of added insulin on brain tissue $^{14}CO_2$ production with palmitate-1-^{14}C as substrate in the SZ fetus and in the normal with glucose-U-^{14}C as substrate, has not been previously described in the same species although the muscle of the fetus responds to the addition of insulin.[44] Although insulin may have a role in controlling the lipid metabolism of the fetal brain, it must be noted that the amount of insulin added to the incubation medium in these experiments is greatly in excess of that measured in normal monkey fetal plasma.[25]

It is concluded that induced glucose intolerance in the pregnant rhesus monkey produces metabolic and physiological changes in the conceptus that resemble those observed in the human newborn infant of the diabetic mother.[8, 25, 41, 45] A more extensive use of this model will help to define the physiological and biochemical changes that occur in pregnancy demonstrating abnormalities in carbohydrate metabolism.

SUMMARY

Rhesus monkeys were placed in a state of carbohydrate intolerance by the administration of streptozotocin (SZ) either prior to or after conception. Nine fetuses delivered by cesarean section at an average of 139.5 days of gestation from monkeys in such a diabetic-like state were shown to be significantly heavier than six control fetuses (mean age 148 days) that were obtained from normal pregnancies.

Although the SZ fetuses were some 8.5 days younger than the controls, liver and muscle samples from these animals exhibited values either more mature or equal to control values while brain tissue was less mature than from control fetuses in most instances. Lipid:nitrogen ratios were approximately equal to or above control levels for all four tissues, supporting the notion that enhanced growth in the fetus accompanies maternal hyperglycemia.

The various phospholipid components were increased in quantity in the control tissues except for phosphatidylethanolamine in brain and liver and monopalmitin in brain, which were greater in the SZ fetuses.

The metabolism of lipids in fetal tissue of streptozotocin-induced glucose-intolerant rhesus monkeys has been studied *in vitro*. The incorporation of palmitate-1-^{14}C into triglycerides and the conversion of the same substrate to $^{14}CO_2$ are greater in fetal tissue from the SZ-treated mother than from the untreated control. Enhanced glucose-U-^{14}C incorporation into lipids is present in the placenta and $^{14}CO_2$ production from the same substrate is markedly increased in the fetal brain and heart of the SZ group. This observation correlated with the increased concentration of triglycerides and ^{16}C fatty acids found in phospholipids measured in fetal placenta, liver, and lung from the SZ-treated mothers.

In the diabetic-like state, an increase in beta oxidation and Krebs-cycle activity is demonstrated by the increased conversion of palmitate-1-^{14}C and glucose-U-$^{14}CO_2$. The addition of insulin to the incubation medium stimulates lipids, triglyceride synthesis, and $^{14}CO_2$ production from palmitate-1-^{14}C to a much greater extent in fetal tissue of SZ-treated animals than in the fetal tissue from normal mothers. Therefore, there is a distinct difference in fetal tissue insulin response in the diabetic-like condition.

REFERENCES

1. Miller, M., and Black, M. E.: In: Danowski, T. S. (Ed.): *Pregnancy in Diabetes Mellitus: Diagnosis and Treatment*. American Diabetes Association, New York, 1964.

2. Sack, R. A.: The large infant. *Am. J. Obstet. Gynecol.* **104**: 195–204, 1969.

3. Pedersen, J.: In: *The Pregnant Diabetic and Her Newborn*. Scandinavian University Books, Copenhagen, 1967, p. 219.

4. Chen, C. H., Adam, P. A. J., Laskowski, D. E., McCann, M. L., and Schwartz, R.: The plasma free fatty acid composition and blood glucose of normal and diabetic pregnant women and of their newborns. *Pediatrics* **36**; 843–855, 1961.

5. Svanberg, A., and Vikrot, O.: Plasma lipids during the first week after delivery. *Acta Med. Scand.* **178**: 631–965, 1965.

6. Osler, M.: Body water of newborn infants of diabetic mothers. *Acta Endocrinol.* **34**: 261–276, 1960.

7. Osler, M.: Body fat of newborn infants of diabetic mothers. *Acta Endocrinol.* **34**: 277–286, 1960.

8. Fee, B. A., and Weil, W. B.: Body composition of infants of diabetic mothers by direct analysis. *Ann. N.Y. Acad. Sci.* **110**: 869–897, 1963.

9. Navarrete, V. N., Paniagua, H. E., Alger, C. R., and Manzo, P. B.: The significance of metabolic adjustment before a new pregnancy. *Am. J. Obstet. Gynecol.* **107**: 250–253, 1970.

10. Beard, R. W., Turner, R. C., and Oakley, N. W.: An investigation into the control of blood glucose in fetuses of normal and diabetic mothers. *Proc. Second Congr. Perinatal Med.*, 114, 1971.

11. Conklin, J. L.: Cytogenesis of the human fetal pancreas. *Am. J. Anat.* **111**: 181–193, 1962.

12. Steinke, J., and Driscoll, S. G.: The extractable insulin content of pancreas from fetuses and infants of diabetic and control mothers. *Diabetes* **14**: 573, 1965.

13. Heinze, E., and Steinke, J.: Glucose metabolism of isolated pancreatic islets: Difference between fetal, newborn, and adult rats. *Endocrinology* **88**: 1259–1263, 1971.

14. Espinosa, A., Driscoll, S. G., and Steinke, J.: Insulin release from isolated human fetal pancreatic islets. *Science* **168**: 1111–1112, 1970.

15. Wells, L. J., and Lazarow, A.: Organ cultures of pancreases of fetuses from diabetic rats. *Diabetes* **16**: 846–851, 1967.

16. Adam, P., Teramo, K., Raiha, N., Gitlin, D., and Schwartz, R.: Human fetal insulin metabolism early in gestation. *Diabetes* **18**: 409–416, 1969.

17. Paterson, P., Page, D., Taft, P., Phillips, L., and Wood, C.: Study of fetal and maternal insulin levels during labor. *J. Obstet. Gynecol. Br. Commonw.* **75**: 917–921, 1968.

18. Tobin, J. D., Roux, J. F., and Soeldner, J. S.: Human fetal insulin response after acute maternal glucose administration during labor. *Pediatrics* **44**: 668–671, 1969.

19. Cordero, L., Jr., Grunt, J. A., and Anderson, G. G.: Hypertonic glucose infusion during labor. *Am. J. Obstet. Gynecol.* **107**: 560–564, 1970.

20. Willes, R. F., Boda, J. M., and Manns, J. G.: Insulin secretion by the ovine fetus *in utero*. *Endocrinology* **84**: 520–527, 1969.

21. Mintz, D. H., Chez, R. A., and Hutchinson, D. L.: The effect of theophylline on glucagon and glucose mediated plasma insulin responses in the subhuman primate fetus and neonate. *Metabolism* **20**: 805–815, 1971.

22. Little, W. A., Nasser, D., and Spellacy, W. N.: Carbohydrate metabolism in the primate fetus. *Am. J. Obstet. Gynecol.* **109**: 732–743, 1971.

23. Obenshain, S. S., Adam, P., King, K., Teramo, K., Raivo, K., Raiha, N., and Schwartz, R.: Human fetal insulin response to sustained maternal hyperglycemia. *N. Engl. J. Med.* **283**: 566–570, 1970.

24. Pitkin, R. M., and Reynolds, W. A.: Diabetogenic effects of streptozotocin in rhesus monkeys. *Diabetes* **19**: 35–90, 1970.

25. Mintz, D. H., Chez, R. A., and Hutchinson, D. L.: Subhuman primate pregnancy complicated by streptozotocin-induced diabetes mellitus. *J. Clin. Invest.* **51**: 837–847, 1972.

26. Reynolds, W. A., Chez, R. A., Bhuyan, B. K., and Neil, G. L.: Placental transfer of streptozotocin in the rhesus monkey. Submitted to *Diabetes*, 1974.

27. Hill, D. E., Holt, A. B., Reba, R., and Cheek, D. B.: Alterations in the growth pattern of fetal rhesus monkeys following the *in utero* injection of streptozotocin. *Pediatr. Res.* **336**: 76, 1972.

28. Chez, R. A., and Hutchinson, D. L.: Unpublished observations.

29. Golob, E. K., Rishi, S., Becker, K. L., Moore, C., and Shah, N.: Effect of streptozotocin-induced diabetes on pancreatic insulin content of the fetus. *Diabetes* **19**: 610–613, 1970.

30. Novak, M.: Colorimetric ultramicro method for the determination of free fatty acids. *J. Lipid Res.* **6**: 431, 1965.

31. Sandesai, W. M., and Manning, J. A.: The determination of triglycerides in plasma and tissues. *Clin. Chem.* **14**: 156–161, 1968.

32. Frings, C. S., and Dunn, R. T.: A colorimetric method for determinations of total serum lipids based on the sulfo-phospho-vanillin reaction. *J. Clin. Pathol.* **53**: 89–91, 1970.

33. Debuch, H., and Mertens, W.: Quantitative determination of phospholipids in small tissue samples. *Add. Int. Arch. Allergy* **36**: 665–671, 1969.

34. Picon, L.: Effect of insulin on growth and biochemical composition of the rat fetus. *Endocrinology* **81**: 1419–1421, 1967.

35. Pitkin, R. M., Plank, C. J., and Filer, L. J.: Fetal and placental composition in experimental maternal diabetes. *Proc. Soc. Exp. Biol. Med.* **138**: 163–166, 1971.

36. Roux, J. F., and Yoshioka, T.: Lipid metabolism in the fetus during development. *Clin. Obstet. Gynecol.* **13**: 595–620, 1970.

37. Nelson, G. H., Kenimer, B. K., and Jones, A. E.: Thin-layer chromatography of placental phospholipids. *Am. J. Obstet. Gynecol.* **99**: 262–265, 1967.

38. Cheek, D. B., Maddison, T. G., Malinek, M., and Coldbeck, J. H.: Further observations on the corrected bromide space of the neonate and investigation of water and electrolyte status in infants born of diabetic mothers. *Pediatrics* **28**: 861, 1961.

39. Baird, J. D.: Some aspects of carbohydrate metabolism in pregnancy with special reference to the energy metabolism and hormonal status of the infant of the diabetic woman and the diabetogenic effect of pregnancy. *J. Endocrinol.* **44**: 139, 1969.

40. Fain, J. N., and Scow, R. O.: Fatty acid synthesis *in vivo* in maternal and fetal tissues in the rat. *Am. J. Physiol.* **210**: 19, 1966.

41. Mueller, P. S., Solomon, F., and Brown, R.: Free fatty acid concentration in maternal plasma and fetal body fat content. *Am. J. Obstet. Gynecol.* **88**: 196, 1964.

42. Yoshioka, T., and Roux, J. F.: *In vitro* metabolism of palmitic acid in human fetal tissue. *Pediatr. Res.* **6**: 675, 1972.

43. Roux, J. F., Takeda, Y., and Grigorian, A.: Lipid concentration and composition in human fetal tissue during development. *Pediatrics* **48**: 540, 1971.

44. Beatty, C. H., and Bock, R. M.: Interrelation of carbohydrate and palmitate metabolism in skeletal muscle. *Am. J. Physiol.* **220**: 1928, 1971.

45. Osler, M., and Pedersen, J.: The body composition of newborn infants of diabetic mothers. *Pediatrics* **26**: 985, 1960.

CHAPTER 20

Amino Acids in the Plasma, Muscle, and Liver During Fetal Growth and the Effects of Prenatal Hormonal and Nutritional Imbalance

Claude Bachmann, William L. Nyhan, Stanko Kulovich, and Mary Etta Hornbeck

INTRODUCTION

Physiologic growth in the soma implies an obligatory synthesis of new cellular proteins and any condition in which growth is inhibited should ultimately be reflected in a diminution in this synthetic process. The free amino acids from which proteins are formed are found in two general pools: the extracellular pool, which may be sampled by analysis of the plasma, and the intracellular pool.

A number of mechanisms for growth inhibition can be postulated that would involve these amino acid pools. Thus decreased growth could be associated with lowered concentrations of amino acids in both pools; it could also be associated with increased concentrations in both pools with a concomitant block in the processes involved in converting amino acids to proteins. A defect in the transport of amino acids into cells may produce low cellular concentrations and normal or high concentrations in the plasma. An imbalance could arise in the concentrations of the various amino acids. For instance, a single amino acid might occur in very high or very low concentration without parallel changes in other amino acids, leading to a decrease in the rate of synthesis of cellular proteins. Changes in conditions such as the supply of a single substrate might influence the content or activity of an enzyme or enzymes, which might then influence amino acid concentrations.

We are grateful to Dr. Inez Beitins who carried out the cortisol determinations.

With these hypotheses in mind, a study was undertaken of the concentrations of amino acids in the plasma, liver, and skeletal muscle of the primate, *Macaca mulatta*. The primates studied were the same groups discussed in Chapter 10. Normal animals were examined during the period of growth from midgestation to 120 days postnatally. The effects on amino acid levels of some nutritional and hormonal interventions were also studied.

METHODS

Aliquots of liver and muscle were stored frozen immediately after weighing. For analysis, muscle and liver were homogenized in ice-cold 0.2 N perchloric acid (100–800 mg tissue in 6 ml $HClO_4$) using a Lourdes Instruments Model MM1 homogenizer at approximately 8,000 rpm for 5 to 15 minutes. Plasma was deproteinized using 4% sulfosalicylic acid (1:4).

For the calculations the original blotted wet weight was used. Computations were performed as described in Chapter 10. Consideration was given to the statistical distribution of the concentrations of amino acids about the means.[1] Since the number of individuals that could be studied in each group was small, a meaningful analysis of distribution could not be performed. Therefore, for the first group processed, the comparisons of amino acid concentrations in tissues of animals with intrauterine growth retardation and of their controls were done in two different ways. The data were first compared by the conventional unpaired t-test, and second, this test was done on the decadic logarithms of the single concentrations in order to determine if significant differences would appear if a log-normal distribution was assumed. This was not the case; therefore the rest of the data were analyzed on the assumption of a normal distribution.

NORMAL ANIMALS

Results

The groups studied have been described elsewhere. Briefly, the animals were divided into six groups as follows:

Group 1.   75 to 112 days of gestation.
Group 2.   122 to 140 days of gestation.
Group 3.   145 to 160 days of gestation.
Group 4.   Postnatal 12 hours to 32 days.
Group 5.   Postnatal 60 to 122 days.
Group 6.   Adult animals.

Changes in amino acid concentrations in the course of normal development were compared (Figure 20.1). There was a tendency for amino acid concentrations in plasma to be relatively high early in fetal life, and to decrease to a minimum in postnatal life in groups 4 and 5, rising thereafter to the adult level. This pattern was seen in the case of taurine, threonine, serine, glutamine, alanine, valine, methionine, isoleucine, leucine, phenylalanine, ornithine, and lysine. For most of these amino acids the ultimate adult level was lower than the early fetal level. For isoleucine they were about the same and for leucine the adult level was the highest observed.

PLASMA

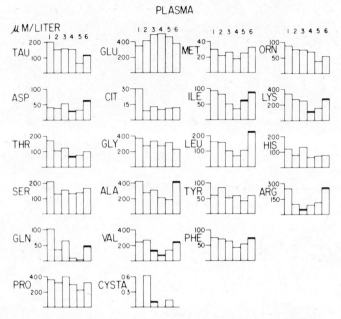

Fig. 20.1. Concentrations of amino acids (μM/l) in plasma during development. The numbers 1 to 6 refer to groups of animals of increasing age (see text). The heavy bars indicate changes that were significant when compared to the first or the second preceding group.

Glycine and histidine concentrations followed the general pattern but failed to rise in adult plasma. Arginine reached a minimum in group 3. Glutamic acid rose progressively in fetal and early neonatal life, falling somewhat thereafter.

The developmental pattern may also be seen by inspection of the ratios in Figure 20.2 and the concentrations recorded for plasma in Table 20.1. In the latter it is seen that group 4 showed a pronounced rise (early postnatal period). There was, in general, a predominance of nonessential amino acids, particularly of glycine and alanine in early postnatal life.

PLASMA

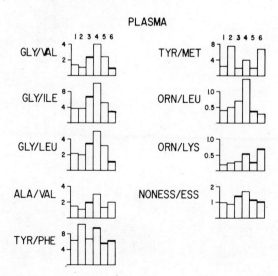

Fig. 20.2. Ratios of amino acid concentrations in plasma. The numbers 1 to 6 refer to groups of animals of increasing age (see text).

TABLE 20.1
Concentrations of Amino Acids Per Unit Volume in Primate Plasma During Development*

(μmoles/liter)

	GROUP 1 MEAN	GROUP 1 S.E.M.	GROUP 1 N	GROUP 2 MEAN	GROUP 2 S.E.M.	GROUP 2 N	GROUP 3 MEAN	GROUP 3 S.E.M.	GROUP 3 N	GROUP 4 MEAN	GROUP 4 S.E.M.	GROUP 4 N	GROUP 5 MEAN	GROUP 5 S.E.M.	GROUP 5 N	GROUP 6 MEAN	GROUP 6 S.E.M.	GROUP 6 N
TAURINE	196.5	72.9	4	152.6	24.2	8	158.5	22.5	10	104.3	22.6	8	65.6	15.3	7	114.8	11.3	5
ASPARTIC ACID	38.8	14.8	4	37.0	6.1	8	53.2	8.6	10	30.6	4.4	8	31.4	9.8	7	64.8	13.0	5
THREONINE	168.2	54.2	4	103.0	20.2	8	122.2	16.7	10	67.5	7.8	8	69.8	17.9	7	97.2	17.3	5
SERINE	211.9	62.8	4	130.9	16.9	8	156.1	19.2	10	134.5	7.7	8	136.3	29.0	7	166.3	28.5	5
GLUTAMINE	103.3	46.2	3	37.4	11.4	8	65.7	27.3	9	10.5	5.0	8	3.4	3.1	7	48.8	12.1	5
PROLINE	362.9	144.3	3	322.3	79.1	8	395.7	81.1	9	297.3	23.8	8	227.0	69.0	7	320.0	89.2	5
GLUTAMIC ACID	345.3	91.8	4	411.8	53.9	8	486.6	72.6	10	495.5	50.8	8	454.2	92.7	7	375.6	62.4	5
CITRULLINE	30.2	27.3	4	8.0	3.6	8	14.5	7.3	10	8.9	3.2	7	11.4	5.3	7	13.6	5.0	5
GLYCINE	374.6	121.7	4	275.3	38.7	8	335.8	47.0	10	267.6	15.9	8	309.1	55.8	7	228.3	36.2	5
ALANINE	421.6	204.2	4	275.1	41.0	8	307.2	43.3	10	209.2	22.7	8	190.0	37.2	7	422.3	77.3	5
VALINE	247.6	75.8	4	263.2	50.3	8	146.6	22.8	10	80.0	9.5	8	141.7	28.9	7	255.7	65.6	5
CYSTATHIONINE	0.0	0.0	4	0.6	0.1	8	0.1	0.1	10	0.0	0.0	8	0.1	0.1	7	0.0	0.1	5
METHIONINE	28.9	8.6	4	22.2	5.8	8	26.1	4.6	9	17.9	2.7	8	25.2	6.0	7	33.5	10.7	5
ISOLEUCINE	91.7	26.3	4	81.3	17.1	8	50.6	7.6	10	34.6	4.9	8	62.9	11.1	6	89.0	21.4	5
LEUCINE	164.6	53.6	4	157.3	35.2	8	103.1	16.6	10	74.8	12.5	8	105.7	22.4	7	233.7	55.0	5
TYROSINE	60.4	15.0	4	85.1	16.4	8	53.1	6.5	10	57.3	8.3	8	44.0	12.7	7	60.5	12.6	5
PHENYLALANINE	74.8	19.9	4	69.5	11.0	8	63.8	8.1	10	43.8	3.0	8	54.1	9.7	7	74.6	15.4	5
ORNITHINE	87.8	46.1	4	76.3	18.8	8	76.3	15.1	10	68.5	10.3	7	37.8	11.2	7	54.8	18.8	5
LYSINE	343.7	104.7	4	272.7	33.3	8	254.5	25.7	10	121.5	12.6	8	158.5	42.2	7	279.8	76.4	5
HISTIDINE	119.6	60.0	4	79.6	12.2	8	131.6	34.5	10	66.8	13.2	8	72.2	16.4	7	73.2	10.0	5
ARGININE	252.8	110.9	4	91.7	25.0	8	55.3	13.8	10	103.4	31.1	8	116.6	35.6	7	265.7	58.2	5
HOMOCARNOSINE	0.0	0.0	4	0.0	0.0	8	0.0	0.0	10	0.0	0.0	8	0.0	0.0	7	0.0	0.0	5
GLY/VAL	1.4	0.1	4	1.1	0.1	8	2.4	0.3	9	4.0	0.8	8	2.4	0.2	7	1.0	0.2	5
GLY/ILE	3.8	0.6	4	3.7	0.4	8	6.9	1.1	9	10.2	2.5	8	5.2	0.4	6	2.9	0.5	5
GLY/LEU	2.1	0.3	4	1.9	0.2	8	3.5	0.6	9	4.9	1.2	8	3.2	0.3	7	1.1	0.2	5
ALA/VAL	1.5	0.3	4	1.1	0.1	8	2.1	0.2	8	3.0	0.7	8	1.4	0.2	7	2.0	0.5	5
TYR/PHE	2.2	0.2	4	7.8	3.1	8	2.1	0.2	9	4.0	1.3	8	2.0	0.3	7	6.8	5.0	5
TYR/MET	0.4	0.1	4	0.5	0.1	8	0.7	0.1	9	1.4	0.4	7	0.3	0.1	7	0.3	0.1	5
ORN/LEU	0.2	0.06	4	0.2	0.03	8	0.2	0.03	10	0.5	0.08	7	0.2	0.07	7	0.7	0.5	5
ORN/LYS	1.4	0.1	4	1.1	0.1	8	2.4	0.3	9	4.0	0.8	8	2.4	0.2	7	1.0	0.2	5
NONESS/ESS	1.0	0.08	4	0.9	0.04	8	1.3	0.2	9	1.7	0.1	7	1.1	0.1	6	1.0	0.2	5

* The groups were as follows: 1, 75-112 days of fetal life; 2, 122-149 days of fetal life; 3, 145-169 days of fetal life; 4, 12 hours-32 days of postnatal life; 5, 60-122 days of postnatal life; and 6, adult monkeys. The data were the means, the standard errors of the means (S.E.M.), and the number of animals (N). Abbreviations employed in this and subsequent tables are as follows: GABA, γ-aminobutyric acid; GLY/VAL, ratio of glycine to valine; ILE, isoleucine; LEU, leucine; ALA, alanine; TYR, tyrosine; PHE, phenylalanine; MET, methionine; ORN, ornithine; LYS, lysine; NONESS/ESS, the ratio of nonessential to essential amino acids.

During the fetal growth period a certain number of statistically significant changes in the plasma concentrations of amino acids were observed (Table 20.2). The concentrations of valine and the other branched-chain amino acids decreased as pregnancy progressed. The differences in valine concentrations between groups 2 and 3 and between 3 and 4 were significant statistically. The significance of the other changes is indicated by the fact that the glycine:isoleucine and glycine:leucine, as well as the alanine:valine and glycine:valine ratios, were significantly different in groups 2 and 3. The change of arginine concentration from a group 1 level to a group 3 level was also significant.

The differences in concentrations of valine, aspartic acid, threonine, and lysine were significantly lower in the immediately postnatal group 4 than in the fetal plasma of group 3 before birth. The concentrations of many amino acids were significantly higher in the adults than in either group of young monkeys (group 4 or 5). These included valine, leucine, isoleucine, phenylalanine, lysine, arginine, aspartic acid, glutamine, alanine, and taurine, all of which were significantly higher in concentration in the adults.

TABLE 20.2
Statistical Analysis of Data Shown in Tables 20.1*

Groups compared	1/3	2/3	3/4	4/5	5/6	4/6
TAURINE					0.05	
ASPARTIC ACID			0.05			0.02
THREONINE			0.02			
SERINE						
GLUTAMINE					0.005	0.01
PROLINE						
GLUTAMIC ACID						
CITRULLINE						
GLYCINE						
ALANINE					0.02	0.01
VALINE		0.05	0.05			0.01
CYSTATHIONINE		0.02				
METHIONINE						
ISOLEUCINE				0.05		0.02
LEUCINE					0.05	0.005
TYROSINE						
PHENYLALANINE						0.05
ORNITHINE						
LYSINE			0.001			0.025
HISTIDINE						
ARGININE	0.02				0.05	0.025
HOMOCARNOSINE						
GLY/VAL		0.01			0.01	0.025
GLY/ILE		0.025			0.02	
GLY/LEU		0.05			0.005	0.05
ALA/VAL		0.01				
TYR/PHE			0.005	0.005		0.02
TYR/MET						
ORN/LEU				0.05		
ORN/LYS			0.005	0.05	0.01	
NONESS/ESS		0.05		0.02		0.05

* The data shown are values (P < .05, etc). Where no values are given the differences were not significant. Comparisons made were per liter of plasma.

The ratios between glycine or alanine and the branched-chain amino acids showed a significant rise before birth in group 3, as did the ratio of nonessential to essential amino acids. Most of these ratios rose further in immediate postnatal life and then decreased during later extrauterine life. Most of these ratios were significantly lower in the adults.

Few of the amino acid concentrations were significantly correlated with fetal corticosteroid concentrations (Table 20.3). A significant difference ($P < 0.001$) in corticosteroid concentration was found between groups 3 and 4.

The pattern of changes in amino acid concentrations in muscle (Figure 20.3) was very different from that seen in the plasma; most amino acids were present in fetal muscle in much lower concentration than at the adult level. Most of them did not change appreciably in concentration throughout pregnancy and even into the first postnatal group (group 4). Thereafter, concentrations rose considerably in either group 5 or 6, or both. Figure 20.3 and Table 20.4 present amino acid concentrations in muscle as amino acid concentration per gram of DNA, which is a measure of the amount of free amino acid per cell. The concentration of glutamine increased significantly toward the end of pregnancy, but this was not a major change in view of the difference in magnitude of all of the fetal glutamine levels from the adult values. The fetal changes in proline, citrulline, ornithine, and lysine were also significant, but their biological significance appears to be similar to that of glutamine. When the amino acid concentrations were compared relative to tissue weight (Tables 20.5 and 20.6), prenatal increases in most of the amino acids between 122 and 140 days and 145 and 160 days were significant statistically. Glutamic acid was again an exception to the usual trend. Levels were relatively high early in fetal life, falling to a minimum in groups 3 and 4 and rising thereafter. Proline was another exception. After birth proline concentration went down. Furthermore, the adult level was significantly lower than the level of the younger monkeys.

The most dramatic changes occurred between the two postnatal age groups of 0 to 32 days and 60 to 122 days. Almost all of the amino acids showed highly significant increases in their cellular concentrations. When expressed as concentrations per kilogram of tissue weight, all of the amino acids were lower in concentration in the adults than in the young monkeys 60 to 122 days of age.

Examination of the ratios (Figure 20.4) did not reveal major changes during fetal life. Most of the ratios showed little change in fetal life, rising with birth in group 4 and falling significantly thereafter. The ratios between glycine and the branched-chain amino acids were significantly higher in the adults than in the preceding group (group 5), as was the ratio of alanine to valine. The tyrosine:phenylalanine ratio and the quotient of nonessential to essential amino acids followed the same pattern.

The concentration of ornithine was positively correlated with the plasma corticosteroid concentrations in fetal monkeys.

In the liver (Figure 20.5, Tables 20.7–20.9) the cellular concentrations of most amino acids were at their lowest concentrations early in fetal life, falling after delivery and then rising considerably in the older animals. For most amino acids there was a fetal maximum in group 3 (145–160 days). This pattern was exemplified by aspartic acid. It was also seen in threonine, serine, glutamine, proline, glutamic acid, alanine, valine, methionine, isoleucine, leucine, tyrosine, phenylalanine, ornithine, and lysine. The pattern for glycine was essentially the same except that postnatally the decrease was not found. The concentrations of amino acids in liver

TABLE 20.3
Correlation Coefficients Between Corticosteroid Concentrations in Fetal Plasma and the Concentrations of Amino Acids in Plasma and Tissues*

	MUSCLE GROUP	CC	DF	P	LIVER GROUP	CC	DF	P	FETAL PLASMA GROUP	CC	DF	P
TAURINE									4&5 /L	0.63	11	0.025
ASPARTIC ACID									2 /L	0.70	6	0.05
									11&13 /L	0.99	2	0.005
									2 /L	0.75	6	0.05
									2 /L	0.80	6	0.02
SERINE					5 /DNA	0.77	5	0.05				
					5 /kg	0.78	5	0.05				
PROLINE					11&13 /kg	0.99	1	0.025				
GLUTAMIC ACID					1 /kg	0.96	2	0.05	11 /L	0.99	1	0.05
					5 /DNA	0.76	5	0.05				
					5 /kg	0.79	5	0.05				
GLYCINE												
CYSTATHIONINE	1 /DNA	0.98	2	0.02					11&13 /L	0.98	2	0.02
	1 /kg	0.98	2	0.001								
ISOLEUCINE					5 /kg	0.76	5	0.05	3 /L	0.64	8	0.05
LEUCINE					5 /DNA	0.93	4	0.01	11&13 /L	0.97	2	0.025
TYROSINE					5 /kg	0.95	4	0.005	11 /L	0.99	1	0.001
									1 /L	-0.98	2	0.02
PHENYLALANINE					5 /DNA	0.79	5	0.05				
					5 /kg	0.80	5	0.05				
ORNITHINE	3 /kg	0.66	8	0.05	5 /kg	0.81	5	0.05				
HISTIDINE	2 /DNA	0.81	6	0.02	5 /kg	0.76	5	0.05				
	2 /kg	0.80	6	0.02								
	2 /DNA	0.72	6	0.05								
	2 /kg	0.72	6	0.05								
ARGININE									11 /L	-0.99	1	0.025
GLY/VAL									3	-0.75	7	0.02
GLY/ILE					2	0.72	6	0.05	3	0.69	7	0.05
					11&13	-0.99	1	0.02	5	0.81	4	0.05
									11	0.99	1	0.02
GLY/LEU					11&13	-0.99	1	0.02				
ALA/VAL					2	0.79	6	0.02				
TYR/MET									3	0.79	6	0.02
									5	-0.81	5	0.05
									11	0.99	1	0.05
TYR/PHE	10	-0.84	4	0.05	2	0.71	6	0.05	4&5	0.55	11	0.05
					4&5	0.61	6	0.05				
ORN/LEU	10&12	-0.74	6	0.05	11&13	-0.99	1	0.05	5 /L	-0.81	5	0.05
NONESS/ESS									4&5	0.70	9	0.02

* Only those coefficients that were significant statistically are shown. The designations CC and DF indicate correlation coefficient and degrees of freedom, respectively. The designations /kg and /DNA indicate that the values compared were those of the concentrations of the amino acid in micromoles per kilogram of tissue and per gram of DNA respectively.

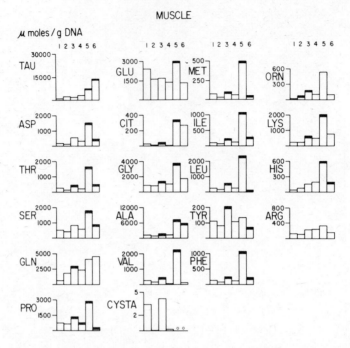

Fig. 20.3. Concentrations of amino acids in muscle during development. The numbers 1 to 6 refer to groups of animals of increasing age (see text).

reached their peak values in the young postnatal monkeys (60–122 days). In this series no determinations could be performed on the livers of adults. The pattern for taurine was slightly different in that the maximum was in group 2, after which there was a progressive decrease with age. Cystathionine showed the same pattern. Citrulline was in high concentration in the youngest fetuses (group 1) and low in concentration in groups 2 to 5.

Summary of Changes during Normal Growth

The results are listed in detail in Tables 20.1 to 20.9, and in Figures 20.1 to 20.6. Summarized below are the main significant changes that were observed.

1. In general the concentrations of amino acids were considerably higher in fetal plasma than in maternal, often by a factor of 8, concentrations falling as gestation proceeded. The effect was equal for essential and nonessential amino acids so that the ratios of these two groups did not differ in fetal and maternal plasma.

2. There was a tendency for amino acid concentrations in plasma to be relatively high early in fetal life and to decrease to a minimum in postnatal life in groups 4 and 5. Concentrations then increased to the adult level, which was lower than the early fetal level.

3. The concentrations of most amino acids were considerably higher in fetal liver and in fetal muscle than in fetal plasma. Concentrations in plasma rarely exceeded 0.5 mM; most concentrations in liver and muscle exceeded this level, concentrations from 1 to 20 mM/kg being not unusual.

TABLE 20.4

Concentrations of Amino Acids per Unit of DNA in Primate Muscle During Development

(μmoles/g DNA)

	GROUP 1			GROUP 2			GROUP 3			GROUP 4			GROUP 5			GROUP 6		
	MEAN	S.E.M.	N	MEAN	S.E.M.	N	MEAN	S.E.M.	N	MEAN	S.E.M.	N	MEAN	S.E.M.	N	MEAN	S.E.M.	N
TAURINE	1359.2	481.7	7	2396.2	409.1	9	2191.7	273.8	10	3330.3	517.6	9	7368.5	829.3	3	13621.0	9109.1	3
ASPARTIC ACID	173.7	36.4	7	140.4	11.6	8	547.9	247.1	10	311.3	109.3	9	1500.7	380.1	6	425.6	158.0	5
THREONINE	263.6	77.9	7	169.7	16.6	9	445.3	103.6	10	276.4	75.3	9	1698.9	357.9	6	489.6	210.9	5
SERINE	521.8	139.3	7	437.1	73.9	9	885.1	206.1	10	595.6	111.9	9	1773.9	313.6	6	881.7	449.3	5
GLUTAMINE	692.2	218.5	7	1184.8	121.6	9	2893.3	472.3	10	2440.8	457.8	9	4238.8	1023.0	6	4577.0	2484.1	5
PROLINE	692.0	139.0	7	674.3	142.6	8	1256.8	210.4	10	653.3	116.7	8	2917.6	547.5	6	210.8	87.7	5
GLUTAMIC ACID	2155.6	444.3	7	1676.7	188.8	9	1660.5	149.1	10	1409.9	253.0	9	3020.6	655.5	6	1303.0	585.2	5
CITRULLINE	13.1	12.8	7	0.1	-0.07	9	39.8	17.4	10	8.0	7.6	9	338.1	98.3	6	270.8	259.1	5
GLYCINE	947.3	192.5	7	773.3	90.2	9	1441.0	209.1	10	1048.5	150.0	9	3715.8	656.3	6	1684.2	661.1	5
ALANINE	1196.0	312.0	7	837.6	79.3	9	1564.0	270.0	10	1463.1	205.6	9	7189.1	1674.3	6	5725.7	2669.9	5
VALINE	247.6	58.5	7	179.2	15.8	9	424.3	108.8	10	212.8	71.8	9	2273.6	506.0	6	457.4	149.7	5
CYSTATHIONINE	3.4	2.1	7	0.04	0.04	9	4.0	3.8	10	0.1	0.09	9	0.0	0.0	6	0.0	0.0	5
METHIONINE	70.0	19.1	7	30.5	4.6	9	105.3	26.7	10	60.2	20.4	9	498.9	158.1	6	41.0	9.9	5
ISOLEUCINE	103.8	23.5	7	77.8	7.1	9	214.7	52.3	10	125.8	41.0	9	1099.9	295.0	6	271.3	104.7	5
LEUCINE	254.2	64.1	7	175.0	15.2	9	547.1	146.1	10	269.1	87.4	9	2363.0	586.1	6	473.5	189.0	5
TYROSINE	111.0	27.7	7	83.3	9.0	9	205.1	45.3	10	109.5	35.0	9	135.0	16.9	4	65.3	17.3	4
PHENYLALANINE	127.2	31.9	7	92.4	8.8	9	262.3	60.7	10	137.2	40.7	9	1093.0	239.6	6	217.6	88.3	5
ORNITHINE	24.9	1.9	4	82.6	9.3	9	171.2	28.8	10	126.2	17.8	9	563.1	262.9	6	97.8	48.2	4
LYSINE	257.9	67.1	7	276.0	28.2	9	697.1	156.6	10	526.3	232.2	9	2021.7	591.4	6	795.6	220.1	5
HISTIDINE	57.0	11.1	7	71.2	9.9	9	157.9	42.9	10	173.7	63.2	9	603.8	159.7	6	184.6	50.7	5
ARGININE	146.9	50.5	7	110.0	17.4	9	242.6	64.2	10	254.0	106.1	9	351.8	85.1	6	165.3	67.5	5
HOMOCARNOSINE	0.0	0.0	7	0.0	0.0	9	0.0	0.0	10	0.0	0.0	9	0.0	0.0	6	0.0	0.0	5

MUSCLE

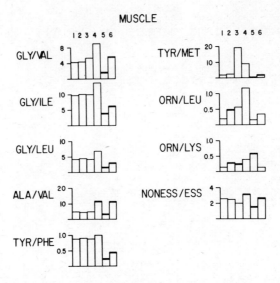

Fig. 20.4. Ratios of amino acid concentrations in muscle. The numbers 1 to 6 refer to groups of animals of increasing age (see text).

LIVER

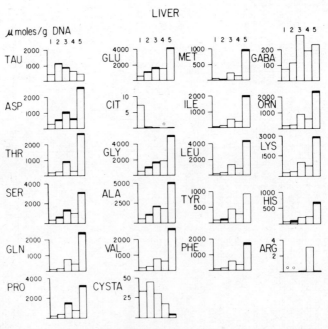

Fig. 20.5. Concentrations of amino acids (μM/g DNA) in liver during development. The numbers 1 to 6 refer to groups of animals of increasing age (see text).

LIVER

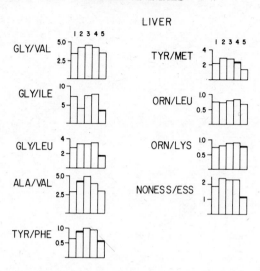

Fig. 20.6. Ratios of amino acid concentrations in liver, per gram of DNA. The numbers 1 to 6 refer to groups of animals of increasing age (see text).

4.   Most amino acids were present in fetal muscle in concentrations that were much lower than those found in adult muscle. The amino acid concentration per cell did not change appreciably throughout pregnancy or even into the first prenatal group: thereafter concentrations increased, the most dramatic increase occurring between the two postnatal age groups of 0 to 32 days and 60 to 122 days (Figure 20.3). When expressed as concentrations per kilogram of tissue, there was a significant increase between groups 2 and 3, and all of the amino acids were lower in concentration in the adults than in the young monkeys 60 to 122 days of age.

5.   In the liver the cellular concentrations of most amino acids were at their lowest earliest in fetal life, falling again after delivery and then rising considerably in the older animals (Figure 20.5). For most amino acids there was a fetal maximum in group 3 (145 –160 days) and a peak value in young animals (60–122 days). The changes in ratios of nonessential to essential amino acids reflect the fact that though both types increased significantly in group 5, the essential amino acids increased more than did the nonessential.

6.   Few of the amino acid concentrations were significantly correlated with fetal corticosteroid concentrations. A significant difference ($P < 0.001$) in corticosteroid concentration was found between groups 3 and 4.

Discussion

The changes in amino acid concentration in plasma and other tissues during normal development were impressive, as had been demonstrated in the brain (Chapter 10). Each had a discrete pattern. The plasma concentrations observed in this series were slightly lower than the values reported by Kerr[6] but the relationships were the same. Concentrations in fetal plasma were always higher than those in adult plasma. The prenatal drop in the concentrations of branched-chain amino acids was more pronounced in our study. In both series the concentrations of several amino acids were higher in adults than in the prenatal animals.

TABLE 20.5
Concentrations of Amino Acids per Unit Tissue Weight in Primate Muscle During Development

(μmoles/kg.)

	GROUP 1			GROUP 2			GROUP 3			GROUP 4			GROUP 5			GROUP 6		
	MEAN	S.E.M.	N	MEAN	S.E.M.	N	MEAN	S.E.M.	N	MEAN	S.E.M.	N	MEAN	S.E.M.	N	MEAN	S.E.M.	N
TAURINE	2807.1	596.2	7	5929.2	1176.5	9	4855.8	614.1	10	6642.6	939.6	9	9998.8	2139.6	3	4380.4	778.3	5
ASPARTIC ACID	4331.1	108.2	7	340.0	36.1	9	1262.1	599.4	10	653.9	224.5	9	2239.6	600.1	6	219.5	778.3	5
THREONINE	582.8	138.9	7	414.8	54.2	8	969.0	221.9	10	562.6	154.9	9	2502.6	550.1	6	231.8	27.0	5
SERINE	1177.4	253.5	7	1060.2	197.2	9	1916.2	433.7	10	1177.6	195.0	9	2600.0	477.1	6	372.8	36.4	5
GLUTAMINE	1447.2	188.1	7	2867.7	335.9	9	6325.1	986.5	10	4760.6	682.8	9	6209.7	1463.8	6	1826.7	249.0	5
PROLINE	1651.5	328.3	7	1608.1	340.9	8	2757.2	443.5	10	1297.4	232.2	8	4190.6	720.1	6	192.9	80.1	5
GLUTAMIC ACID	4951.8	710.9	7	4031.5	484.0	9	3662.0	337.2	10	2831.8	497.6	9	4504.1	1050.5	6	604.2	101.9	5
CITRULLINE	42.6	41.9	7	0.3	0.1	9	84.4	37.4	10	17.4	16.6	9	526.8	164.0	6	33.8	24.5	4
GLYCINE	2150.8	258.4	7	1873.1	248.7	9	3153.4	437.7	10	2084.6	236.5	9	5476.0	1013.8	6	840.4	111.0	5
ALANINE	2646.7	428.3	7	2022.5	225.6	9	3422.3	566.6	10	2954.2	403.0	9	10629.6	2414.0	6	2589.6	266.6	5
VALINE	588.1	146.1	7	431.8	43.8	9	918.0	228.5	10	437.8	152.5	9	3348.9	775.7	6	250.0	48.9	5
CYSTATHIONINE	10.3	6.4	7	0.1	0.1	9	9.2	8.7	10	0.3	0.1	9	0.0	0.0	6	0.0	0.0	5
METHIONINE	171.1	52.7	7	74.5	12.0	9	228.8	56.7	10	122.7	41.7	9	733.1	239.4	6	35.8	9.9	5
ISOLEUCINE	241.4	47.9	7	188.6	21.5	9	464.6	110.6	10	257.8	86.0	9	1624.5	452.6	6	137.3	23.5	5
LEUCINE	588.5	136.2	7	422.9	45.0	9	1184.0	312.1	10	551.5	185.0	9	3530.8	930.6	6	234.8	34.4	5
TYROSINE	260.9	63.1	7	202.0	25.8	9	445.5	98.8	10	219.9	70.5	9	214.0	18.1	4	57.9	16.4	5
PHENYLALANINE	296.2	69.9	7	224.2	25.8	9	566.6	128.0	10	280.2	85.9	9	1624.1	379.2	6	106.6	14.9	5
ORNITHINE	73.6	8.3	7	197.7	24.2	9	380.4	63.9	10	260.1	39.0	9	839.1	401.3	6	90.6	43.1	4
LYSINE	565.0	81.9	7	660.8	71.0	9	1527.0	327.6	10	1103.4	508.2	9	3177.7	917.1	6	460.7	77.8	5
HISTIDINE	132.7	22.6	7	170.4	24.0	9	347.9	91.6	10	360.4	140.3	9	918.5	252.7	6	171.1	47.7	5
ARGININE	338.8	123.8	7	264.2	40.8	9	533.1	139.9	10	533.9	232.5	9	493.7	95.2	6	153.8	63.6	5
HOMOCARNOSINE	0.0	0.0	7	0.0	0.0	9	0.0	0.0	10	0.0	0.0	9	0.0	0.0	6	0.0	0.0	5
GLY/VAL	4.2	0.5	7	4.3	0.3	9	5.2	0.9	10	9.0	2.1	9	1.8	0.2	6	3.6	0.4	5
GLY/ILE	9.7	0.8	7	10.1	1.0	9	10.0	2.0	10	13.8	2.8	9	4.0	0.6	6	6.3	0.5	5
GLY/LEU	4.3	0.6	7	4.4	0.3	9	4.2	0.8	10	6.7	1.5	9	1.8	0.2	6	3.6	0.2	5
ALA/VAL	4.9	0.3	7	4.7	0.2	9	4.9	0.6	10	11.9	2.7	9	3.6	0.7	6	11.7	1.8	5
TYR/PHE	0.8	0.02	7	0.8	0.03	9	0.8	0.08	10	0.9	0.1	9	0.2	0.1	4	0.4	0.1	5
TYR/MET	2.0	0.4	7	2.5	0.1	8	19.1	17.2	10	8.8	6.9	9	0.5	0.1	4	1.4	0.1	5
ORN/LEU	0.1	0.04	4	0.5	0.08	9	0.5	0.1	10	1.1	0.5	9	0.2	0.04	6	0.3	0.1	4
ORN/LYS	0.1	0.02	4	0.3	0.03	9	0.2	0.03	9	0.4	0.07	9	0.5	0.3	4	0.1	0.07	4
NONESS/ESS	2.6	0.2	4	2.4	0.2	9	2.0	0.2	10	3.1	0.4	9	1.5	0.2	4	2.6	0.08	4

TABLE 20.6
Statistical Comparison of the Data Shown in Tables IV and V

Groups compared	1/2 µmoles/kg	1/2 /gDNA	1/3 µmoles/kg	1/3 /gDNA	2/3 µmoles/kg	2/3 /gDNA	3/4 µmoles/kg	3/4 /gDNA	4/5 µmoles/kg	4/5 /gDNA	5/6 µmoles/kg	5/6 /gDNA	4/6 µmoles/kg	4/6 /gDNA
TAURINE	0.05		0.05											0.05
ASPARTIC ACID									0.02	0.005	0.02	0.05		
THREONINE					0.05	0.05			0.005	0.001	0.005	0.025	0.02	
SERINE									0.01	0.005	0.005		0.01	
GLUTAMINE	0.005		0.005	0.005	0.01	0.05			0.005	0.001	0.001	0.005	0.005	0.025
PROLINE						0.05	0.02	0.05			0.01		0.01	
GLUTAMIC ACID										0.025	0.01			
CITRULLINE					0.05	0.05			0.005	0.005	0.05			
GLYCINE					0.025	0.02			0.005	0.001	0.005		0.005	0.05
ALANINE					0.05	0.025			0.005	0.005	0.02			
VALINE						0.05			0.001	0.001	0.01	0.02		
CYSTATHIONINE		0.05												
METHIONINE					0.025	0.02			0.01	0.005	0.05	0.05		
ISOLEUCINE					0.05	0.05			0.005	0.005	0.02	0.05		
LEUCINE					0.05	0.05			0.005	0.001	0.02	0.025		
TYROSINE					0.05	0.025					0.001	0.05		
PHENYLALANINE					0.025	0.02			0.005	0.001	0.01	0.02	0.05	
ORNITHINE	0.01	0.005	0.02	0.05										
LYSINE										0.02	0.05			
HISTIDINE										0.02	0.05	0.05		
ARGININE											0.02			
HOMOCARNOSINE														
GLY/VAL									0.02		0.005			
GLY/ILE									0.02		0.05			
GLY/LEU									0.025		0.001			
ALA/VAL									0.05		0.005			
TYR/PHE							0.02		0.005					
TYR/MET											0.005		0.05	
ORN/LEU	0.05													
ORN/LYS	0.05		0.05						0.02					
NONESS/ESS							0.05		0.05		0.005			

* The data shown are P values. Where no values were given the differences were not significant.

351

TABLE 20.7
Concentrations of Amino Acids per Unit of DNA in Primate Liver During Development

(μmoles/gDNA)

	GROUP 1			GROUP 2			GROUP 3			GROUP 4			GROUP 5		
	MEAN	S.E.M.	N	MEAN	S.E.M.	N	MEAN	S.E.M.	N	MEAN	S.E.M.	N	MEAN	S.E.M.	N
TAURINE	448.0	63.5	7	1158.0	191.1	9	931.8	126.1	11	654.5	133.8	9	465.4	70.3	7
ASPARTIC ACID	307.3	61.7	6	558.9	41.9	9	1076.2	261.2	11	669.0	63.4	7	2638.5	714.6	6
THREONINE	233.9	54.3	5	293.6	14.0	9	986.6	308.3	9	322.6	25.1	7	2732.8	791.5	6
SERINE	353.9	60.5	7	679.4	34.8	9	1442.2	382.4	11	1027.7	278.8	9	3154.5	870.1	7
GLUTAMINE	139.1	30.1	5	190.9	15.7	9	778.2	264.6	11	490.7	215.1	9	2496.5	901.6	7
PROLINE	229.4	25.1	5	404.6	57.6	9	1691.9	364.4	6	797.4	230.7	8	3324.3	916.4	6
GLUTAMIC ACID	561.4	87.9	7	1207.7	141.0	9	1771.3	348.7	11	1656.2	274.0	9	4222.1	1178.3	7
CITRULLINE	7.2	7.2	7	0.1	0.04	8	0.02	0.02	11	0.0	0.0	9	0.03	0.03	7
GLYCINE	578.0	80.1	7	1107.2	113.8	9	1770.0	357.8	11	1825.5	315.9	9	5108.6	1257.6	7
ALANINE	536.8	85.8	7	1129.5	73.0	9	2236.0	549.2	11	1913.5	426.2	9	5199.1	1499.4	7
VALINE	208.6	40.1	7	268.9	12.0	9	788.5	272.2	11	647.5	295.1	9	2722.5	848.9	7
CYSTATHIONINE	34.1	7.2	7	46.1	12.9	9	31.0	8.5	11	18.7	2.3	8	5.0	2.6	6
METHIONINE	51.3	15.0	7	47.8	5.8	9	233.7	80.5	11	137.4	68.4	8	979.2	293.3	7
ISOLEUCINE	97.1	19.1	7	127.8	6.7	9	567.8	199.7	11	402.2	218.2	9	2018.1	622.3	7
LEUCINE	282.9	73.4	7	358.3	40.5	9	1355.5	479.6	11	913.1	495.3	9	4420.6	1407.1	7
TYROSINE	81.7	20.9	7	124.3	4.9	9	471.5	156.1	11	297.4	129.0	9	927.2	380.4	6
PHENYLALANINE	124.1	27.7	7	144.0	8.2	9	600.9	206.9	11	392.4	214.9	9	1784.7	551.4	7
ORNITHINE	211.8	58.8	6	246.9	21.9	9	901.5	301.3	11	677.0	327.2	9	2361.3	560.3	7
LYSINE	258.5	51.6	7	329.5	47.6	9	1017.3	340.4	11	747.2	348.3	9	3059.6	709.6	7
HISTIDINE	66.3	14.6	7	116.4	14.2	9	208.7	58.8	11	220.1	72.9	9	701.9	167.5	7
ARGININE	0.0	0.0	7	0.0	0.0	9	0.05	0.03	11	3.7	3.7	9	0.06	0.04	7
HOMOCARNOSINE	0.0	0.0	7	0.0	0.0	9	0.0	0.0	11	0.0	0.0	9	0.0	0.0	7

TABLE 20.8

Concentrations of Amino Acids per Unit Tissue Weight in Primate Liver During Development

(μmoles/kg)

	GROUP 1			GROUP 2			GROUP 3			GROUP 4			GROUP 5		
	MEAN	S.E.M.	N	MEAN	S.E.M.	N	MEAN	S.E.M.	N	MEAN	S.E.M.	N	MEAN	S.E.M.	N
TAURINE	3804.6	449.5	7	5310.3	881.9	9	3903.8	422.1	11	2447.9	444.6	9	1919.1	324.0	7
ASPARTIC ACID	2591.2	439.1	6	2557.6	251.9	9	4373.9	1007.2	11	2508.1	217.7	7	11086.7	3351.0	6
THREONINE	1921.8	406.4	5	1348.3	120.4	9	3862.5	1206.0	9	1209.7	88.2	9	11503.1	3717.8	6
SERINE	2960.0	438.6	7	3120.4	278.6	9	5785.8	1456.5	11	4076.3	1288.8	9	13265.3	3987.6	7
GLUTAMINE	1157.1	236.6	7	870.5	84.5	9	3054.4	1018.5	11	2007.6	980.6	8	10638.2	4141.8	7
PROLINE	1944.1	195.4	5	1809.7	226.9	9	6595.6	1542.6	6	3119.3	1059.7	8	13998.2	4293.8	6
GLUTAMIC ACID	4777.2	653.7	7	5434.1	580.3	9	7329.6	1333.1	11	6365.3	1196.9	9	17678.8	5368.7	7
CITRULLINE	72.4	72.1	7	0.5	0.1	8	0.09	0.09	11	0.0	0.0	9	0.1	0.1	7
GLYCINE	4892.3	557.0	7	5010.1	500.8	9	7300.5	1392.5	11	7128.3	1493.6	9	21487.6	5879.0	7
ALANINE	4494.4	609.1	7	5098.6	322.6	9	9127.1	2111.1	11	7462.2	1931.2	9	21959.2	6974.6	7
VALINE	1731.2	309.4	7	1250.8	139.5	9	3150.1	1093.4	11	2653.4	1342.7	9	11462.2	3902.7	7
CYSTATHIONINE	293.1	64.3	7	202.1	51.2	9	139.4	39.3	11	72.0	8.7	8	21.0	10.8	7
METHIONINE	422.0	122.6	7	212.9	21.6	9	919.0	318.2	11	572.2	310.8	8	4149.1	1376.2	6
ISOLEUCINE	805.9	145.9	7	595.1	70.9	9	2260.1	797.6	11	1673.7	987.9	9	8505.4	2856.3	7
LEUCINE	2334.8	571.3	7	1641.7	212.0	9	5393.4	1919.5	11	3796.4	2240.0	9	18666.3	6459.7	7
TYROSINE	679.6	167.7	7	577.9	61.2	9	1876.7	623.0	11	1213.9	588.6	9	3792.6	1680.5	6
PHENYLALANINE	1025.1	216.7	7	673.1	83.8	9	2382.7	824.8	11	1629.9	972.3	9	7516.4	2530.9	7
ORNITHINE	1728.8	454.4	6	1142.3	132.9	9	3572.6	1162.7	11	2779.4	1486.3	9	9735.2	2478.0	7
LYSINE	2124.7	375.3	7	1511.7	230.4	9	4042.5	1318.7	11	3062.0	1583.1	9	12557.1	3099.6	7
HISTIDINE	543.1	105.3	7	516.1	49.4	9	859.8	231.6	11	871.2	330.1	9	2852.9	717.1	7
ARGININE	0.0	0.0	7	0.0	0.0	9	0.18	0.12	11	16.6	16.6	9	0.2	0.1	7
HOMOCARNOSINE	0.0	0.0	7	0.0	0.0	9	0.0	0.0	11	0.0	0.0	9	0.0	0.0	7
GLY/VAL	3.3	0.6	7	4.2	0.5	9	4.4	0.9	11	4.1	0.5	9	3.5	1.4	7
GLY/ILE	7.2	1.2	7	8.8	1.0	9	7.5	1.6	11	7.9	1.0	9	3.7	0.8	7
GLY/LEU	2.8	0.5	7	3.2	0.4	9	3.2	0.8	11	3.5	0.4	9	1.7	0.4	7
ALA/VAL	2.9	0.3	7	4.2	0.3	9	4.8	1.0	11	4.0	0.4	9	2.9	0.9	7
TYR/PHE	0.6	0.06	7	0.8	0.03	9	0.99	0.1	11	0.9	0.07	9	0.6	0.07	6
TYR/MET	2.3	0.5	7	2.8	0.3	9	2.8	0.4	11	2.4	0.2	8	1.3	0.1	5
ORN/LEU	0.7	0.1	6	0.7	0.09	9	0.8	0.07	11	0.8	0.07	9	0.6	0.08	7
ORN/LYS	0.7	0.1	6	0.7	0.04	9	0.8	0.02	11	0.8	0.02	9	0.7	0.03	7
NONESS/ESS	1.8	0.3	6	2.4	0.1	9	2.3	0.3	11	2.2	0.2	8	1.2	0.1	5

TABLE 20.9
Statistical Comparison of the Data Shown in Tables 20.7 and 20.8

Groups Compared	μmoles /kg 1/2	μmoles /gDNA 1/2	μmoles /kg 1/3	μmoles /gDNA 1/3	μmoles /kg 2/3	μmoles /gDNA 2/3	μmoles /kg 3/4	μmoles /gDNA 3/4	μmoles /kg 4/5	μmoles /gDNA 4/5
TAURINE		0.01		0.02			0.05			
ASPARTIC ACID		0.005							0.02	0.02
THREONINE						0.05			0.02	0.01
SERINE		0.001		0.05					0.05	0.025
GLUTAMINE									0.05	0.05
PROLINE			0.025	0.01	0.005	0.001			0.02	0.02
GLUTAMIC ACID		0.005		0.02					0.05	0.05
CITRULLINE					0.05					
GLYCINE		0.005		0.02					0.02	0.02
ALANINE		0.001		0.05					0.05	0.05
VALINE									0.05	0.025
CYSTATHIONINE			0.05						0.005	0.005
METHIONINE									0.02	0.01
ISOLEUCINE									0.05	0.02
LEUCINE									0.05	0.025
TYROSINE		0.05								
PHENYLALANINE									0.05	0.025
ORNITHINE									0.025	0.02
LYSINE									0.02	0.01
HISTIDINE		0.05							0.02	0.02
ARGININE										
HOMOCARNOSINE										
GLY/VAL										
GLY/ILE									0.02	
GLY/LEU									0.025	
ALA/VAL	0.02									
TYR/PHE	0.005								0.02	
TYR/MET										
ORN/LEU										
ORN/LYS									0.05	
NONESS/ESS									0.01	

The general pattern in muscle was of a gradual increase during prenatal life followed by a large increase 60 days after birth. Thereafter most amino acids decreased in concentration until adulthood.

Kipnis and colleagues[3] found a decrease in the ability of rat muscle to concentrate amino acids with increasing age. The age groups studied were 40 and 125 days. These observations are consistent with the difference in *in vivo* concentrations that we observed in monkeys between groups 5 and 6, and could point to a low rate of protein synthesis in the adult than in the younger age group. However, the concentrations in both of these groups were considerably larger than those found in fetal and early postnatal samples of muscle, when rates of protein synthesis are presumably highest. Possibly, rapid synthesis of proteins may deplete cellular concentrations of amino acids.

The very large increase in taurine concentration in adult muscle is of interest (Figure 20.3). In cat muscle and liver, Tallan et al[4] found a decrease of a peak eluting in the taurine position after the tissue extract had been hydrolyzed in acid. Thus a part of the taurine peak was due to an unidentified ninhydrin-positive compound. Although the chromatographic system used by these authors differed somewhat from the one we employed, this possibility should be kept in mind.

During fetal life, liver amino acids (per unit DNA) were, as previously stated, highest prior to birth (group 3), then reduced immediately after birth but increasing again 2 months after birth (group 5). It was in this group that muscle also showed high values.

In liver polyploidy of cells might be considered to introduce problems in the proportionality of DNA concentration to cell number. It appears likely that this can be neglected, since there is probably still the usual proportionality between cytoplasm and nucleus. In a polyploid tissue, concentrations of amino acids per unit DNA reflect concentrations per nucleus or cellular unit rather than strictly per cell. The concentration of glutamine and glutamic acid may vary because of the conversion of glutamine to glutamic acid and to pyroglutamic acid.[2]

In the liver, taurine was also an exception to the general pattern, but in this tissue the adult value was very low instead of very high (Figure 20.5). Taurine is an end product of the metabolism of sulfur-containing amino acids and the steady decrease in values in liver could point to an increasing diversion of these intermediates into other synthetic pathways. On the other hand, an increase in taurine concentration in adult muscle could reflect a decrease in the need for those synthetic pathways.

Sturman and colleagues[5] have recently reported metabolic studies on the sulfur-containing amino acids in fetal rhesus monkeys. They found, as we did, relatively high concentrations of cystathionine in fetal liver, and this was consistent with their findings in human fetal liver. In this series of experiments they did find some cystathionase activity in contrast to other results, but it appeared that this was somehow induced by the conditions of the experiment. Their data, which were obtained using ^{35}S-labeled methionine, indicated that the fetus accumulates this amino acid from the mother against a concentration gradient. Isotope of methionine accumulated in fetal hepatic cystathionine, indicating a diminished metabolism of cystathionine.

FETAL BETA-CELL ABLATION

The monkeys used for these investigations were the same animals described in Chapter 9. Briefly, the groups were as follows:

Group	Treatment	Delivery
10	Streptozotocin at 110 days gestation	Cesarean
3	None	Cesarean
11	Streptozotocin at 110 days gestation	Natural
12	Streptozotocin at 130 days gestation	Cesarean
13	Streptozotocin at 130 days gestation	Natural

For analysis, group 12 was combined with group 10, and group 13 with group 11. The results are listed in Tables 20.10 to 20.16 and the following is a summary of the overall changes.

Results

1. The plasma concentration of nearly every amino acid was higher in group 10 than in group 3, while in the liver the concentrations of most amino acids were lower in group 10 than in group 3. Most amino acid concentrations in muscle were unchanged except for some branched-chain amino acids where there was a decrease in concentration.

2. The ratios of nonessential to essential amino acids were unchanged in the experimental animals.

3. In naturally born animals the plasma concentration of many amino acids was lower and the corticosteroid concentration was higher than in animals delivered by cesarean section.

Discussion

The overall pattern of amino acid concentration change following direct fetal beta-cell ablation is of an increase in concentration of nearly every amino acid in plasma and no meaningful change in the pattern of essential and nonessential amino acids. In contrast, in the liver most of the amino acid concentrations were lower in the experimental animals, but the essential amino acid concentrations were more severely depressed, so that the ratios of nonessential to essential amino acids were increased. The net pattern in muscle was similar; the ratios were also increased, but in this tissue most amino acid concentrations were unchanged, while the concentrations of the branched-chain amino acids were decreased.

These observations suggest that the insulin deficiency of these fetuses is reflected predominantly in the transport of amino acids into tissues. In the face of diminished transport, the amino acid concentrations of plasma increase, and those of the tissues decrease, the effect being most marked in the case of the branched-chain amino acids. These findings in the case of muscle are consistent with those of Wool,[7] who concluded that insulin influences the transport of amino acids into muscle and the incorporation of amino acids into protein. However, if its influence on transport is greater than its influence on protein synthesis, a lack of insulin would be expected to be manifest by a decrease in cellular concentrations of amino acids and an increase in their concentrations in plasma.

In these studies the mean concentration of alanine was lower in the liver of streptozotocin-treated animals than in the controls, whereas in plasma of treated animals it was higher than in the controls. Bloxam [8] has reported an increase of the branched-chain amino acids in the liver of streptozotocin-diabetic rats starved for 1 day. These findings reported here are in the opposite direction, possibly due to the fact that fetal animals were studied. It seems unlikely that such findings could be related to different nutritional backgrounds or to the starvation in Bloxam's study. It may well be that this reflects a species variation in the differential effect of insulin on transport and on increased incorporation of amino acids into proteins. The increase in the plasma concentrations of branched-chain amino acids was also seen in Bloxam's rats.

ABLATION OF THE PANCREATIC BETA CELLS OF THE
MATERNAL MONKEY

Results

In the experimental series streptozotocin was given to the mother as described in Chapter 9. The mean data for this group (group 9) are set out in Table 20.17.

TABLE 20.10

Concentrations of Amino Acids per Unit Volume in Primate Plasma of Streptozotocin-Treated Fetuses*

(μmoles/liter)

	GROUP 10			GROUP 11			GROUP 10+12			GROUP 11+13		
	MEAN	S.E.M.	N	MEAN	S.E.M.	N	MEAN	S.E.M.	N	MEAN	S.E.M.	N
TAURINE	173.2	29.9	6	187.7	49.9	3	195.1	31.6	8	182.3	48.6	5
ASPARTIC ACID	46.6	7.7	6	24.1	4.2	3	44.2	5.8	8	23.5	5.1	5
THREONINE	139.8	20.3	6	74.2	18.0	3	141.6	16.7	8	80.4	16.4	5
SERINE	201.0	26.8	6	137.8	22.1	3	214.4	27.1	8	131.9	25.2	5
GLUTAMINE	136.8	22.4	5	26.8	14.7	3	275.3	129.9	7	41.6	13.9	5
PROLINE	511.2	80.9	5	257.8	52.1	3	499.7	56.6	7	238.5	36.1	5
GLUTAMIC ACID	517.2	99.7	6	436.6	57.7	3	499.5	74.1	8	387.3	54.1	5
CITRULLINE	4.9	2.7	6	1.0	0.0	3	6.5	3.0	8	6.3	5.3	5
GLYCINE	491.0	76.0	6	277.8	39.7	3	513.9	68.6	8	287.6	50.5	5
ALANINE	472.4	88.3	6	247.4	96.9	3	497.4	71.4	8	281.6	88.3	5
VALINE	271.9	25.3	6	74.2	17.7	3	262.3	21.9	8	96.2	27.1	5
CYSTATHIONINE	1.2	1.0	6	.0.0	0.0	3	0.9	0.7	8	0.0	0.0	5
METHIONINE	46.4	9.0	6	17.8	2.8	3	41.7	7.5	8	17.8	1.7	5
ISOLEUCINE	85.8	7.5	6	29.8	1.4	3	82.5	7.2	8	36.1	8.5	5
LEUCINE	142.4	13.1	6	70.2	.4.9	3	250.6	104.1	8	77.3	16.7	5
TYROSINE	79.0	14.0	6	77.2	20.2	3	78.6	10.6	8	68.5	13.2	5
PHENYLALANINE	89.7	6.4	6	67.0	6.4	3	85.5	5.9	8	65.8	4.5	5
ORNITHINE	77.5	17.6	6	128.0	54.2	3	96.3	24.1	8	94.4	36.6	5
LYSINE	289.2	38.2	6	194.4	82.5	3	307.6	40.9	8	180.3	52.2	5
HISTIDINE	155.4	44.3	6	63.2	28.0	3	155.5	32.5	8	61.3	16.2	5
ARGININE	59.1	30.1	6	44.5	24.8	3	59.5	23.2	8	26.9	17.3	5
HOMOCARNOSINE	0.0	0.0	6	0.0	0.0	3	0.0	0.0	8	0.0	0.0	5
GLY/VAL	1.8	0.2	6	4.0	0.7	3	2.0	0.2	8	3.4	0.5	5
GLY/ILE	5.9	0.9	6	9.5	1.8	3	6.4	0.7	8	8.4	1.2	5
GLY/LEU	3.5	0.5	6	3.9	0.2	3	3.2	0.6	8	3.8	0.2	5
ALA/VAL	1.7	0.2	6	3.2	0.7	3	1.9	0.2	8	2.9	0.4	5
TYR/PHE	0.8	0.1	6	1.1	0.1	3	0.9	0.08	8	1.0	0.1	5
TYR/MET	1.8	0.2	6	4.8	1.7	3	2.1	0.2	8	4.1	1.0	5
ORN/LEU	0.5	0.1	6	1.8	0.8	3	0.6	0.1	8	1.3	0.5	5
ORN/LYS	0.2	0.05	6	0.8	0.4	3	0.2	0.04	8	0.5	0.2	5
NONESS/ESS	1.2	0.1	6	1.7	0.08	3	1.2	0.1	8	1.6	0.1	5

* The groups were as follows: 10, fetal monkeys injected with streptozotocin at 110 days of gestation and delivered by cesarean section at 154-160 days; group 11, fetuses injected at the same time but born naturally; group 12, fetuses injected at 130 days and delivered by cesarean section at 157 and 158 days; and group 13, fetuses injected at 139 days and born naturally.

357

TABLE 20.11

Concentrations of Amino Acids per Unit DNA in Primate Liver of Streptozotocin-Treated Fetuses

(µmoles/g DNA)

	GROUP 10			GROUP 11			GROUP 10+12			GROUP 11+13		
	MEAN	S.E.M.	N	MEAN	S.E.M.	N	MEAN	S.E.M.	N	MEAN	S.E.M.	N
TAURINE	887.7	147.5	5	1042.3	118.6	4	1137.9	195.0	7	996.1	102.8	5
ASPARTIC ACID	985.0	403.7	5	680.0	58.3	4	857.6	290.6	7	590.2	100.5	5
THREONINE	679.4	453.0	5	349.8	54.0	4	568.4	321.7	7	304.5	61.7	5
SERINE	1161.4	566.9	5	899.7	130.9	4	1041.2	401.1	7	777.8	158.5	5
GLUTAMINE	577.2	370.1	5	373.8	89.6	4	527.3	266.7	7	328.6	82.8	5
PROLINE	1024.8	570.9	4	506.2	127.6	4	824.5	382.6	6	-428.3	125.8	5
GLUTAMIC ACID	2178.9	395.4	5	1582.8	228.7	4	1931.4	319.0	7	1433.0	232.0	5
CITRULLINE	0.0	0.0	5	0.0	0.0	4	0.06	0.04	7	0.0	0.0	5
GLYCINE	1899.1	576.9	5	1231.2	243.4	4	1818.6	319.4	7	1142.8	208.2	5
ALANINE	1705.7	698.2	5	1184.4	110.7	4	1657.7	493.1	7	1073.7	140.0	5
VALINE	740.7	551.3	5	340.6	81.4	4	590.0	393.2	7	294.6	78.0	5
CYSTATHIONINE	80.7	37.2	5	16.3	1.9	4	63.2	28.1	7	14.2	2.6	5
METHIONINE	144.4	98.7	5	86.6	30.0	4	117.1	70.7	7	77.2	25.1	5
ISOLEUCINE	471.0	370.4	5	178.0	33.4	4	371.9	263.8	7	154.8	34.7	5
LEUCINE	479.1	249.8	5	434.3	95.8	4	417.6	179.2	7	375.3	94.8	5
TYROSINE	416.6	322.7	5	180.8	40.4	4	333.6	229.4	7	158.2	38.6	5
PHENYLALANINE	396.4	305.0	5	216.2	51.5	4	318.3	217.0	7	187.5	49.1	5
ORNITHINE	620.0	360.2	5	366.6	96.0	4	541.0	255.3	7	332.9	81.6	5
LYSINE	725.8	438.8	5	475.0	95.1	4	618.5	311.9	7	430.6	86.0	5
HISTIDINE	263.0	46.4	5	149.7	38.3	4	231.3	39.2	7	138.6	31.6	5
ARGININE	2.3	2.3	5	0.0	0.0	4	1.7	1.7	7	0.0	0.0	5
HOMOCARNOSINE	0.0	0.0	5	0.0	0.0	4	0.0	0.0	7	0.0	0.0	5

TABLE 20.12

Concentrations of Amino Acids per Unit Tissue Weight in Primate Liver of Streptozotocin-Treated Fetuses

(μmoles/kg)

	GROUP 10			GROUP 11			GROUP 10+12			GROUP 11+13		
	MEAN	S.E.M.	N	MEAN	S.E.M.	N	MEAN	S.E.M.	N	MEAN	S.E.M.	N
TAURINE	3589.7	556.0	5	4721.7	695.9	4	4741.8	860.8	7	4631.1	546.6	5
ASPARTIC ACID	4191.7	1886.8	5	3002.8	113.7	4	3657.9	1347.2	7	2645.3	368.1	5
THREONINE	2960.7	2071.6	5	1584.0	295.2	4	2471.2	1467.9	7	1396.9	295.4	5
SERINE	4979.7	2626.6	5	4068.0	705.1	4	4465.9	1850.6	7	3559.9	746.0	5
GLUTAMINE	2503.2	1690.9	5	1659.7	373.1	4	2277.4	1212.1	7	1483.4	338.5	5
PROLINE	4409.3	2650.2	4	2223.7	480.8	4	3549.3	1762.2	6	1902.0	492.1	5
GLUTAMIC ACID	9061.9	1949.4	5	7018.8	870.6	4	8087.0	1493.7	7	6492.1	855.6	5
CITRULLINE	0.0	0.0	5	0.0	0.0	4	0.2	0.1	7	0.0	0.0	5
GLYCINE	8008.2	2746.9	5	5673.8	1341.7	4	7702.2	1969.8	7	5369.4	1082.9	5
ALANINE	7301.5	3265.1	5	5384.9	748.2	4	7101.4	2293.4	7	4971.6	711.8	5
VALINE	3251.8	2513.5	5	1553.7	417.0	4	2583.7	1789.2	7	1359.7	376.8	5
CYSTATHIONINE	318.4	140.9	5	73.2	10.0	4	251.4	106.7	7	64.6	11.6	5
METHIONINE	629.3	450.1	5	392.0	140.7	4	508.8	321.7	7	355.2	115.0	5
ISOLEUCINE	2079.5	1685.7	5	803.8	166.2	4	1637.3	1198.9	7	708.4	160.2	5
LEUCINE	2048.0	1148.7	5	1972.2	487.3	4	1785.4	819.4	7	1724.5	451.5	5
TYROSINE	1836.7	1469.1	5	821.1	205.9	4	1466.4	1043.0	7	728.2	184.5	5
PHENYLALANINE	1742.9	1387.8	5	985.8	264.4	4	1395.1	986.1	7	865.0	237.7	5
ORNITHINE	2666.1	1642.8	5	1643.6	436.2	4	2325.3	1160.7	7	1523.3	358.7	5
LYSINE	3137.2	2007.1	5	2114.6	415.2	4	2669.7	1422.1	7	1957.8	357.8	5
HISTIDINE	1063.2	184.9	5	658.3	149.6	4	945.7	153.4	7	626.0	120.3	5
ARGININE	8.9	8.9	5	0.0	0.0	4	6.4	6.4	7	0.0	0.0	5
HOMOCARNOSINE	0.0	0.0	5	0.0	0.0	4	0.0	0.0	7	0.0	0.0	5
GLY/VAL	7.0	1.9	5	4.3	1.2	4	7.2	1.3	7	4.9	1.1	5
GLY/ILE	13.1	3.7	5	7.3	1.3	4	13.3	2.6	7	8.4	1.4	5
GLY/LEU	6.2	1.5	5	3.3	0.8	4	6.3	1.1	7	3.7	0.8	5
ALA/VAL	5.4	1.5	5	5.2	2.5	4	6.0	1.1	7	5.3	1.9	5
TYR/PHE	1.2	0.1	5	0.8	0.03	4	1.1	0.1	7	0.8	0.03	5
TYR/MET	2.5	0.2	5	67.1	65.1	4	2.7	0.3	7	54.0	52.1	5
ORN/LEU	1.1	0.1	5	0.8	0.09	4	1.2	0.1	7	0.9	0.1	5
ORN/LYS	0.8	0.05	5	0.7	0.07	4	0.8	0.04	7	0.7	0.05	5
NONESS/ESS	2.9	0.6	5	2.4	0.6	4	3.1	0.4	7	2.4	0.4	5

TABLE 20.13
Statistical Comparison of the Data Shown in Tables 20.10, 20.11, and 20.12*

The table columns are grouped under LIVER (μmoles/kg, μmoles/gDNA, and pmoles/gDNA measures) and PLASMA (μmoles/liter). The "Groups compared" are indicated in the header.

	LIVER								PLASMA (μmoles/liter)					
	μmoles/kg	μmoles/gDNA	μmoles/kg	μmoles/gDNA	μmoles/kg	μmoles/gDNA	pmoles/gDNA	pmoles/gDNA						
Groups compared	10+12/3	10+12/3	14/15	14/15	9/3	9/3	10+12/11+13	15/3	10/3	10+11/3	10+12/3	10+12/11+13	10/11	9/3
TAURINE														
ASPARTIC ACID					0.05	0.05						0.05		
THREONINE					0.025	0.025						0.05		
SERINE					0.05	0.05								
GLUTAMINE					0.05	0.05								
PROLINE			0.02	0.005	0.005	0.001					0.02	0.01		
GLUTAMIC ACID														
CITRULLINE														
GLYCINE											0.05	0.05		
ALANINE					0.05	0.05					0.05			
VALINE									0.005		0.005	0.001	0.005	
CYSTATHIONINE														
METHIONINE					0.05	0.05						0.05		
ISOLEUCINE					0.05	0.05			0.01		0.01	0.005	0.005	
LEUCINE					0.05	0.05							0.01	
TYROSINE					0.05	0.05			0.05		0.05	0.05		
PHENYLALANINE					0.05	0.05								
ORNITHINE														
LYSINE														
HISTIDINE														
ARGININE														
HOMOCARNOSINE														
GLY/VAL					0.05									
GLY/ILE	0.05				0.05						0.02	0.025	0.02	
GLY/LEU														
ALA/VAL														
TYR/PHE							0.05						0.05	
TYR/MET								0.02						
ORN/LEU	0.02				0.001								0.05	
ORN/LYS								0.01					0.02	
NONESS/ESS														
CORTICOIDS									0.05	0.02	0.02	0.005	0.001	

* Groups 3, 10, 11, and 12 are those described in previous tables. Group 9 consisted of fetuses delivered following injection of the maternal monkeys with streptozotocin in order to induce ablation of the maternal beta cells.

360

TABLE 20.14

Concentrations of Amino Acids per Unit DNA in Primate Muscle of Streptozotocin-Treated Fetuses

(μmoles/gDNA)

	GROUP 10			GROUP 11			GROUP 10+12			GROUP 11+13		
	MEAN	S.E.M.	N	MEAN	S.E.M.	N	MEAN	S.E.M.	N	MEAN	S.E.M.	N
TAURINE	2135.2	284.1	6	1732.1	452.9	4	2319.8	264.0	8	1706.6	287.4	6
ASPARTIC ACID	274.1	118.9	6	120.0	30.3	4	234.9	91.0	8	160.1	54.7	6
THREONINE	375.0	164.8	5	184.5	48.5	4	300.6	123.5	7	190.2	39.2	6
SERINE	751.0	235.5	6	405.6	85.5	4	634.7	188.5	8	384.9	68.2	6
GLUTAMINE	2717.6	250.4	6	2637.8	598.9	4	2603.1	200.3	8	2405.0	409.9	6
PROLINE	1203.7	232.8	6	554.9	113.4	4	1114.4	191.8	8	436.5	103.7	6
GLUTAMIC ACID	1727.3	260.8	6	821.5	208.7	4	1538.6	237.3	8	715.2	154.4	6
CITRULLINE	26.5	26.4	6	0.2	0.1	4	19.9	19.8	8	0.16	0.1	5
GLYCINE	1529.4	288.2	6	829.2	162.2	4	1365.1	236.9	8	791.5	110.5	6
ALANINE	1541.7	344.6	6	1244.0	262.5	4	1391.6	273.3	8	1081.2	198.2	6
VALINE	354.9	188.3	6	114.6	25.5	4	288.8	144.5	8	95.3	20.5	6
CYSTATHIONINE	0.1	0.09	6	0.2	0.1	4	0.1	0.07	8	0.15	0.09	6
METHIONINE	82.5	44.5	6	35.1	8.0	3	61.9	35.2	8	30.7	7.4	5
ISOLEUCINE	177.7	100.2	6	61.3	10.1	4	142.3	76.9	8	60.2	9.3	6
LEUCINE	369.3	204.1	6	129.9	27.2	4	295.6	157.0	8	117.6	21.6	6
TYROSINE	160.2	82.3	6	89.4	19.2	4	130.7	63.3	8	81.4	14.7	6
PHENYLALANINE	178.2	91.4	6	83.1	21.0	4	143.5	70.6	8	75.8	14.2	6
ORNITHINE	178.7	32.2	6	128.0	7.3	4	177.0	23.9	8	125.6	17.0	6
LYSINE	720.1	191.5	6	400.6	75.2	4	668.5	151.8	8	338.8	66.3	6
HISTIDINE	157.6	44.6	6	57.6	11.3	4	153.2	33.1	8	54.6	11.3	6
ARGININE	262.2	76.4	6	85.4	29.3	3	225.3	64.6	8	78.1	19.2	5
HOMOCARNOSINE	0.0	0.0	6	0.0	0.0	4	0.0	0.0	8	0.0	0.0	6

TABLE 20.15

Concentrations of Amino Acids per Unit Tissue Weight in Primate Muscle of Streptozotocin-Treated Fetuses

(μmoles/kg)

	GROUP 10			GROUP 11			GROUP 10+12			GROUP 11+13		
	MEAN	S.E.M.	N	MEAN	S.E.M.	N	MEAN	S.E.M.	N	MEAN	S.E.M.	N
TAURINE	4197.8	584.8	6	3990.5	1215.2	4	4569.2	521.2	8	3733.4	797.3	6
ASPARTIC ACID	558.4	260.3	6	270.9	79.5	4	476.5	198.3	8	321.5	92.7	6
THREONINE	753.2	364.6	5	414.0	117.9	4	603.3	269.5	7	398.4	82.5	6
SERINE	1527.1	525.8	6	898.5	198.4	4	1288.2	415.6	8	808.1	148.3	6
GLUTAMINE	5272.7	471.3	6	5808.4	1260.7	4	5078.2	368.5	8	5140.4	930.4	6
PROLINE	2443.0	547.3	6	1270.6	334.4	4	2247.1	436.9	8	977.0	282.1	6
GLUTAMIC ACID	3395.6	581.2	6	1841.3	501.5	4	3024.1	504.4	8	1537.9	374.4	6
CITRULLINE	56.8	56.6	6	0.5	0.2	4	42.7	42.4	8	0.4	0.2	5
GLYCINE	3016.9	637.2	6	1855.8	410.4	4	2698.9	511.8	8	1688.5	281.0	6
ALANINE	3022.5	736.6	6	2801.3	664.6	4	2732.2	574.6	8	2344.3	510.4	6
VALINE	723.1	407.9	6	257.7	62.3	4	587.1	311.6	8	207.2	50.8	6
CYSTATHIONINE	0.3	0.2	6	0.5	0.2	4	0.2	0.1	8	0.3	0.2	6
METHIONINE	168.5	95.2	6	82.1	22.8	3	126.5	74.9	8	66.3	17.9	5
ISOLEUCINE	362.7	216.5	6	138.3	28.7	4	290.0	165.4	8	127.5	21.5	6
LEUCINE	755.8	440.8	6	294.7	72.0	4	604.1	337.5	8	252.8	54.5	6
TYROSINE	328.0	178.5	6	201.7	49.6	4	267.0	136.8	8	174.6	36.7	6
PHENYLALANINE	361.1	197.9	6	189.5	54.1	4	290.3	152.1	8	165.1	37.5	6
ORNITHINE	355.3	70.7	6	283.4	25.8	4	352.8	52.8	8	261.7	32.1	6
LYSINE	1436.7	426.1	6	892.1	182.9	4	1339.2	334.6	8	725.7	160.0	6
HISTIDINE	313.5	98.7	6	130.3	31.1	4	305.6	73.3	8	115.6	25.6	6
ARGININE	530.5	170.8	6	202.9	80.8	3	452.6	141.2	8	171.3	50.4	5
HOMOCARNOSINE	0.0	0.0	6	0.0	0.0	4	0.0	0.0	8	0.0	0.0	6
GLY/VAL	7.3	1.4	6	7.8	1.1	4	8.1	1.2	8	9.5	1.2	6
GLY/ILE	17.1	3.9	6	13.6	1.8	4	18.9	3.1	8	13.8	1.5	6
GLY/LEU	7.9	1.9	6	6.7	0.8	4	8.9	1.5	8	7.4	0.9	6
ALA/VAL	6.8	1.0	6	11.4	1.1	4	7.7	0.9	8	12.1	0.9	6
TYR/PHE	0.9	0.1	6	1.1	0.1	4	1.0	0.09	8	1.0	0.1	6
TYR/MET	18.9	17.0	6	3.5	1.2	3	28.9	17.5	7	3.6	0.7	5
ORN/LEU	1.1	0.3	6	1.2	0.4	4	1.4	0.3	8	1.2	0.2	6
ORN/LYS	0.3	0.07	6	0.3	0.08	4	0.3	0.06	8	0.4	0.06	6
NONESS/ESS	2.5	0.3	6	3.1	0.3	3	2.6	0.2	8	3.4	0.3	5

TABLE 20.16
Statistical Comparison of the Data Shown in Tables 20.14 and 20.15

Groups compared	μmoles /kg 10+11/3	μmoles /gDNA 10+11/3	μmoles /kg 10+12/3	μmoles /gDNA 10+12/3	μmoles /kg 10+12/11+13	μmoles /gDNA 10+12/11+13	μmoles /kg 10/11	μmoles /gDNA 10/11	μmoles /kg 9/3	μmoles /gDNA 9/3
TAURINE										
ASPARTIC ACID										
THREONINE										
SERINE										
GLUTAMINE										
PROLINE					0.05					
GLUTAMIC ACID						0.02		0.05		
CITRULLINE										
GLYCINE										
ALANINE										
VALINE										
CYSTATHIONINE										
METHIONINE										
ISOLEUCINE									0.05	0.05
LEUCINE									0.05	
TYROSINE									0.02	0.05
PHENYLALANINE									0.02	0.02
ORNITHINE										
LYSINE										
HISTIDINE						0.05				
ARGININE										
HOMOCARNOSINE										
GLY/VAL	0.05		0.05							
GLY/ILE	0.01		0.02							
GLY/LEU			0.05						0.01	
ALA/VAL					0.01				0.05	
TYR/PHE							0.025			
TYR/MET										
ORN/LEU	0.05		0.02						0.02	
ORN/LYS									0.025	
NONESS/ESS									0.05	

TABLE 20.17
Concentrations of Amino Acids in Primate Muscle, Liver, and Plasma of the Fetus Following Maternal Beta Cell Ablation with Streptozotocin (Group 9)

	MUSCLE (μmoles/kg.)			MUSCLE (μmoles/g DNA)			LIVER (μmoles/kg.)			LIVER (μmoles/g DNA)			PLASMA (μmoles/liter)		
	MEAN	S.E.M.	N	MEAN	S.E.M.	N	MEAN	S.E.M.	N	MEAN	S.E.M.	N	MEAN	S.E.M.	N
TAURINE	3971.7	227.2	8	2166.5	221.2	8	4767.6	999.1	9	1124.9	225.1	9	193.1	44.1	8
ASPARTIC ACID	669.8	374.9	9	361.5	204.1	9	1719.0	211.2	9	400.9	30.0	9	40.9	6.6	8
THREONINE	899.4	365.6	9	470.9	180.7	9	830.6	71.2	9	198.9	14.7	9	112.6	14.0	8
SERINE	1347.1	171.4	9	722.1	98.5	9	2121.7	248.7	9	504.9	47.4	9	175.5	25.1	8
GLUTAMINE	4611.3	527.1	9	2528.7	362.0	9	625.4	85.2	9	146.7	14.4	9	47.9	12.9	8
PROLINE	1877.4	202.3	7	1025.2	128.6	7	1032.0	184.6	8	251.8	52.4	8	364.2	106.9	7
GLUTAMIC ACID	3047.0	1020.8	9	1658.2	561.3	9	4444.7	551.2	9	1047.7	104.6	9	517.0	62.1	8
CITRULLINE	41.9	35.2	9	23.7	19.4	9	0.2	0.1	9	0.05	0.04	9	11.5	4.9	8
GLYCINE	2567.5	232.1	9	1393.0	151.2	9	4112.2	453.7	9	976.9	92.7	9	336.2	43.1	8
ALANINE	2755.1	184.1	9	1511.0	154.5	9	3600.8	319.8	9	858.4	64.0	9	354.1	71.0	8
VALINE	403.3	81.7	9	217.6	45.8	9	657.2	53.2	9	158.6	13.6	9	191.4	33.5	8
CYSTATHIONINE	22.2	22.0	9	12.0	12.0	9	146.3	32.6	7	31.7	6.5	7	0.2	0.1	8
METHIONINE	112.0	27.9	9	59.9	15.1	9	172.8	15.9	9	41.0	3.0	9	20.6	3.6	8
ISOLEUCINE	200.0	38.7	9	106.6	20.9	9	343.5	26.3	9	82.3	6.3	9	65.1	15.3	8
LEUCINE	391.2	90.6	9	210.5	49.6	9	702.0	46.7	9	170.3	12.9	9	112.4	19.4	8
TYROSINE	157.3	33.4	9	85.6	19.0	9	293.9	22.0	9	71.8	6.6	9	71.5	7.9	8
PHENYLALANINE	165.2	32.8	9	89.6	18.6	9	255.6	21.3	9	61.7	5.6	9	70.9	8.0	8
ORNITHINE	406.5	56.1	9	217.3	32.3	9	1272.0	177.4	9	307.3	39.1	9	149.9	56.8	7
LYSINE	1050.5	189.6	9	563.9	112.1	9	1652.3	249.5	9	386.5	47.8	9	326.3	61.6	8
HISTIDINE	253.6	94.4	9	142.4	60.8	9	923.2	188.1	9	233.1	52.9	9	129.2	25.1	7
ARGININE	352.6	108.1	9	187.4	60.3	9	0.0	0.0	9	0.0	0.0	9	34.7	22.0	8
HOMOCARNOSINE	0.0	0.0	9	0.0	0.0	9	0.0	0.0	9	0.0	0.0	9	0.0	0.0	8
GLY/VAL	7.3	0.7	9				6.4	0.7	9				1.9	0.2	8
GLY/ILE	14.6	1.5	9				12.1	1.1	9				6.9	1.5	8
GLY/LEU	7.8	0.8	9				5.9	0.7	9				3.2	0.3	8
ALA/VAL	8.3	1.3	9				5.6	0.5	9				1.8	0.1	8
TYR/PHE	0.9	0.1	9				1.1	0.09	9				1.0	0.09	8
TYR/MET	1.4	0.1	9				1.8	0.2	9				3.6	0.2	8
ORN/LEU	1.3	0.2	9				1.8	0.2	9				1.4	0.5	7
ORN/LYS	0.4	0.05	9				0.8	0.1	9				0.4	0.1	7
NONESS/ESS	3.1	0.3	9				2.5	0.3	9				1.2	0.07	6

Statistical comparisons with the controls are shown in Tables 20.13 and 20.16. The main changes are summarized below.

1. In the plasma there were very few differences between the two groups and those differences that were found did not conform to a pattern.

2. After ablation of the beta cells in the mother, most of the concentrations of amino acids in the fetal liver were significantly lower. Most of the ratios of specific amino acids were higher in the experimental group, indicating a greater lowering of the essential amino acids.

3. In muscle, many of the amino acid concentrations, as in the plasma, were about the same in the control and experimental groups.

Discussion

When beta-cell ablation is produced by administering streptozotocin to the mother, a compensating hyperinsulinism is presumed to develop in the fetus. It is therefore surprising that there were not more changes in amino acid content in the plasma. However, there were major changes in the amino acids of the liver. The decrease, particularly in the essential amino acids, and the elevation of the ratios of non-essential to essential amino acids, which was also true of muscle, suggest that increased amounts of insulin lead to increased cellular synthesis of proteins. Since insulin also promotes transport of these amino acids into the cell, these data indicate that the balance is in favor of protein synthesis.

Insulin is thought to stimulate the peripheral formation of alanine,[9] but there was no evidence of an increase in the concentration of this amino acid in muscle.

Comparison of the effects of beta-cell ablation in the mother with beta-cell ablation in the fetus is interesting. In both instances the concentrations of the branched-chain amino acids were decreased in muscle and liver. Thus the changes must be due to mechanisms other than the simple excess or lack of insulin. One hypothesis is that in maternal diabetes an increased release of growth hormone might follow hyperinsulinemia and hypoglycemia, with increased protein synthesis. Maternal hormonal imbalance could interfere with placental transfer of amino acids even though those influences of maternal diabetes were not apparent in the fetal plasma.

MATERNAL NUTRITIONAL DEPRIVATION

Results

The details of the maternal diets are given in Chapter 6. There were four groups:

Group	Calories	Protein	Maternal Weight Gain
1	Normal	Normal	Normal
2	Sufficient	Deficient	Normal
3	Deficient	Sufficient	None
4	Deficient	Deficient	None

The means and standard deviations for each amino acid in each of the groups are set out in Tables 20.18 to 20.23. The results are summarized below.

1.   For fetuses on the low protein diet (group 2) the ratios of some nonessential to essential amino acids increased in maternal plasma (glycine to valine, alanine to valine, ornithine to leucine, and ornithine to lysine). The overall ratio of nonessential to essential amino acids was not different in the two groups. With a few exceptions (valine and isoleucine, which were lower, and ornithine, which was higher) the individual amino acids were present in virtually the same concentration in the control and experimental animals.

2.   For fetuses in group 3, the concentration of ornithine was significantly decreased but the other amino acid concentrations of maternal plasma were not greatly altered. Most of the ratios calculated were lower.

3.   For fetuses in group 4, the amino acid concentrations were very similar to those of the controls. It appeared that the effects of low calorie and low protein intake tended to cancel each other.

4.   In fetal plasma (Table 20.19) the concentrations of amino acids did not simply parallel the changes observed in maternal plasma. There was throughout a tendency for an increase in the concentrations of nonessential amino acids in fetal plasma. Many of the essential amino acids also increased in concentration. The ratios tended to be higher. The concentration of ornithine in fetal plasma was considerably higher in each of the experimental groups than in the controls. However, unlike the situation in maternal plasma, none of the changes observed in fetal plasma was significant statistically.

5.   In liver the changes were not great and few were significant statistically, the greatest occurring in the low calorie group (group 3).

6.   In muscle (Tables 20.22 and 20.23) there was a significant elevation of ornithine concentration in the protein-restricted group. The concentrations of valine, isoleucine, and leucine were significantly lower in group 4, whereas the concentrations of these amino acids tended to be higher in groups 2 and 3.

Discussion

High concentrations of ornithine were observed throughout this series of experiments. The higher concentration of ornithine in muscle with protein restriction could reflect the elevated concentrations in plasma and liver, the maternal plasma level being also considerably higher than in the control mothers. In the liver the enzyme ornithine transcarbamylase is known to be active during pregnancy, but it shows a marked adaptation to protein supply. Changes in the hepatic concentrations of this enzyme in fetus and in mother might follow protein restriction and might account for all of the changes observed in ornithine.

There was a tendency for the mean values of the essential amino acids to increase in the fetal liver, muscle, and plasma. This was reflected in the statistically significant change in the ratio of nonessential to essential amino acids. On the other hand, in maternal plasma most of these amino acids decreased in concentration. The changes in maternal plasma may be less complex. Unlike most of the changes in fetal concentrations, they were statistically significant.

An important byproduct of these studies might be the development of reliable chemical indicators of either the type of malnutrition or of the effects on growth. The glycine:valine and alanine:valine ratios increased in maternal protein restriction, whereas the total ratio of nonessential to essential amino acids was unchanged. The tyrosine:phenylalanine ratio, which Arroyave and colleagues[10] regard as being useful in kwashiorkor, was also unchanged.

These observations might clarify the highly variable ornithine concentrations and arginine:ornithine ratios that have been reported in the plasma of children with kwashiorkor.[10, 11] It is possible that maternal plasma concentrations of ornithine, or the ratios of glycine or alanine to valine in combination with ratios of ornithine to valine, might act as indicators of protein malnutrition and may help its differentiation from calorie malnutrition.

PLACENTAL INSUFFICIENCY

Results

Intrauterine growth retardation was established by ligation of the vessels to one disc of the placenta at 100 days of gestation, control fetuses being sham-operated without ligation of the vessels. The procedures have been described in detail in Chapter 7. The results are shown in Tables 20.24 to 20.28 and are summarized below.

1. In general, plasma amino acid concentrations were higher in the growth-retarded group (group 15). Significantly higher concentrations were found for taurine, serine, tyrosine, and phenylalanine. The lysine and ornithine concentrations also tended to be high.
2. The concentrations of amino acids in the liver were generally lower in the growth-retarded fetuses but the variability of amino acid concentrations about the mean was considerably larger, and therefore data of statistical significance were rare.
3. In the muscle the amino acid concentrations were usually lower in the fetuses with intrauterine growth retardation than in the control group, although none of the differences was statistically significant.

Discussion

In this series of experiments (unlike the results of a previous series concerning protein and caloric restriction of the mother), lower concentrations of amino acids in tissues were regularly observed. This is the result one would expect with a decrease of supply of nutrients to the fetus, the restriction to the circulation being of sufficient magnitude to influence growth. The data point to the importance of the placental transport of amino acids in the process of normal fetal growth and homeostasis.

It is probable that under these experimental conditions which led to intrauterine growth retardation, the supply of precursors of protein was extensively limited. The elevation in taurine concentrations suggests the probability of breakdown of protein in muscle. Methylhistidine was also found to be increased in concentration, which is consistent with this hypothesis.

TABLE 20.18
Concentrations of Amino Acids per Unit Volume in the Plasma of Nutritionally Deprived Maternal Monkeys[a]

(μmoles/liter)

	GROUP 1			GROUP 2			GROUP 3			GROUP 4			SIGNIFICANCE P ≤		
	MEAN	S.D.	N	MEAN	S.D.	N	MEAN	S.D.	N	MEAN	S.D.	N	RESTRICTION OF PROTEIN	WEIGHT GAIN	INTERACTION
TAURINE	102.0	27.1	4	73.6	23.2	3	133.0	94.5	4	67.5	31.2	6			
ASPARTIC ACID	22.6	2.4	4	29.1	13.7	3	21.7	17.1	4	20.6	10.0	6			
THREONINE	88.3	18.5	4	94.5	40.0	3	117.8	89.3	4	86.0	22.5	6			
SERINE	157.0	49.5	4	153.0	73.9	3	157.5	58.7	4	151.0	33.7	6			
GLUTAMINE	386.0	92.1	4	374.0	139.0	3	291.0	91.6	4	345.0	85.8	6			
PROLINE	193.0	87.3	4	142.0	30.1	3	99.2	41.7	4	146.0	82.3	6			
GLUTAMIC ACID	113.0	18.9	4	137.0	45.7	3	176.0	67.1	4	121.0	33.2	6			
CITRULLINE	6.5	9.2	2	0.0	0.0	2	8.8	6.8	4	8.1	15.3	6			
GLYCINE	313.0	65.8	4	293.0	107.0	3	322.0	145.0	4	319.0	109.0	6			
ALANINE	277.0	38.0	4	250.0	102.0	3	214.0	120.0	4	224.0	79.0	6			
VALINE	132.0	22.6	4	103.0	50.0	3	161.0	30.0	4	104.0	19.3	6	0.025		
METHIONINE	20.8	8.3	4	18.2	4.8	3	16.2	9.0	4	14.9	6.1	6			
ISOLEUCINE	66.5	17.4	4	55.2	8.8	3	87.0	17.6	4	59.3	14.2	6	0.025		
LEUCINE	96.7	18.9	4	99.7	50.2	3	121.0	31.5	4	88.5	21.5	6			
TYROSINE	41.1	8.7	4	34.4	14.9	3	48.0	20.2	4	31.3	9.5	6			
PHENYLALANINE	50.7	14.3	4	44.2	12.5	3	56.0	17.7	4	43.0	16.3	6		0.025	
ORNITHINE	39.3	14.8	4	68.0	10.1	3	28.2	6.4	3	46.6	12.0	6	0.005		
LYSINE	180.0	56.4	4	157.0	71.6	3	126.0	33.5	3	185.0	117.0	6			
HISTIDINE	79.9	16.1	4	97.1	39.4	3	54.2	23.6	3	88.1	41.7	6			
ARGININE	79.5	51.6	4	43.3	16.7	3	28.9	8.5	3	81.1	35.5	5			0.05
GLY/VAL	2.3	0.45	4	3.0	0.58	3	2.0	0.85	3	3.0	0.76	6	0.05		
GLY/ILE	4.7	1.6	4	5.2	1.4	3	3.6	1.1	3	5.4	1.7	6			
GLY/LEU	3.4	1.0	4	3.1	0.79	3	2.6	0.6	3	3.7	1.5	6			
ALA/VAL	2.1	0.3	4	2.5	0.26	3	1.3	0.63	3	2.1	0.52	6	0.05	0.05	
TYR/PHE	0.82	0.13	4	0.76	0.11	3	0.83	0.1	3	0.75	0.11	6			
TYR/MET	2.2	0.18	4	1.8	0.52	3	3.1	0.52	4	2.3	0.88	6			
ORN/LEU	0.42	0.17	4	0.83	0.5	3	0.27	0.05	3	0.56	0.21	6	0.025		
ORN/LYS	0.22	0.05	4	0.51	0.21	3	0.23	0.07	3	0.31	0.12	6	0.025		
NONESS/ESS	1.2	0.12	4	1.2	0.35	3	0.93	0.18	4	1.1	0.18	6			

* Groups were as follows: 1, controls; 2, protein restriction; 3, calorie restriction; and 4, calorie and protein restriction. Significant differences from the control group are indicated by the P values at the right. S.D.: standard deviation.

TABLE 20.19

Concentrations of Amino Acids per Unit Volume of Plasma of Fetuses of Nutritionally Deprived Maternal Monkeys

(μmoles/liter)

	GROUP 1			GROUP 2			GROUP 3			GROUP 4		
	MEAN	S.D.	N	MEAN	S.D.	N	MEAN	S.D.	N	MEAN	S.D.	N
TAURINE	375.0	503.0	4	128.0	80.6	3	138.0	18.4	4	122.0	59.1	6
ASPARTIC ACID	16.5	2.4	4	13.5	0.0	1	49.2	37.2	4	22.1	5.0	4
THREONINE	115.0	6.7	4	167.0	57.8	3	154.0	48.4	4	180.0	76.6	6
SERINE	180.0	40.6	4	255.0	79.6	3	270.0	105.0	4	291.0	114.0	6
GLUTAMINE	451.0	165.0	4	510.0	162.0	3	641.0	281.0	4	648.0	103.0	6
PROLINE	322.0	88.7	4	289.0	98.4	3	225.0	67.0	3	301.0	101.0	6
GLUTAMIC ACID	170.0	79.2	4	219.0	70.4	3	234.0	86.5	3	232.0	119.0	6
CITRULLINE	9.1	8.1	3	29.5	14.9	3	19.4	24.4	3	14.1	15.2	6
GLYCINE	307.0	70.1	4	409.0	65.7	3	429.0	159.0	4	457.0	169.0	6
ALANINE	359.0	18.1	4	443.0	115.0	3	402.0	101.0	4	458.0	137.0	6
VALINE	205.9	18.9	4	282.0	79.0	3	301.0	57.6	4	277.0	93.0	6
METHIONINE	32.3	3.7	4	37.2	14.5	3	28.0	8.1	4	41.3	16.8	6
ISOLEUCINE	80.6	7.3	4	100.0	39.8	3	123.0	33.8	4	121.0	44.7	6
LEUCINE	117.0	20.8	4	126.0	47.5	3	179.0	62.4	4	167.0	66.9	6
TYROSINE	80.5	13.6	4	96.0	47.7	3	76.5	3.3	4	104.0	42.1	6
PHENYLALANINE	75.4	10.2	4	107.0	48.3	3	91.5	19.9	4	108.0	41.5	6
ORNITHINE	65.6	22.3	4	86.3	25.3	3	111.4	45.4	4	96.3	55.0	6
LYSINE	400.0	102.0	4	347.0	100.0	3	456.0	162.0	4	402.0	186.0	6
HISTIDINE	193.0	54.7	4	219.0	88.0	3	159.0	64.2	4	217.0	106.0	6
ARGININE	132.0	439.0	4	104.0	14.6	3	104.0	40.8	4	115.0	80.4	6
GLY/VAL	1.4	0.28	4	1.4	0.24	3	1.4	0.30	4	1.7	0.56	6
GLY/ILE	3.6	0.68	4	4.3	1.11	3	3.6	1.77	4	3.9	1.16	6
GLY/LEU	2.8	0.86	4	3.4	0.87	3	2.7	1.73	4	2.9	1.03	6
ALA/VAL	1.7	0.18	4	1.5	0.38	3	1.3	0.22	4	1.7	0.41	6
TYR/PHE	1.0	0.15	4	0.8	0.07	3	1.0	0.40	4		0.07	6
TYR/MET	2.4	0.21	4	2.5	0.30	3	2.9	0.67	4	2.5	0.69	6
ORN/LEU	0.55	0.15	4	0.7	0.39	3	0.7	0.46	4	0.6	0.38	6
ORN/LYS	0.16	0.05	4	0.2	0.06	3	0.2	0.03	4	0.2	0.09	6
NONESS/ESS	0.82	0.11	4	0.9	0.08	3	0.8	0.23	4	0.9	0.23	6

TABLE 20.20

Concentrations of Amino Acids per Unit DNA in the Liver of Fetuses of Nutritionally Deprived Maternal Monkeys

(μmoles/gDNA)

	GROUP 1			GROUP 2			GROUP 3			GROUP 4		
	MEAN	S.D.	N	MEAN	S.D.	N	MEAN	S.D.	N	MEAN	S.D.	N
TAURINE	809.0	443.0	4	1430.0	982.0	3	1350.0	701.0	4	1150.0	805.0	6
ASPARTIC ACID	566.0	273.0	4	440.0	88.0	3	418.0	192.0	4	469.0	187.0	6
THREONINE	176.0	54.0	4	398.0	424.0	3	238.0	82.0	4	205.0	61.0	6
SERINE	587.0	185.0	4	457.0	174.0	3	693.0	212.0	4	599.0	157.0	6
GLUTAMINE	731.0	300.0	4	650.0	193.0	3	515.0	194.0	4	570.0	187.0	6
PROLINE	215.0	104.0	3	320.0	148.0	3	292.0	59.0	4	292.0	87.0	6
GLUTAMIC ACID	1356.0	631.0	4	1635.0	416.0	3	1446.0	454.0	4	1346.0	510.0	6
GLYCINE	946.0	386.0	4	1068.0	334.0	3	1198.0	352.0	4	1001.0	268.0	6
ALANINE	1103.0	408.0	4	1014.0	342.0	3	999.0	266.0	4	876.0	217.0	6
VALINE	100.0	44.0	4	130.0	42.0	3	127.0	38.0	4	122.0	45.0	6
CYSTATHIONINE	60.0	53.0	4	42.0	24.0	3	18.0	17.0	4	22.0	11.0	6
METHIONINE	20.0	12.0	4	29.0	11.0	3	28.0	8.0	4	34.0	16.0	6
ISOLEUCINE	45.0	14.0	4	64.0	23.0	3	56.0	18.0	4	63.0	19.0	6
LEUCINE	97.0	30.0	4	125.0	30.0	3	121.0	29.0	4	128.0	39.0	6
TYROSINE	72.0	18.0	3	73.0	13.0	3	63.0	10.0	4	72.0	30.0	6
PHENYLALANINE	43.0	9.0	3	51.0	13.0	3	41.0	8.0	4	43.0	12.0	6
ORNITHINE	89.0	74.0	4	149.0	51.0	3	177.0	63.0	4	183.0	96.0	6
LYSINE	146.0	99.0	4	182.0	49.0	3	222.0	71.0	4	218.0	105.0	6
HISTIDINE	201.0	154.0	4	245.0	67.0	3	176.0	33.0	4	232.0	102.0	6

TABLE 20.21

Concentrations of Amino Acids per Unit Tissue Weight in the Liver of Fetuses of Nutritionally Deprived Maternal Monkeys

(μmoles/kg)

	GROUP 1			GROUP 2			GROUP 3			GROUP 4			SIGNIFICANCE P RESTRICTION OF PROTEIN	WEIGHT GAIN	INTERACTION
	MEAN	S.D.	N	MEAN	S.D.	N	MEAN	S.D.	N	MEAN	S.D.	N			
TAURINE	3242.0	1198.0	4	5209.0	2833.0	3	5809.0	2995.0	4	4507.0	3367.0	6			
ASPARTIC ACID	2227.0	786.0	4	1717.0	569.0	3	1669.0	340.0	4	1688.0	497.0	6			
THREONINE	725.0	187.0	4	1403.0	1314.0	3	993.0	320.0	4	784.0	270.0	6			
SERINE	2390.0	529.0	4	1837.0	965.0	3	2876.0	608.0	4	2281.0	643.0	6			
GLUTAMINE	3057.0	1120.0	4	2529.0	974.0	3	2098.0	557.0	4	2144.0	596.0	6			
PROLINE	942.0	362.0	3	1204.0	458.0	3	1292.0	468.0	4	1143.0	483.0	6			
GLUTAMIC ACID	5404.0	2053.0	4	6240.0	1487.0	3	5933.0	485.0	4	5000.0	1546.0	6			
GLYCINE	3794.0	1160.0	4	4076.0	1215.0	3	4944.0	673.0	4	3813.0	1112.0	6			
ALANINE	4482.0	1379.0	4	3825.0	955.0	3	4164.0	729.0	4	3351.0	1042.0	6			
VALINE	407.0	144.0	4	501.0	170.0	3	526.0	82.1	4	471.0	200.0	6			
CYSTATHIONINE	228.0	160.0	4	155.0	68.0	3	80.2	81.1	4	89.6	56.9	6		0.05	
METHIONINE	86.2	49.7	4	118.0	60.9	3	119.0	25.5	4	135.0	69.3	6			
ISOLEUCINE	187.0	50.7	4	247.0	84.6	3	233.0	31.3	4	242.0	84.8	6			
LEUCINE	406.0	121.0	4	485.0	145.0	3	505.0	53.5	4	490.0	176.0	6			
TYROSINE	278.0	84.0	3	283.0	62.8	3	272.0	53.4	4	282.0	134.0	6			
PHENYLALANINE	170.0	49.8	4	198.0	60.9	3	175.0	18.0	4	170.0	71.7	6			
ORNITHINE	356.0	274.0	4	580.0	240.0	3	811.0	495.0	4	714.0	416.0	6			
LYSINE	583.0	345.0	4	716.0	297.0	3	1030.0	595.0	4	843.0	423.0	6			
HISTIDINE	781.0	475.0	4	932.0	192.0	3	791.0	335.0	4	864.0	322.0	6			
GLY/VAL	9.6	2.3	4	8.2	0.4	3	9.4	0.8	4	8.6	1.8	6			
GLY/ILE	20.6	5.4	4	16.7	1.0	3	21.5	4.0	4	16.5	3.6	6	0.05		
GLY/LEU	9.6	2.8	4	8.4	0.9	3	9.8	1.2	4	8.1	1.8	6			
ALA/VAL	11.6	4.5	4	7.8	1.2	3	7.9	0.7	4	7.7	2.2	6			
TYR/PHE	1.6	0.2	3	1.4	0.1	3	1.5	0.2	4	1.6	0.4	6			
TYR/MET	3.4	1.0	3	2.6	0.6	3	2.3	0.5	4	2.1	0.3	6			
ORN/LEU	0.8	0.5	4	1.1	0.1	3	1.6	0.9	4	1.3	0.3	6		0.05	
ORN/LYS	0.5	0.2	4	0.8	0.1	3	0.8	0.1	4	0.8	0.1	6			
NONESS/ESS	3.6	1.0	3	2.3	0.4	3	3.0	0.6	4	2.7	0.6	6	0.05		

TABLE 20.22
Concentrations of Amino Acids per Unit DNA in the Muscle of Fetuses of Nutritionally Deprived Maternal Monkeys

(μmoles/gDNA)

	GROUP 1			GROUP 2			GROUP 3			GROUP 4			SIGNIFICANCE P ≤		
	MEAN	S.D.	N	MEAN	S.D.	N	MEAN	S.D.	N	MEAN	S.D.	N	RESTRICTION OF PROTEIN	WEIGHT GAIN	INTERACTION
TAURINE	2030.0	1303.0	4	3988.0	162.0	3	2863.0	1859.0	4	5464.0	5371.0	6			
ASPARTIC ACID	197.0	76.0	4	222.0	21.0	3	171.0	63.0	3	148.0	78.0	5			
THREONINE	217.0	62.0	4	285.0	74.0	3	279.0	72.0	4	295.0	230.0	6			
SERINE	569.0	110.0	4	682.0	178.0	3	583.0	129.0	4	667.0	399.0	6			
GLUTAMINE	2784.0	784.0	4	3225.0	514.0	3	3718.0	399.0	4	6133.0	6651.0	6			
PROLINE	1044.0	260.0	4	1152.0	299.0	3	799.0	305.0	4	1286.0	1287.0	6			
GLUTAMIC ACID	950.0	413.0	4	1118.0	292.0	3	906.0	323.0	4	1215.0	1099.0	6			
GLYCINE	1418.0	693.0	4	1472.0	355.0	3	1529.0	291.0	4	1635.0	1048.0	6			
ALANINE	1161.0	665.0	4	1325.0	418.0	3	1328.0	223.0	4	1366.0	1016.0	6			
VALINE	144.0	40.0	4	207.0	40.0	3	179.0	79.0	4	163.0	158.0	6			
METHIONINE	29.0	10.0	4	56.0	25.0	3	31.0	11.0	4	38.0	47.0	6			
ISOLEUCINE	56.0	28.0	4	84.0	15.0	3	73.0	15.0	4	76.0	67.0	6			
LEUCINE	89.0	51.0	4	110.0	12.0	3	118.0	27.0	4	132.0	109.0	6			
TYROSINE	67.0	18.0	4	98.0	33.0	3	67.0	25.0	4	92.0	96.0	6			
PHENYLALANINE	61.0	28.0	4	96.0	25.0	3	66.0	17.0	4	91.0	81.0	6		0.025	
ORNITHINE	125.0	50.0	4	268.0	77.0	3	196.0	38.0	4	226.0	70.0	6			
LYSINE	435.0	189.0	4	588.0	200.0	3	723.0	278.0	4	664.0	436.0	6			
HISTIDINE	109.0	47.0	4	204.0	74.0	3	110.0	89.0	4	186.0	101.0	6			
ARGININE	74.0	61.0	4	105.0	42.0	3	162.0	168.0	4	87.0	59.0	6			

TABLE 20.23

Concentrations of Amino Acids per Unit Tissue Weight in the Muscle of Fetuses of Nutritionally Deprived Maternal Monkeys

(μmoles/kg)

	GROUP 1			GROUP 2			GROUP 3			GROUP 4			SIGNIFICANCE P↓ RESTRICTION OF		
	MEAN	S.D.	N	MEAN	S.D.	N	MEAN	S.D.	N	MEAN	S.D.	N	PROTEIN	WEIGHT GAIN	INTERACTION
TAURINE	4960.0	3550.0	4	9097.0	676.0	3	6252.0	4174.0	4	6362.0	4908.0	6			
ASPARTIC ACID	470.0	192.4	4	508.7	71.1	3	357.0	145.4	4	292.6	165.2	6			
THREONINE	514.3	119.6	4	652.9	182.1	3	611.5	200.8	4	406.3	195.6	6			
SERINE	1346.0	198.3	4	1559.0	422.6	3	1259.0	298.1	4	1170.0	353.5	6			
GLUTAMINE	6659.0	1930.0	4	7377.0	1419.0	3	8066.0	1524.0	4	6586.0	2057.0	6			
PROLINE	2473.0	520.9	4	2634.0	713.7	3	1693.0	516.5	4	2000.0	1126.0	6			
GLUTAMIC ACID	2242.0	882.6	4	2559.0	705.7	3	1919.0	594.2	4	1627.0	309.8	6			
GLYCINE	3301.0	1329.0	4	3370.0	883.4	3	3311.0	734.3	4	2755.0	619.7	6			
ALANINE	2699.0	1318.0	4	3044.0	1059.0	3	2872.0	563.8	4	2151.0	518.4	6			
VALINE	343.0	94.4	4	472.9	96.2	3	388.0	176.0	4	206.2	61.7	6			0.025
METHIONINE	69.7	26.9	4	129.9	57.4	3	67.1	25.2	4	53.8	39.0	6			0.025
ISOLEUCINE	134.3	62.8	4	194.1	36.9	3	158.3	36.2	4	99.2	40.2	6			
LEUCINE	210.3	115.7	4	252.6	29.3	3	256.5	62.4	4	180.2	117.4	6			
TYROSINE	157.9	34.1	4	225.1	82.3	3	146.8	57.1	4	108.6	64.1	6			
PHENYLALANINE	143.8	58.6	4	220.5	61.6	3	143.3	39.9	4	119.5	80.1	6			
ORNITHINE	294.3	100.8	4	607.7	152.7	3	428.8	117.7	4	473.8	156.6	6	0.025		
LYSINE	1013.0	376.9	4	1330.0	404.0	3	1599.0	779.7	4	1387.0	931.1	6			
HISTIDINE	259.5	114.2	4	463.4	155.1	3	248.9	228.1	4	387.4	201.3	6			
ARGININE	173.3	136.2	4	237.4	86.4	3	372.2	419.7	4	182.0	119.5	6			
GLY/VAL	10.1	4.0	4	7.0	0.6	3	9.4	3.1	4	14.5	5.9	6			
GLY/ILE	27.0	9.6	4	17.2	1.4	3	21.2	3.5	4	29.8	12.0	6			
GLY/LEU	18.4	7.5	4	13.2	2.3	3	13.1	2.4	4	23.7	17.9	6			
ALA/VAL	8.1	3.3	4	6.3	1.4	3	8.2	2.7	4	10.8	2.9	6			
TYR/PHE	1.2	0.4	4	0.9	0.06	3	1.0	0.1	4	0.9	0.09	6			
TYR/MET	2.4	0.7	4	1.8	0.4	3	2.1	0.4	4	2.0	1.1	5			
ORN/LEU	1.8	1.1	4	2.4	0.9	3	1.6	0.3	4	3.5	2.2	6			
ORN/LYS	0.3	0.08	4	0.4	0.06	3	0.2	0.08	4	0.4	0.1	6			
NONESS/ESS	2.8	0.4	4	2.3	0.6	3	2.4	0.5	4	2.5	0.6	6	0.05		

TABLE 20.24
Concentrations of Amino Acids per Unit Volume in Fetal Plasma Following Placental Insufficiency*

(μmoles/liter)

	GROUP 14			GROUP 15				
	MEAN	S.E.M.	N	MEAN	S.E.M.	N	t	p<
TAURINE	145.0	7.4	6	207.6	24.9	4	2.50	0.05
ASPARTIC ACID	48.0	5.7	6	58.2	8.7	4	0.19	
THREONINE	107.9	11.5	6	161.2	19.6	4	2.23	0.05
SERINE	149.8	14.0	6	205.6	16.0	4	2.31	
GLUTAMINE	37.4	19.9	6	96.9	54.3	4	1.05	
PROLINE	444.3	130.0	6	410.7	24.5	4	-0.18	
GLUTAMIC ACID	608.6	34.7	6	594.5	44.7	4	-0.22	
CITRULLINE	16.5	5.2	6	17.3	9.4	4	0.07	
GLYCINE	367.5	19.3	6	446.4	49.9	4	1.49	
ALANINE	322.5	29.3	6	541.6	96.3	4	2.26	
VALINE	226.8	16.4	6	297.0	24.8	4	2.19	
CYSTATHIONINE	0.1	0.1	6					
METHIONINE	30.2	3.8	6	40.5	8.9	4	1.06	
ISOLEUCINE	71.4	7.5	6	94.0	12.9	4	1.43	
LEUCINE	113.6	9.2	6	176.2	26.8	4	2.27	
TYROSINE	54.5	7.0	6	99.8	12.8	4	2.98	0.02
PHENYLALANINE	83.5	8.0	6	120.6	10.1	4	2.57	0.05
ORNITHINE	72.5	11.3	6	120.5	16.6	4	2.21	
LYSINE	285.3	59.7	6	451.1	49.3	4	1.77	
HISTIDINE	124.9	16.0	6	156.8	18.4	4	1.15	
ARGININE	102.1	14.4	6	121.7	20.6	4	0.71	
HOMOCARNOSINE	0.0	0.0	6					
GLYCINE/VALINE	1.6	0.08	6					
GLYCINE/ISOLEUCINE	5.3	0.4	6					
GLYCINE/LEUCINE	3.3	0.3	6					
ALANINE/VALINE	1.4	0.07	6					
TYROSINE/PHENYLALANINE	0.6	0.07	6					
TYROSINE/METHIONINE	1.8	0.09	6					
ORNITHINE/LEUCINE	0.6	0.06	6					
ORNITHINE/LYSINE	0.2	0.04	6					
NONESSENTIAL/ESSENTIAL	1.0	0.05	6					

* Group 14, controls; group 15, monkeys with intrauterine growth retardation.

TABLE 20.25
Concentrations of Amino Acids per Unit DNA in Fetal Liver Following Placental
Insufficiency

(μmoles/gDNA)

	GROUP 14			GROUP 15		
	MEAN	S.E.M.	N	MEAN	S.E.M.	N
TAURINE	921.5	132.0	7	1271.5	316.7	5
ASPARTIC ACID	913.7	370.5	7	504.1	62.2	5
THREONINE	858.5	385.9	7	338.7	53.7	4
SERINE	1381.8	514.5	7	699.0	60.6	5
GLUTAMINE	1124.7	467.8	7	276.8	100.8	5
PROLINE	1847.7	187.2	3	516.3	125.7	3
GLUTAMIC ACID	2272.4	509.0	7	1693.5	323.2	5
CITRULLINE	0.0	0.0	7	0.05	0.05	5
GLYCINE	1916.5	555.6	7	1338.2	173.8	5
ALANINE	2433.7	650.5	7	1520.8	336.7	5
VALINE	1279.7	544.3	7	266.7	56.3	5
CYSTATHIONINE	33.0	7.2	7	35.4	22.6	5
METHIONINE	302.8	174.0	7	28.0	6.2	5
ISOLEUCINE	623.7	311.4	7	143.5	34.0	5
LEUCINE	1453.9	708.3	7	374.0	80.3	5
TYROSINE	567.5	230.3	7	142.0	16.0	5
PHENYLALANINE	758.7	328.5	7	139.0	35.2	5
ORNITHINE	1110.4	466.0	7	263.2	49.3	5
LYSINE	1361.3	582.3	7	351.1	56.4	5
HISTIDINE	354.9	128.3	7	148.8	21.5	5
ARGININE	0.03	0.03	7	0.0	0.0	5
HOMOCARNOSINE	0.0	0.0	7	0.0	0.0	5

* Group 14, controls; group 15, monkeys with intrauterine growth retardation.

GENERAL DISCUSSION

The data obtained in this study indicate that the processes of fetal growth as they
relate to amino acid composition are complex. Highly significant changes and discrete tissue-specific patterns were found in the course of the procession from one
stage of normal growth to the next. In our view, these were impressive and unexpected findings.

Against this background of normal developmental change the results of interventions were almost invariably less impressive, with complex patterns emerging.
Probably the simplest pattern of change was that occurring in intrauterine growth
retardation induced by the placental insufficiency. In this instance the fetuses did
manifest growth retardation, and their amino acids were increased in the plasma
pool but decreased in the intracellular pool, suggesting a reduced transfer of
amino acids into the cell. A similar situation pertained following ablation of the
fetal beta cells.

Insulin is known to be important in transferring amino acids into the cell. In the
fetuses thought to be secreting an excess of insulin, the change in the ratio of essential
to nonessential amino acids in the liver was in favor of protein synthesis.

The results of maternal nutritional deprivation were provocative and, of course,
could be relevant to a large segment of the human population. Changes in actual
growth were small. However, there were some definite and interesting changes in
amino acid content that should stimulate further, more definitive experiments.

TABLE 20.26

Concentrations of Amino Acids per Unit Tissue Weight in Fetal Liver Following Placental Insufficiency (μmoles/kg)

	GROUP 14			GROUP 15		
	MEAN	S.E.M.	N	MEAN	S.E.M.	N
TAURINE	3880.0	638.7	7	5062.8	1077.7	5
ASPARTIC ACID	4022.8	1638.0	7	2120.3	241.8	5
THREONINE	3851.1	1731.4	7	1524.9	265.8	4
SERINE	6100.0	2335.6	7	2973.4	307.2	5
GLUTAMINE	4907.0	2016.1	7	1249.4	527.4	5
PROLINE	8410.0	1299.6	3	2487.8	735.4	3
GLUTAMIC ACID	9732.8	2315.5	7	6909.5	1062.3	5
CITRULLINE	0.0	0.0	7	0.2	0.2	5
GLYCINE	8330.0	2526.5	7	5570.4	579.1	5
ALANINE	10645.7	3061.0	7	6410.9	1355.4	5
VALINE	5585.2	2839.4	7	1175.3	315.9	5
CYSTATHIONINE	129.7	21.3	7	147.3	90.9	5
METHIONINE	1243.9	701.7	7	123.8	34.2	5
ISOLEUCINE	2819.7	1402.2	7	630.9	186.5	5
LEUCINE	6590.1	3210.2	7	1656.0	453.6	5
TYROSINE	2464.8	982.4	7	614.8	101.9	5
PHENYLALANINE	3314.1	1412.8	7	620.2	195.5	5
ORNITHINE	4893.1	2055.7	7	1163.2	283.8	5
LYSINE	5969.7	2530.6	7	1541.2	333.1	5
HISTIDINE	1461.5	512.0	7	618.2	74.6	5
ARGININE	0.1	0.1	7	0.0	0.0	5
HOMOCARNOSINE	0.0	0.0	7	0.0	.0.0	5
GLYCINE/VALINE	3.8	1.0	7	5.8	1.0	5
GLYCINE/ISOLEUCINE	8.6	2.4	7	11.0	2.0	5
GLYCINE/LEUCINE	2.9	0.7	7	4.1	0.8	5
ALANINE/VALINE	5.3	1.6	7	6.3	1.4	5
TYROSINE/PHENYLALANINE	0.8	0.06	7	1.1	0.1	5
TYROSINE/METHIONINE	50.9	47.4	6	6.0	1.5	5
ORNITHINE/LEUCINE	0.8	0.02	7	0.7	0.03	5
ORNITHINE/LYSINE	0.8	0.02	7	0.7	0.02	5
NONESSENTIAL/ESSENTIAL	2.4	0.5	7	2.9	0.4	5

* Group 14, controls; group 15, monkeys with intrauterine growth retardation.

TABLE 20.27
Concentrations of Amino Acids per Unit DNA in Fetal Muscle Following Placental Insufficiency

(μmoles/gDNA)

	GROUP 14				GROUP 15		
	MEAN	S.E.M.	N		MEAN	S.E.M.	N
TAURINE	2580.9	512.2	7		3200.0	363.6	5
ASPARTIC ACID	388.8	129.8	7		237.3	114.2	5
THREONINE	522.2	154.2	7		353.2	170.0	5
SERINE	1033.0	260.3	7		683.2	282.5	5
GLUTAMINE	3422.1	670.2	7		2747.8	914.0	5
PROLINE	1677.3	332.5	7		1376.5	775.1	4
GLUTAMIC ACID	1732.8	240.8	7		1491.0	229.6	5
CITRULLINE	7.5	7.2	7		0.2	0.1	5
GLYCINE	1776.5	248.0	7		1347.8	226.3	5
ALANINE	2134.2	292.3	7		1393.1	478.5	5
VALINE	583.1	186.5	7		359.7	208.6	5
CYSTATHIONINE	9.4	6.0	7		4.6	4.6	5
METHIONINE	106.7	44.5	7		98.4	56.8	5
ISOLEUCINE	288.9	85.9	7		182.6	107.6	5
LEUCINE	692.5	222.7	7		427.8	268.6	5
TYROSINE	262.5	72.4	7		168.5	103.0	5
PHENYLALANINE	346.8	107.5	7		204.5	125.5	5
ORNITHINE	250.5	95.2	7		244.6	28.3	5
LYSINE	599.9	173.8	7		856.8	214.9	5
HISTIDINE	175.9	61.2	7		162.2	76.7	5
ARGININE	259.5	79.0	7		296.4	130.6	5
HOMOCARNOSINE	0.0	0.0	7		0.0	0.0	5

* Group 14, controls; group 15, monkeys with intrauterine growth retardation.

TABLE 20.28

Concentrations of Amino Acids per Unit Tissue Weight in Fetal Muscle Following Placental Insufficiency*   (µmoles/kg)

	GROUP 14				GROUP 15		
	MEAN	S.E.M.	N		MEAN	S.E.M.	N
TAURINE	5425.7	1013.1	7		7352.3	1317.2	5
ASPARTIC ACID	798.5	252.6	7		468.7	169.1	5
THREONINE	1073.7	287.1	7		704.3	250.8	5
SERINE	2152.8	511.0	7		1395.8	411.3	5
GLUTAMINE	7100.0	1171.1	7		5753.7	1329.2	5
PROLINE	3480.0	634.3	7		2694.5	1172.2	4
GLUTAMIC ACID	3614.2	368.7	7		3346.4	511.3	5
CITRULLINE	13.2	12.7	7		0.4	0.2	5
GLYCINE	3753.7	474.3	7		2964.2	394.2	5
ALANINE	4504.2	532.4	7		2932.4	698.6	5
VALINE	1200.2	356.6	7		686.3	315.5	5
CYSTATHIONINE	17.6	11.3	7		7.4	7.4	5
METHIONINE	219.0	82.6	7		190.0	86.1	5
ISOLEUCINE	594.0	160.2	7		348.4	163.0	5
LEUCINE	1421.5	421.1	7		804.8	410.4	5
TYROSINE	542.4	135.1	7		318.3	156.9	5
PHENYLALANINE	716.1	209.1	7		386.6	191.4	5
ORNITHINE	494.0	165.2	7		541.2	70.7	5
LYSINE	1206.0	303.9	7		1773.6	274.2	5
HISTIDINE	347.4	111.2	7		317.7	112.1	5
ARGININE	519.5	140.6	7		596.9	191.7	5
HOMOCARNOSINE	0.0	0.0	7		0.0	0.0	5
GLYCINE/VALINE	5.0	1.2	7		6.4	1.1	5
GLYCINE/ISOLEUCINE	8.7	1.7	7		12.7	2.3	5
GLYCINE/LEUCINE	4.1	1.0	7		6.0	1.1	5
ALANINE/VALINE	5.8	1.2	7		5.4	0.8	5
TYROSINE/PHENYLALANINE	0.8	0.05	7		0.8	0.03	5
TYROSINE/METHIONINE	5.6	3.4	7		1.6	0.09	5
ORNITHINE/LEUCINE	0.5	0.1	7		1.1	0.2	5
ORNITHINE/LYSINE	0.3	0.06	6		0.3	0.04	5
NONESSENTIAL/ESSENTIAL	2.3	0.2	7		2.0	0.2	5

* Group 14, controls; group 15, monkeys with intrauterine growth retardation.

It is, of course, difficult to obtain a successful gestation with nutritional deprivation and it is this balance that must be studied further.

Now that the normal patterns of growth in amino acid concentration are known, it should be possible to design further experiments in such a way that alteration of specific patterns is the objective.

REFERENCES

1. Wick, H., Brechbuhler, T., Bachmann, C., and Baumgartner, R.: The statistical distribution of amino acid concentrations in plasma. *Pediatr. Res.* **6**: 56, 1972.

2. Nyhan, W. L., Yujnovsky, A. O., and Wehr, R. F.: Amino acids and cell growth. In: Cheek, D. B. (Ed.): *Human Growth*. Lea & Febiger, Philadelphia, 1968, p. 396.

3. Kipnis, D. M., Galvao, P. A. A., Greene, G., and Daughaday, W. H.: The significance of amino acid transport in protein synthesis. *J. Lab. Clin. Med.* **54**: 914, 1959.

4. Tallan, H. H., Moore, S., and Stein, W. H.: Studies on the free amino acids and related compounds in the tissues of the cat. *J. Biol. Chem.* **221**: 927, 1974.

5. Sturman, J. A., Niemann, W. H., and Gaull, G. E.: Metabolism of ^{35}S-methionine and ^{35}S-cystine in the pregnant rhesus monkey. *Biol. Neonate* **22**: 16, 1973.

6. Kerr, G. R.: The free amino acids of serum during development of *Macaca mulatta*. II. During pregnancy and fetal life. *Pediatr. Res.* **2**: 493, 1968.

7. Wool, I. G.: Relation of effects of insulin on amino acid transport and on protein synthesis. *Fed. Proc.* **24**: 1960, 1965.

8. Bloxam, D. L.: Nutritional aspects of amino acid metabolism. III. The effects of diabetes on blood and liver amino acid concentrations in the rat. *Br. J. Nutr.* **27**: 249, 1972.

9. Felig, P.: The glucose-alanine cycle. *Metabolism* **22**: 179, 1973.

10. Arroyave, G.: Comparative sensitivity of specific amino acid ratios versus "essential to nonessential" amino acid ratios. *Am. J. Clin. Nutr.* **23**: 703, 1970.

11. Arroyave, G., Wilson, D., De Funes, C., and Behar, M.: The free amino acids in blood plasma of children with kwashiorkor and marasmus. *Am. J. Clin. Nutr.* **11**: 517, 1962.

12. Holt, L. E., Snyderman, S. E., Norton, P. M., and Rotiman, E.: The plasma aminogram as affected by protein intake. In: Leathem, J. H. (Ed.): *Protein Nutrition and Free Amino Acid Patterns*. Rutgers University Press, New Brunswick, 1968, p. 32.

CHAPTER 21

Assessment of the Biological
Age Index in the Fetal Primate

E. David Mellits

INTRODUCTION

The concept of biological age in man has been presented in the past as a means of describing the growth process. Crampton defined pubertal age in 1908,[1] and in 1944[2] expanded this definition into a dissertation on the fundamental principle of physiological age. Other investigators have described growth as a process punctuated by the activation of "physiological clocks." An eloquent exposition of this concept, complete with an extensive bibliography, is presented by Brody.[3] The use of data concerning body composition and body length to predict "maturation age index" in boys and girls was discussed in a previous book.[4] The inclusion of bone age into such equations is important.[5]

Brody characterized physiological time by the rate of change of an organism. He proposed that while physical time is assumed to progress on a uniform scale, physiological time is variable. This variability exists between species, between different individuals of the same species, and between different tissues within the same individual. The various tissues have been examined separately in the past, leading, for example, to expressions of bone age, dental age, mental age, and pubertal age.

In an earlier effort we attempted to relate chronological age in boys to testosterone excretion, as a means of biochemically appraising Crampton's thesis of pubertal age. It became clear to us, however, that a helpful assessment of maturational age depends on the consideration of many parameters. Therefore an integration of information into one system of equations was accomplished and presented[4] (for example, body length, bone age, and body water could be integrated into a single equation). Such equations can be used to assess delayed growth or excess growth.[4,5] Little information is available concerning the prediction of age in the primate fetus. In 1920 Streeter published some information concerning the use of weight, sitting height, and head size to predict the age of the human fetus.[6]

In order to derive an expression that would adequately describe the growth process of the primate fetus we have used an approach similar to that used previously. The many determinants measured and documented in this book were inspected and assessed regarding the estimation of known time from conception. The objective is to ascertain a system or multivariate equation by which the theoretical gestational age of a rhesus monkey may be determined. This theoretical age should represent the expected time of gestation if the animal is normal. The calculated theoretical age is defined as the biological fetal age index (BFA).

The crucial decision in deriving the BFA involves the criteria by which the expression is derived. If the biological fetal age of an individual monkey defines its progress in terms of a normal biological clock, then the BFA should theoretically be equivalent to the gestational age of a normal monkey that has growth to its biological equivalent. Thus, one would expect a normal monkey's BFA to represent its true time from conception. It is impossible to derive a scheme in which each normal monkey's BFA is equivalent to the actual gestational age. The method of defining the BFA should minimize the expected difference in the two ages on some sound statistical basis. If gestational age is viewed as a dependent random variable, resulting from some set of biological parameters, then multiple regression analysis (which minimizes the sum of squares of the differences between the predicted and the actual dependent variable) constitutes such a reasonable basis. Additionally, the mathematical expectation of a variable derived in this manner is equal to the true value of the dependent variable. We are therefore defining the BFA as the predicted gestational age, estimated from multiple regression equations, which apply to normal fetuses. In such a scheme, for a large number of normal animals, the mean BFA would be equal to the mean gestational age, and the error in prediction would be minimized.

In deriving multiple regression equations, the evaluation of the contribution of each variable, relative to the other variables in the scheme, to the overall reduction of variance is usually of prime importance. In representing biological development, however, other considerations must be applied. The final equation should represent as many areas of growth as is feasible, so long as each area makes some contribution.

Expressions derived by this procedure may be applied to any normal fetus, in which the variables included in the expression are calculated, in order to estimate the theoretical gestational age. Additionally, nonnormal conditions may be examined by calculating the difference between the BFA and the actual gestational age. This difference may be thought of as an estimate of the difference in biological maturity between normal growth and that of the fetus being examined, that is, undermaturity or overmaturity. The BFA should prove to be useful as a dependent outcome variable in future research that is controlled adequately.

RESULTS

Biochemical and anthropometric data were available on 26 of the normal rhesus monkey fetuses studied in this book. Their gestational age ranged from 75 to 160 days.

After analyzing all variables with respect to their correlation with gestational age, a multiple regression equation was derived for the 75- to 160-day gestational age period.

A key for the variables used, with appropriate units in parentheses, is as follows:

BFA	=	biological fetal age (days, ie, the predicted gestational age for normal tissues)
Tot. Body Wt.	=	total body weight (g)
Mu H_2O/Prot	=	water:protein ratio in muscle (ml/g)
Cb Tot. H_2O	=	total water in the cerebellum (g)
Cr DNA FC	=	DNA concentration in fresh cerebrum (mg/g)
Cr H_2O DS	=	water per 100 g dry solid in cerebrum (ml/100 g)

The BFA equation,* derived from the 26 fetuses, is

$$\text{BFA} = 184.8361 + 0.0353 \text{ (Tot. Body Wt.)} - 1.8948 \text{ (Mu } H_2O/\text{Prot)}$$
$$+ 4.4153 \text{ (Cb Tot. } H_2O) - 7.8178 \text{ (Cr DNA FC)}$$
$$- 0.0581 \text{ (Cr } H_2O \text{ DS)}$$

The standard deviation about the fitted equation is 4.0 days.

All included variables made a significant contribution to the equation. An example of how to use the equation is now given.

The following set of values were those of a fetus with an actual gestational age of 156 days.

$$\text{Tot. Body Wt.} = 421.7$$
$$\text{Mu } H_2O/\text{Prot} = 4.95$$
$$\text{Cb Tot. } H_2O = 2.711$$
$$\text{Cr DNA FC} = 1.323$$
$$\text{Cr } H_2O \text{ DS} = 662.7$$

$$\text{BFA} = 184.8361 + 0.0353(421.7) - 1.8948(4.95)$$
$$+ 4.4153(2.711) - 7.8178(1.323) - 0.0581(662.7)$$
$$= 153.5 \text{ days}$$

In actual use for normal monkeys, the real gestational age would not be known and the BFA would be a good estimate of what it should be. For nonnormal situations the BFA may be used as a measure of the departure from normal growth.

For example, if we apply the BFA equation to the two series of fetal monkeys described in Chapter 9—that is, (a) fetuses injected with streptozotocin after the 100th day of gestation, and (b) fetuses whose mothers were injected with streptozotocin at 60 days of gestation—we can demonstrate departures in BFA in both overdevelopment and underdevelopment.

---

* A simplified equation is provided for investigators who are unable to determine the variables required for the BFA equation.

Only two variables, which are simply determined, are required—total body weight (g) of the fetus, and the percentage of water in the carcass ($\%H_2O$) determined by weight difference.
The equation is

$$\text{predicted age (in days)} = 256.1526 + 0.1165 \text{ (Tot. Body Wt.)}$$
$$- 2.0949 \text{ (}\%H_2O)$$
$$\text{SD} = 5.2 \text{ days}$$

The larger SD simply means that the equation provides a less precise estimate of fetal age and will therefore be subject to larger errors of prediction.

In Table 21.1, the fetuses injected with streptozotocin have been divided into two groups on the basis of adrenal weight for body size. The rationale and use of this division have been described in Chapter 9. In both groups the actual gestational age has been compared with the BFA for each individual fetus and the differences (in respect to actual gestational age) obtained have been analyzed by a t-test for any apparent deviation from zero. The individual fetuses in the group that had a "normal" adrenal weight for body size all showed a BFA that was less than the actual gestational age. As a group their predicted biological age was retarded 4 days ($P = 0.05$).

On the other hand, the individual fetuses in the group that had enlarged adrenal weight for body size showed a BFA that was the same or in advance of the actual gestational age. Although the mean difference is small ($+2.27$ days) it is significant at the 95% level.

Similarly, it can be clearly demonstrated that the BFA is advanced in respect to actual gestational age for all infants born to diabetic mothers (Table 21.2). As a group their predicted biological age index was advanced approximately 6 days ($P < 0.001$).

All these findings are consistent with the results in Chapter 9. Thus the evidence indicates support for the use of the BFA equation for assessment of delayed and advanced maturity.

Table 21.1   A comparison of Actual Gestational Age with Predicted Fetal Age in Fetuses injected with Streptozotocin.

Group	Actual Gestational Age (days) (GA)	Predicted Fetal Age (days) (BFA)	(BFA)-(GA)
Normal adrenal weight for body size.	160	155.3	-4.7
	158	148.9	-9.1
	159	158.5	-0.5
	157	151.8	-5.2
	157	156.2	-0.8
Mean	158.20	154.14	-4.06
SD	1.30	3.79	3.55
t			2.56
p			=0.05
Enlarged adrenal weight for body size.	160	162.6	+2.6
	158	158.7	+0.7
	160	165.9	+5.9
	149	153.1	+4.1
	154	157.1	+3.1
	158	158.0	0
	158	157.5	+2.6
Mean	156.71	158.98	+2.27
SD	3.95	4.13	2.33
t			2.57
p			<0.05

Table 21.2   A comparison of Actual Gestational
Age with Predicted Total Age in
Infants born of Diabetic Mothers.

No.	Actual Gestational Age (days) (GA)	Predicted Fetal Age (days) (BFA)	(BFA) - (GA)
1	143	150.2	+ 7.2
2	154	163.4	+ 9.4
3	151	155.4	+ 4.4
4	155	159.9	+ 4.9
5	152	154.5	+ 2.5
6	150	153.5	+ 3.5
7	145	155.2	+10.2
8	142	149.5	+ 7.5
9	153	156.9	+ 3.9
M	149.4	155.4	+ 5.94
SD	4.88	4.37	2.72
t			6.54
p			< 0.001

SUMMARY

The biological fetal age (BFA) equation is derived from data concerning 26 normal fetuses. The equation is constructed to assess fetal age or degree of maturation. The equation utilizes fetal weight and data from biochemical measurements concerning muscle, cerebrum, and cerebellum. An application of the equation to assess the age of fetuses in experimental circumstances is presented.

This equation, if applied to fetuses that are normal but of unknown gestation will accurately predict gestational age. In experimental situations overdevelopment or underdevelopment can also be documented.

REFERENCES

1. Crampton, W. C.: *Am. Phys. Educ. Rev.* **13:** 144 and 268, 1908.

2. Crampton, W. C.: Physiological age—A fundamental principle. *Child Dev.* **15:** 3, 1944.

3. Brody, S.: *Bioenergetics and Growth.* Van Nostrand-Reinholt, Princeton, New Jersey, 1945, p. 712.

4. Cheek, D. B., Migeon, C. J., and Mellits, E. D.: The concept of physiological age. In: Cheek, D. B. (Ed.): *Human Growth.* Lea & Febiger, Philadelphia, 1968, p. 541.

5. Mellits, E. D., Dorst, J. P., and Cheek, D. B.: Bone age: Its contribution to the prediction of maturational or biological age. *Am. J. Phys. Anthropol.* **35:** 3, 1971.

6. Streeter, G. L.: Weight, sitting height, head size, foot length and menstrual age of the human embryo. *Contrib. Embryol. Carnegie Inst.* **11:** 143, 1920.

PART III

POSTNATAL GROWTH

CHAPTER 22

Growth and Body Composition

Donald B. Cheek

INTRODUCTION

Traditionally the appraisal of postnatal growth in the clinic has been through anthropometric methods and assessment of maturation has usually been by the measurement of bone age; in other words, inspection of a major but single tissue. For more than a decade we have been involved in study of normal and abnormal growth in children. The growth of cell mass (metabolic size) in the body as a whole has been studied, as well as the growth of individual tissues such as muscle and adipose tissue. The change in function with change in time has been noted and where possible the opportunity has been taken to develop better methods for the assessment of maturational age, whether this be by the measurement of hormone secretions or by the appraisal of cell numbers. Much of the work was published in 1968 in a previous book[1] and it is pertinent to review here and in subsequent chapters the work done in the last decade. Subsequent chapters deal with the role of nutrition and hormones in cellular growth.

THE MEASUREMENT OF EXTRACELLULAR AND INTRACELLULAR VOLUME

Increments in body weight represent the growth of many tissues growing at different rates, reaching a steady state at different times and having different metabolic rates at rest. Complicated mathematical expressions fitting weight data are of academic and limited interest. The study of growth in individual tissues and organs is more useful but difficult to document in the live individual. The time period over which tissue growth is studied often determines the order of an equation that fits the data best.

We have drawn attention to the differences between primate and nonprimate growth in the prenatal period; in the postnatal period this difference is still evident. The pattern of growth for mammals that are nonprimates fits a simple sigmoid curve and characteristically the pause between infancy and adolescence is minimal. The growth curve of the human child from birth to maturity follows the primate curve.

Figure 22.1 is taken from the observations of Laird[2] and is based on data of Bayley.[3, 4] The data were fitted by computer and by the method of least squares using the Gompertz model or method. This approach considers growth as a multiplicative phenomenon with a linear component, or growth in cell size and in cell number. In the male up to 3 years, there is an accelerated increase in weight, then a slower rate until 9 years when the adolescent growth spurt begins. The growth of the female is not dissimilar but the adolescent growth spurt is less and (as will be discussed) is more related to fat increments than to muscle.

We have endeavored to establish determinants that describe growth more accurately than do anthropometric measurements (eg, body weight), experience showing that certain parameters are highly informative. One of these is the intracellular mass which is equivalent to the cell mass of muscle plus viscera. Although active muscle accounts for a major part of oxygen utilization, resting muscle represents only about 17% of the active tissue mass.

In the conclusion of our previous book[1] we considered major components of body composition (cell mass, muscle mass, extracellular volume) in children from 4 to 17 years of age. Figure 22.2 illustrates the increments in intracellular water

EVOLUTION OF THE HUMAN GROWTH CURVE

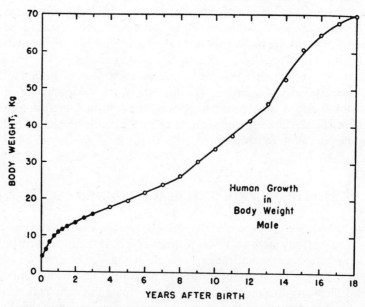

Fig. 22.1. Growth in body weight of male children selected according to age of maturation. (Reprinted from Laird, *Growth* **31**: 345, 1967, with permission of the Editor.)

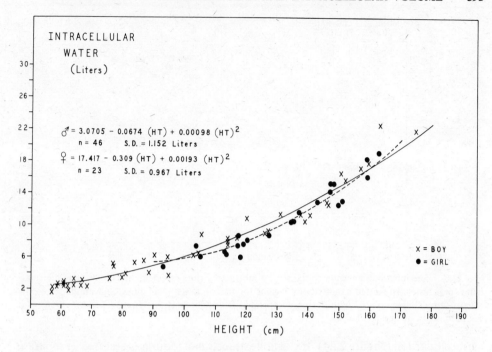

Fig. 22.2. Intracellular water is plotted against body length for infants, boys and girls (1 month to 17 years of age). The relationships are quadratic. No sex difference is demonstrable. [Reprinted from Reba et al: *Pediatr. Nucl. Med.*, James, E. (Ed.), 458, 1974, with the permission of W. B. Saunders.]

(metabolically active tissue) for human males and females from 0.2 to 17 years old. There is no sex difference. The points for girls could also have been expressed as a linear function, but additional data obtained recently from older girls indicate that a quadratic fit is more appropriate. However, the upward sweep of the quadratic is always more extended in the male. If additional data from infants are included, a cubic function may unfold, as, for example, when the growth of muscle mass is considered (Chapter 24). The abscissa records height as this is more significant as an index of maturation than chronological age.

Admittedly, for normal children body weight per se is an excellent measure of metabolic size, as pointed out by Darrow years ago.[5] In Figure 22.3 it is shown that intracellular water in normal children holds a strong correlation with body weight during growth. The slope of the lines for infant boys and girls is the same. During adult life (20–60 years) the slope changes while in the autumn of existence (60–90 years) the metabolic mass comprises less of the body weight. The data for adults have been obtained from the work of others.[6] It is known that BMR per unit weight decreases with senility as does calorie intake. [7, 8]

Extracellular tissues (eg, collagen) contain extracellular fluid as does plasma and the interstitial space. All comprise the extracellular compartment. When extracellular volume is subtracted from the total body water one obtains the parameter intracellular water (ICW). This index is a measure of total cell mass. The extracellular fluid contains a low concentration of potassium and a high concentration of chloride, as reviewed previously.[9] The extracellular phase is well described by the distribution of chloride (or bromide) provided allowance is made for the non-

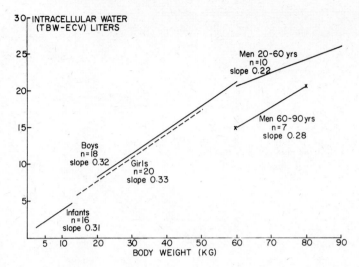

Fig. 22.3. The intracellular water (obtained by subtracting the corrected chloride or bromide space from total water) is plotted against body weight for male infants, girls, boys, and adults. Note the loss of intracellular volume with ageing. [Reprinted from Cheek (Ed.): *Human Growth*, 1968, with the permission of Lea & Febiger.]

extracellular ion (Figure 22.4). If the nonextracellular sodium is assessed in separate experiments, the corrected sodium space equals the corrected chloride space.[10] During 1950 to 1960 much work was devoted to the definition of the limits of this compartment. In both rats[10] and man[11] it was found that about 12% of chloride was nonextracellular (in red cells, gastric mucosa, renal tubular cells). Thus it has been the custom to reduce the chloride space by 10% to allow for nonextracellular chloride. The amount of chloride or bromide injected minus 10%, divided by the concentration of chloride or bromide in a plasma ultrafiltrate, yields a volume that is anatomically and biochemically acceptable as a close approximation of the extracellular phase of the entire body. Subtraction of this volume from total water closely reflects the protoplasmic mass of muscle and visceral cells.

However, it should be cautioned that the question of whether significant amounts of chloride are present within the intracellular phase of muscle remains unanswered. Walser and Barrat[12] drew attention to the earlier observation[13] that the distribution of sulfate did not agree with the value for the distribution of chloride in muscle. While this may be due to inadequate penetration of sulfate into connective tissue surrounding the muscle fibers, this may not be the entire explanation.[12] Other workers have shown that the transverse longitudinal canals within the sarcoplasm, which are important in muscle contraction, are selectively permeable to Cl and continuous with the extracellular phase,[14] but are impermeable to nitrate[15] and sulfate. Hence, an explanation exists for the disparity.

The extracellular phase, as defined above, makes up 40% of the total body water from infancy to adolescence, and the intracellular phase accounts for 60% (Figure 22.5).

Under conditions of disease, in our experience the ratio of cell protein to cell water tends to remain constant. Increased hydration within the cell gives rise to water intoxication and it is probably only in the last stages of malnutrition, cardiac failure or cachexia, or in sodium depletion, that the ratio of cell water to cell protein

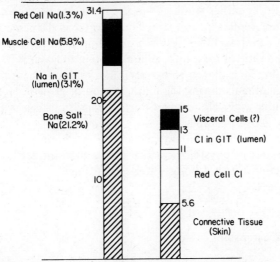

Fig. 22.4. By experiment the amount of chloride in red cells, connective tissue, and visceral cells has been determined in 220-g rats. Up to 15% of chloride is nonextracellular. Similar experiments revealed that up to 30% of body sodium is outside the extracellular volume. However, the sodium space and the volume of distribution of chloride, when corrected for nonextracellular electrolyte, yield volumes that are very similar. Such spaces account for true extracellular volume. (The figure is calculated on the basis of data published by Cheek et al: *J. Clin. Invest.* **36**: 340, 1957.)

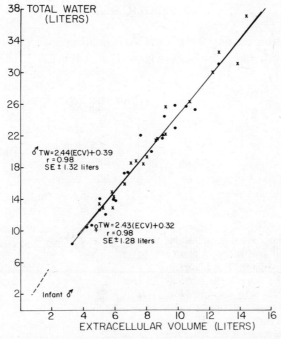

Fig. 22.5. Total water for infant males, children, and adolescents is plotted against the extracellular volume. Note that the E.C.V. makes up a constant fraction of the total body water, whereas the line for the male (x) is almost identical with the line for the female (●). [Reprinted from Cheek (Ed.): *Human Growth*, 1968, with the permission of Lea & Febiger.]

in muscle changes. From earlier studies[10] in the rat it can be shown that the ratio of extracellular protein (collagen) to extracellular water is the same as the ratio of intracellular protein to intracellular water. For example, in the mature rat (220 g Sprague-Dawley), the ratio of total intracellular protein to water is 27g to 100 g and a similar ratio pertains for collagen to extracellular volume. These ratios probably remain constant in mammals during the major period of growth. Hence, the measurement of intracellular water alone under normal conditions is a satisfactory index of the metabolically active protoplasm.

Most investigators have been content to use lean body mass (LBM) or fat-free body weight as an index of physiological size rather than intracellular mass. Lean body mass is a function of total body water (TW) thus:

$$\frac{TW}{0.72} = LBM$$

where 0.72 is the Pace constant. Also

$$\text{body weight} - LBM = \text{body fat}$$

However, since, as we have seen, TW has a linear relationship with extracellular volume (ECW), it follows that extracellular protein (mainly collagen) should hold a relationship (probably linear) with intracellular protein.

THE RELATION BETWEEN INTRACELLULAR MASS (ICW) AND METABOLIC RATE

The overall equation relating BMR to ICW is quadratic with a reduction of BMR as the growth of cell mass continues (Figure 22.6, Table 22.1). The investigation of

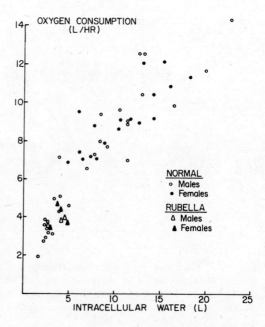

Fig. 22.6. The oxygen consumption for infant males, boys, and girls is shown plotted against intracellular volume. The linear regressions in Table 22.1 describe the relationships for infants and for older children. Note that children with congenital rubella (who have previously undergone a loss of cell mass) have an oxygen consumption which is normal if related to cell mass but low if related to body length. [Reprinted from Reba et al: Pediatr. Nucl. Med., James, E. (Ed.), 468, 1974, with the permission of W. B. Saunders.]

Table 22.1   Relationship between oxygen
              consumption and intracellular
              water in normal children.

	Male Infants 0.18 - 1.54 yrs Sample size 14	Boys & Girls 2.50-17.08 yrs Sample size 33
Oxygen Consumption $(L.O_2/hr)$	0.2080 + 1.1112 ICW	4.9801 + 0.3795 ICW
SD	1.094	1.200
r	0.70	0.80
p=less than	0.01	0.001
Calorie Expenditure (Cals/hr)	0.9394 + 5.3522 ICW	25.0265 + 1.17195 ICW
SD	5.159	5.794
r	0.70	0.78
p=less than	0.01	0.001

children 1 to 3 years of age with congenital rubella and superimposed congenital heart disease revealed that these children were growth retarded and their cell mass and muscle mass were significantly reduced for body length. The BMR was reduced for height, weight, or age and a diagnosis of hypothyroidism might be considered. However, as seen in Figure 22.6 their basal oxygen consumption was commensurate with their cell mass and no aberration of heat production could be defined. The investigation of these patients is reported in detail elsewhere[16] but the point is made here that reduction of cell mass was accompanied by a reduction of BMR.

A similar reduction in metabolic rates has been found in situations where cell mass or ICW is reduced due to protein-calorie restriction.[17, 18] On rehabilitation one would expect rapid growth of the intracellular phase, particularly of the visceral cell mass, which could account for increased metabolic rate.[19, 20]

Holliday et al[8] in a reappraisal or reconsideration of basal metabolic rate pointed out that with respect to body weight or surface area no satisfactory mathematical relationships could be obtained: "In humans the comparative rates of increase of weight and BMR do not conform precisely either to the surface area or to any other simple function of body size over the total range." They formulated three postulates:

1. The BMR of an organism is derived from the metabolic activity of the internal organs (e.g, brain, liver, lungs, and kidneys).

2. The reason that BMR decreases as body size increases is related to the fact that the vital organs are reduced in size relative to the other body constituents.

3. The decrease in BMR per kilogram in the individual during growth is due to a slower growth of the highly active organs.

The first of these postulates is supported by a consideration of individual organs which revealed that 80% of the BMR could be accounted for in visceral organs. Also, it is known that muscle accounts for only 17% of the total BMR for the human at rest.[7, 21]

Munro[22] found that in the mature mammal irrespective of size, muscle mass is always 45% of body weight, but visceral mass (as illustrated by the liver) is not always a constant proportion. For example, in the elephant, liver mass is only 1% of body weight while in man it is 7%. These findings support the second postulate. Holliday et al considered the organ-weight:body-weight ratios in nine species and found that the differences in relative weight of active organs would account for some, but not all, the differences in BMR per kilogram observed from species to species. They reviewed the observations of many workers on tissue oxygen consumption in different organs. It would appear that at least some decrease in tissue oxygen consumption occurs in liver as the animal increases in size. However, the weight of evidence indicates that little change occurs in tissue oxygen consumption in the various visceral organs during growth. The decline in BMR in the human at $1\frac{1}{2}$ years is related mainly to the increasing growth and expansion of the musculature. Holliday et al concluded that the intracellular phase of the body could be considered as two entities, the visceral organs which affect the BMR and the muscle which plays a small part.

Figure 22.7 demonstrates the relationship between the intracellular water of the body and the intracellular water of the muscle.[23] At 4 years of age, muscle accounts for 30% of the total ICW and at adolescence 70%. While muscle is an important tissue with respect to body metabolism and protein reserves and turnover, it accounts for only a small proportion of the resting metabolic rate, the situation altering markedly, of course, with activity. The contribution of muscle to the total ICW can be measured; in our studies muscle mass was measured from creatinine excretion, and intracellular and extracellular water was partitioned by measurement of muscle chloride in each subject. Since total water (TW) and extracellular water (ECW) were also measured in each individual it is possible to obtain a value for visceral water (or mass) during growth by the following calculation:

TW − (ECW + intracellular water within the muscle mass)
    = visceral cell water (mass)

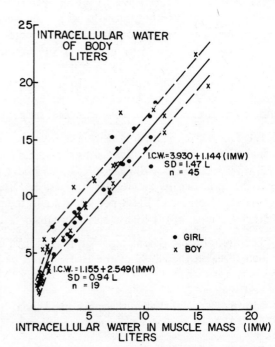

Fig. 22.7. The total intracellular water of the body is plotted against the intracellular water within the muscle mass for male infants, boys, and girls. Note that by 17 years about 70 percent of the intracellular volume (mass) is constituted by muscle. [Reprinted from Reba et al: *Pediatr. Nucl. Med.*, James, E. (Ed.), 468, 1974, with the permission of W. B. Saunders.]

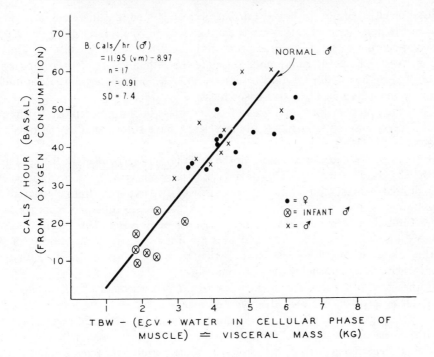

Fig. 22.8. Visceral cell plotted against basal heat production; a linear relationship from infancy to adolescence for the male is revealed. [Reprinted from Cheek (Ed.): *Human Growth*, 1968, with the permission of Lea & Febiger.]

Alternatively

$$\text{ICW (total)} - \text{ICW (muscle)} = \text{ICW (viscera)}$$

When the basal metabolic rate is plotted against visceral mass (Figure 22.8) a strong linear relationship is obtained which adds strength to the arguments of Holliday et al. No other parameter will yield a linear relationship with BMR from infancy through adolescence. We would argue that changes in visceral mass account for the changes in basal oxygen consumption during growth. For the assessment of metabolic activity in situations where growth retardation is severe, however, the measurement of total ICW is clearly a meaningful parameter.

A NOTE ON MEASUREMENT OF INTRACELLULAR MASS WITH ⁴⁰K

⁴⁰K is a natural isotope occurring in the body in low concentration, but proportional to ³⁹K or stable potassium. The total body potassium can thus be determined by a sensitive body counter that monitors ⁴⁰K.

Almost all of the body's potassium is located intracellularly[6] so measurement of this electrolyte yields a direct index of cell mass. The division of total body potassium by the net potassium concentration in the cell water (146 meq/l)[10] yields the intracellular water (ICW).

If the value for ICW as determined by volume difference is compared with ICW as determined by ⁴⁰K for the sexes, there is some difference between the two ICW values for girls but not for boys.[24] It has been suggested that this finding could be due to the deposition of fat which is characteristic in the adolescent girl, adipose tissue appearing to act as a shield preventing the detection of all the ^{40}K. Thus in the girl with ^{40}K method may underestimate the cellular mass. This suggestion is supported by our finding[25] that in obesity the ^{40}K method certainly does underestimate the metabolically active tissue mass.

Thus the apparent increased growth of cell mass in the boy relative to the girl after 9 years may be an artifact. Flynn et al[26] have shown that at the outset of adolescence for the boy or at a stature of 135 cm the accretion of new cell mass (as monitored by ^{40}K) accelerates more in the boy than in the girl, length being plotted on the abscissa (Figure 22.9). Our own work in previous years[27] showed that if ^{40}K was plotted against body water during growth two separate lines appeared for boys and girls. This was difficult to understand since no sex difference appears when other total electrolyte values are plotted against body water. Our recent data for obese subjects suggest that the departures are due to incorrect monitoring of ^{40}K in the adolescent girl. Hence we suspect that a single line should pertain for both sexes when ^{40}K is considered against total water.

Forbes,[28] who has devoted much work to the measurement of ^{40}K in boys and girls during growth, has recently reviewed available data on the growth of LBM and sets out a sigmoid curve with documentation of the 25th centile and the 75th centile. These data also reveal the increased growth of lean tissue in the male with an actual negative growth of fat tissue for short period between 17 and 18 years of age. On the other hand, the growth of adipose tissue in the female is clearly documented. It would appear from this information that postpubertal growth of lean tissue ceases in the male at about 20 to 21 years and at 17 to 18 years in the female.

MUSCLE AND ADIPOSE TISSUE GROWTH THROUGH ADOLESCENCE

As we discussed at the beginning of the chapter, growth of the soma in postnatal life in the primate does not conform to a sigmoid curve when weight is plotted against time. A period of slow growth occurs after infancy. By contrast, growth in the rodent is rapid from weaning into sexual maturation, the steepest point on the sigmoid curve representing sexual maturation in the male or the first estrus in the female.[29] In the primate also the point of maximal growth velocity (eg, height velocity) in postnatal life corresponds to the time of sexual maturation (puberty).

Over the years we have been concerned with approaches to assess just how far along the road of life a child has traveled, anatomically, physiologically, and biochemically, the so-called maturational age of biological age index.[30,31] Children mature at various ages, sexual maturation occurring at 10 years in one girl or 13 years in another. For this reason chronological age per se has limited significance and any stated time for sexual maturation only reflects mean maturational age for a large group of subjects. The degree of maturation may be reflected by hormonal levels, cell number, bone age, or simply by body length. "Height age" has long been appreciated as a better maturational index than chronological age. A combination of body length and bone age (multivariate equation) predicts well the biological age index.[31]

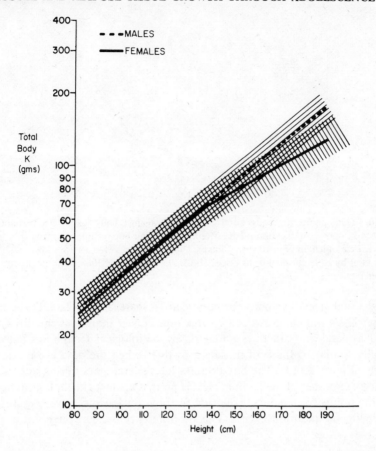

Fig. 22.9. Regression line for the mean and tolerance region for 68 percent of the population for the log of body K versus height for 432 children age 3 to 18 years. Note the departure of the male and female populatons at 130 to 140 cm. The significance of this sex difference is discussed in the test. (Reprinted from Flynn et al: *Pediatr. Res.* **6:** 239, 1972, with the permission of the Editor.)

At the onset of prepubertal growth an acceleration of tissue growth occurs. When increase in body water or lean body mass (LBM) was plotted versus body length, two quadratic equations evolved, one for boys and another for girls.[32] Application of the Mellits "breaking line technique"[33] revealed that a break occurred at about 137 cm of length for boys (or at 9 to 10 years of age) and at about 113 cm for girls (or at 6 to 7 years). The break in the line for girls was less marked (Figures 22.10 and 22.11). It was considered that these breaking points indicated the onset of pre-pubertal growth. The second line for boys was steeper than for girls, indicating a more rapid growth of lean body mass (LBM) in the male.

Inspection of other determinants of body composition such as muscle mass (creatinine excretion), extracellular volume (corrected bromide space), or cell mass (^{40}K) revealed quadratic equations when the data were considered against body length with the breaking-line technique, again indicating a distinct change in growth rate for the male between 137 and 140 cm of stature. Our own data on muscle mass indicate that the boy doubles his muscle mass from prepuberty to postpuberty and

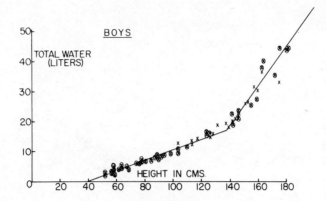

Fig. 22.10. Data points for body water are plotted against body length from infancy through adolescence in males. Application of the Mellits' "breaking line technique" reveals an intersection at about 137 cm of length (9 to 10 years of age). The data of Friis Hansen are shown by ⊗ and those of Cheek et al by X. [Reprinted from Cheek (Ed.): *Human Growth*, 1968, with the premission of Lea & Febiger.]

has a maximal growth velocity for muscle at 14 years (Figure 22.12). The boy in the 13th year has a muscle growth rate three times faster than does the girl.[34] Assessment of skeletal mass in boys and girls by radiological techniques shows curves essentially similar to those of muscle growth[23] when the data are plotted agaitns height[35] (Figure 22.13). The boy doubles his skeletal mass during adolescence.

When the number of nuclei in muscle is plotted against chronological age (Figure 22.14) the points form a cubic equation for boys (cf Laird's curve, Figure 22.1) and a simple linear equation for girls. The sex difference is clear, the point of departure

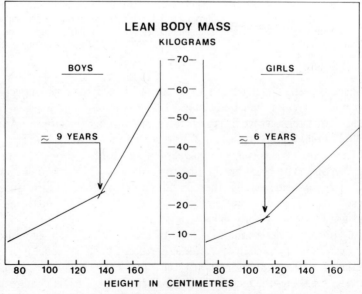

Fig. 22.11. Intersecting lines have been drawn to express the relationship of LBM (which is TW/0.72) to body length for boys and girls. Note the sex difference.

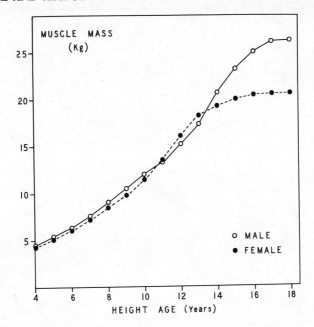

Fig. 22.12. Muscle mass (calculated from creatinine excretion) for adolescent boys and girls is plotted against height age. The points have been corrected on the basis that the length of each subject is on the 50th centile of the growth chart for age. Note the significant increase in muscle mass for the adolescent boy. [Reprinted from Grumbach (Ed.): *Control of Onset of Puberty*, 1974, with the permission of John Wiley and Sons.]

again being 9 years of age, at which time nuclear replication accelerates in the boy. We are aware of course that a limit has to be reached for both boys and girls and would speculate that with further data the curve for girls would probably become quadratic. These data demonstrate a limit for boys close to 3.8×10^{12} nuclei and for girls 2×10^{12}, or only half the number in males.

The growth of cytoplasmic mass in muscle also shows a strong sex difference. The protein relative to the DNA can be considered against organ size, muscle mass, or body size (body water) (Figures 22.15 and 22.16). The protein:DNA ratio increases faster for the female than for the male but ultimately the male values

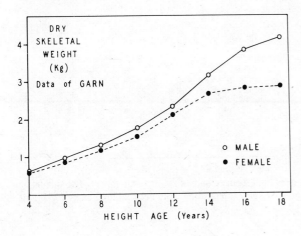

Fig. 22.13. Dry skeletal weight is plotted against height age [from the data of Garn[35]]. Note the greater increase in weight for the adolescent male. [Reprinted from Grumbach (Ed.): *Control of Onset of Puberty*, 1974, with the permission of John Wiley and Sons.]

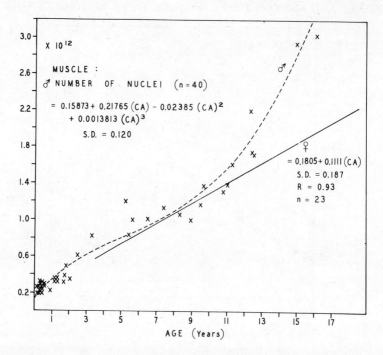

Fig. 22.14. Relationship between nuclear number in the musculature is shown with chronological age (CA) for boys and girls. For males the relationship is cubic, suggesting three phases of muscle cell growth postnatally. Clearly the male adolescent growth spurt is more remarkable and associated with increase of nuclear number. (Reprinted from Cheek et al: *Fed. Proc.* **29:** 1503, 1970, with the permission of the Editor.)

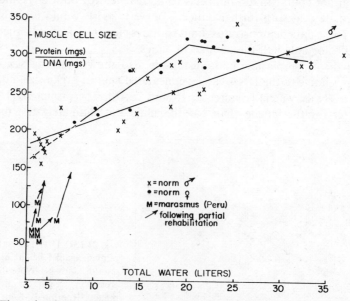

Fig. 22.15. The ratio of protein:DNA is plotted against body size (or total water). The quadratic equation for the female has been expressed as two intersecting lines. Note that points for infant males with protein-calorie malnutrition (M) fall well below the normal.

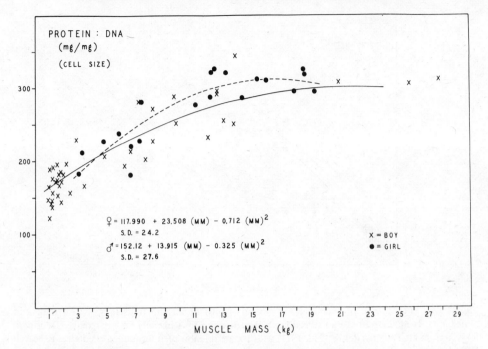

PROTEIN : DNA
(mg/mg)
(CELL SIZE)

$♀ = 117.990 + 23.508 \, (\text{MM}) - 0.712 \, (\text{MM})^2$
S.D. = 24.2

$♂ = 152.12 + 13.915 \, (\text{MM}) - 0.325 \, (\text{MM})^2$
S.D. = 27.6

X = BOY
● = GIRL

MUSCLE   MASS (kg)

Fig. 22.16. Muscle cell size (protein:DNA) is plotted against muscle mass for boys and girls from infancy to adolescence. (Reprinted from Cheek et al: *Pediatr. Res.* **5**: 312, 1971, with the permission of the Editor.)

catch up and probably exceed those of the female, as indeed happens in the rat (Figure 22.17). While the female does gain lean tissue, growth of adipose tissue is considerable and characteristic. Consideration of our own data indicates that the female reaches a maximum rate of adipose tissue growth in the 12th year[34] or at the time the girl reaches sexual maturation (Figure 22.18).

HORMONES: INSULIN AND GROWTH HORMONE AND ADOLESCENCE

A separate chapter is set aside for the discussion of hormonal influences on growth but here the influence of hormones on adolescent growth is discussed briefly.

Adequate nutrition is mandatory for the proper action of hormones. We have put forward the thesis that the two major hormones for postnatal muscle growth are insulin and growth hormone, growth hormone being concerned with nuclear replication and insulin with cytoplasmic growth. To a large extent, the predominating action of one hormone over the other can be gauged by inspection of the nuclear number in the musculature versus the ratio of protein to DNA.[23]

Other hormones including sex hormones would appear to be of secondary importance with respect to childhood and adolescent growth. The evidence can be briefly discussed. The elevation of testosterone which occurs at 9 to 10 years[30, 36, 37] stimulates the production of growth hormone.[30, 36—38]

Castration of the female rat at weaning causes a pattern of muscle growth similar to that of the male.[39] Estrogens inhibit the peripheral action of growth hor-

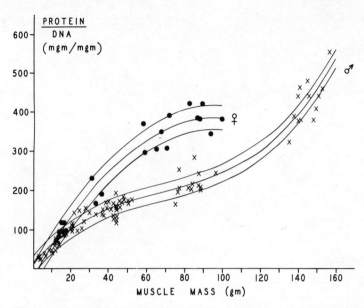

Fig. 22.17. The ratio of protein:DNA is plotted against organ size (muscle mass) for male and female rats. Note the more rapid secretion of protein/unit DNA initially for the female. (Reprinted for Cheek et al: *Pediatr. Res.* **5**: 312, 1971, with the permission of International Pediatric Research Foundation.)

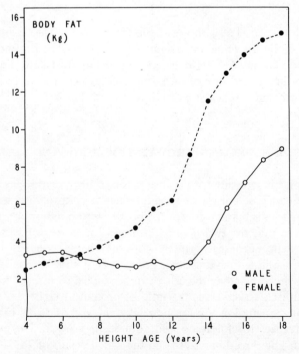

Fig. 22.18. Body fat is plotted against height age for boys and girls. Note the sex difference. [Reprinted from Grumbach (Ed.): *Control of Onset of Puberty*, 1974, with the permission of John Wiley and Sons.]

404

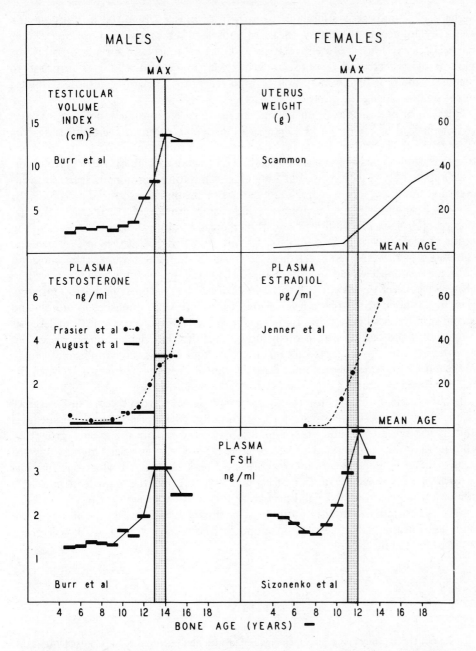

Fig. 22.19. Various indices of sexual maturation in the human have been plotted against bone age and peak height velocity (V_{max}) is indicated in each figure. The significance of this figure is discussed in the text. [Reprinted from Grambach (Ed.): Control of Onset of Puberty, 1974, with the permission of John Wiley and Sons.]

405

mone.[40, 41] Androgens stimulate the growth of muscles involved in reproduction and may influence protein synthesis in muscle after sexual maturation.[42] The increased accretion of protein relative to DNA in muscle in girls is possibly explained by a decreased response to growth hormone and a greater response to insulin in the girl. Insulin may well be involved in the growth of adipose tissue fat in the female during the adolescent period.

Some information concerning changes in sex hormone production during puberty is summarized in Figure 22.19. Changes in testicular volume have been studied by Burr et al.[43] The range of data is shown by the horizontal bars. Bone age (maturational age index) has been used on the abscissa (where available). Testicular volume rises appreciably at $10\frac{1}{2}$ years, but follicular stimulating hormone is secreted in increasing amounts from 9 years. Testosterone secretion rises at the same time. The data of Scammon[44] demonstrate the increasing growth of the uterus from $10\frac{1}{2}$ years while plasma estradiol[45] and follicular stimulating hormone[46] escalate in terms of secretion from 8 to 9 years. It is noteworthy that at the time of maximal somatic growth velocity (V_{max}) the FSH reaches its highest value, then subsides.

In conclusion, it would seem that there is a radical departure between boys and girls with respect to growth at 9 to 10 years. The male becomes more responsive to growth hormone at the tissue level. Rapid cell multiplication ensues in muscle and in the epiphyses, some visceral tissues being similarly involved. Growth of LBM is remarkable and calorie and protein intake escalate. Fat deposition increases but at a lesser rate. Androgen secretion increases and augments cytoplasmic growth in the muscle and possibly accounts for a continued growth of protein : DNA in the male to some 30 years of age when testosterone secretion diminishes.

In the female, follicular stimulating hormone escalates from 8 years and estradiol from 9 years. The estrogens restrict the action of growth hormone at the tissue level and the response to insulin predominates. This may explain the greater growth of adipose tissue and accelerated growth of protein : DNA in muscle. Thus the upward growth of lean tissue is less remarkable (no break is detected when one inspects growth of lean tissue versus height around 9 years), but the growth of muscle is somewhat increased and skeletal growth follows muscle growth (as in the male).

Growth hormone would thus appear to be the major adolescent hormone for the male and insulin the adolescent hormone for the female. Future work will prove or disprove the thesis.

REFERENCES

1. Cheek, D. B.: Body composition, energy, cell growth and intelligence. In: Cheek, D. B. (Ed.): *Human Growth*. Lea & Febiger, Philadelphia, 1968.
2. Laird, A. K.: Evolution of the human growth curve. *Growth* **31**: 345, 1967.
3. Bayley, N.: Growth curves of height and weight by age for boys and girls, scaled according to physical maturity. *J. Pediatr.* **48**: 187, 1956.
4. Bayley, N., and Davis, F.: Growth changes in bodily size and proportions during the first three years: A developmental study of 61 children by repeated measurements. *Biometrika* 27: 26, 1935.
5. Darrow, D. C.: The significance of body size. *Am. J. Dis. Child.* **93**: 416, 1959.
6. Moore, F. D., Olesen, K. H., McMurrey, J. D., Parker, H. V., Ball, M. R., and Boyden, C. M.: *The Body Cell Mass and Its Supporting Environment*. Saunders, Philadelphia, 1963.

7. Brozek, J., and Grande, F.: Body composition and basal metabolism in man: Correlation analysis versus physiological approach. *Human Biol*. **27**: 22, 1955.

8. Holliday, M. A., Potter, D., Jarrah, A., and Bearg, S.: The relation of metabolic rate to body weight and organ size. *Pediatr. Res*. **1**: 185, 1967.

9. Cheek, D. B., and Talbert, J. B.: Extracellular volume (and sodium) and body water in infants. In: Cheek, D. B. (Ed.): *Human Growth*. Lea & Febiger, Philadelphia, 1968.

10. Cheek, D. B., West, C. D., and Golden, C. C.: The distribution of Na and Cl and the extracellular fluid volume in the rat. *J. Clin. Invest*. **36**: 340, 1957.

11. Edelman, I. S., and Leibman, J.: Anatomy of body water and electrolytes. *Am. J. Med*. **27**: 256, 1959.

12. Walser, M., and Barrat, T. M.: Extracellular fluid in individual tissues and in whole animals: The distribution of radio-sulfate and radio-bromide. *J. Clin. Invest*. **48**: 56, 1969.

13. Walser, M., Seldin, D. W., and Grollman, A.: An evaluation of radiosulfate for the determination of extracellular fluid in man and dogs. *J. Clin. Invest*. **32**: 299, 1953.

14. Huxley, H. E.: Evidence for continuity between the central elements of the triads and extracellular space in frog sartorium muscle. *Nature* **202**: 1067, 1964.

15. Girardier, L., Reuben, J. P., Brandt, P. W., and Grundfest, H.: Evidence for anion-permselection membrane in crayfish muscle fibers and its possible role in excitation-contraction coupling. *J. Gen. Physiol*. **47**: 189, 1963.

16. Hill, D. E., Arellano, C. P., Izukawa, T., Holt, A. B., and Cheek, D. B.: Studies in infants and children with congenital rubella: Oxygen consumption, body water, cell mass, muscle mass and adipose tissue composition. *Johns Hopkins Med. J*. **127**: 309, 1970.

17. Varga, F.: The respective effects of starvation and changed body composition on energy metabolism in malnourished infants. *Pediatrics* **23**: 1085, 1959.

18. Monckeberg, F., Beas, F., Horwitz, I., Dabacens, A., and Gonzalez, M.: Oxygen consumption in infant malnutrition. *Pediatrics* **33**: 554, 1964.

19. Montgomery, R. D.: Changes in the basal metabolic rate of the malnourished infant and their relation to body composition. *J. Clin. Invest*. **41**: 1655, 1962.

20. Levine, S., Wilson, J., and Gottschall, G.: The respiratory metabolism in infancy and childhood. VIII. The respiratory exchange in marasmus: Basal metabolism. *Am. J. Dis. Child*. **35**: 615, 1928.

21. Aschoff, J.: In: Smith, R. E., and Hoyer, D. J. (Eds.): Metabolism and cellular function in cold acclimation. *Physiol. Rev*. **42**: 60, 1962.

22. Munro, H. N.: Evolution of protein metabolism in mammals: In: Munro, H. N., and Allison, J. R. (Eds.): *Mammalian Protein Metabolism*, Vol. 3. Academic Press, New York, 1969.

23. Cheek, D. B., Holt, A. B., Hill, D. E., and Talbert, J. L.: Skeletal muscle cell mass and growth: The concept of the deoxyribonucleic acid unit. *Pediatr. Res*. **5**: 312, 1971.

24. Reba, R. C., Cheek, D. B., and Mellits, E. D.: Body composition studies: Growth of intracellular mass and metabolic size and the assessment of maturational age. In: James, A. E. (Ed.): *Symposium on Nuclear Medicine*. The Johns Hopkins Hospital, Baltimore, 1972 (in press).

25. Cheek, D. B., Schultz, R. B., Parra, A., and Reba, R. C.: Overgrowth of lean and adipose tissues in adolescent obesity. *Pediatr. Res*. **4**: 268, 1970.

26. Flynn, M. A., Woodruff, C., Clark, J., and Chase, G.: Total body potassium in normal children. *Pediatr. Res*. **6**: 239, 1972.

27. Reba, R. C., Cheek, D. B., and Leitnaker, F. C.: Body potassium and lean body mass. In: Cheek, D. B. (Ed.): *Human Growth*. Lea & Febiger, Philadelphia, 1968, Chapter 11, p. 165.

28. Forbes, G. B.: Growth of the lean tissue mass in man. *Growth* **36**: 325, 1972.

29. Cheek, D. B., and Holt, A. B.: Growth and body composition of the mouse. *Am. J. Physiol*. **205**: 913, 1963.

30. Cheek, D. B., Migeon, C. J., and Mellits, E. D.: In: Cheek, D. B. (Ed.): *Human Growth*. Lea & Febiger, Philadelphia, 1968, p. 541.

31. Mellits, E. D., Dorst, J. D., and Cheek, D. B.: Bone age: Contribution to the prediction of maturational and biological age. *Phys. Anthropol*. **35**: 381, 1971.

32. Cheek, D. B., Mellits, E. D., and Elliot, D.: Body water height and weight during growth in normal children. *Am. J. Dis. Child.* **112:** 312, 1966.

33. Mellits, E. D., and Cheek, D. B.: In: Cheek, D. B. (Ed.): *Human Growth.* Lea & Febiger, Philadelphia, 1968, p. 141.

34. Cheek, D. B.: Body composition, hormones, nutrition, and adolescent growth. In: *Control of Onset of Puberty*, Grumbach, M. M., Grave, G. D. and Mayer, F. E. (Eds.). Wiley, New York, 1974, p. 426.

35. Garn, S. M.: *The Earlier Gain and the Later Loss of Cortical Bone in Nutritional Perspective.* Thomas, Springfield, Illinois, 1970.

36. Frasier, S. D., Gafford, F., and Horton, R.: Plasma androgens in childhood and adolescence. *J. Clin. Endocrinol.* **29:** 1404, 1969.

37. August, G. P., Grumbach, M. M., and Kaplan, S. L.: Hormonal changes in puberty: III. Correlation of plasma testosterone, LH, FSH, testicular size, and bone age with male pubertal development. *J. Clin. Endocrinol.* **34:** 319, 1972.

38. Illig, R., and Prader, A.: Effect of testosterone on growth hormone secretion in patients with anorchia and delayed puberty. *J. Clin. Endocrinol.* **30:** 615, 1970.

39. Cheek, D. B., Brasel, J. A., and Graystone, J. E.: In: Cheek, D. B. (Ed.): *Human Growth.* Lea & Febiger, Philadelphia, 1968, p. 306.

40. Wiedemann, E., and Schwartz, E.: Suppression of growth hormone-dependent human serum sulfation factor by estrogen. *J. Clin. Endocrinol.* **34:** 51, 1972.

41. Merimee, T. J., and Fineberg, S. E.: Studies of the sex based variation of human growth hormone secretion. *J. Clin. Endocrinol.* **33:** 896, 1971.

42. Kochakian, C. D.: *The Physiology and Biochemistry of Muscle as a Food.* University of Wisconsin Press, Madison, 1966.

43. Burr, I. M., Sizonenko, P. C., Kaplan, S. L., and Grumbach, M. M.: Hormonal changes in puberty. I. Correlation of serum luteinizing hormone and follicle stimulating hormone with stages of puberty, testicular size, and bone age in normal boys. *Pediatr. Res.* **4:** 25, 1970.

44. Scammon, R. E.: *Proceedings of the Second International Congress on Sex Research.* Oliver & Boyd, Edinburgh, 1931, p. 118.

45. Jenner, M. R., Kelch, R. P., Kaplan, S. L., and Grumbach, M. M.: Hormonal changes in puberty: IV. Plasma estradiol, LH, and FSH in prepubertal children, pubertal females, and in precocious puberty, premature thelarche, hypogonadism, and in a child with a feminizing ovarian tumor. *J. Clin. Endocrinol. Metab.* **34:** 521, 1972.

46. Sizonenko, P. C., Burr, I. M., Kaplan, S. L., and Grumbach, M. M.: Hormonal changes in puberty: II. Correlation of serum luteinizing hormone and follicle stimulating hormone with stages of puberty and bone age in normal girls. *Pediatr. Res.* **4:** 36, 1970.

CHAPTER 23

Prepubertal and Postpubertal Growth

Alex F. Roche and Gail Davila

The evidence presented in the preceding chapter suggested that the prepubertal growth spurt began at 9 to 10 years for the boys and 6 to 7 years for the girls and adolescent growth ended at about 20 years for the male and 17 to 18 years for the female. Analyses of anthropometric and longitudinal data gathered at the Fels Institute over a period of years are presented in this chapter. The analysis has been carried out with the aid of recently developed computer programs applied to the height and weight data of 200 normal subjects studied from birth to 22 years. A program for piecewise regression analysis divided the serial data *for individuals* into earlier and later subsets.[1, 2] Mathematically determined curves were fitted to each subset, and all possible junctions between these subsets were examined to determine the junction at which the goodness of fit was maximized for the two lines combined. This analysis should be used only if a preliminary examination of the data indicates that a change in the rate of growth occurs for the variable being studied during the age range considered. The effective use of the method depends also on the selection of suitable curves to fit the early and later subsets.

The method can be used to determine when these subjects ceased to grow in stature.[3] Preliminary analysis showed it was appropriate to fit a second-degree polynomial curve to the earlier subset and a zero-degree polynomial (horizontal straight line) to the later subset. Data recorded before the age of peak height velocity (PHV) were excluded so that very early data would not influence the result. Data recorded after 28 years were omitted because stature decreases at these ages.

The levels of these junctions provided excellent estimates of adult stature for individuals. The ages at these junctions provided more accurate estimates of the ages of growth cessation than those previously available. The ages for cessation of growth in stature were considerably later in the boys than the girls, whether considered on the basis of chronological age or the interval after peak height velocity (PHV). As expected, there were marked differences between individuals in these

Table 23.1 Centiles for ages at which adult stature was reached in 50 boys and 45 girls.

Ages	Boys			Girls		
	10	50	90	10	50	90
Chronological age (yr)	18.4	21.2	23.5	15.8	17.3	21.1
Years after PHV	4.4	7.8	10.3	4.6	6.0	9.8
Years after menarche	ND	ND	ND	3.8	4.8	6.7
Years after SA* 13 years	4.8	8.1	10.9	ND	ND	ND
Years after SA* 11 years	ND	ND	ND	4.7	6.3	9.7

* SA = skeletal age   ND = not determined

ages (Table 23.1). The girls grew for a considerable period after menarche but not for as long as boys after comparable Greulich-Pyle levels of skeletal maturity (13 years, boys; 11 years, girls). Stature increments after particular growth and development landmarks were larger in the girls than the boys but they varied markedly in each sex (Table 23.2). This occurred even for increments after the completion of epiphyseodiaphyseal fusion at the distal end of the femur or the proximal end of the tibia. The latter small but consistent sex-associated differences probably reflect variations between the sexes in late adolescent elongation of the trunk.[4-6] These data are important in stature prediction, patient management, and growth study design.

Table 23.2 Centiles for total increments in stature after growth and developmental landmarks.

Landmarks	Boys			Girls		
	10	50	90	10	50	90
16 years	1.2	2.8	7.2	- 0.1	1.1	2.7
18 years	- 0.3	0.8	2.3	- 0.4	0.6	1.4
PHV	11.6	17.8	23.7	10.8	15.8	22.3
Menarche	ND	ND	ND	4.3	7.4	10.6
Femur mature	0.6	1.4	2.7	0.3	1.0	2.0
Tibia mature	0.3	1.2	2.3	0.1	1.1	2.2

ND = not determined

Table 23.3   Centiles for ages of intersection
of polynomial lines for weight in 57
boys and 58 girls.

Ages	Boys			Girls		
	10	50	90	10	50	90
Chronological age (yr)	16.9	21.2	25.1	15.8	18.4	24.6
Years after PHV	4.0	8.2	11.5	3.5	7.3	12.8
Years after menarche	ND	ND	ND	2.5	5.6	11.8
Years after SA* 13 years	3.9	8.4	12.3	ND	ND	ND
Years after SA* 11 years	ND	ND	ND	4.3	7.3	14.0

* SA = skeletal age   ND = not determined

A preliminary analysis of serial weight data for the same group of children showed that discontinuities occurred when the decelerating rates of weight gain after PHV became relatively constant in late adolescence and early adulthood.[7] It was shown that it was appropriate to fit a second-degree polynomial to the earlier subset of data for each child and a first-degree polynomial to the later subset.

In the boys, the median ages of the junctions at which the fit was maximized for these two lines combined were the same as for stature (21.2 years). In the girls, the junctions occurred 1 year later (medians) for weight than for statute (18.4 years) (Table 23.3).

As expected, the total weight increments for particular growth and development landmarks to the ages of the junctions varied markedly (Table 23.4). The median

Table 23.4   Medians for total increments in
weight (kg) after soma growth and
developmental landmarks.

Landmarks	To intersection		To last weight	
	Boys	Girls	Boys	Girls
C.A. 16 years	7.5	1.6	14.0	3.9
C.A. 18 years	3.2	- 0.3	7.9	2.5
PHV	24.2	15.5	28.0	18.5
Menarche	ND	10.4	ND	11.2
Femur mature	5.5	0.7	14.2	3.4
Tibia mature	6.1	0.7	13.2	5.2

C.A.=Chronological age   ND=not determined

increments were much larger in the boys than the girls; this difference was particularly large after the femur and the tibia were mature. To compensate for sex-associated differences in rates of maturation, the total increments for girls after 16 years can be compared with those in boys after 18 years. Even after these corresponding maturity levels, the total increments were larger in the boys. Presumably, this reflects the occurrence of greater late adolescent growth in both trunk length and circumference in boys than in girls.[4-6] These normal data for individuals can assist the definition of nutritional needs during adolescence and the management of children with unusual body weights.

A different approach was used to analyze serial recumbent lengths from 1 to 18 years from many of the same children.[8] Previous attempts to fit mathematically defined curves to serial growth data have been successful but only for comparatively short age ranges, for example, birth to 3 years. It is not difficult to fit curves over any range using higher order polynomials; the problem is that the parameters of such curves cannot be interpreted biologically. The analysis to be described was an attempt to summarize 17 years of growth, *for each individual*, in a few parameters that had clear biological meanings.

The curve fitted was the sum (total) of two logistic components; these have been called the prepubertal and adolescent components (Figure 23.1). This concept was used because there is good cause to consider adolescent growth as something added to the typical primate growth curve in human beings.

Each component has three parameters with clear interpretations: maximum velocity (centimeters per year), age at the maximum rate (years), and the upper limit or complete contribution (centimeters). Because the sum of the two upper limits is known (recumbent length at 18 years), the total contribution of one component can be obtained by subtraction. Therefore, five parameters are needed to summarize an individual growth record. The total fitted curve fits the observed data points so closely that the addition of other parameters to the model is not justified.

According to the model, the final period of linear prepubertal growth is due to an approximate balance between deceleration of the prepubertal component and acceleration of the adolescent component. The asymmetry of the total spurt is due to the addition of the symmetric adolescent component to the decelerating phase of the prepubertal component.

The modal ages of 10 years for boys and 7 years for girls for the onset of the adolescent component closely match the ages for junctions between pairs of regression lines fitted to earlier and later cross-sectional data subsets for total body water, extracellular volume, total body potassium, and muscle cell population.[9-12] At these ages, there are increases in circulating gonadotropins and even earlier there are histological changes in gonads indicating pubescence.[13,14] The onset of the spurt in the total curve is masked by the balance between acceleration and deceleration in the two components.

The contribution of the prepubertal component varied similarly in each sex but the adolescent component was much more variable in the girls. The prepubertal component is the primary determinant of adult length. However, age at which the maximum velocity of the adolescent component occurs has a small but significant effect so that a delay is associated with greater adult length. According to the model, sex differences in adult length reflect differences in the prepubertal component.

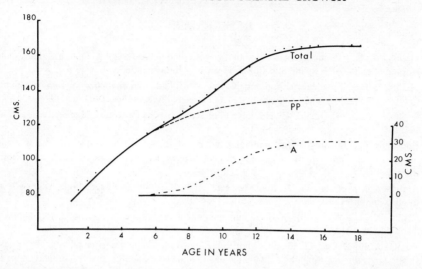

Fig. 23.1. Serial recumbent length data for a model girl in the Fels sample graphed against chronological age. The dots represent the observed data, many of which are hidden by the fitted curve labeled "Total." This is the sum of the two logistic curves: prepubertal (PP) and adolescent (A).

There is considerable interest in the mean values for some parameters of these curves (Table 23.5). The contribution of the prepubertal component is considerably larger in boys than in girls but the contribution of the adolescent component is similar in each sex. The age at maximum velocity of the adolescent component shows the familiar sex difference in timing; the sex difference in the maximum velocity of this component is small but real. There are negative correlations between the contributions of the prepubertal and adolescent components to final length. This homeostatic mechanism may be due to differential contributions by the trunk and lower extremities to the logistic components.

Existing stores of serial growth data can now provide more useful and more important information than was the case previously. When methods such as these described above are applied to other variables, and to groups of variables observed serially on the same children, understanding of growth and development will be markedly increased.

Table 23.5   Mean values for selected parameters of double logistic curves for recumbent length.

Parameters	Boys	Girls
Prepubertal component upper limit (cm)	149.7	138.0
Adolescent component upper limit (cm)	31.1	30.0
maximum velocity (cm /yr)	6.9	6.4
age at maximum velocity (yr)	13.0	11.0

REFERENCES

1. Mellits, E. D.: Estimation and design for intersecting regressions, Doctoral Thesis. Johns Hopkins School of Hygiene and Public Health, Baltimore, 1965.

2. Mellits, E. D.: Statistical methods. In: Cheek, D. B. (Ed.): *Human Growth; Body Composition, Cell Growth, Energy and Intelligence*. Lea & Febiger, Philadelphia, 1968, pp. 19–38.

3. Roche, A. F., and Davila, G. H.: Late adolescent growth in stature. *Pediatrics* **50**: 874–880, 1972.

4. Hansman, C.: Anthropometry and related data, anthropometry skinfold thickness measurements. In: McCammon, R. W. (Ed.): *Human Growth and Development*. Thomas, Springfield, Illinois, 1970, pp. 103–154.

5. Anderson, M., Green, W. T., and Messner, M. B.: Growth and predictions of growth in the lower extremities. *J. Bone Jt. Surg.* **45-A**: 1–14, 1963.

6. Roche, A. F.: The elongation of the human cervical vertebral column. *Am. J. Phys. Anthropol.* **36**: 221–228, 1972.

7. Roche, A. F., Davila, G. H., and Mellits, E. D.: Weight changes after puberty. In: Fuchs, E. (Ed.): *International Research Conference on Adolescence*. Mouton Press, The Hague, in press.

8. Bock, R. D., Wainer, H., Petersen, A., Thissen, D., Murray, J., and Roche, A.: A parametrization for individual human growth curves. *Human Biol.* **45**: 63–80, 1973.

9. Mellits, E. D., and Cheek, D. B.: Growth and body water. In: Cheek, D. B. (Ed.): *Human Growth; Body Composition, Cell Growth, Energy and Intelligence*. Lea & Febiger, Philadelphia, 1968, pp. 135–149.

10. Cheek, D. B., and Graystone, J. E.: Intracellular and extracellular volume (and sodium), and exchangeable chloride in children. In: Cheek, D. B. (Ed.): *Human Growth; Body Composition, Cell Growth, Energy and Intelligence*. Lea & Febiger, Philadelphia, 1968, pp. 150–164.

11. Reba, R. C., Cheek, D. B., and Leitnaker, F. C.: Body potassium and lean body mass. In: Cheek, D. B. (Ed.): *Human Growth; Body Composition, Cell Growth, Energy and Intelligence*. Lea & Febiger, Philadelphia, 1968, pp. 165–181.

12. Cheek, D. B.: *Human Growth; Body Composition, Cell Growth, Energy and Intelligence*. Lea & Febiger, Philadelphia, 1968.

13. Sniffen, R. C.: The testis. I. The normal testis. *Arch. Pathol. (Lab. Med.)* **50**: 259–284, 1950.

14. Blizzard, R. M., Johanson, A., Guyda, H., Baghadassarian, A., Raiti, S., and Migeon, C. J.: Recent developments in the study of gonadotropin secretion in adolescence. In: Heald, F. P., and Hung, W. (Eds.): *Adolescent Endocrinology*. Appleton-Century-Crofts, New York, 1970.

CHAPTER 24

Postnatal Cellular Growth:
Hormonal Considerations

Donald B. Cheek and Robert G. Wyllie

INTRODUCTION

In this chapter information on cellular growth in the human and the role of hormones during postnatal life are reviewed with particular reference to our own work.[1-11] Mention has already been made of hormonal influences on adolescent growth.[6] The study of the growth of muscle and its cellular components and the influence of hormones has occupied much of our time in recent years. The role of hormones in cell growth has been reviewed[3, 4], especially with respect to muscle and liver cells.[5] The growth of adipocytes and adipose tissue will be considered in the section on overnutrition (Chapter 26). Much information has been deleted in order to achieve brevity.

In our previous book, a major thesis was proposed, namely that the action of growth hormone is mainly involved in DNA replication while insulin stimulates cytoplasmic growth. Subsequent work has supported this contention, particularly with respect to the distinct actions of insulin and growth hormone on muscle growth. During puberty growth hormone is probably the major hormone for male adolescent growth, while in the female, insulin may prove to be of greater importance (Chapter 22). In the present chapter the action of these hormones in terms of nuclear replication and cytoplasmic growth is reviewed. A section of the chapter reports histometric studies on liver cells with simultaneous biochemical analyses. In other sections the actions and properties of thyroxine and somatomedin are discussed.

THE ACTION OF GROWTH HORMONE AND INSULIN ON MUSCLE

Some years ago, we found that when rats were hypophysectomized at 21 days there was not only cessation of DNA replication in muscle but a loss of DNA content (Figure 24.1). Clearly, the nuclear number in the muscle was less than the expected value at 21 days for intact rats. The protein : DNA ratio in muscle increased with time whether cell size was plotted against organ size (muscle mass) or against time (Figures 24.2 and 24.3). The growth of muscle mass following hypophysectomy was highly significant (Figure 24.1). It has been suggested that weight increase is mainly related to the fat deposition in pituitary insufficiency. It is possible that endogenous insulin, in the absence of growth hormone in hypophysectomized rats, may divert carbohydrate toward fat storage while insulin also increases the total protein within the musculature.

That endogenous insulin does play a role in the growth of the hypophysectomized rat is supported but not proven by the finding that the injection of streptozotocin[12] prevented increments in body weight following removal of the pituitary[4] (Figure 24.4). If no such intervention was carried out, the body weight reached a constant value at about 38 days postnatally or 17 days following hypophysectomy. If at that time the rat received exogenous insulin for 11 days, further growth occurred in the

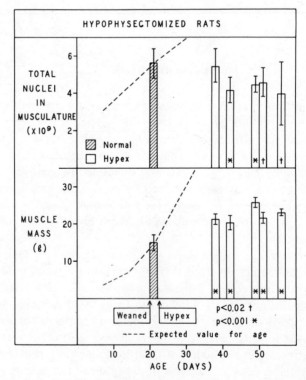

Fig. 24.1. Hypophysectomized (hypex.) rats, greater than 38 days of age are compared with normal 21-day-old animals. Note the reduction in total muscle nuclei and the small but significant increase in muscle mass.

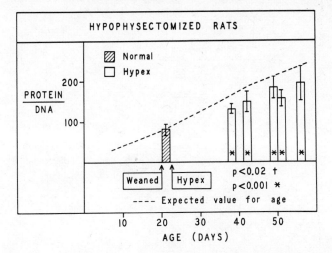

Fig. 24.2. Hypophysectomized (hypex.) rats, greater than 38 days of age are compared with normal 21-day-old animals. Note the significant increase in the ratio of protein to DNA.

liver, but almost no increase in muscle mass was found.[1] No further loss of muscle DNA was seen, however, and no diminution in the high protein:DNA ratio occurred (Figures 24.5 and 24.6).

It was found that DNA replication did increase in muscle in hypophysectomized rats given growth hormone with or without epinephrine. Moreover, with growth hormone and epinephrine injections the protein:DNA ratio fell below the level achieved by growth hormone per se, suggesting that the suppression of endogenous

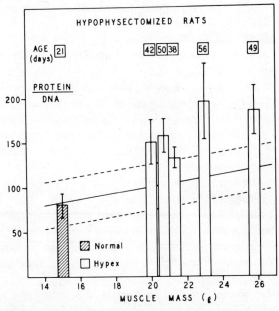

Fig. 24.3. The ratios of Protein:DNA are plotted against muscle mass in rats hypophysectomized (hypex.) at 21 days and subsequently examined at ages greater than 38 days. The lines represent the values for the normal animal.

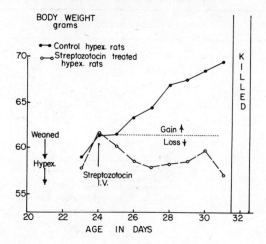

Fig. 24.4. The effect of hypophysectomy at 21 days together with injection of streptozotocin at 24 days on the body weight of the rat until 32 days of age. The body-weight curve for control hypophysectomized rats is also shown.

insulin by epinephrine caused reduced protein accretion. Insulin had no effect on muscle DNA content, hence the protein:DNA ratio in muscle remained elevated (Figure 24.5).

In an attempt to differentiate the actions of exogenous growth hormone and endogenous insulin on muscle cells, a group of hypophysectomized rats were given these hormones for 11 days as stated above, one group receiving injections of long-acting epinephrine in addition.[1] The latter hormone is known to block insulin release.[16] In the intact rat given protamine zinc insulin (PZ insulin) from the 24th to 38th day, food intake increases and muscle mass enlarges.[21] This expansion of muscle mass is accompanied by an accretion of protein relative to DNA as demonstrated in Figure 24.7. Body weight changes are shown in Figure 24.8 for these hormonal experiments.

The evidence just discussed leads us to suggest that insulin is primarily involved in the accretion of protein within the myofiber. In the absence of the pituitary such accretion continues for a time, perhaps until the cytoplasmic nuclear ratio reaches a limit. It has been shown that for some cells cytoplasmic size is limited. The failure of other workers[14,15] to appreciate the role of insulin in muscle growth in the absence of growth hormone may be due to the finding that growth continues in the hypophysectomized animal prior to the injection of exogenous insulin, presumably as a result of endogenous insulin.

The finding that nuclear replication in muscle and an increase in DNA can be achieved with growth hormone in the hypophysectomized rat or in the hypopituitary human dwarf, again supports the hypothesis that growth hormone stimulates DNA synthesis. Presumably, the satellite cells of muscle, discussed in Chapter 13, are involved in this sequence of events.

While an extensive discussion could be made concerning the relative merits of insulin versus growth hormone in protein accretion,[4,17] we prefer to take the view that for muscle, growth hormone is primarily responsible for cell number increase and insulin is concerned mainly with cytoplasmic growth.[4]

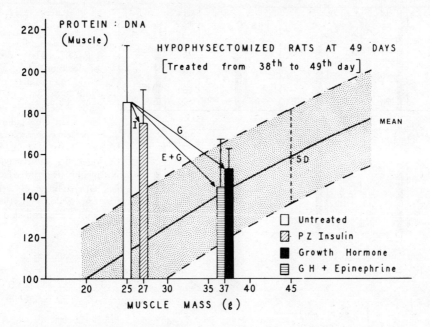

Fig. 24.5. Rats were hypophysectomized at 21 days. This figure shows the effect of subsequent administration of insulin (I), growth hormone (G), and long-acting epinephrine (to block endogenous insulin) together with growth hormone (E&G). The protein:DNA ratios in muscle were determined at 49 days.

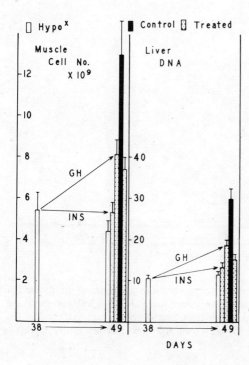

Fig. 24.6. Following hypophysectomy at 21 days the weight of the rat stabilizes by 38 days. If growth hormone is injected at this time until the 49th day, DNA replication in muscle occurs in the presence or absence of long-acting epinephrine (columns 2 and 5 on the right-hand side of the Figure). Untreated rats (clear column) lose DNA, whereas the injection of P. Z. insulin prevents this loss. In the liver insulin as well as growth hormone stimulates DNA replication.

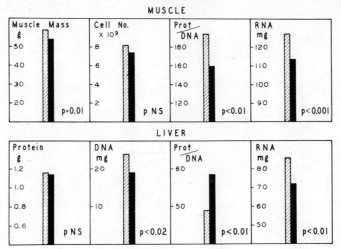

Fig. 24.7. The effect of injecting P.Z. insulin into the intact rats (26th–38th day) is shown for muscle and liver. The dark column represents control rats and the shaded column refers to rats receiving insulin. (Reprinted from Graystone et al: *Pediatr. Res.* **3**: 66, 1969, with the permission of the Editor.)

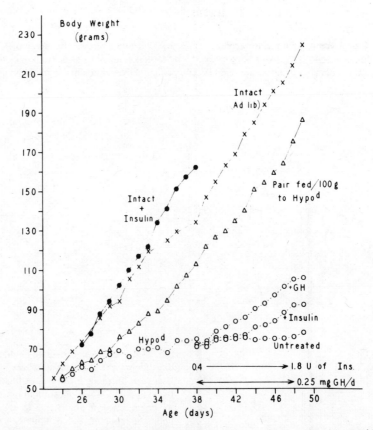

Fig. 24.8. Changes in body weight for different groups of rats are shown. The intact ad libitum fed rat is shown by the crosses. Data from intact rats receiving insulin are also shown (black dots); the weight of hypophysectomized rats is shown by the open circles. The weight changes as a result of the injection of insulin or growth hormone are also shown. Data from rats pair-fed to the hypophysectomized rats are shown by the triangles.

THE ACTION OF GROWTH HORMONE AND INSULIN ON LIVER

Biochemical Considerations

The amount of DNA may be used as a measure of cell number in the tissues with diploid cells. However, organs such as liver contain polyploid cells with 4N, 8N, 16N, or even 32N nuclei.[18-21] Parenchymal cells represent about 90% of the liver weight but have been said to contain only half the total organ content of DNA.[22] In some mammals such as mice as many as 70% of liver cells may contain two nuclei. Man and rat usually have liver cells with nuclei not exceeding 8N.[23] In binucleate cells the nuclei are of the same order, and the mass of cytoplasm within the cell is directly related to the degree of ploidy[23, 24] so that the ratio of protein to DNA may be used to monitor aspects of parenchymal cell growth. It has also been stated that the nucleolar volume is proportional to nuclear ploidy,[25] suggesting that a high-order cell is functionally equivalent to a group of smaller cells with the same total ploidy. The multiplication of diploid mononucleate cells is the major mode of liver growth until puberty in man[26] or until a weight of 8 to 10 g is reached in the mouse.[18] After that stage binucleate diploid cells appear, followed by polyploid cells, with little further increase in the total number of parenchymal cells. Polyploidy is evident as sexual maturation approaches. This is particularly true for the male and moreover castration of the male rat reduces the degree of polyploidy[19].

Snell-Smith mice have hereditary pituitary insufficiency and a lack of growth hormone and TSH[27] due to a recessive gene.[28] They stop growing at 14 days of postnatal life. The ratio of organ weight to body weight reaches a constant but infantile proportions exist. Only diploid cells are present in the liver and pancreas. Growth hormone is necessary for the higher ploidy cells to develop.[21] Such mice are unduly sensitive to insulin,[29] being subject to hypoglycemia, and some growth can be achieved by the injection of glucagon or growth hormone.[30] The latter hormone has the action of increasing pancreatic cells and the production of insulin.[31] However, most organs show a failure of DNA replication[32] in the absence of growth hormone and a reduction of protein relative to DNA.[33] The latter finding may be ascribed to concomitant cretinism and/or insulin insufficiency.[31]

The protein:DNA ratio tends to be higher in the liver of hypophysectomized rats. Both hypophysectomy and thyroidectomy halt the development of higher class cells while appropriate hormonal treatment restores the situation.[34, 35] In the untreated rat hypophysectomized at weaning, liver protein content increases from about 400 to 650 mg from 22 to 49 days postnatally. No increase in DNA is detectable and the RNA content remains decreased. We have studied the effects of intervention with either growth hormone or insulin (P.Z. insulin) in increasing doses as recommended by Salter and Best[14] and have demonstrated a significant increase in liver weight and of protein and RNA content.[1] The DNA content increased markedly with growth hormone but there was also some increase in DNA with the injection of insulin (Table 24.1).

These differences are unrelated to food intake, which was equal for all groups studied. The increase in protein relative to DNA in the liver of rats receiving insulin suggests that there is more cytoplasm relative to nucleus than in the normal liver cell. Attempts to block endogenous insulin with epinephrine in the presence of growth hormone did not prevent the DNA increase but did prevent the accretion of protein (not shown in Table 24.1).

Table 24.1   The effect of hormones on the liver composition of hypophysectomised rats (Animals hypex day 21, studied at day 38-50). The results of two experiments are shown, see text for explanation.

	Experiment 1			Experiment 2		
	Untreated	Insulin	Growth Hormone	Untreated	Insulin	Growth Hormone
Age (days)	50	50	50	49	49	49
N	8	18	9	9	8	8
Weight (g)	3.46 (0.17)	6.33* (1.14)	5.64* (0.42)	3.12 (0.36)	4.45** (0.76)	4.61** (0.40)
DNA (mg)	12.97 (1.80)	17.02* (2.83)	18.71* (2.17)	11.41 (0.81)	13.21** (0.93)	18.70** (1.32)
RNA (mg)	31.76 (3.39)	56.22* (8.67)	59.61* (8.20)	30.80 (3.57)	45.99*** (3.72)	49.66** (1.53)
Protein (g)	0.784 (0.047)	1.074* (0.129)	1.163* (0.085)	0.641 (0.044)	0.903** (0.042)	0.964** (0.051)
Prot/DNA	61.14 (6.27)	63.94 (7.71)	62.52 (5.00)	56.32 (3.96)	68.88*** (5.81)	51.70* (3.55)
RNA/DNA	2.48 (0.31)	3.34* (0.43)	3.22* (0.59)	2.71 (0.28)	3.50** (0.43)	2.66 (0.18)
Non Protein Dry Solid (g)	0.244 (0.050)	0.859* (0.345)	0.477* (0.057)	0.259 (0.067)	0.431 (0.227)	0.369 (0.105)

Values are means with SD in parenthesis. When compared with controls, * P = less than 0.005 and **P = less than 0.001.

The ratios of zinc to DNA and RNA to DNA were greater when insulin was injected, thus supporting the hypothesis that insulin (more than growth hormone) is active in producing protein accretion. The evidence led us to suggest that in the liver, insulin produces cytoplasmic growth while growth hormone is more likely to produce polyploidy.

This experiment has now been repeated with the same protocol[1] with the difference that the final doses of insulin necessary to ensure weight gain were much greater than in the previous experiment (Figure 24.9). In the second experiment, the rate of increase in liver weight was greater (Table 24.1). Rats receiving growth hormone gained in liver weight, DNA, RNA, and protein content. These findings differed from those of the first experiment: the increase in DNA was far greater in the insulin-treated rats, giving the same protein:DNA ratio as the control value. In the first experiment, however, the ratio was greater than the control value.

In the second experiment the nonprotein dry solid of the liver was greater than that for the controls in both groups treated with hormones. There was a difference between the two hormone-treated groups, the hypophysectomized rats receiving insulin having double the value for dry solid found for rats receiving growth hormone. In view of the fact that the fat content was the same in the liver of both of these groups of rats, a further component such as carbohydrate must have been present (see discussion later in this chapter).

In summary, from chemical analysis very little difference was found in liver between the effects of growth hormone and those of insulin when the dose of insulin was maximal.

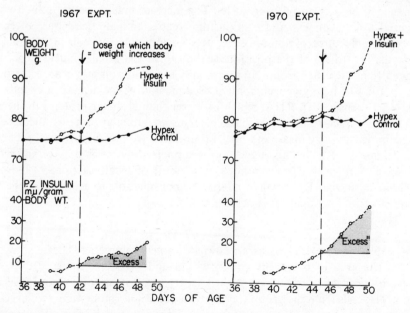

Fig. 24.9. A comparison of two experiments is shown in which P.Z. insulin was injected into hypophysectomized rats. The weight increase was greater in the 1970 experiment as was the amount of P.Z. insulin injected to produce the weight increase (or weight increase relative to control or untreated rats).

Histometric Considerations

These findings were extended by measurements made by interference microscopy on isolated liver cells and nuclei, and by use of a variety of histochemical reactions performed on fresh frozen sections of liver. Cell area and the diameter of cell nuclei were also measured.

The Nucleus

Statistical analysis of the data showed that if individual cell variances were used (pooling the data from cell counts rather than from individual rats) the dry mass of liver nuclei from rats given growth hormone or insulin were significantly higher than the value obtained for controls (Figures 24.10 and 24.11, Table 24.2). The nuclear volume was greater in cells of rats receiving growth hormone. If average cell values for each rat were used, the P value fell to less than 0.05. There is thus evidence to support the conclusion that higher ploidy cells developed in rats treated with growth hormone. This is compatible with the significant rise shown by these rats in DNA content in liver—a finding well established in the literature. Changes in volume of the nucleus correlate with changes in ploidy.[23, 24, 34—36] The increase in volume of the nuclei from rats receiving growth hormone may also be related to increments in nuclear protein that would be expected when nuclear volume increases in the presence of growth hormone.[37]

The higher mass and unchanged volume of nuclei from liver cells exposed to exogenous insulin are consistent with the finding of an increase of density. The distribution of nuclear dry mass about a mean of 2N, as found in the experiment with insulin, and the absence of any trace of localization about points of higher ploidy, argues strongly against a change in ploidy being responsible for the predominance of heavier and denser nuclei. The increase must have been due to some compound other than DNA. In the insulin-treated animals there were often two and occasionally three pyronin-positive RNA-containing nucleoli in the nuclei of many cells, regardless of the position of the cell in the lobule. Nucleoli occurred infrequently in the other groups and were only found in cells adjacent to the portal triads or areas of high glycogen content. Sedimentation coefficients have indicated that DNA is denser than RNA, which is denser than globular proteins in the ratio 30:20:5. Since nuclear acidic and basic proteins are globular proteins, the observed increase in density, dry mass, and nucleoli in nuclei from insulin-treated rats could be due to nuclear RNA. This suggestion is supported by the finding of an increase in the rate of nuclear RNA synthesis as a result of insulin action.[38] However, increments in nuclear RNA would have to be considerable to account for the findings and further investigation is needed.

The Cytoplasm

It is possible to use cell areas as an estimate of cell volume as Delesse showed in 1848.[39] The area of liver cells varied within and between groups (Table 24.2). Cells from the insulin group were slightly larger and less uniform than those from the controls; cells from the group treated with growth hormone were the largest.

The glycogen content, demonstrated as diastase-sensitive PAS-positive material, was elevated in all liver cells in the group of rats treated with insulin. The maximum amounts of glycogen were evenly distributed throughout the cytoplasm without any evidence of a gradient across the lobule (which was such a conspicuous feature in the other groups). This may explain the elevation of liver fat-free dry solid.

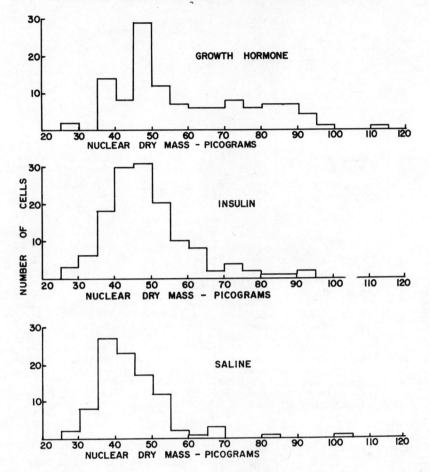

Fig. 24.10. The dry mass of liver cell nuclei is shown. These nuclei are taken from hypophysectomized rats receiving growth hormone, P.Z. insulin, or saline. Note the wide range of values shown by the group receiving growth hormone.

The distribution of RNA in the cytoplasm, estimated by the amount of pyronin-positive material, differed between groups. RNA in the control material was evenly dispersed in the cytoplasm and present in greatest amounts in cells near the portal triad. Liver cells from rats treated with growth hormone contained more pyronin-positive RNA, the concentration being highest in cells near the portal triads. The RNA in cells containing the most glycogen was not evenly dispersed but gathered into small discrete masses that were for the most part randomly distributed in the cytoplasm. Liver cells from rats treated with insulin contained less pyronin-positive RNA. Here the RNA was distributed about the nucleus with only an occasional fleck located more peripherally.

Discussion of Histometric Observations

The liver of the hypophysectomized rat is hypoplastic and has a reduced capacity to synthesize protein[40–42] and RNA. The defect in protein synthesis may be due to failure in the formation of peptide chains as suggested recently.[43] The nature of the defect in RNA synthesis is not known. The increase in gluconeogenesis

Table 24.2 The effect of hormones on the liver
           cell nuclei of hypophysectomised rats.

GROUP	Surface area u^2	Volume u^3	Dry mass pg	Density pg/u^3
A CONTROL				
Mean	712.2	1789.2	44.1	.0247
SE	17.7	66.5	1.6	.0012
B GROWTH HORMONE				
Mean	824.7	2244.4	58.2	.0262
SE	53.3	220.0	4.7	.0008
t, between A & B	2.0	1.98	2.85 $p<0.02$	1.02
C INSULIN				
Mean	720.1	1819.2	49.1	.0271
SE	16.5	61.1	1.4	.0008
t, between A & C	0.33	0.33	2.40 $p<0.05$	1.64

For statistical analyses of individual cells
(nuclei or cytoplasm) irrespective of which rat in
the group the cells come from, n=100 for GROUP A,
120 for GROUP B and 140 for GROUP C. The data are
significantly different for surface area, volume,
density, and dry mass, when GROUP B or C is
compared with A. However, for this table the mean
values from groups of rats are used for statistical
purposes and not the number of observations.

could be due to an increase in the amount of substrate available due to increased transport of amino acids or increased transamination, or both, with a concomitant diminution of activity in alternate metabolic pathways governing the synthesis of fatty acids, proteins, glycogen, and oxidation to CO_2 as suggested by Jefferson et al.[43]

Treatment with growth hormone has a marked effect on these metabolic defects. In the hypophysectomized rat, growth hormone increases the incorporation of orotic acid into nuclear and microsomal RNA and amino acids into protein,[44] and increases the number of polysomes in proportion to the amount of growth hormone administered.[42] Hybridization experiments showed that no new species of RNA were formed following the exposure to growth hormone.[45] The newly formed RNA resembled in all respects that produced by the liver nucleus of the untreated hypophysectomized rat.[46] There was no change in the chromatin template activity during these events.[45] Apparently in the hypophysectomized rat, growth hormone stimulates the synthesis of nuclear and microsomal RNA, the aggregation of polysomes, and the synthesis of protein by stimulating a mechanism that is already primed to function or already active, and which does not require additional information by transcription from DNA. This is in contrast to most other anabolic hormones (eg, estrogens), which require an increase in DNA template activity to fulfill their function.[47] Studies in the hypophysectomized rat involving the injection of growth hormone leave doubt as to the action of this hormone versus the action of endogenous insulin stimulated by growth hormone.

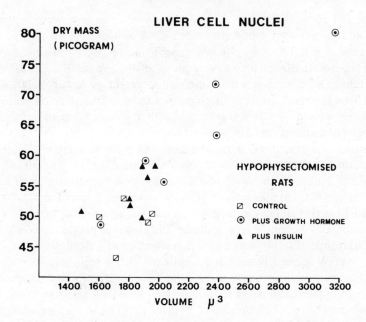

Fig. 24.11. The relationship of dry mass to volume for liver cell nuclei is shown. Groups of hypophysectomized rats receiving insulin, growth hormone, or saline are identified.

SOMATOMEDIN

Salmon and Daughaday in 1957[48] reported that growth hormone had the capacity to increase the incorporation of sulfate into the cartilage of hypophysectomized rats. This action was shown to be due not to the hormone itself but to an intermediate factor generated or released by growth hormone. This factor was called the sulfation factor and was nondialyzable. In March of 1965 at a Ross Conference, Daughaday[49] reviewed the data on sulfation factor. He emphasized that linear growth depended on proliferation of cartilage and the incorporation of protein into hydroxyproline. He showed convincingly that the "factor" was not growth hormone and that it could be sedimented if placed in a gravitational field of 100,000 g for 24 hours. At the same conference Cheek[50] reported that he and his co-workers had found that growth hormone was necessary for DNA replication in the muscle of hypophysectomized rats or in the muscle of Snell-Smith mice or for nuclear replication in the muscle of children with hypopituitarism. Subsequently, Beach and Kostoyo[51] showed that the increased incorporation of thymidine into DNA in muscle did not occur for several hours after the injection of growth hormone in the presence of pituitary insufficiency. Daughaday and Reeder[52] in similar experiments showed a delay in the incorporation of thymidine into DNA of cartilage of hypophysectomized rats. It has been suggested that the "sulfation factor" and "thymidine factor" may be the same peptide.[53] The factor responsible for sulfate incorporation into cartilage or tritium-labeled thymidine into DNA has been designated "somatomedin."[54]

Evidence now points to a family of closely related growth-stimulating peptides. The production of some of these may be stimulated by growth hormone. Levi-

Montalcini and co-workers[55,56] showed some years ago that nerve growth factor (NGF) from the maxillary gland stimulates RNA and protein synthesis in sensory and sympathetic ganglia. An epithelial growth factor (EGF) distinct from NGF has also been isolated from the salivary gland of the mouse.[57-61] EGF is a heat-stable, nondialyzable peptide with a molecular weight of about 6,500, and is responsible for epidermal growth. In epidermis from cultured chick embryo EGF will stimulate protein and RNA synthesis with the formation of activated polysomes. Erythropoietin stimulates production of red blood cells. Metcalf describes a colony-stimulating factor (CSF) in the clones of leukemic cells;[62] bone marrow cells do not undergo cell replication *in vitro* unless this factor is present, while in the acute phase of leukemia the level of CSF is increased significantly. Hall et al[63] and Bozovic et al[64] have isolated a growth-promoting factor from muscle which if subjected to high-voltage electrophoresis locates in a region similar to somatomedin. Pierson and Temin[65] have isolated a heat-stable protein (molecular weight about 5,000) from calf serum which causes replication of fibroblasts in tissue culture.

Initially Van Wyk used plasma from patients with acromegaly to isolate somatomedin. The method of bioassay was by the incorporation of sulfate into cartilage or the uptake of tritium-labeled thymidine into DNA of cartilage taken from the hypophysectomized rat. The uptake of both of these isotopes was inhibited if the sample to be tested had been exposed to proteolytic digestion with Pronase®. Anion exchange chromatography on DEAE cellulose allowed some separation from other plasma proteins. Investigation revealed that the molecular weight of somatomedin was in the region of 50,000 daltons, but subsequent work has suggested that such high values were due to aggregation or adsorption to larger proteins, the molecular weight probably being 4,000 to 8,000.[66] Acid ethanol extraction and Sephadex G-100 equilibrated with ammonium bicarbonate have been used in purification. Further purification by isoelectric focusing, ion exchange chromatography, and other electrophoretic separations has allowed Hall and Uthne[67] to purify somatomedin 1 millionfold. It is heat stable.

Somatomedin is not only involved in cell replication but in cartilage is responsible for the incorporation of uridine into RNA, proline into hydroxyproline, and the stimulation of amino acid transport. This is well seen in muscle also.[68,69] Both puromycin and actinomycin inhibit the action of somatomedin, suggesting that somatomedin is involved directly in protein synthesis. Somatomedin has insulin-like activity.[70,71,66,67] It enhances the transport of glucose across the cell membrane, the formation of glycogen in muscle, and the incorporation of fat into adipocytes; it also inhibits glycerol release.[72,73] Indeed, it has been postulated that somatomedin is identical to so-called nonsuppressible insulin-like activity (NSILA) in serum.[66] (NSILA is that insulin fraction not suppressed by antiinsulin antibodies.) No evidence exists to the contrary. It has been shown that somatomedin binds to the insulin receptors of adipocytes, liver cells, and chondrocytes, thus indicating structural homology with insulin.[73] It has been suggested that somatomedin is produced mainly by the liver and kidney.[74,75] In acromegaly high levels of somatomedin are found; in hypopituitarism there are low levels.[76] It is thought that in certain growth disorders, previously not well understood, there may be a disturbance of production of somatomedin (Laron dwarf, Turner's syndrome, the African pygmies).[77-80]

THYROXINE

Thyroid hormone is important to early postnatal growth. Cretinism can lead to permanent growth retardation and failure of protein accretion.[81] There is a marked reduction of protein relative to DNA in the muscle of patients with congenital hypothyroidism. In acquired hypothyroidism there is a reduction of DNA in the muscle mass and therefore a relative increase in the protein:DNA ratio.[82] It is known that growth hormone secretion is reduced in hypothyroidism.[83-87] In the growing rodent, thyroid ablation causes slowing of DNA replication[82, 88] and triiodothyronine can enhance the DNA replication in the hypothyroid rat.[89] Thus it is not clear whether the changes in cell growth are related to thyroid insufficiency or lack of growth hormone.

In infancy, both thyroid hormone and insulin must have an important role in protein synthesis but subsequently this role would appear to be undertaken by insulin per se: Leblond and Carriere[90] showed that the number of dividing cells in the intestinal mucosa (a tissue of rapid cell renewal) was reduced by thyroidectomy or hypophysectomy but returned to normal with growth hormone therapy. This supports once again the thesis that thyroxine acts to increase cell number through endogenous growth hormone.[91] Sesso and Valeri[92] in 1958 showed that growth hormone could increase the DNA content in the pancreas of rats previously subjected to hypophysectomy.

Removal of the pituitary produces arrest of bone growth in rhesus monkeys[93] and in rats.[94-97] Maturation continues (probably due to continued activity of thyroxine[93]), transformation of chondrocytes ceases and the epiphyseal plate narrows with eventual sealing by a transverse lamina of bone.[98] These changes can be reversed by growth hormone and enhanced by exogenous thyroid hormone. Thyroid hormone alone will increase bone growth in the hypophysectomized rat but not to expected levels and only for a limited time. Thyroid ablation early in postnatal life does not cause complete cessation of cell proliferation and the cartilage plate is not sealed by a lamina of bone.[99] The situation is reversed by administration of thyroxine which restores growth hormone release.[100] The action of growth hormone then is to promote chondrogenesis and to increase linear growth. Thyroxine stimulates maturation, but both hormones are necessary for chondrogenesis and osteogenesis.

SUMMARY

Evidence has shown that insulin can cause protein accretion in muscle in the presence or absence of the pituitary, while growth hormone is capable of producing nuclear replication and may not require insulin to produce this effect in muscle. Thyroid insufficiency may cause a depression of growth hormone release. The hypothesis has been made that the accretion of protein relative to DNA is characteristic of insulin activity and increments of DNA within the muscle mass are characteristic of growth hormone activity.

As we turn to liver cells the picture is less clear. The work of many investigators indicates that both insulin and growth hormone are involved in protein synthesis and in DNA replication. The increment in DNA found in the liver of the hypophysectomized rat with high doses of exogenous insulin does not signify that insulin is responsible for DNA replication within liver cell nuclei in physiological doses. The fact that protein accumulates in liver tissue following removal of the pituitary in rats is perhaps a more significant indicator of the role of insulin.

Histometric and histochemical techniques indicated the development of higher nuclear class cells in rats receiving growth hormone. The increase in mass of liver nuclei for rats receiving insulin was accompanied by an increase in density. It was suggested that increased RNA synthesis occurred in the nucleus following exogenous insulin. The finding of increased glycogen in the liver cells of insulin-treated rats may suggest alterations in metabolic processes.

Evidence indicates that somatomedin is a factor of central importance in growth. While we have drawn attention to the role of insulin in influencing cytoplasmic growth (of muscle for example) and growth hormone as activating nuclear replication, it is possible that somatomedin can achieve both actions.

In conclusion, optimal growth occurs when endocrine balance is achieved. For example, the anabolic actions of insulin and growth hormone are interdependent.[101–104] However, distinction should be drawn regarding whether growth hormones such as insulin exert effects on cytoplasmic growth primarily, or on nuclear replication. Thus the term "growth hormone" may be a misnomer and possibly future research will indicate that growth hormone should be designated nuclear growth hormone and insulin the cytoplasmic growth hormone.

Such thinking is true for adipose tissue (Chapter 26) where Bonnet et al.[105] have shown recently that growth hormone is responsible for fat cell multiplication while, as is well known, insulin increases fat cell size. In terms of organs such as liver the role of insulin versus growth hormone can only be differentiated in a mammal with isolated growth hormone deficiency in which one could also ablate B islet cells with streptozotocin. The recent discovery of the lit/lit mouse at The Jackson Laboratories by Dr. Eicher may well provide such a model where the action of each hormone can be studied separately.

REFERENCES

1. Cheek, D. B., and Graystone, J. E.: The action of insulin, growth hormone and epinephrine on cell growth in liver, muscle, and brain of the hypophysectomized rat. *Pediatr. Res.* **3**: 77, 1969.

2. Graystone, J. E., and Cheek, D. B.: The effects of reduced caloric intake and increased insulin-induced caloric intake on the cell growth of muscle, liver, and cerebrum and on skeletal collagen in the postweanling rat. *Pediatr. Res.* **3**: 66, 1969.

3. Cheek, D. B., Holt, A. B., Hill, D. E., and Talbert, J. L.: Skeletal muscle cell mass and growth: The concept of the deoxyribonucleic acid unit. *Pediatr. Res.* **5**: 312, 1971.

4. Cheek, D. B., and Hill, D. E.: The effect of growth hormone on cell and somatic growth. *Handbook of Physiology*, Section 7, Greep, R. O. and Astwood, E. B. (Eds.): *Endocrinology.* IV Part 2, Chapter 28, page 159, 1974.

5. Cheek, D. B., and Hill, D. E.: Muscle and liver cell growth: Role of hormones and nutritional factors. *Fed. Proc.* **29**: 1503, 1970.

6. Cheek, D. B.: Body composition, hormones, nutrition and adolescent growth. In: *Control of Onset of Puberty*, Grumbach, M. M., Grave, G. D. and Mayer, F. E. (Eds.): Wiley, New York, 1974, p. 424.

7. Parra, A., Schultz, R. B., Graystone, J. E., and Cheek, D. B.: Correlative studies in obese children and adolescents concerning body composition and plasma insulin and growth hormone levels. *Pediatr. Res.* **5**: 605, 1971.

8. Cheek, D. B., Graystone, J. E., and Read, M. S.: Cellular growth, nutrition and development. *Pediatrics* **45**: 315, 1970.

9. Cheek, D. B., Hill, D. E., Cordano, A., and Graham, G. G.: Malnutrition in infancy: Changes in muscle and adipose tissue before and after rehabilitation. *Pediatr. Res.* **4**: 135, 1970.

10. Cheek, D. B., and Graystone, J. E.: Changes in enzymes (GOT and GDH) and metals (Zn, Mn, and Mg) in liver of rats during endocrine imbalance and calorie restriction. *Pediatr. Res.* **3**: 433, 1969.

11. Graham, G. G., Cordano, A., Blizzard, R. M., and Cheek, D. B.: Infantile malnutrition: Changes in body composition during rehabilitation. *Pediatr. Res.* **3**: 579, 1969.

12. Pitkin, R. M., and Reynolds, W. A.: Diabetogenic effects of streptozotocin in rhesus monkeys. *Diabetes* **19**: 85, 1970.

13. Graystone, J. E., and Cheek, D. B.: The effects of reduced caloric intake and increased insulin-induced caloric intake on the cell growth of muscle, liver, and cerebrum and on skeletal collagen in the post-weanling rat. *Pediatr. Res.* **3**: 66, 1969.

14. Salter, J., and Best, C. H.: Insulin as a growth hormone. *Br. Med. J.* **2**: 353, 1953.

15. Wagner, E. M., and Scow, R. O.: Effect of insulin on growth in force-fed hypophysectomized rats. *Endocrinology* **61**: 419, 1957.

16. Porte, D.: A receptor mechanism for the inhibition of insulin release by epinephrine in man. *J. Clin. Invest.* **46**: 86, 1967.

17. Knobil, E., and Hotchkiss, J.: Growth hormone. *Ann. Rev. Physiol.* **26**: 47, 1964.

18. Leuchtenberger, C., Helweg-Larsen, H. F., and Murmanis, L.: Relationship between hereditary pituitary dwarfism and the formation of multiple desoxyribose nucleic acid (DNA) classes in mice. *Lab. Invest.* **3**: 245, 1954.

19. Schwartz, F. J.: Chemical and cytological aspects of rat liver growth. *Growth* **26**: 167, 1962.

20. Helweg-Larsen, H. F.: Nuclear class series. *Acta Pathol. Microbiol. Scand. Suppl.* 92, 1952.

21. Helweg-Larsen, H., and Nielson, E. L.: Studies on hereditary dwarfism in mice. X. Significance of the pituitary growth hormone to the relation between organ weight and body weight. *Acta Pathol. Microbiol. Scand.* **27**: 119, 1950.

22. Bucher, N. L. R.: Experimental aspects of hepatic regeneration. *N. Engl. J. Med.* **277**: 686, 1967.

23. Epstein, C. J.: Cell size, nuclear content, and the development of polyploidy in the mammalian liver. *Proc. Natl. Acad. Sci. U.S.A.* **57**: 327, 1967.

24. Epstein, C. J., Moses, H. L., Epstein, L. B., and Garrison, N. M.: A structural analysis of hepatomegaly induced by a hormone-secreting tumor. *Exp. Mol. Pathol.* **7**: 304, 1967.

25. Mironescu, S., and Dragomir, C.: Number, volume, surface and inner structure of the rat liver cells nucleoli. *Exp. Cell Res.* **48**: 140, 1967.

26. Schwartz, F. J.: The development in the human liver of multiple deoxyribose nucleic acid (DNA) classes and their relationship to the age of the individual. *Chromosoma* **8**: 52, 1956.

27. Elftman, H., and Wogelius, O.: Anterior pituitary cytology of the dwarf mouse. *Anat. Rec.* **135**: 43, 1959.

28. Carsner, R. L., and Rennels, E. G.: Primary site of gene action in anterior pituitary dwarf mice. *Science* **131**: 829, 1960.

29. Mirand, E. A., and Osborn, C. M.: Effect of fasting on blood sugars in hereditary hypopituitary dwarf mice. *Proc. Soc. Exp. Biol. Med.* **81**: 706, 1952.

30. Cavallero, C.: Glucagon and body growth in dwarf mice. *Lancet* **1**: 521, 1959.

31. Like, A. A., and Soeldner, J. S.: Pancreatic studies in hereditary pituitary dwarf mice. *Fed. Proc.* (*Abstr.*) **24**: 307, 1965.

32. Winick, M., and Grant, P.: Cellular growth in the organs of the hypopituitary dwarf mouse. *Endocrinology* **83**: 544, 1968.

33. Cheek, D. B., Powell, G. K., and Scott, R. E.: Growth of muscle cells (size and number) and liver DNA in rats and Snell-Smith mice with insufficient pituitary, thyroid or testicular function. *Bull. Johns Hopkins Hosp.* **117**: 306, 1965.

34. DiStefano, H. S., and Diermeir, H. F.: Effects of hypophysectomy and growth hormone on ploidy distribution and mitotic activity of rat liver. *Proc. Soc. Exp. Biol. Med.* **92**: 590, 1956.

35. Schwartz, F. J., and Ford, J. D., Jr.: Effect of thyroidectomy on development of polyploid nuclei in rat liver. *Proc. Soc. Exp. Biol. Med.* **104**: 756, 1960.

36. DiStefano, H. S., and Diermeir, H. F.: Effects of restricted food intake and growth hormone on rat liver proteins and nucleic acids. *Endocrinology* **64**: 448, 1959.

37. Korner, A.: Growth hormone control of biosynthesis of protein and ribonucleic acid. *Recent Progr. Horm. Res.* **21**: 205, 1965.

38. Steiner, D. F., and King, J.: Insulin-stimulated ribonucleic acid synthesis and RNA polymerase activity in alloxan-diabetic rat liver. *Biochim. Biophys. Acta* **119**: 510, 1966.

39. Delesse, A.: Pour determiner le composition des roches. *Ann. Mines., Paris*, 4th Series **13**: 379, 1848.

40. Simpson, M. E., Evans, H. M., and Li, C. H.: The growth of hypophysectomized female rats following chronic treatment with pure pituitary growth hormone. I. General growth and organ changes. *Growth* **13**: 151, 1949.

41. Talwar, G. P., Panda, N. C., Sarin, G. S., and Tolani, A. J.: Effects of growth hormone on ribonucleic acid metabolism. I. Incorporation of radioactive phosphate into ribonucleic acid fractions of rat liver. *Biochem. J.* **82**: 173, 1962.

42. Korner, A.: The effects of the administration of insulin to the hypophysectomized rat on the incorporation of amino acids into liver proteins *in vivo* and in a cell free system. *Biochem. J.* **74**: 471, 1960.

43. Jefferson, L. S., Robertson, J. W., and Tolman, E. L.: Effects of hypophysectomy on protein and carbohydrate metabolism in the perfused rat liver. In: Pecile, A., and Müller, E. E. (Eds.): *Growth and Growth Hormone Proc. 2nd Int. Symposium on Growth Hormone, Milan, 1971.* Excerpta Medica, The Netherlands, 1972.

44. Jefferson, L. S., and Korner, A.: A direct effect of growth hormone on the incorporation of precursors into protein and nucleic acids of perfused rat liver. *Biochem. J.* **104**: 826, 1967.

45. Gupta, S. L., and Talwar, G. P.: Effects of growth hormone on ribonucleic acid metabolism. The template activity of the chromatin and molecular species of ribonucleic acid synthesized after treatment with hormone. *Biochem. J.* **110**: 401, 1969.

46. Drewes, J., and Brawerman, G.: Messenger RNA patterns in rat liver nuclei before and after treatment with growth hormone. *Science* **156**: 1385, 1967.

47. Teng, C.-S., and Hamilton, T.: Role of chromatin in estrogen action in the uterus. II. Hormone induced synthesis of nonhistone acidic proteins which restore histone-inhibited DNA-dependent RNA synthesis. *Proc. Natl. Acad. Sci. U.S.A.* **63**: 465, 1971.

48. Salmon, W. D., Jr., and Daughaday, W. H.: A hormonally controlled serum factor which stimulates sulfate incorporation by cartilage *in vitro. J. Lab. Clin. Med.* **49**: 825, 1957.

49. Daughaday, W. H.: Studies on the effects of growth hormone on cartilage. In: Blizzard, R. M. (Ed.): *Human Pituitary Growth Hormone.* 54th Ross Conference, March 1965.

50. Cheek, D. B.: The effect of growth hormone on cell multiplication and cell size. In: Blizzard, R. M. (Ed.): *Human Pituitary Growth Hormone.* 54th Ross Conference, March 1965.

51. Beach, R. K., and Kostoyo, J. L.: Effect of growth hormone on the DNA content of muscles of young hypophysectomized rats. *Endocrinology* **82**: 882, 1968.

52. Daughaday, W. H., and Reeder, C.: Synchronous activation of DNA synthesis in hypophysectomized rat cartilage by growth hormone. *J. Lab. Clin. Med.* **68**: 357, 1966.

53. Van Wyk, J. J., Hall, K., Van den Brande, J. L., Weaver, R. P., Uthnea, K., Hintz, R. L., Harrison, J. H., and Mathewson, P.: Partial purification from human plasma of a small peptide with sulfation factor and thymidine factor activities. In: Pecile, A., and Müller, E. (Eds.): *Proceedings of the 2nd International Symposium on Growth Hormone.* Excerpta Medica, The Netherlands, 1972, p. 148.

54. Daughaday, W. H., Hall, K., Raben, M. S., Salmon, W. D., Jr., Van den Brande, J. L., and Van Wyk, J. J.: Somatomedin: Proposed designation for sulphation factor. *Nature (London)* **235:** 107, 1972.

55. Levi-Montalcini, R., and Cohen, S.: Effects of the extract of the mouse submaxillary salivary glands on the sympathetic system of mammals. *Ann. N.Y. Acad. Sci.* **85:** 324, 1960.

56. Angeletti, P. U., Gandini-Attardi, D., Toschi, G., Salvi, M. L., and Levi-Montalcini, R.: Metabolic aspects of the effect of nerve growth factor on sympathetic and sensory ganglia: Protein and ribonucleic acid synthesis. *Biochim. Biophys. Acta* **95:** 111, 1965.

57. Cohen, S.: Isolation of a mouse submaxillary gland protein accelerating incisor eruption and eyelid opening in the new-born animal. *J. Biol. Chem.* **237:** 1555, 1962.

58. Cohen, S., and Stastny, M.: Epidermal growth factor. III. The stimulation of polysome formation in chick embryo epidermis. *Biochim. Biophys. Acta* **166:** 427, 1968.

59. Hoober, J. K., and Cohen, S.: Epidermal growth factor. I. The stimulation of protein and ribonucleic acid synthesis in chick embryo epidermis. *Biochim. Biophys. Acta* **138:** 347, 1967.

60. Hoober, J. K., and Cohen, S.: Epidermal growth factor. II. Increased activity of ribosomes from chick embryo epidermis for cell-free protein synthesis. *Biochim. Biophys. Acta* **138:** 357, 1967.

61. Byyny, R. L., Orth, D. N., and Cohen, S.: Radioimmunoassay of epidermal growth factor. *Endocrinology* **90:** 1261, 1972.

62. Metcalf, D.: The colony stimulating factor (CSF). *Aust. J. Exp. Biol. Med. Sci.* **50:** 547, 1972.

63. Hall, K., Holmgren, A., and Lindahl, U.: Purification of a sulphation factor from skeletal muscle of rat. *Biochim. Biophys. Acta* **201:** 398, 1970.

64. Bozovic, M., Bostrom, H., Uthne, K., Berntsen, K., and Bozovic, L.: Effect of a growth-promoting factor from calf muscles on the weight gain of hypophysectomised rats. *Experientia* **26:** 156, 1970.

65. Pierson, R. W., and Temin, H. M.: The partial purification from calf serum of a fraction with multiplication-stimulating activity for chicken fibroblasts in cell culture and with non-suppressible insulin-like activity. *J. Cell Physiol.* **79:** 319, 1972.

66. Hall, K.: Human somatomedin. Determination, occurrence, biological activity and purification. *Acta Endocrinol. Suppl.* 163, 1972.

67. Hall, K., and Uthne, K.: Some biological properties of purified sulfation factor (SF) from human plasma. *Acta Med. Scand.* **190:** 137, 1971.

68. Adamson, L. F., and Anast, C. S.: Amino acid, potassium and sulphate transport and incorporation by embryonic chick cartilage: The mechanism of the stimulatory effects of serum. *Biochim. Biophys. Acta* **121:** 10, 1966.

69. Bozovic, M., Bostrom, H., and Bozovic, L.: Effect of a growth-promoting factor on protein synthesis and amino acid transport *in vitro*. *Experientia* **26:** 1194, 1970.

70. Salmon, W. D., Jr., and Duvall, M. R.: A serum fraction with "sulfation factor activity" stimulates *in vitro* incorporation of leucine and sulfate into protein-polysaccharide complexes, uridine into RNA, and thymidine into DNA of costal cartilage from hypophysectomized rats. *Endocrinology* **86:** 721, 1970.

71. Salmon, W. D., Jr., and Duvall, M. R.: *In vitro* stimulation of leucine incorporation into muscle and cartilage protein by a serum fraction with sulfation factor activity: Differentiation of effects from those of growth hormone and insulin. *Endocrinology* **87:** 1168, 1970.

72. Froesch, E. R., Müller, W. A., Burgi, H., Waldvogel, M., and Labhart, A.: Non-suppressible insulin-like activity of human serum. II. Biological properties of plasma extracts with non-suppressible insulin-like activity. *Biochim. Biophys. Acta* **121:** 360, 1966.

73. Hintz, R. L., Clemmons, D. R., Underwood, L. E., and Van Wyk, J. J.: Competitive binding of somatomedin to the insulin receptors of adipocytes, chondrocytes and liver membranes. *Proc. Natl. Acad. Sci. U.S.A.* **69:** 2351, 1972. See also Underwood, L. E., Hintz, R. L., Voina, S. J., and Van Wyk, J. J.: Human somatomedin, the growth hormone dependent sulfation factor, is antilipolytic. *J. Clin. Endocrinol. Metab.* **35:** 194, 1972.

74. McConaghey, P.: The production of "sulphation factor" by rat liver. *J. Endocrinol.* **52:** 1, 1972.

75. McConaghey, P., and Dehnel, J.: Preliminary studies of "sulphation factor" production by rat kidney. *J. Endocrinol.* **52:** 587, 1972.

76. Mayberry, H. E., Van den Brande, J. L., Van Wyk, J. J., and Waddell, W. J.: Early localization of 125-I-labelled human growth hormone in adrenals and other organs of immature hypophysectomized rats. *Endocrinology* **88:** 1309, 1971.

77. Laron, Z., Karp, M., Pertzelan, A., Kauli, R., Keret, R., and Doron, M.: The syndrome of familial dwarfism and high plasma immunoreactive human growth hormone (IR-HGH). In: Pecile, A., and Muller, E. E. (Eds.): *Growth and Growth Hormone.* Excerpta Medica, The Netherlands, 1972, p. 458.

78. New, M. I., Schwartz, E., Parks, G. A., Landey, S., and Wiedmann, E.: Pseudohypopituitary dwarfism with normal plasma growth hormone and low serum sulfation factor. *J. Pediatr.* **80:** 620, 1972.

79. Almquist, S., Lindsten, J., and Lindvall, N.: Linear growth, sulfation factor activity and chromosome constitution in 22 subjects with Turner's syndrome. *Acta Endocrinol.* **42:** 168, 1963.

80. Finkelstein, J. W., Kream, L., Ludan, A., and Hellman, L.: Sulphation factor—Somatomedin?: An explanation for continued growth in the absence of immunoassayable growth hormone in patients with hypothalamic tumors. *J. Clin. Endocrinol. Metab.* **35:** 13, 1972.

81. Sokoloff, L.: Action of thyroid hormones and cerebral development. *Am. J. Dis. Child.* **114:** 498, 1967.

82. Cheek, D. B.: Cellular growth, hormones, nutrition and time. Borden Award Address. *Pediatrics* **41:** 30, 1968.

83. Brauman, H., and Corvilain, J.: Growth hormone response to hypoglycemia in myxoedema. *J. Clin. Endocrinol.* **28:** 301, 1968.

84. Fink, C. W.: Thyrotropin deficiency in a child resulting in secondary growth hormone deficiency. *Pediatrics* **40:** 881, 1967.

85. Iwatsubo, H., Omori, K., Okada, Y., Fuchuchi, M., Miyai, K., Abe, H., and Kumahara, Y.: Human growth hormone secretion in primary hypothyroidism before and after treatment. *J. Clin. Endocrinol.* **27;** 1951, 1967.

86. Katz, H. P., Youlton, R., Kaplan, S. L., and Grumbach, M. M.: Growth and growth hormone. III. Growth hormone release in children with primary hypothyroidism and thyrotoxicosis. *J. Clin. Endocrinol.* **29:** 346, 1969.

87. MacGillivray, M. H., Aceto, T., and Frohman, L. H.: Plasma growth hormone responses and growth retardation of hypothyroidism. *Am. J. Dis. Child.* **115:** 273, 1968.

88. Brasel, J. A., Ehrenkranz, R. A., and Winick, M.: DNA polymerase activity in rat brain during ontogeny. *Dev. Biol.* **23:** 424, 1970.

89. Lee, K. L., Sun, S. C., and Miller, O. N.: Stimulation of incorporation by triiodothyronine of thymidine-methyl-^{3}H into hepatic DNA of the rat. *Arch. Biochem. Biophys.* **125:** 751, 1968.

90. Leblond, C. P., and Carriere, R.: The effect of growth hormone and thyroxine on the mitotic rate of the intestinal mucosa of the rat. *Endocrinology* **56:** 261, 1955.

91. Eartly, H., and Leblond, C. P.: Identification of the effects of thyroxine mediated by the hypophysis. *Endocrinology* **54:** 249, 1954.

92. Sesso, H., and Valeri, V.: Nucleic acid patterns in the pancreas of hypophysectomized rats after administration of growth hormone and of thyroxine. *Exp. Cell Res.* **14:** 201, 1958.

93. Knobil, E., Morse, A., Wolf, R. C., and Greep, R. O.: The action of bovine, porcine, and simian growth hormone preparations on the costochondral junction in the hypophysectomized rhesus monkey. Endocrinol **62:** 348, 1957.

94. Becks, H., Kibrick, E. A., Marr, W., and Evans, H. M.: The early effect of hypophysectomy and of immediate growth hormone therapy on endochondral bone formation. *Growth* **5:** 449, 1941.

95. Becks, H., Simpson, M. E., and Evans, H. M.: Ossification at proximal tibial epiphysis in the rat: Changes in females at progressively longer intervals following hypophysectomy. *Anat. Rec.* **92:** 121, 1945.

96. Ingalls, T. H., and Hayes, D. R.: Epiphyseal growth: The effect of removal of the adrenal and pituitary glands on the epiphysis of growing rats. *Endocrinology* **29**: 720, 1941.

97. Walker, D. G., Asling, C. W., Simpson, M. E., Li, C. H., and Evans, H. K.: Structural alterations in rats hypophysectomized at six days of age and their correction with growth hormone. *Anat. Rec.* **114**: 19, 1952.

98. Becks, H., Simpson, M. E., and Evans, H. M.: Ossification at proximal tibial epiphysis in the rat: Changes in females with increasing age. *Anat. Rec.* **92**: 109, 1945.

99. Simpson, M. E., Asling, C. W., and Evans, H. M.: Some endocrine influences on skeletal growth and differentiation. *Yale J. Biol. Med.* **23**: 1, 1950.

100. Koneff, A. A., Scow, R. O., Simpson, M. E., Li, C. H., and Evans, H. M.: Response by the rat thyro-parathyroidectomized at birth to growth hormone and to thyroxin given separately or in combination. II. Histological changes in the pituitary. *Anat. Rec.* **104**: 465, 1949.

101. Ketterer, B., Randle, P. J., and Young, F. G.: The pituitary growth hormone and metabolic processes. *Ergebn. Physiol.* **49**: 127, 1957.

102. Knobil, E.: The pituitary growth hormone: Some physiological considerations. In: Zarrow, M. X. (Ed.): *Growth in Living Systems.* Basic Books, New York, 1961, p. 353.

103. Korner, A., and Manchester, K. L.: Insulin and protein metabolism. *Br. Med. Bull.* **16**: 233, 1960.

104. Wagle, S. R.: The influence of growth hormone, cortisol and insulin on the incorporation of amino acids into protein. *Arch. Biochem.* **102**: 373, 1963.

105. Bonnet, F., Vanderschueren-Lodeweyckx, M., Eeckels, R. and Malvaux, P.: Subcutaneous adipose tissue and lipids in blood in growth hormone deficiency before and after treatment with human growth hormone. *Pediat. Res.*, **8**: 800, 1974.

CHAPTER 25

Nutrition and Restricted Nutrition

Joan Graystone and Donald B. Cheek

CALORIE INTAKE

It is stated that mammals grow fastest when they are youngest.[1] There is a mathematical basis for this statement, insofar as the total cellular growth conforms to Huxley's differential growth equation.[2] This means that cellular growth can be expressed as an allometric formula. Implicit in this concept of growth is the notion that the organism is in a state of positive energy and nitrogen balance to allow for the deposition of new tissue. Indeed during infancy and adolescence, the growth rate of an individual is used as the criterion for assessment of the nutritional status of that individual. That is, maximum growth implies optimum nutrition.

What is maximum growth? This concept is difficult to define, and problems of oversize are manifest in affluent societies of the world (Chapter 26). Waterlow[3] has expressed the opinion that the size explosion resulting from the assumption that the "bigger the better" is as dangerous for the future of the human species as the population explosion. Hence, his definition of "satisfactory" growth: "In a given population the growth rate of those who are well off and known to be well fed presumably represents the fulfillment of their genetic potential, and any rate which falls between the 10th and 90th percentiles for that group could be regarded as satisfactory." On this basis it should be possible to calculate the nutritional requirements for the maintenance of a satisfactory growth rate for any population and compare these values to the observed intake under normal environmental conditions.

Fomon et al[4] in recent work defined the calorie and protein requirement of the infant from 8 to 111 days postnatally, using a variety of diets each providing 67 cal/100 ml, and protein from fat-free cow's milk. They described the changes in body weight and length and, for the first time, showed a definite relationship between weight gain and calorie intake at various intervals during this age period.

Their data indicated that calorie expenditure for growth at that time is as high as one-third of the intake (or one-third of 525 cal/day). Implicit from their data is the conclusion that the composition of the diet may alter the rate of growth.

Earlier work by Holt and Snyderman[5] established the requirement of essential amino acids for infants. Using their data, Waterlow has calculated that essential amino acids must constitute about 33% of the total protein intake in the 2-month-old infant to satisfy the minimum requirement for maintenance and growth. Milk protein contains approximately 50% of essential amino acids and appears to be utilized with an efficiency of about 80% in well-nourished infants fed ad libitum.[4] Therefore diets based on milk protein should provide the essential amino acid requirements with a reasonable margin of safety.

Rose and Mayer[6] concluded from their study of infants 4 to 6 months of age, that activity was a greater determinant of total calorie intake than growth. The relationship between calorie intake and growth became apparent only when the influence of activity was removed from the analysis of variance. They calculated that the average infant of their study expended only 7% of his total calorie intake on growth and 27% on activity. It is of interest to note that, if the assumptions made by Fomon relating to the composition of the weight gain[5] are applied to their data, the percentage of total calories required for growth is increased to 16% and the energy expenditure of activity is reduced to 18%, suggesting that approximately equal percentages of the total calorie intake are required for activity and growth during this age period. Again referring to Waterlow's calculations,[3] partitioning of calorie requirements for infants 3 to 6 months of age using recommended calorie intake data from the Food and Agricultural Organization,[7] results in the requirement of equal calories for growth (15.5 cal/kg/day) and for activity (15 cal/kg/day). The percentage of total calorie intake available for activity increases to 15% by 1 year of age.

A close relationship is apparent between growth and basal calorie requirement curves in infancy. Heald et al[8] have reviewed the available information on dietary intake from childhood through adolescence under normal environmental conditions. The data indicate that a similar relationship exists between the increments in ad libitum intake and increments in growth. A difference between the sexes emerges at puberty. The calorie demands parallel the adolescent growth spurt in boys. These needs diminish from 16 to 19 years coincident with the diminishing growth rate. In girls, calorie intake steadily rises to age 12 then gradually declines to a plateau level around age 18. The combined data confirm the observations of Wait and Roberts[9] in 1932 that increments in calorie intake relate precisely to increments in body length up to the time of sexual maturation.

Heald[8] states that although a decreased demand for nutrients essential for growth may be responsible for the reduction in calorie intake in late adolescence, diminished physical activity could also reduce the total energy requirements at that time. Because of the lack of data relating to physical activity he finds it impossible to differentiate between decelerated growth and decreased physical activity as the major factor contributing to the reduction of calorie consumption.

Our own work has shown that positive correlations are obtained when lean body mass, cell mass, and nuclear number in the muscle are related to calorie intake from infancy to adolescence in normal children.[10] Recently, Forbes[11] demonstrated that adolescent boys had a much higher ratio of lean body mass to height than did adolescent girls. The slope of the regression relating the two parameters was also greater for boys. These differences did not exist prior to adolescence. Since lean body mass comprises the bulk of the actively metabolizing tissues of the body,[12] the greater nutritional requirements of the adolescent boy are only an indication of the demands of the growth process.

The accumulated data demonstrate that there is a relationship between total body potassium content (an index of lean body mass) and body length in the infant, through childhood and adolescence and in both young and old adult individuals[10,13-15]. Forbes suggested that because of the relationship between height and lean body mass (developed from his data), nutritional requirements should be related to the velocity of growth in length.

Earlier, the 1930 White House Conference Committee on Nutrition[16] found that the best prediction of calorie needs for both boys and girls was that expressed in terms of calorie requirement as a function of height. On the basis of the information obtained from body composition studies on normal subjects, the nutritional and concomitant calorie requirements of an individual are directly related to the amount of actively metabolizing tissue associated with length according to the age and sex of the individual.

This approach may be applied to situations of abnormal growth. In overnutrition and obesity, the lean body mass and intracellular mass are increased relative to age and body length. Excess nutritional intake produces excess growth and early maturation. Conversely, the reduced cell mass demonstrable in the growth-retarded child resulting from maternal rubella infection[73] or from congenital heart disease is associated with a reduced food intake.

The infant or child with congenital heart disease exhibits reduced protein-calorie intake whether or not cardiac failure is present. The first year of life may be associated with multiple episodes of cardiac failure resulting in prolonged periods of hypoxia. Sympathetic overactivity is evident as demonstrated by excessive catechol excretion during cyanosis,[17] the metabolic rate is high, and protein intake low with a resulting negative nitrogen balance. The hypoxic episodes can vary in severity and can recur for years. It is known that hypoxia upsets the balance between epinephrine, cortisol, and insulin and retards cell multiplication.[18-21]

It is not surprising that the cell mass, muscle mass, and extracellular mass are significantly reduced for body length up to the time of sexual maturation in these children. The number of nuclei in their muscle is reduced. A priori, one would suspect growth retardation of soft tissues. The reduced nutrition coupled with endocrine imbalance, hypoxia, and poor delivery of substrates to tissues leads, no doubt, to permanent changes. While these investigations were mentioned in our earlier book there are no detailed studies during and after adolescence in the child with congenital heart disease. Sexual maturation if delayed may allow adequate "catchup growth."

Growth retardation is apparent in children with congenital heart disease even in the absence of cyanotic episodes, indicating that nutrition and other factors are of importance. Calorie intake is reduced but activity is also reduced and, in the absence of cardiac failure, the basal metabolic rate is normal. There is evidence of a significant nitrogen leak occurring in these patients[21] but the route of loss has not been found.

Scrimshaw[22] states that normal growth in children is interrupted, not only during a period of negative nitrogen balance, but also during both the catabolic and anabolic stages of the stress reaction. A depression of appetite leading to reduced food intake is the result of stress. There can be an alteration in the type of food consumed with a resultant imbalanced intake. Other effects are reduced serum levels of various vitamins and negative calcium balance. Such findings may be relevant to the child with congenital heart disease.

RESTRICTED NUTRITION IN HUMANS: CELL MASS

In the development of clinical malnutrition, while a low total calorie intake is obviously important, alterations in the protein:calorie ratio in the diet are also considered to be of significance. A deficiency of protein with more than adequate calories results in kwashiorkor characterized by the presence of edema in the child whose body weight is more than 60% of that expected. Deficiencies of both protein and calories lead to marasmus in which there is no edema and body weight is less than 60% of expected weight.[23]

We have measured the intracellular mass (ICW) in Peruvian infants with marasmus (Figure 25.1).[24, 25] Intracellular mass is disproportionally reduced relative to body length and does not reach expected values even after 5 months of rehabilitation. Initially all infants had severe growth deficits. On the average, the "height age" was 40% below expected and "weight age" was only 15% of that expected for chronological age. There were losses of cell mass and body fat. Rehabilitation of patients did result in accelerated growth and after 5 months, height age was 60% of that expected for chronological age. There was an obvious increase in the amount of adipose tissue; however, the lipid per cell was still lower than expected. It was noteworthy that the smaller infants (under 11 months of age) showed reduced growth of both muscle and intracellular mass.

Changes in muscle mass are shown in Figure 25.2 before and during rehabilitation. Figure 25.3 documents the ratio of hydroxyproline to creatinine excretion. In general, while both of these indices increased, the increment in hydroxyproline was greatest. This suggests a greater growth of collagen than of muscle. (Hydroxyproline excretion, recently reviewed by Teller et al,[26] is considered to be a direct index for the proliferation of cartilage cells and collagen turnover. The work of Waterlow et al[27] and our own work support the thesis that creatinine excretion reflects muscle mass even under conditions of undernutrition.)

Muscle is a tissue of major importance in protein restriction. Waterlow states: "Reduction of muscle mass is probably the best available indicator of the extent of protein depletion in the body as a whole."[27] Inspection of muscle tissue (obtained by biopsy) demonstrated a large reduction in the protein:DNA ratio especially relative to body size (or body water). (See Chapter 22.) At the same time the RNA:DNA and magnesium:DNA ratios were reduced and did not reach expected levels after 5 months. The zinc:DNA ratio was reduced initially but was at the level expected at the later date. There was some reduction in the number of muscle nuclei for age but this reduction was not impressive. This statement of course assumes that the small muscle sample is representative of the entire muscle mass. Under these conditions, the relative increase in collagen and fibrous tissue containing DNA might well contribute significantly to the amount of DNA outside the myofiber; usually only 25% of nuclei are outside the myofiber.

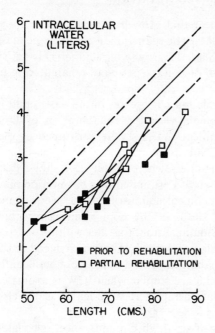

Fig. 25.1. The intracellular water (ICW), an index of intracellular mass is shown in infants with protein-calorie malnutrition (PCM) before rehabilitation (filled-in squares) and after 5 months of rehabilitation (open squares). Note that in these infants proportional relationships between intracellular mass and body length are not restored after 5 months.

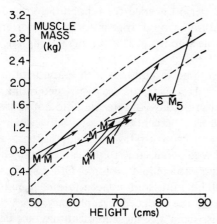

Fig. 25.2. Muscle mass (from creatinine excretion) is plotted against body length. Muscle mass (a component of cell mass) is not restored after 5 months of rehabilitation.

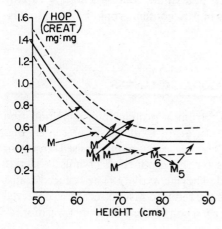

Fig. 25.3. The ratio of urinary hydroxyproline to urinary creatinine is shown in infants with PCM before and 5 months after rehabilitation. Note that in general the ratio is increased after rehabilitation, indicating that connective tissue growth is greater than that of metabolically active protoplasm (muscle).

From the discussion just presented it is clear that growth retardation is disproportional in protein-calorie malnutrition (PCM). The reduction of cytoplasmic mass is far greater than that of the skeletal mass. Also, the growth of metabolically active tissue is small relative to the increase in length during the period of rehabilitation in the younger infant.

The hypothesis that accretion of cytoplasmic mass is greater in the older child is supported by studies carried out in Guatemala with the collaboration of Drs. J. Habicht, J. Berall, and J. Viteri. The chemical analyses were performed by our laboratory while Dr. L. Novak of the Mayo Clinic assisted with the interpretation of data. These studies will be published in detail elsewhere. Table 25.1 shows data pertinent to this discussion. Intracellular water was estimated in a hospital population of boys admitted for reasons other than clinical malnutrition, the group being considered representative of the nutritional status of the population as a whole. The results from boys suffering from clinical malnutrition, together with those from children at two stages of rehabilitation, are also presented. ICW was reduced in the malnourished group and increased with rehabilitation to a value not significantly different from the reference group. The results are similar when ICW is expressed as a percentage of total body water. The relationship of ICW to length is depicted in Figure 25.4.

Anthropometric measurements, such as calf or thigh circumference, correlated well with measurements of ICW. Clearly the period needed for rehabilitation and restoration to "proportional growth retardation" would appear to be of shorter duration in older children, notwithstanding the importance of the magnitude and duration of the insult in protein restriction.[28, 29]

There was an expansion of extracellular volume in children with malnutrition. This has also been demonstrated by Alleyne.[30] However, the use of ^{40}K determinations to assess the cellular mass of children after 20 days of refeeding did not show any changes in ICW when this was expressed as a percentage of total body water.

Reba et al[12] have found that, in normal and growth-retarded children, the use of total body potassium underestimates ICW when compared to the value obtained from the measurement of total body water and extracellular volume. Other studies indicate that there is a reduction of intracellular potassium concentration in malnourished children[31–33] which, together with the reduced cytoplasmic size,[25] could mean that interpretation of cellular mass from ^{40}K measurement may not be reliable. It would appear that intracellular potassium concentration is rapidly corrected with therapy so that later increases in ^{40}K content would reflect cytoplasmic expansion.[34]

METABOLIC AND HORMONAL CHANGES

The metabolic changes associated with the spectrum of protein-calorie malnutrition are the subject of a recent review by Alleyne et al.[35] Evidence is presented that indicates some impairment in glucose tolerance, presumably caused by poor transport into the cell. *In vitro* experiments on the production of muscle lactate do not indicate any abnormality in glycolytic enzyme activity. The reduced transport of glucose into the cell may be related to the reduced insulin secretion observed by many workers.[36, 37] The relatively higher carbohydrate intake in kwashiorkor

Table 25.1 Anthropometric data and intracellular water (ICW) measurements in normal and malnourished children.

GROUP		AGE (yr)	HEIGHT (cm)	WEIGHT (kg)	ICW (L)	CIRCUMFERENCE CALF (cm)	CIRCUMFERENCE UPPER ARM (cm)	I.C.W. as % T.B.W.
I No history of clinical malnutrition	Mean	3.61	88.6	12.81	5.48	19.3	15.3	59.9
	SD	0.99	4.9	1.98	1.32	1.5	1.2	5.1
	N	14	14	14	14	12	12	14
II Clinically malnourished	Mean	4.35	84.2	10.90	3.86**	15.9**	12.0**	51.7**
	SD	1.42	8.0	2.46	0.67	2.2	1.2	4.0
	N	8	8	8	8	8	8	8
III Malnourished rehabilitation period 1 to 4 months	Mean	4.02	85.2	11.57	4.37*	17.0**	13.1**	52.6**
	SD	1.07	7.1	1.65	1.07	1.4	0.9	6.0
	N	12	12	12	12	12	12	12
IV Malnourished fully rehabilitated	Mean	3.27	83.1*	12.21	4.74	18.3	15.1	60.2
	SD	1.47	8.7	2.10	0.74	1.5	1.9	4.8
	N	14	14	14	14	14	14	14

When compared with Group I values using student t test; * P is less than 0.05
** P is less than 0.005

443

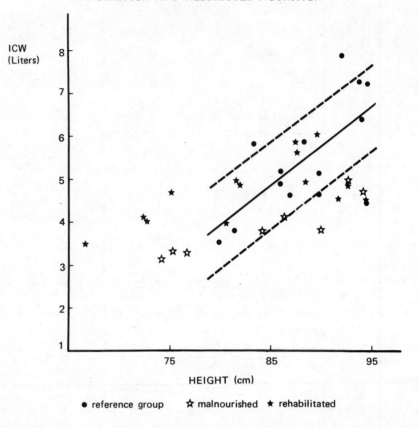

Fig. 25.4. The ICW or intracellular mass index is plotted against body length for boys in Guate-mala. Control data are shown by filled-in circles and the regression line with ± one standard deviation. Boys rehabilitated for 2 months with an adequate diet (shown by stars) elevate their ICW relative to length while boys malnourished without an adequate diet show a disproportionate ICW relative to length (stars with a central open circle). Thus malnutrition causes retardation in body weight and body length but when protein deprivation is present the reduction in cell mass is dis-proportionately low relative to body length. In older children the presence of an adequate diet causes rapid restoration to a proportional situation (cf Fig. 25.1).

may be associated with a high incidence of fatty liver, possibly due to decreased manufacture of low-density lipoproteins.

Waterlow, Alleyne, and associates have contributed much information toward our understanding of protein turnover in malnutrition.[35, 38, 39] In the malnourished child, both protein synthesis and catabolism are increased compared with the findings after rehabilitation. The hormonal changes observed in marasmus or PCM may be an index of the adaptive changes of the child to the reduced protein intake. As mentioned previously, insulin secretion is reduced, therefore the output of amino acids from the muscle could be expected to increase. The high or normal levels of circulating growth hormone[37, 40] and cortisol,[35, 39] both of which are insulin antagonists, may exert similar effects. At the same time, very little nitrogen is lost as urea. This adaptation to a reduced protein intake has been observed over many years[41] and is a phenomenon of importance to the fetus restricted in protein, as we have discussed earlier in this book with reference to renal growth (Chapter 17).

The hormonal changes in marasmus or PCM are of considerable interest. Conflicting reports appear about the response of these infants to the stimulus of arginine infusion. Beas and co-workers[42] found low levels of circulating growth hormone in marasmic infants aged 6 to 13 months and little or no response to arginine stimulation. Parra et al[43] reported that their subjects aged 2.5 to 9 months exhibited a normal growth hormone response to stimulus but the immunoreactive insulin level was significantly depressed. Similar findings with regard to insulin have been reported by other workers.[24, 44] This finding may explain why many months of rehabilitation are required for the infant to return to normal levels of growth since, as we have emphasized, insulin is important to cytoplasmic growth.[24] However, it is known that 25% of adult Australian aboriginals have diabetes mellitus and PCM is common in infancy.

It would appear that tissue insensitivity to growth hormone occurs in PCM or, as with insulin, hormonal levels are significantly reduced. The argument can be presented that lipolysis or gluconeogenesis predominates and that hormones are playing a purely metabolic role with no relationship to growth.

At the clinical level the situation is complex. Factors such as trace metal deficiencies,[25, 45-47] vitamins,[22] immunologic aberrations,[48] and various infections accentuate the already precarious nutritional state resulting from impoverished environmental conditions.

Monckeberg et al[49] claim to have accelerated growth in malnourished infants with human growth hormone during rehabilitation, a finding not supported by Hadden and Rutishauser.[50] The latter workers found that growth hormone given during rehabilitation did not have a significant effect on nitrogen retention or fatty acid mobilization. Experimental studies, to be discussed later, indicate that the proportion of protein to calories in the diet producing clinical malnutrition is an important factor in determining the effect of exogenous growth hormone during rehabilitation.

Further research into the mechanisms of hormonal response to malnutrition is necessary. Enquiry into the endocrine pancreatic response must include investigations into the interaction between insulin and glucagon. Glucagon is considered to play an important role in the metabolic adaptations of the adult to periods of fasting.[51] Recent reports by Becker et al suggest that an impaired gut betacytotrophic mechanism is involved in the diminished release of insulin to the stimulus of oral glucose. Following the improvement in nutritional status, there is a disproportionate increase in the response to oral glucose compared with that from intravenous glucose administration.[52, 53]

RESTRICTED NUTRITION IN RODENTS

An increase in the understanding of the metabolic processes that precede and accompany human nutritional disease syndromes, such as beri-beri, scurvy, rickets, and pellagra, followed the development of experimental animal models that enabled extensive laboratory investigations to be performed. The syndromes produced were the result of single nutritional deficiencies. A different situation exists in protein-calorie malnutrition which results from a complex insult seldom, if ever, related to a diet deficient in calories or protein alone. For example, concomitant deficiencies in the calcium, magnesium, potassium, and vitamin content are usual.

The key to the understanding of the metabolism of protein deficiency is the "differentiation between the effects of the normal adaptation by an organism to an abnormal diet and the pathological effects resulting from dietary abnormality.[41]"

Considerable information is available about the effects of restricted nutrition on the developing rat. The timing of the dietary insult is important in the effect produced in the growing animal. The effect of food restriction on the cellular growth of rats has been shown to be dependent on the phase of growth of the tissue at the time of restriction.[54, 55] No attempt was made in the study of Winick and Noble[55] to separate the effects of protein restriction from calorie restriction on cellular growth.

Food restriction in the preweaning period, obtained by increasing the litter size, results in both protein and calorie restriction and causes permanent growth retardation. A full complement of cells is not attained (see Cheek et al[56] for review). In the postweaning period it is possible to present diets varying in the degree of protein restriction. Only a moderate reduction in calories can be investigated, since a severe restriction will result in the use of protein for energy requirements rather than for growth.

Calorie restriction without protein restriction causes a slowing of cell multiplication and a delay in sexual maturation,[57] but eventually a full complement of cells is present in muscle and liver.[58] The experiment of Hill et al[59] indicated that a severe calorie plus protein restriction leads to almost complete cessation of growth. These rats gained only 10 to 15 g in body weight from 23 to 48 days of age compared with the control gain of 150 g. The ratio of muscle mass to skeletal mass was reduced (Table 25.2). Other findings included a decreased circulating insulin level and a reduction in the protein:DNA ratio of the muscle and liver cells.

If the weanling rat receives a 40% casein diet but is given only 60% by weight of the control ad libitum intake, then the rat receives a protein-sufficient but calorie-deficient diet. This diet produces growth retardation but, in this case, the reduction in muscle mass to skeletal mass is proportional (Table 25.2). The change in tissues suggests a slowing of cell multiplication but no reduction in cytoplasmic mass. The reduction in circulating insulin levels was not as marked as that of the protein-calorie-restricted group. This study demonstrated the striking differences in effect of the two diets. Other workers have shown that if calorie restriction is sustained for the major part of the life span, growth is compromised and the expected levels of cell number are not reached.[60]

Further investigations have been carried out using the rat fed a protein-sufficient, calorie-deficient diet (unpublished data). One group of these rats was given 250 μg of bovine growth hormone (GH) per rat per day and another group injected with saline, the diet remaining calorie deficient. The only difference that could be detected 2 weeks later was a decrease of carcass collagen (Table 25.3). The inference from the data is that the rats receiving growth hormone were insensitive to the hormone. By contrast it is known that if a normal diet is fed to rats previously fed a

Table 25.2 Changes in muscle mass and skeletal mass in rats subjected to dietary restriction.

	Control	Protein/ Calorie Deficient	Protein Sufficient/ Calorie Deficient
	27% casein 59% sucrose	6% casein 80% sucrose	40% casein 46% sucrose
Muscle Mass (MM) g	72	23*	53*
Skeletal Mass (SM) g	32	13.1*	23.3*
MM/SM ratio	2.09	1.81*	2.44

* P is less than 0.02

calorie-deficient diet and growth hormone is administered, then accelerated growth is produced.[61] These results are comparable with those found by Monckeberg in the human.[49] Moreover, it is claimed that intact rats fed isocaloric diets accelerate growth if given growth hormone.[62] Howarth[63] used diets similar in casein composition to that used by Hill et al.[59] Howarth supplemented his diet with 0.5% methionine and demonstrated that protein synthesis had priority over DNA synthesis when muscle growth was impaired by feeding a protein-deficient diet. Insulin

Table 25.3 The effect of growth hormone administration on the body composition of protein sufficient/calorie deficient rats.

	Control	Growth Hormone Treated
Muscle Mass g	58.8	59.0
Nuclear No. x 10^9	8.8	9.0
Carcass		
Protein mg/g FFDS	730	733
Collagen mg/g FFDS	111	101*
Non Coll. Prot. mg/g FFDS	619	632

* P is less than 0.02   FFDS = fat free dry solid

levels were not reported. Earlier work by Noda[64] demonstrated a significant elevation in the level of circulating insulin when rats were fed a low casein diet supplemented with 0.3% methionine. The inference that can be drawn from these studies using diets supplemented with methionine is that insulin is exerting a demonstrable effect on the mechanisms of protein synthesis in the muscle of protein-depleted rats.

The weanling rat would appear to be the most suitable model for the study of mechanisms of metabolic processes in protein-calorie malnutrition, because this period is more closely related to the time of onset of overt clinical malnutrition in the human child.[65] Indeed a recent report[66] indicates that signs of protein depletion are apparent within 4 days of feeding weanling rats a diet containing 4% casein. By contrast several months are required for 100-g postweanling rats to exhibit similar effects.[67–69] The observation of a high variability in the response of the young rats and the suggestion that this may reflect individual variation in metabolic adaptation to the protein-deficient diet could prove to be of value in studies relating to epidemiology of the clinical syndrome.

Anthony and Faloona[70] have described alterations in the insulin:glucagon molar ratio in rats fed a low protein diet for several months. During the period of study, there was a rise in the plasma glucagon level similar to that found in well-nourished control rats of the same age, but the plasma insulin was significantly reduced. It appears that insulin synthesis and secretion are impaired whereas glucagon metabolism is unaffected in keeping with the increase in the proportion of alpha cells in the islets of the pancreas of protein-malnourished rats described by Heard and Stewart.[71] It has been suggested that the insulin:glucagon ratio is more important in determining the homeostatic function of the two hormones than the absolute concentration of either.[72] The relevance of these findings to the demonstrated abnormal glucose tolerance in clinical protein-calorie malnutrition warrants further investigation.

To summarize, it becomes apparent that sufficient evidence is available to justify the use of the rat as an experimental model for studies relating to the alterations in metabolism induced by the protein deficiency syndrome. All the features of the disease can be produced by malnutrition alone, using diets that approximate the level of protein intake common in developing countries. Thus the rat is in our opinion a suitable model for the study of PCM and the mechanisms involved in somatic growth in the presence of PCM.

CONCLUSION

The appearance of clinical malnutrition is considered to occur when adverse environmental conditions result in the breakdown of the mechanisms of adaptation to minimal nutrition. Many observations suggest that the smallness of stature evident in communities subsisting on a low level of protein intake could be a useful adaptation to the limited diet. The small individual requires fewer calories and less protein to maintain the integrity of metabolizing tissue.

The changes in body size produced by the introduction of a generous food supply to a population previously deprived are dramatic. This is exemplified by the Japanese experience. The height of Japanese children diminished sharply due to the dietary restriction of World War II, but the prewar growth rate was surpassed by 1955. At present the growth rate is similar to that of children in Mediterranean countries.[54]

However, to suggest that upgrading of the quantity or quality of the diet alone will be effective in the cure or prevention of malnutrition is an oversimplification of the problem. Many factors are involved in the attainment of normal growth and development. Controlled studies into the relative importance of nutrition, control of infectious disease, and the psychological effects of an impoverished environment in this process are necessary. Assessment of the results of these studies may lead to the definition of the type of intervention program that will be effective in the amelioration of the widespread human misery evident in the world at this time.

REFERENCES

1. Forbes, G. B.: Chemical growth in infancy and childhood. *J. Pediatr.* **41**: 202, 1952.
2. Huxley, J. S.: *Problems of Relative Growth.* Methuen, London, 1932.
3. Waterlow, J. C.: Protein and energy requirements of children. *Bibl. Nutr. Dieta* **18**: 6, 1973.
4. Fomon, S. J., Thomas, L. N., Filer, L. J., Jr., Ziegler, E. E., and Leonard, M. T.: Food consumption and growth of normal infants fed milk-based formulas. *Acta Paediatr. Scand. Suppl.* 223, 1971.
5. Holt, L. E., and Snyderman, S. E.: The amino acid requirements of infants. *J.A.M.A.* **175**: 100, 1961.
6. Rose, H. E., and Mayer, J.: Activity, calorie intake, fat storage and the energy balance of infants. *Pediatrics* **41**: 18, 1968.
7. Food and Agricultural Organization: Calorie requirements. *Report of Second Committee on Calorie Requirements.* FAO Nutritional Studies No. 15. FAO, Rome, 1957.
8. Heald, F. P., Remmell, P. S., and Mayer, J.: Calorie, protein and fat intakes in children and adolescents. In: Heald, F. P. (Ed.): *Adolescent Nutrition and Growth.* Appleton-Century-Crofts, New York, 1969, p. 17.
9. Wait, B., and Roberts, J. J.: Studies in food requirements of adolescent girls: Energy intake of well-nourished girls 10 to 16 years of age. *J. Am. Diet. Assoc.* **8**: 209, 1932.
10. Cheek, D. B.: In: Cheek, D. B. (Ed.): *Human Growth.* Lea & Febiger, Philadelphia, 1968, p. 565.
11. Forbes, G. B.: Relation of lean body mass to height in children and adolescents. *Pediatr. Res.* **6**: 32, 1972.
12. Reba, R. C., Cheek, D. B., and Mellits, E. D.: Body composition studies in pediatrics. In: James, E. (Ed.): *Pediatric Nuclear Medicine.* Saunders, Philadelphia, 1974, p. 458.
13. Novak, L. P., Hamamoto, K., Orvis, A. L., and Burke, E. C.: Total body potassium in infants. *Am. J. Dis. Child.* **119**: 419, 1970.
14. Sagild, U.: Total exchangeable potassium in normal subjects with special reference to changes with age. *Scand. J. Clin. Lab. Invest.* **8**: 44, 1956.
15. da Costa, F., and Moorhouse, J. A.: Protein nutrition in aged individuals on self-selected diets *Am. J. Clin. Nutr.* **22**: 1618, 1969.
16. White House Conference. *Report of the Committee on Growth and Development of the Child.* Part III, *Nutrition.* The Century Co., New York, 1932.
17. Folger, G. M., Jr., and Hollowell, J. G.: Excretion of catecholamine in urine by infants and children with cyanotic congenital heart disease. *Pediatr. Res.* **6**: 151, 1972.
18. Cheek, D. B., Graystone, J. E., and Rowe, R. D.: Hypoxia and malnutrition in newborn rats: Effects on RNA, DNA, and protein in tissues. *Am. J. Physiol.* **217**: 642, 1969.

19. Cheek, D. B., and Rowe, R. D.: Aspects of sympathetic activity in the newborn, including the respiratory distress syndrome. *Pediatr. Clin. North Am.* **13**: 863, 1966.

20. Harrison, T. S., and Seaton, J.: The relative effects of hypoxia and hypercarbia on adrenal medullary secretion in anaesthetized dogs. *J. Surg. Res.* **5**: 560, 1965.

21. Iber, F. L., Cheek, D. B., and Wolf, K. P.: Nitrogen metabolism in children with congenital cardiac defects and severe growth retardation. *Am. J. Clin. Nutr.* **20**: 1166, 1967.

22. Scrimshaw, N.: The effect of stress on nutrition in adolescents and young adults. In: Heald, F. P. (Ed.): *Adolescent Nutrition and Growth.* Appleton-Century-Crofts, New York, 1969, p. 101.

23. Classification of infantile malnutrition. *Lancet* **2**: 302, 1970.

24. Graham, G. D. C., Cordano, A., Blizzard, R., and Cheek, D. B.: Infantile malnutrition: Changes in body composition during rehabilitation. *Pediatr. Res.* **3**: 579, 1969.

25. Cheek, D. B., Hill, D. E., Cordano, A., and Graham, G.: Malnutrition in infancy: Changes in muscle and adipose tissue before and after rehabilitation. *Pediatr. Res.* **4**: 135, 1970.

26. Teller, W. M., Genscher, U., Burkhardt, H., and Rommel, K.: Hydroxyproline excretion in various forms of growth failure. *Arch. Dis. Child.* **48**: 127, 1973.

27. Waterlow, J. C., Neale, R. J., Rowe, L., and Palin, I.: Effects of diet and infection on creatine turnover in the rat. *Am. J. Clin. Nutr.* **25**: 371, 1972.

28. Garrow, J. S., Fletcher, K., and Halliday, D.: Body composition in severe infantile malnutrition. *J. Clin. Invest.* **44**: 417, 1965.

29. Metcoff, J.: Biochemical effects of protein-calorie malnutrition in man. *Recent Adv. Med.* **18**: 377, 1967.

30. Alleyne, G. A. O.: Studies on total body potassium in infantile malnutrition: The relation to body fluids, spaces, and urinary creatinine. *Clin. Sci.* **34**: 199, 1968.

31. Alleyne, G. A. O.: Studies on total body potassium in malnourished infants. Factors affecting potassium repletion. *Br. J. Nutr.* **24**: 205, 1970.

32. Hansen, J. D. L.: Electrolyte and nitrogen metabolism in kwashiorkor. *S. Afr. Lab. Clin. Med.* **2**: 206, 1956.

33. Nichols, B. L., Alvarado, J. M., Hazelwood, C. F., and Viteri, F. E.: Clinical significance of muscle potassium depletion in protein-calorie malnutrition. *J. Pediatr.* **80**: 319, 1972.

34. Alleyne, G. A. O., Viteri, F., and Alvarado, J.: Indices of body composition in infantile malnutrition: Total body potassium and urinary creatinine. *Am. J. Clin. Nutr.* **23**: 875, 1970.

35. Alleyne, G. A. O., Flores, H., Picou, D. I. M., and Waterlow, J. C.: Metabolic changes in children with protein-calorie malnutrition. In: Winick, M. (Ed.): *Nutrition and Development.* Wiley, New York, 1972.

36. Milner, R. D. G. Insulin secretion in human protein-calorie deficiency. *Proc. Nutr. Soc.* **31**: 219, 1972.

37. Milner, R. D. G.: Metabolic and hormonal response to glucose and glucagon in patients with infantile malnutrition. *Pediatr. Res.* **5**: 33, 1971.

38. Waterlow, J. C., Cravioto, J., and Stephen, J. M. L.: Protein malnutrition in man. *Adv. Protein Chem.* **15**: 131, 1960.

39. Whitehead, R. G., and Alleyne, G. A. O.: Pathophysiological factors of importance in protein-calorie malnutrition. *Br. Med. Bull.* **28**: 72, 1972.

40. Pimstone, G. L., Barbezat, G., Hansen, J. D. L., and Murray, P.: Studies on growth hormone secretion in protein-calorie malnutrition. *Am. J. Clin. Nutr.* **21**: 482, 1968.

41. Waterlow, J. C.: Observations on the mechanism of adaptation to low protein intakes. *Lancet* **ii**: 1091, 1968.

42. Beas, F., Contreras, I., Maccioni, A., and Arenas, S.: Growth hormone in infant malnutrition: The arginine test in marasmus and kwashiorkor. *Br. J. Nutr.* **26**: 169, 1971.

43. Parra, A., Garza, C., Garza, Y., Saravia, J. L., Hazelwood, C. F., and Nichols, B. L.: Changes in growth hormone, insulin, and thyroxine values, and in energy metabolism of marasmic infants. *J. Pediatr.* **82**: 133, 1973.

44. Hadden, D. R.: Glucose, free fatty acid and insulin interrelations in kwashiorkor and marasmus. *Lancet* **2**: 589, 1967.

45. Graham, G. G., and Cordano, A.: Copper depletion and deficiency in the malnourished infant. *Johns Hopkins Med. J.* **124**: 139, 1969.

46. Mehtar, S., Chaparwal, B. C., Vijayvargiya, R., Singh, S. D., and Mathur, P. S.: Some aspects of magnesium and zinc metabolism in protein-calorie malnutrition. *Indian Pediatr.* **9**: 216, 1972.

47. Leading article: Magnesium and malnutrition. *Lancet* **1**: 712, 1967.

48. Jose, D. G., Stutman, O., and Good, R. A.: Long term effects on immune function of early nutritional deprivation. *Nature* **241**: 57, 1973.

49. Monckeberg, F., Dunoso, G., Oxman, S., Pak, N., and Meneghello, J.: Human growth hormone in infant malnutrition. *Pediatrics* **31**: 58, 1963.

50. Hadden, D. R., and Rutishauser, I. H. E.: Effect of human growth hormone in kwashiorkor and marasmus. *Arch. Dis. Child.* **42**: 29, 1967.

51. Cahill, G. F., Jr.: Starvation in man. *N. Engl. J. Med.* **282**: 668, 1970.

52. Becker, D. J., Pimstone, B. L., Hansen, J. D. L., and Hendricks, S.: Insulin secretion in protein-calorie malnutrition. *Diabetes* **20**: 542, 1971.

53. Becker, D. J., Pimstone, B. L., Hansen, J. D. L., MacHutchen, B., and Drysdale, A.: Patterns of insulin response to glucose in protein-calorie malnutrition. *Am. J. Clin. Nutr.* **25**: 499, 1972.

54. Munro, H. N.: Report of a conference on protein and amino acid needs for growth and development. *Am. J. Clin. Nutr.* **27**: 55, 1974.

55. Winick, M., and Noble, A.: Cellular response in rats during malnutrition at various ages. *J. Nutr.* **89**: 300, 1966.

56. Cheek, D. B., Graystone, J. E., and Read, M. S.: Cellular growth, nutrition and development. *Pediatrics* **45**: 315, 1970.

57. Graystone, J. E., and Cheek, D. B.: The effects of reduced caloric intake and increased insulin-induced caloric intake on the cell growth of muscle, liver, and cerebrum and on skeletal collagen in the postweanling rat. *Pediatr. Res.* **3**: 66, 1969.

58. Durand, G., Fauconneau, G., and Penot, E.: Croissance des tissus du rat et reduction de l'apport energetique de la ration: Influence sur la taneur en acides nucleiques. *Ann. Biol. Anim. Biochim. Biophys.* **7**: 145, 1967.

59. Hill, D. E., Holt, A. B., Parra, A., and Cheek. D. B.: The influence of protein-calorie versus calorie restriction on the body composition and cellular growth of muscle and liver in weanling rats. *Johns Hopkins Med. J.* **127**: 146, 1970.

60. Durand, G., and Penot, E.: Restoration of cellular multiplication and growth in the young rat previously maintained at constant weight. Paper presented at IXth International Congress of Nutrition, Mexico City, Sept. 1972.

61. Hruza, Z., and Fabry, P.: Some metabolic and endocrine changes due to long lasting caloric undernutrition. *Gerontologia* **1**: 279, 1957.

62. Lee, M. O., and Schaffer, N. K.: Anterior pituitary growth hormone and the composition of growth. *J. Nutr.* **7**: 337, 1934.

63. Howarth, R. E.: Influence of dietary protein on rat skeletal muscle growth. *J. Nutr.* **102**: 37, 1972.

64. Noda, K.: The influence of insulin, hydrocortisone and thyroxine on fatty liver of rats fed a low casein diet supplemented with methionine. *J. Nutr.* **101**: 1391, 1971.

65. Widdowson, E. M.: The place of experimental animals in the study of human malnutrition. In: McCance, R. A. and Widdowson, E. M. (Eds.): *Calorie Deficiencies and Protein Deficiencies.* Little, Brown, Boston, 1968.

66. Stead, R. H., and Brock, J. F.: Experimental protein-calorie malnutrition. Rapid induction of protein depletion signs in early-weaned rats. *J. Nutr.* **102**: 1357, 1972.

67. Kirsch, R. E., Brock, J. F., and Saunders, S. J.: Experimental protein-calorie malnutrition. *Am. J. Clin. Nutr.* **21**: 820, 1968.

68. Endozien, J. C.: Experimental kwashiorkor and marasmus. *Nature* **220**: 917, 1968.

69. Enwonwu, C. O., and Sreebny, L. M.: Experimental protein-calorie malnutrition in rats: Biochemical and ultrastructural studies. *Exp. Mol. Pathol.* **12**: 332, 1970.

70. Anthony, L. E., and Faloona, G. R.: Plasma insulin and glucagon levels in protein-malnourished rats. *Metabolism* **23**: 303, 1974.

71. Heard, C. R. C., and Stewart, R. J. C.: Protein caloric deficiency and disorders of the endocrine glands. *Hormones* **2**: 40, 1971.

72. Unger, R. H.: Glucagon physiology and pathophysiology. *N. Engl. J. Med.* **285**: 443, 1971.

73. Hill, D. E., Arellano, C. P., Izukawa, T., Holt, A. B., and Cheek, D. B.: Studies in infants and children with congenital rubella: Oxygen consumption, body water, cell mass, muscle and adipose tissue composition. *Johns Hopkins Med. J.* **127**: 309–322, 1970.

CHAPTER 26

Overnutrition

Donald B. Cheek, Adalberto Parra, and John White

INTRODUCTION

In this chapter, the subject of overnutrition is briefly discussed. Its relative effects on muscle and adipose tissue are described and the effects of early nutrition on the amount of adipose tissue are considered. The study of a single patient can be inconclusive; however, a single patient well studied can provide considerable insight into a metabolic problem. Hence, we report here the findings obtained after the operation of ileal bypass on a patient with gross obesity and studied over a 5-year period. There is a brief note on overnutrition and longevity. The chapter ends with a discussion of the role played in obesity by hormones.

BODY COMPOSITION AND OBESITY

The pathogenesis of obesity (defined as excess adipose tissue) is complex, involving hormones, psychological factors, nutrition, and genetic factors. It is not known which factors predominate and which are secondary. Several types of obesity may exist.

We have been able to establish quadratic equations for the prediction of body fat from body length[1] (Figure 26.1). Such equations are derived from data on body water (D_2O determinations) and body length (height and age) from infancy to 30 years, length being a better index of development than chronological age. While no physiological implications can be drawn, the expected fat for an individual may be assessed. The measurement of lean body mass (from the distribution of D_2O) allows the prediction of actual or total body fat. The difference between actual fat and expected fat yields what we call "excess fat." We have also investigated the body

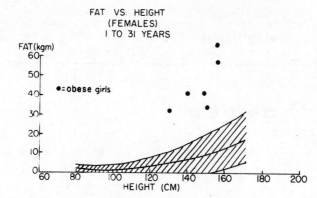

FAT VS. HEIGHT
(FEMALES)
I TO 31 YEARS

Fig. 26.1. The relationship between body fat and height for normal females from 1 to 31 years of age is shown with an approximate 95 percent confidence area (shaded). Points for 6 obese females are shown. (Reprinted from *Monogr. Soc. Res. Child Dev.* Serial No. 140, No. 7., October 1970, with the permission of the Society for Research in Child Development Inc.)

composition of 24 preadolescent or adolescent females and males[2, 3] who were regarded clinically as grossly obese.

Figures 26.2 to 26.4 depict the fat mass, lean body mass, intracellular mass, and muscle mass of normal and obese boys and girls when height was used as a measure of maturation. This approach is important since the majority of these adolescents had an excessive height for age. The finding of increased lean body mass, intracellular mass, and muscle mass for length supports the concept that overnutrition leads to excess growth of lean tissues as well as adipose tissue, in man as well as in the rat. In muscle (the major lean tissue) the number of nuclei within the muscle mass was excessive, particularly in the case of girls (Figure 26.5). If the data are plotted against chronological age, a striking difference is again seen for girls, especially if advanced bone age is considered (Figure 26.6). The excess muscle growth was not related to increase in cytoplasmic growth as is clear from inspection of the ratio of protein to DNA in the musculature (Figure 26.7). Of interest was the finding that in girls with an excess number of nuclei in the musculature there was also an increase of bone age of at least 2 years as well as an increase in muscle mass. These studies on preadolescent and adolescent obese females and males show advanced growth of lean tissues for age in the presence of excess adipose tissue.

Our investigations did not support the use of ^{40}K to assess the lean body mass. Part of the problem lies in the fact that in obesity, ^{40}K may not monitor the lean body mass correctly, the adipose tissue probably acting as a shield.[3, 4] The measurement of body water to predict body fat is more reliable.[5]

ADIPOSE TISSUE GROWTH

Knittle has reviewed the subject of adipose tissue growth.[6] He points out that fat increases steadily during the first 9 months of postnatal life, reaching a plateau about that time with no further acceleration until 9 years[7] when the prepubertal growth spurt commences. In obese subjects this spurt may occur earlier (from 5 to 7 years). Adipose tissue growth may result from increments in size or number of fat cells. When adult life is reached fat cell number is fixed and fluctuations in adipose tissue weight occur only by changes in fat cell size. A similar constancy is found in the epididymal fat pads of Sprague-Dawley rats where fat cell numbers increase rapidly in early life but reach a constancy at 10 to 15 weeks of age. Thus the obese

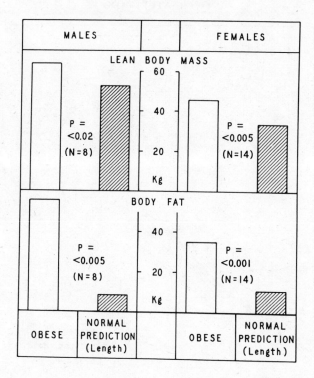

Fig. 26.2. The numerical relationship of length to body fat and lean body mass (LBM) makes it possible to predict the amount of "normal" LBM and fat in an obese individual. In this figure it can be shown that the estimated values for fat but also LBM in the obese patients significantly exceed the predicted value.

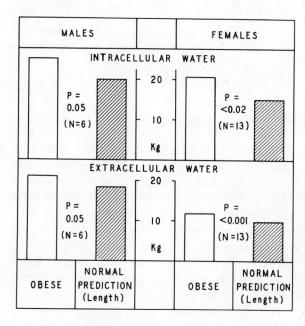

Fig. 26.3. The numerical relationship of length to intracellular (ICW) and extracellular water (ECV) makes it possible to predict the "normal" amount of these components in an obese individual. This figure shows that the estimated values for ICW and ECV in the obese patient significantly exceed the predicted values.

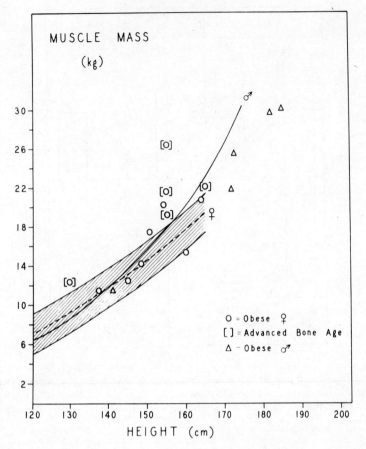

Fig. 26.4. The quadratic equations for muscle mass versus body length are shown by the solid line (males) and by the dashed line (females). The shaded area around the line for females represents ± two standard deviations. Note that obese females have an excess muscle mass for length, especially if bone age is advanced by 2 years or more. Obese males tend to have a proportionate increase in muscle mass for length. (Reprinted from Cheek et al: *Pediatr. Res.* **4**: 268, 1970, with the permission of the Editor.)

individual can only reduce adipose tissue by loss of intracellular lipid (reduction of fat cell size).

Grinker and Hirsch[8] presented data for cell size and number from individuals of normal weight, obese, and reduced obese individuals (Table 26.1). In addition to demonstrating the fixation of fat cell number these workers showed that in rodents, obesity is usually associated with an increase in cell size. However the Zucker obese rat and the ob/ob mouse do demonstrate an abnormally prolonged increase in fat cell number during growth. Moreover for the Zucker rat nutritional deprivation in early life does not prevent the occurrence of excess fat cell number later in life.[9] Thus genetic influences are important. In the normal rat if nutrition is restricted in early postnatal life but an ad libitum intake is given after weaning, the rats remain lean.[10] Thus environmental factors are also important.

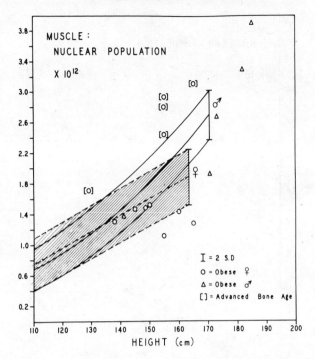

Fig. 26.5. The equations for nuclear number within the muscle mass are shown for adolescent boys and girls against body length. Note that the data for girls with obesity indicate advanced growth in nuclear number, especially if bone age is advanced. The shaded area represents ± two standard deviations. (Reprinted from Cheek et al: *Pediatr. Res.* **4**: 268, 1970, with the permission of the Editor.)

Our approach to the measurement of fat cell number has been to analyze a small sample of adipose tissue for water, fat, collagen, and noncollagen protein.[3,11] If the cytoplasmic protein within the adipocyte remains constant, then the percentage of noncollagen protein present in a sample should reflect the number of cells per gram of adipose tissue (Figure 26.8). Recent data of Salans and Dougherty confirm the thinking.[12] In the Hirsch method [13,14] fat cells are freed with osmium tetroxide and counted with a Coulter counter. The noncollagen protein (NCP) method agrees closely with the Hirsch method as a measure of fat cell number.[11]

Knittle and Hirsch [13,14] have suggested that the growth of fat cell number within the adipose tissue in early infancy may be a key to the induction of obesity. They estimate that the obese adolescent has three to four times the normal number of adipocytes. Application of the NCP method to the study of obese children and adolescents together with the measurement of excess fat has allowed us to confirm the three- to fourfold increase in fat cell number in obese subjects claimed by Knittle and Hirsch (Figure 26.9). Indeed most of the obese preadolescents had a fat cell number equivalent to that of a normal adult.

Changes in adipose tissue would be expected in malnutrition. However, it is difficult to obtain data relating to adipose tissue in malnourished children by the Hirsch method, because little fat is contained within the adipocyte and the cells are not completely or easily freed by osmium tetroxide. Thus in infancy many adipocytes may not be counted as they contain insufficient lipid.

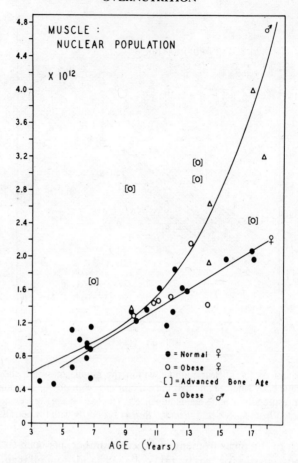

Fig. 26.6. The equations for nuclear number within the muscle mass are plotted for adolescent boys and girls against age. Note the gross departure of data points for obese girls where bone age is advanced.

The NCP method can be used in such cases. The percentage of water, fat, protein, and collagen was documented in nine Peruvian infants suffering from protein-calorie malnutrition.[15] The mean value of lipid per cell was 0.266 ± 0.209 μg whereas after treatment (which did not restore these infants to normal) the value increased to 0.463 ± 0.174 μg per cell. The difference is significant statistically. An increase in fat was detected clinically after partial rehabilitation. Previously it was not possible to assess these data since expected lipid levels in cells were not available until recently.[11]

This finding has lead us recently to consider whether a population of fat cells might be small in size in the adipose tissue during infancy. The acquisition of a precise determinator for particle size has revealed that such a population of fat cells does exist in the first 2 years of life.[152]

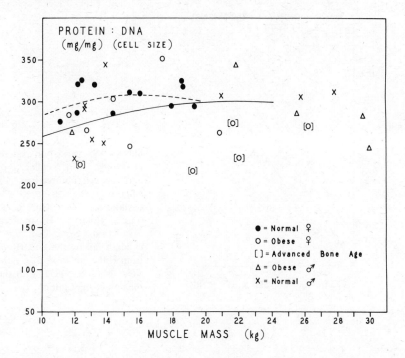

Fig. 26.7. The ratio of protein to DNA (index of cell size) is shown for adolescent boys and girls when muscle mass (organ size) forms the abscissa. Note that for obese adolescents the ratio of protein to DNA is usually reduced. (Reprinted from Cheek et al: *Pediatr. Res.* **4:** 268, 1970, with permission of the Editor.)

Table 26.1   Cell size and number in normal and obese individuals. (8)

	Cell size**	Cell number*
Normal weight	0.66 ± 0.06	26 ± 26.8
Juvenile onset obese	0.90 ± 0.05	85 ± 6.9
Adult onset obese	0.98 ± 0.14	62 ± 4.2
Reduced obese***	0.45 ± 0.05	62 ± 5.3

* X 10^9 ** μg lipid/cell   *** each subject had lost 50 Kg in weight

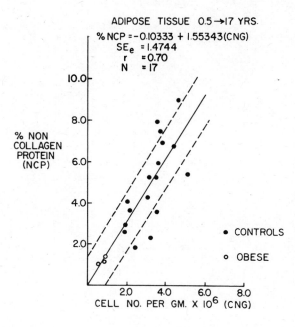

Fig. 26.8. The calculated regression line for the correlation between the percentage of non-collagen protein and the cell number per gram of adipose tissue ± one standard deviation is given. Only data from normal children were used for the calculation. Note that for obese children fall on the line. (Reprinted from Hill et al: *Proc. Soc. Exp. Biol. Med.* 140: 782, 1972, with the permission of the Editor.)

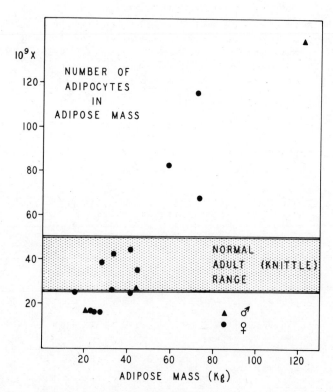

Fig. 26.9. Number of adipocytes for obese children and adolescents is shown. Note that most of the data fall in the adult range or above it. (Normal Adult Range from Knittle and Hirsch, *Fed. Proc.* 29, 1516, 1970.)

460

NUTRITIONAL EFFECTS ON OBESITY

Studies in rodents by Widdowson and McCance[16] left little doubt that if a litter was reduced in size, the generous milk supply available from the mother was consumed by the few offspring and as a result excessive growth was encountered. This growth encompassed not only adipose tissue but also lean tissue and was sustained beyond weaning. Since cell size in general is reasonably constant from mammal to mammal at maturity, as shown by Teissier,[17] the number of cells must be greater in the lean tissues of such rats. This was confirmed by the subsequent experiments of Winick and Noble.[18] The manipulation of diet in neonatal rats has been of particular interest over the years.[19, 20]

Overnutrition can cause excessive cell multiplication prior to sexual maturation. In rodents advanced bone age occurs,[16] as well as increased lean body mass[31, 32] and increased adipocyte cell number.[10] By contrast restricted nutrition during early postnatal life does influence the number of fat cells eventually found in the adipose tissue of rats.[10] It is considered that the findings mentioned here hold for primates.

In the human, Fomon estimates that in the normal infant by 6 months of age 50% of body weight is adipose tissue.[21] Clearly, the growth of fat cells either in number or in size must be remarkable in infancy. No precise data are available. While birth weight has not altered during the last 100 years[22] the period at which birth weight doubles seems to be closer to 3 months than to the expected 6 months. Lightwood[23] in a survey throughout certain parts of the United States found that calorie intake was 200 to 300% above requirements in "well baby clinics." Fomon et al[24] have shown that high-density feeding in the neonatal period leads to excessive somatic and skeletal growth while similar conclusions have been found in the infant baboon given an ad libitum diet and confined to the cage.[25] Thus the primate resembles the rodent in this situation.

Regarding the infant and child, excessive growth may thus be related to overnutrition, children of school age showing an increasing incidence of obesity in the affluent society.[26-30] In high school the incidence varies from 10 to 20%. That this increase in weight for age is not always due to fat increments per se is shown by our own studies[2, 3] and those of Fomon.[21, 24]

ILEAL BYPASS

The procedure of ileal bypass has been performed in many obese patients. One such patient was studied by our group over a period of 5 years. The weight of this male patient was above 200 kg on presentation and when first seen he was almost 17 years of age. His body fat was close to 100 kg, as was his lean body mass. His body length measured 185 cm (Figure 26.10).

Two years after these measurements were made or just prior to 19 years, an ileal bypass was performed. There was a 70-kg loss of fat with a 25-kg loss of lean tissue. Body weight was reduced to a value close to 100 kg. The number of fat cells was determined by assessing the noncollagen protein in the adipose tissue, while total fat was determined by assessing body water from D_2O. The results are shown in Figure 26.11. Clearly the great loss of adipose tissue mass was accompanied by a

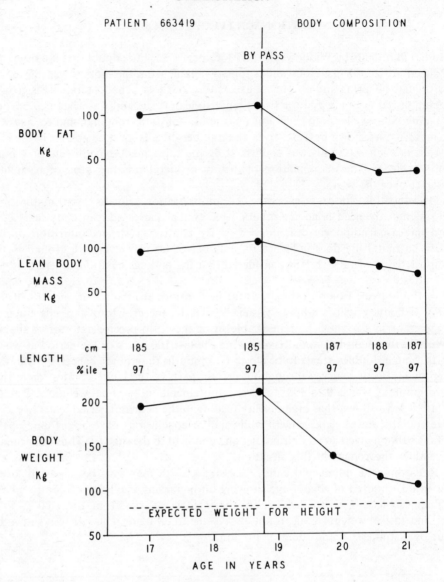

Fig. 26.10. Changes in body fat, lean body mass, and body weight are recorded over a 5-year priod and 3 years after ileal bypass for a grossly obese male.

reduction of adipocyte number from 160×10^9 to 75×10^9. This may be an exceptional result related to the effectiveness of the bypass, since this information has not been reported by other workers. The lipid per cell was also reduced (Figure 26.12).

The changes in lean tissue were just as remarkable following bypass and during the following 2 years. There was a reduction of both intracellular and extracellular volume (Figure 26.13), while the reduction in muscle mass was accompanied by a reduction in DNA content (nuclear number in muscle; Figure 26.14). By contrast there was no increase in protein relative to DNA within the muscle (Figure 26.15).

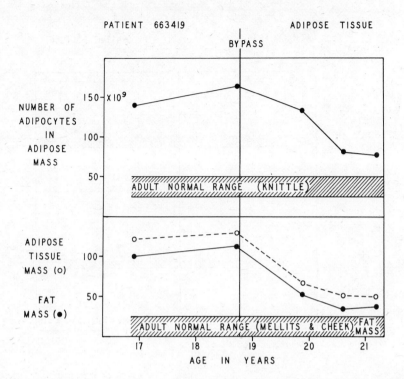

Fig. 26.11. Changes in fat cell number and adipose tissue mass are recorded over a 5-year period and 3 years after ileal bypass for a grossly obese male. [Normal Adult Range for number of adipocytes from Knittle and Hirsch, *Fed. Proc.*, 29, 1516, 1970; Normal Adult range for Fat Mass see ref. (1).]

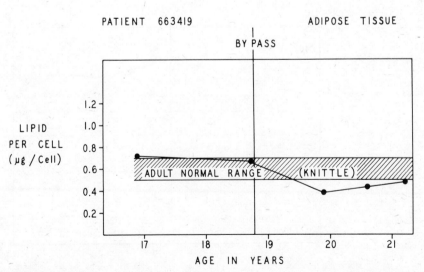

Fig. 26.12. The amount of lipid per adipocyte is recorded over a 5-year period and 3 years after ileal bypass by a grossly obese male. (Normal Adult range from Knittle and Hirsch, *Fed. Proc.* 29, 1516, 1970.)

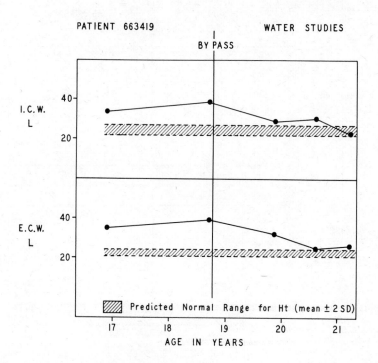

Fig. 26.13. The intracellular and extracellular volumes are recorded over a 5-year period and 3 years after ileal bypass for a grossly obese male.

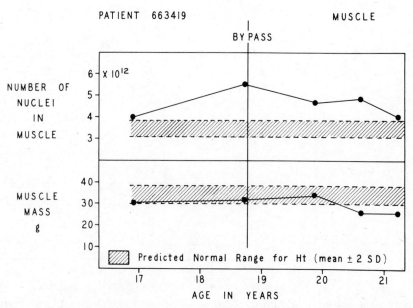

Fig. 26.14. The number of nuclei within the muscle and the changes in muscle mass are recorded over a 5-year period and 3 years after ileal bypass by a grossly obese male.

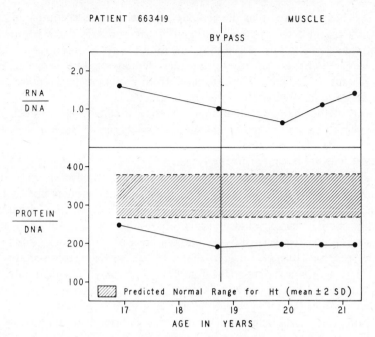

Fig. 26.15. The changes in protein:DNA and RNA:DNA ratios in the muscle are recorded over a 5-year period and 3 years after ileal bypass for a grossly obese male.

This suggests that the insulin insensitivity still persisted with respect to muscle tissue. Indeed the reduction of RNA relative to DNA which occurred supports the thesis that protein synthesis was reduced in muscle and that a situation of protein deprivation exists.[31] Other workers[32, 33] also consider that ileal bypass reduces the patient to a state of protein-calorie deprivation. Amino acid studies in plasma support such thinking. Coincidental loss of lean body mass has been demonstrated by measurement of whole body potassium.[33] Negative growth due to limitation of substrate may be said to occur.

A NOTE ON LONGEVITY AND CALORIE INTAKE

In our previous book we concluded by reviewing the subject of overnutrition and longevity,[34] so only a brief review will be given here.

Many factors have been considered in relation to the process of aging. For example, the loss of essential and nonrenewable cells has been considered to be a factor. Cameron[35] studied thymidine labeling of various tissues in mice and clearly established a decrease in cell turnover with time and aging. Limited information is available for primates. Gelfant and Smith[36] considered aging to be a progressive conversion of cycling to noncycling cells in tissues capable of proliferation, while immune mechanisms may be involved in cellular aging insofar as noncycling cells may be kept in restraint.

Adams[37] has suggested that the cellular basis of aging is accompanied by three events. These are the decline in the functional efficiency and the deterioration or death of specialized cells; a failure of cell multiplication in tissues that have a high rate of cell renewal; and changes in structural protein (collagen). The studies of Hayflick, cited by Adams,[37] indicate that fibroblasts from an infant may replicate 80 times while those from an 80-year-old replicate 20 times.

The thesis of the changing functional efficiency of cells received much attention in earlier years and was reviewed in our previous book.[38] Such a thesis fits well into the concepts of Comfort[39] where exhaustion of cell enzymes and coenzymes is envisaged with involvement of the lysosomes.

Another recent development has been the consideration of a failure or reduction of immunological surveillance. Walford[40] considers that aging is due to a somatic mutation whereby autoimmune processes become stimulated. Burnet[41] has modified this thinking by considering that aging is programmed as a result of evolutionary processes that are also governed by a metabolic state or "time clock" and influenced by genetic processes. Burnet considers that each tissue is compromised at a different time and that the thymus-dependent immune system plays a critical role. Thus he accepts the concept of aging as an immune phenomenon as proposed by Walford,[40] except that the mechanism is visualized as being intimately related to the process of immunological surveillance and the thymus. Fabris et al have also suggested that the thymus might represent the biological clock.[42]

Study of Snell-Bagg dwarf mice is of great interest since these mammals only live until 5 months of age.[42] Growth hormone and thyroid stimulating hormone are absent. A poorly developed thymus, spleen, and lymph glands are present and cell-mediated immune reactions are reduced. The injection of bone marrow or thymocytes does not postpone aging. By contrast, the injection of mature lymphocytes causes the return of cell-mediated immunity and also prolongs life.[43] The usual features of aging at the fifth month do not occur but such mice do not gain weight. The injection of growth hormone and thyroxine can induce a complete maturation of the lymphoid system, prolonging life in these mice to the expected 12 months.[42] The injection of hormones not only prevented aging until the 12th month but also produced growth and gain in body weight. Moreover if thymectomy was performed on the young adult prior to hormone therapy, the life span was not restored nor were the signs of aging delayed.

Thus a combination of the activities of the endocrine system and the lymphatic system would appear to be of great importance to the process of aging. Duquesnoy and Good [44] have shown that if Snell-Bagg mice (dwarfs) receive prolonged nursing they remain immunologically competent, which suggests that a hormone or some factor is present in the milk of the mother which allows maturation of the thymus and lymphocytes.

In spite of the confusion that exists concerning primary and secondary factors in obesity, there is much evidence that obesity is associated with a reduced life span. Recently Nolan[45] fed an enriched well-balanced diet to rats at 80% of ad libitum. He showed that healthier, smaller, and longer living animals resulted. If an unlimited intake was given during the prepuberty period and a restricted diet after puberty (80%), then health and longevity were maximal. Such findings confirm the early observation of McCay[46] that rats subjected to intermittent food deprivation had a longer life span than controls fed ad libitum.

The role of nutrition early in postnatal life has been studied as a factor in obesity and may affect the life span. At present in America 80% of infants are fed commercially prepared formulas whereas only 15% are breast fed.[47] By 110 days after birth, most infants fed commercially prepared formulas have heights and weights close to the 90th percentile, in contrast to breast-fed infants who are around the 50th percentile. Moreover it appears that infants fed a more concentrated formula tend to take a greater volume of formula per day with a resultant higher calorie intake.

Ross has written extensively on the effects of calorie restriction and longevity. In recent work Ross and Bras[48] report a reduced incidence of tumors of various types with calorie restriction from weaning.

In recent times concern has been expressed regarding the feeding of a high cholesterol diet from infancy, since this may be related to the increasing incidence of atherosclerosis. In breast-fed babies females have a higher blood cholesterol concentration. The range for male and female is from 150 to 125 mg/100 ml. Whether cow's milk or human milk is fed, the infant has a higher blood cholesterol than would be the case if corn or coconut oil was the source of fat. It is agreed, however, that an increased level of cholesterol is important for the induction of enzymatic pathways to metabolize cholesterol and to allow for myelination in the central nervous system. By contrast infants with a hereditary predisposition to hyperlipoproteinemia have high levels of lipid from birth. This can be shown even in cord blood in infants with the type II hyperlipoproteinemia.[49, 50]

In certain parts of the world it is claimed that people live to 100 or 130 years. An investigation was made by Dr. Alexander Leaf who visited such areas as Hunza (near Pakistan), Vilcabamba (Equador), and Abkhazia (near the Black Sea). He found that the inhabitants frequently lived to 100 years and some to 130 years.[51] These people have calorie intakes of less than 2,000 per day with restricted animal fats. They often live at high altitudes and maintain an active physical life. Clearly the affluent life of the Western society is in no way programmed for longevity but rather toward overeating and lack of exercise. Of interest is the fact that only now are experimental situations being undertaken to investigate behavior and longevity. For example, Spott[52] reports that mice placed in isolation and fed ad libitum have the shortest life span regardless of genotype. The situation can be partly salvaged by restricting food intake to 80%. If daily exposure to an operant conditioning situation is introduced, an increase in both life span and life expectancy can be anticipated. Clearly we are only at the outset of understanding the process of aging.

THE RELATION BETWEEN HORMONES AND OBESITY

The interrelationships of obesity, overgrowth, and hormones have been reviewed [53—57] and while the papers concerning hormonal aberrations are extensive[58—62] they apply mainly to the adult. Only recently has attention been given to the child and adolescent.[2, 63] Investigations of "excess fat" described earlier in this chapter demonstrated a positive correlation between the amount of excess fat and the circulating insulin level. Attention has been drawn to a relationship between circulating insulin levels and adipocyte size,[64] while others dispute this finding.[65]

Investigation of adipocyte metabolism, particularly with respect to the action of insulin, has shown that insulin sensitivity as reflected by glucose oxidation is dependent on the size of the fat cell. The larger the cell the less responsive it is to insulin. On the other hand, no change in the rate of conversion of fatty acid to triglyceride has been found in adipose tissue from obese subjects, although change in lipogenesis resulting from glucose may occur.[6]

Our own studies in the obese children described earlier in this chapter are relevant to this problem. We have demonstrated a reduced response to arginine infusion as is true also for the adult with obesity. Higher insulin levels existed during fasting and the longer the duration of obesity from birth, the higher the fasting level of insulin (Figure 26.16). As obesity progressed there was a gradual development of an insensitivity to insulin at the tissue level. The transport of [14C]glucose and of amino acids into the muscle cell is compromised.[66–68] The adipose tissue cells became resistant to the action of insulin. The concentration of growth hormone in plasma was depressed, especially following arginine infusion. Whether this is due to decreased release or increased tissue uptake of growth hormone is not known.

Thus we suspect that prior to adolescence or in childhood, substrates initiate excessive release of insulin and growth hormone and, as with the rodent, excess cell multiplication takes place. This occurs especially in muscle although Naeye and Roode point also to visceral tissues.[69] Insulin exerts its effect on adipocyte cell size, but the multiplication of these cells is dependent on growth hormone as shown by Bonnet et al.,[68a] in the hypopituitary patient. We showed a similar action on muscle growth some years ago. Knittle has some evidence to support the thinking.[6] Since the infant with hypopituitarism appears to continue to grow in the early

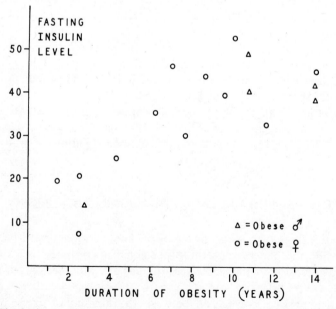

Fig. 26.16. The fasting immunoreactive insulin level for obese patients is plotted against the duration of obesity (years). (Reprinted from Parra et al: *Pediatr. Res.* **5**: 611, 1971, with the permission of the Editor.)

postnatal months, one might conclude that physiological fatness in the infant is due to an increase in fat cell size per se.

In obesity muscle becomes insensitive to the high insulin levels, hence the protein:DNA ratio falls and the transport of amino acids may be directed more out of the cell than into the cell, a situation not unlike calorie-protein deprivation.[68] If one plots the peak of the immunoreactive insulin (as a result of infusion of arginine in such patients), the greater the peak the greater the protein:DNA ratio as though the synthesis of protein is set at a new and higher level in muscle (Figure 26.17).

Zierler and Rabinowitz[70] and Rabinowitz and Merimee[71] drew attention to the sequence of events involving the secretion of insulin and growth hormone following food ingestion. They defined periods of fasting and feasting that could be related to hormonal predominance of either insulin or growth hormone. They suggested periods of maximal protein synthesis.

Sex hormones may play a role in the development of obesity. Adipose tissue growth occurs significantly and is characteristic for the female at puberty.[72] For the boy muscle mass begins to double and at the time of sexual maturation at 14 years, the number of nuclei within the muscle mass has doubled while gain in fat is not remarkable. By contrast the girl shows no such dramatic gain in muscle mass or of DNA within her muscle mass (Chapter 22). However, each tissue reaches a stable or steady state of cell population.

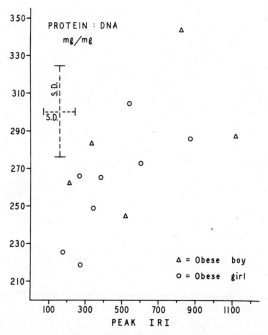

Fig. 26.17. The muscle cell size (protein:DNA) for obese boys and girls is plotted against the peak insulin response produced by a protein glucose meal. Note that the peak insulin levels are higher than expected in most instances and similarly protein:DNA is generally reduced. (On the left side of the figure is shown the cell size for normal children with the standard deviation and also the expected peak insulin response.) (Reprinted from Cheek et al: *Pediatr. Res.* **5**: 605 1971, with the permission of the Editor.)

Adrenal cortical function increases in obesity[73] but the exact role of these hormones is not known. Clearly if the human female shows changes in obesity characteristic of male growth (increased cell number in muscle, for example), the question arises as to why estrogens are not exerting their expected effect with respect to minimizing the action of growth hormone on cell multiplication. Is it that more male hormone is being secreted which directs body growth toward the masculine pattern? Adrenal steroids in small amounts can enhance the release of growth hormone, as does testosterone.[74] Of great importance may be the demonstration of an increased excretion of 17-ketosteroid and 17-ketogenic steroids in obese girls with increased stature.[75]

It is clear from the discussion just presented that the exact role of hormones in obesity is not yet fully understood. It is tempting to assume that both insulin and growth hormone are secreted in excess during the initial phase of the syndrome. It is also possible that adrenal cortical hormones are involved and that estrogen levels in the obese female are not effective in their action. Bray[76] considers that thyroid hormone could be involved by virtue of its role in the glycerophosphate cycle.

REFERENCES

1. Mellits, E. D., and Cheek, D. B.: The assessment of body water and fatness from infancy to adulthood. *Monogr. Soc. Res. Child Dev.* **35**: 7, 1970.

2. Parra, A., Schultz, R. B., Graystone, J. E., and Cheek, D. B.: Correlative studies in obese children and adolescents concerning body composition and plasma insulin and growth hormone levels. *Pediatr. Res.* **5**: 605, 1971.

3. Cheek, D. B., Schultz, R. B., Parra, A., and Reba, R. C.: Overgrowth of lean and adipose tissues in adolescent obesity. *Pediatr. Res.* **4**: 268, 1970.

4. Forbes, G. B., Schultz, F., Cafarelli, G., and Amirhakimi, G. H.: Effects of body size on potassium-40 measurement in the whole body counter (tilt-chair technique). *Health Phys.* **15**: 435, 1968.

5. Babineau, L. M., and Page, E.: On body fat and body water in rats. *Can. J. Biochem.* **33**: 970, 1955.

6. Knittle, J. L.: Obesity in childhood: A problem in adipose tissue cellular development. *J. Pediatr.* **81**: No. 6, 1048–1059, 1972.

7. Mossberg, H. O.: Obesity in children; a clinical prognostical investigation. *Acta Pediatr. Suppl.* **2**, 35, 1948.

8. Grinker, J., and Hirsch, J.: *Metabolic and Behavioral Correlates of Obesity*, Ciba Foundation Symposium No. 8, 1972, p. 350.

9. Johnston, P. R., Stern, J. S., Greenwood, M. R. C., Zucker, L. M., and Hirsch, J.: Effect of early nutrition on adipose cellularity and pancreatic insulin release in the Zucker rat. *J. Nutr.* **103**: 5, 738, 1973.

10. Knittle, J. L., and Hirsch, J.: Effects of early nutrition on the development of rat epididymal fat pads: Cellularity and metabolism. *J. Clin. Invest.* **47**: 2091, 1968.

11. Hill, D. E., Hirsch, J., and Cheek, D. B.: The noncollagen protein in adipose tissue as an index of cell number. *Proc. Soc. Exp. Biol. Med.* **140**: 782, 1972.

12. Salans, L. B., and Dougherty, J. W.: The effect of insulin upon glucose metabolism by adipose cells of different size. Influence of cell lipid, protein content, age and nutritional status. *J. Clin. Invest.* **50**: 1399, 1971.

13. Hirsch, J., Knittle, J. L., and Salans, L. B.: Cell lipid content and cell number in obese and nonobese human adipose tissue. *J. Clin. Invest.* **45**: 1023, 1966.

14. Knittle, J., and Hirsch, J.: Infantile nutrition as a determinant of adult adipose tissue metabolism and cellularity. *Clin. Res.* **15**: 323, 1967.

15. Cheek, D. B., Hill, D. E., Cordano, A., and Graham, G. G.: Malnutrition in infancy: Changes in muscle and adipose tissue before and after rehabilitation. *Pediatr. Res.* **4**: 135–144, 1970.

15a. Boulton, T. J. C., Dunlop, M. and Court, J. M.: Adipocyte growth in the first 2 years of life. *Aust. Pediat. J.* **10**: 301, 1974.

16. Widdowson, E. M., and McCance, R. A.: Some effects on accelerating growth. I. General somatic development. *Proc. Roy. Soc. B* **152**: 188, 1960.

17. Teissier, G.: Biometrie de la cellule. *Tabulae Biol.* **19**: 1, 1939.

18. Winick, M., and Noble, A.: Cellular response with increased feeding in neonatal rats. *J. Nutr.* **91**: 179, 1967.

19. Kennedy, G. C.: The development with age of hypothalamic restraint upon the appetite of the rat. *J. Endocrinol.* **16**: 9, 1957.

20. Heggeness, F. W., Bindshadler, D., Chadwick, J., Conklin, P., Hulnick, S., and Oaks, M.: Weight gain of overnourished and undernourished preweanling rats. *J. Nutr.* **75**: 39, 1961.

21. Fomon, S. J.: Body composition of the male reference infant during the first year of life. *Pediatrics* **40**: 863, 1967.

22. Frost, L. H., and Jackson, R. L.: Growth and development of infants receiving proprietary preparation of evaporated milk with dextrimaltose and vitamin D. *J. Pediatr.* **38**: 585, 1951.

23. Lightwood, R.: Personal communication.

24. Fomon, S. J., Filer, L. J., Thomas, L. M., Rogers, P. R., and Proksch, L. N.: Relationship between formula concentration and rate of growth of normal infants. *J. Nutr.* **98**: 241, 1969.

25. Buss, D. B., and Voss, W. R.: An evaluation of four methods for estimating the milk yield of baboons. *J. Nutr.* **101**: 901, 1971.

26. Canning, H., and Mayer, J.: Obesity—Its possible effect on college acceptance. *N. Engl. J. Med.* **275**: 1172, 1966.

27. Huenemann, R. L., Shapiro, L. R., Hampton, M. C., and Mitchell, B. W.: A longitudinal study of gross body composition and body conformation and their association with food and activity in a teen-age population: Views of teen-age subjects on body composition, food and activity. *Am. J. Clin. Nutr.* **18**: 325, 1966.

28. Johnson, M. L., Burke, B. S., and Mayer, J.: Incidence and prevalence of obesity in a section of school children in the Boston area. *Am. J. Clin. Nutr.* **4**: 231, 1956.

29. Lloyd, J. K., Wolff, O. H., and Whelan, W. S.: Childhood obesity; Long-term study of height and weight. *Br. Med. J.* **2**: 145, 1961.

30. Stefanik, P. A., Heald, F. P., and Mayer, J.: Caloric intake in relation to energy output of non-obese and obese adolescent boys. *Am. J. Clin. Nutr.* **7**: 55, 1959.

31. White, J. J., Cheek, D. B. and Haller, Jr., J. A.: Small bowel bypass is applicable for adolescents with morbid obesity. *The Amer. Surgeon.* **40**: 704, 1974.

32. Shibata, H. R., Mackenzie, J. R., and Shao-nan, H.: Morphologic changes of the liver following small intestinal bypass for obesity. *Arch. Surg.* **103**: 229, 1971.

33. Sandstead, H. H., Brill, A. B., Law, D. H., and Scott, H. W.: Effects of jejuno-ileal shunt on body composition in morbidly obese patients. *Surg. Forum* **23**: 404, 1972.

34. Cheek, D. B. (Ed.): *Human Growth*. Lea & Febiger, Philadelphia, 1968, p. 638.

35. Cameron, I. L.: Cell proliferation in ageing mice. *J. Gerontol.* **27**; 162, 1972.

36. Gelfant, S., and Smith, J. G.: Ageing: Noncycling cells, an explanation. *Science* **178**: 357, 1972.

37. Adams, L. D.: Ageing involution and senescence. *S. Afr. Med. J.* p. 1239, October 1969.

38. Cheek, D. B. (Ed.): *Human Growth*. Lea & Febiger, Philadelphia, 1968, p. 641.

39. Comfort, A.: The prevention of ageing in cells. *Lancet* **2**: 1325, 1966.

40. Walford, R. L.: *Immunologic Theory of Ageing*. Williams & Wilkins, Copenhagen, 1969.

41. Burnet, F. M.: An immunological approach to ageing. *Lancet* **2**: 358, 1970.

42. Fabris, N., Pierpaoli, W., and Sorkin, E.: Lymphocytes, hormones and ageing. *Nature* **240**: 557, 1972.

43. Fabris, N., Pierpaoli, W., and Sorkin, E.: Hormones and the immunological capacity. IV. Restoration effects of developmental hormones or of lymphocytes on the immunodeficiency syndrome of the dwarf mice. *Clin. Exp. Immunol.* **9**: 227, 1971.

44. Duquesnoy, R. J., and Good, R. A.: Prevention of immunologic deficiency in pituitary dwarf mice by prolonged nursing. *J. Immunol.* **104**: 1553, 1970.

45. Nolen, G. A.: Effect of various restricted dietary regimes on the growth, health and longevity of albino rats. *J. Nutr.* **102**: 1477, 1972.

46. McCay, C. M., Maynard, L. A., Sperling, G., and Barnes, L. L.: Retarded growth, life span, ultimate body size and age changes in the albino rat after feeding diets restricted in calories. *J. Nutr.* **18**: 1, 1939.

47. Fomon, S. J.: A pediatrician looks at early nutrition. *Bull. N. Y. Acad. Med.* **47**: 569, 1971.

48. Ross, A. H., and Bras, G.: Lasting influence of early calorie restriction on prevalence of neoplasms in the rat. *J. Nutr. Cancer Inst.* **47**: 1095, 1971.

49. Frederickson, D. S., and Breslow, J. L.: Primary hyperlipoproteinemia in infants. *Ann. Rev. Med.* **24**: 315, 1973.

50. Kwiterovich, P. O., Levy, K. I., and Frederickson, D. S.: Neonatal diagnosis of familial type II hyperlipoproteinemia. *Lancet* **1**: 118, 1973.

51. Leaf, A.: A scientist visits some of the world's oldest people. *Natl. Geogr. Mag.* **143**: 93, 1973.

52. Spott, R. L.: *Age Dependent Behaviour.* Report from the Jackson Laboratory, Bar Harbor, Maine, 1974.

53. Borjeson, J.: Overweight children. *Acta Paediatr. Scand.* **51**: Suppl. 123, 7, 1962.

54. Christian, J. E., Combs, L. W., and Kessler, W. V.: The body composition of obese subjects. *Am. J. Clin. Nutr.* **15**: 29, 1964.

55. Forbes, G. B.: Lean body mass and fat in obese children. *Pediatrics* **34**: 308, 1964.

56. Heald, F. P.: Natural history and physiological basis of adolescent obesity. *Fed. Proc.* **25**: 1, 1966.

57. Stunkard, A. J.: Environment and obesity: Recent advances in our understanding of regulation of food intake in man. *Fed. Proc.* **27**: 1367, 1968.

58. Boshell, B. R., Chandalia, H. B., Kreisberg, R. A., and Roddarn, R. F.: Serum insulin in obesity and diabetes mellitus. *Am. J. Clin. Nutr.* **21**: 1419, 1968.

59. Kreisberg, R. A., Boshell, B. R., DiPlacido, J., and Roddarn, R. F.: Insulin secretion in obesity. *N. Engl. J. Med.* **276**: 314, 1967.

60. Lessof, M. H., and Greenwood, F. C.: Growth hormone secretion in obese subjects. *Guy's Hosp. Rep.* **115**: 65, 1966.

61. Perley, M., and Kipnis, D. M.: Plasma insulin responses to glucose and tolbutamide of norma weight and obese diabetic and non-diabetic subjects. *Diabetes* **15**: 867, 1966.

62. Rabinowitz, D., and Zierler, K. L.: Forearm metabolism in obesity and its response to intra-arterial insulin. Characterization of insulin resistance and evidence for adaptative hyperinsulinism. *J. Clin. Invest.* **41**: 2173, 1962.

63. Paulsen, E. L., Richenderfer, F., and Ginsberg-Fellner, F.: Plasma glucose, free fatty acids and immunoreactive insulin in sixty-six obese children. *Diabetes* **17**: 261, 1968.

64. Stern, J. S., Hollander, N., Batchelor, B. R., Cohn, C. K., and Hirsch, J.: Adipose-cell size and immunoreactive insulin levels in obese and normal-weight adults. *Lancet* **2**: 948, 1972.

65. Brook, C. G. D., and Lloyd, J. K.: Adipose cell size and glucose tolerance in obese children and effects of diet. *Arch. Dis. Child.* **48**: 301, 1973.

66. Stauffacher, W., Crofford, D. B., Jeanrenaud, B., and Renold, A. B.: Comparative studies of muscle and adipose tissue metabolism in lean and obese mice. *Ann. N.Y. Acad. Sci.* **131**: 534, 1965.

67. Felig, P., Marliss, E., and Cahill, G. F.: Plasma amino acid levels and insulin secretion in obesity. *N. Engl. J. Med.* **281**: 811, 1969.

68. Felig, P., Owen, O. E., Wahren, J., and Cahill, G. F.: Amino acid metabolism during prolonged starvation. *J. Clin. Invest.* **48**: 584, 1969.

68a. Bonnet, F., Vanderschueren-Lodeweyckx, M., Eeckels, R. and Malvaux, P.: Subcutaneous adipose tissue and lipids in blood in growth hormone deficiency before and after treatment with human growth hormone. *Pediat. Res.*, **8**: 800, 1974.

69. Naeye, R. L., and Roode, P.: The sizes and numbers of cells in visceral organs in human obesity. *Am. J. Clin. Pathol.* **54**: 251, 1970.

70. Zierler, K. L., and Rabinowitz, D.: Roles of insulin and growth hormone, based on studies of forearm metabolism in man. *Medicine* (Balt) **42**: 385, 1963.

71. Rabinowitz, D., and Merimee, T. J.: Peripheral actions and regulation of insulin and growth hormone secretion in intact man. In: Cheek, D. B. (Ed.): *Human Growth*. Lea & Febiger, Philadelphia, 1968.

72. Cheek, D. B.: Body composition, hormones, nutrition and adolescent growth. In: *Control of Onset of Puberty*, (Eds.) Grumbach, M. M., Grave, G. D. and Mayer, F. E., John Wiley & Sons, Inc., 1974, p. 424.

73. Migeon, C. J., Green, O. C., and Eckert, J. P. Study of adrenocortical function in obesity. *Metabolism* **12**: 718, 1963.

74. Illig, R., and Prader, A.: Effect of testosterone on growth hormone secretion in patients with anorchia and delayed puberty. *J. Clin. Endocrinol. Metab.* **30**: 615, 1970.

75. Jacobson, G., Seltzer, C. G., Bondy, P. K., and Mayer, J.: Importance of body characteristics in the excretion of 17-ketosteroids and 17-ketogenic steroids in obesity. *N. Engl. J. Med.* **271**: 651, 1964.

76. Bray, G.: The myth of diet in the management of obesity. *Am. J. Clin. Nutr.* **23**: 1141, 1970.

CHAPTER 27

Implications and Conclusions

Donald B. Cheek

PRENATAL GROWTH IN THE BRAIN

For the investigator of fetal growth the study of brain development offers the greatest challenge. Protein is distributed in the brain between neuronal and neuroglial cells. Connective tissues and collagen are virtually absent. Much has been written in this book concerning the appraisal of cell number by the use of DNA content, a technique used to a small extent by earlier investigators and by our laboratory in 1962. Biochemists (eg, Kissane and Robins, see Appendix I) have developed methods for the precise determination of DNA in micron slices of brain tissue. Use of this technique by ourselves and other investigators has provided valuable information especially with respect to malnutrition. As stated in the first chapter, the DNA content of tissue from the nervous system only has significance if it can be related to the type of cell involved and the region of the brain concerned. McKhann and co-workers have developed techniques for separating brain tissue into its different cell types.[1]

Of importance in the assessment of function is the study of enzymes. For example, carbonic anhydrase, which regulates the rate of the reaction $H_2CO_3 \rightarrow HCO_3^- + H^+$, is confined to the neuroglial cells. Evidence available suggests that RNA distributes mainly over neuronal cells. Enzymes such as $Na^+K^+ATPase$ are found at the synapse or in neuronal membranes and are involved with ion transport. N-Acetylneuraminic acid (NANA) is also intimately associated with neuronal function.

Cholesterol and phospholipids both characterize myelination. Brain water content can be determined with great precision and by itself hydration provides a sensitive index of maturation, since a reduction in hydration occurs continuously and

---

References to the literature are included in the chapters referred to. If not, they are given at the end of this final chapter.

very gradually during fetal life. Pathological processes may of course produce gross changes in brain hydration, and in such situations the significance of changes in this determinant is destroyed. We have attempted to define the extracellular space from the distribution of chloride in brain tissue.

Adequate evidence has been produced in this book (Chapter 2) to support the thesis that in the primate both brain and somatic growth patterns are different from those of other mammals. For the subprimate the rate of growth is much faster prenatally. Brain growth relative to time follows a sigmoid curve for all mammals, but during development we find that in the primate a common pathway is present for the growth of the brain, when brain size is related to body size. Eventually, with maturity, brain size reaches its limit and these limits vary according to the primate order and hold little relationship to the time of birth. For the human 2 years postnatally is the time when brain size reaches a limit. The brain size of the primate is greater relative to body size (Chapter 2). The larger brain ensures a greater cerebral blood supply (or a greater proportion of the cardiac output). Neuronal growth is defined well before midgestation, in contrast to the rat.

Dobbing mentions, correctly, that birth is only of passing importance relative to brain development. However, it is also true that insults (such as nutritional restriction) can have a greater or lesser effect depending on whether changes in velocity of brain growth occur prenatally or postnatally. The brain has vulnerable periods (we are told) during which insults will produce effects in various biochemical parameters. The maturity of the brain in the newborn rat is equivalent to that reached by the human at the end of the first trimester. A maximum spurt of growth of the rat brain occurs 8 to 10 days after birth. Equivalent times for development in the primate brain differ. Thus insults occurring postnatally in small mammals like the rat may affect the development of the brain. Dobbing points out that neuronal multiplication is complete in the human at 20 weeks. In terms of growth of the brain mass in the human, we find two points that can be identified as periods of maximal growth velocity. At the 32nd week of gestation and at 20 weeks postnatally, a spurt in growth velocity occurs (Figure 1.4). Until recently there was no confirmatory evidence that 32 weeks was a time of significance. However, Conde et al.[2] of Spain find that in the human brain accretion of sphingomyelin, sulfatides, and glycosphingolipids is negligible until the 29th week, but they report that "a very sharp increase in the concentrations of these compounds was seen from the 32nd week."

In the human fetus weight follows an almost linear relationship with time up until the 32nd week. From then on normal fetal growth follows closely an S-shaped curve of acceleration. Thus the spurt of brain growth may precede that of the soma—or may even initiate the somatic spurt.

For the macaque and the human, different biochemical indices reach mature values at different times in development. In Chapters 3 and 4 the biochemical determinants of the brain (cerebrum versus cerebellum) have been defined and mathematically described. The curves are either linear, quadratic, cubic, or quartic with time. Clearly, different indices increase their growth rate at different times, and Figure 27.1 summarizes a small portion of some of the data. For cerebrum and cerebellum the different chemical determinants grow in the same sequence. The development of the cerebellum lags behind that of the cerebrum but from midgestation the rate of cerebellar growth is much faster.

If the velocity of brain growth expressed as a percentage increase is considered for the human (Chapter 1, Figure 1.4) but also for the macaque (Figure 27.2)

PERCENTAGE OF ADULT MACAQUE VALUE

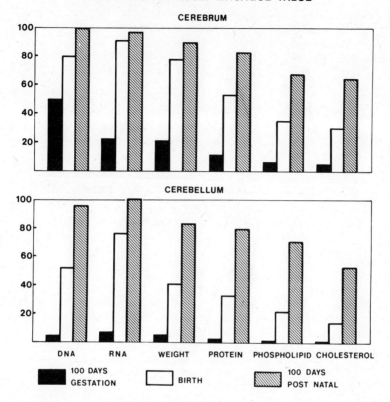

Fig. 27.1. A portion of our data concerning biochemical components of the cerebrum and cerebellum are expressed as a percentage of the mature value at three periods in development (i.e., at 100 days gestation, birth, and 100 days postnatally). It can be seen from this figure that the growth of the cerebellum lags behind that of the cerebrum. However, the rate of growth of the cerebellum from midgestation is faster. Note that the sequence of maturation for the biochemical components is the the same in cerebrum and cerebellum.

it can be seen that the period for accelerated brain growth occurs at exactly the same stage of gestation for both primates. This is the stage when protein and cholesterol concentrations increase and that for water decreases in the macaque. It is also clear that the second period of acceleration occurs just after birth while in the human it does not occur until 20 weeks after birth.

The increase in cell number in the cerebrum of the macaque fetus is almost complete by the end of gestation. Relative to the cerebellum a great deal of cell growth has occurred already in the cerebrum by midgestation (when this study began). Presumably neuroblast growth is complete by midgestation as Dobbing[3] has shown for the human (Chapter 1).

NUTRITION AND THE BRAIN

The data of Riopelle for the fetal macaque and the studies of Zena Stein (Chapter 6) argue against fetal brain damage resulting from maternal protein deprivation in the primate. One would speculate that a restricted protein intake would be needed

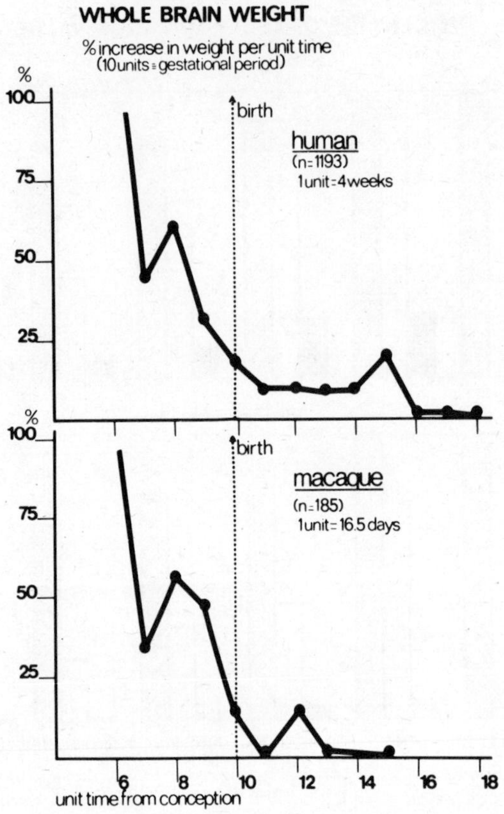

WHOLE BRAIN WEIGHT

Fig. 27.2. The period of gestation for the human and for the monkey is divided into 10 units. The percentage increase in weight gain per unit time is shown. Note that the period of accelerated fetal brain growth for man and monkey is at the same stage of gestation while the second peak is earlier for the macaque occuring soon after birth.

throughout pregnancy and well into the postnatal period if the human fetus was to sustain irreversible changes. Even when nutrition is restricted during the immediate postnatal period, the data of Kerr relating to protein restriction do not indicate brain damage. Infant macaques were reduced in protein intake to 25% of normal for 6 months from the first to the seventh month. Death occurred in some infants but those that survived did not reveal behavioral changes or growth retardation in the soma when maturity was reached.

Intellectual impairment of the human infant does not appear to be solely related to poor nutrition in the early postnatal period. The infant with fibrocystic disease exhibits frank growth failure due to inadequate nutrition in the first year of life but is found to have normal intellectual capabilities later in childhood. These children have an adequate social and psychological environment. In contrast, the combination of poor nutrition and a nonstimulating environment may lead to reduced levels of intellectual ability.

Clearly there is a need for further studies in the pregnant primate to assess the effects of reducing protein intake pre and postnatally. There is also a need to assess the effects of reduction of the placental blood supply to the fetus followed by adequate postnatal nutrition. A careful assessment of the concomitant changes in chemistry and morphology of the brain is needed. Controlled studies are required with deprivation of calories versus protein, or calorie plus protein during pregnancy extending into the postnatal period. The results recorded here demonstrate the potential importance of such future work. All such insults (including hypoxia) will probably produce different patterns of growth arrest in the brain, a suggestion implicit in the results of studies of tissue amino acids made by Nyhan's group.

Whether nutritional restriction is produced by interference with placental circulation (Chapter 7) or by reducing maternal diet (Chapter 6) the growth arrest occurs mainly in the cerebellum and, as we have seen, normal growth is faster in that organ during the latter half of pregnancy. The patterns of change are different. There is no reason to believe that such changes are irreversible. However precise data are not yet available.

When one considers the opposite situation, the infant born of the diabetic mother where some biochemical indices of development are advanced in the brain (eg, protein accretion and carbonic anhydrase activity) and other indices of development are reduced (phospholipid content, cerebral DNA content, Chapters 9 and 19), it becomes clear that differential changes can occur, some representing advanced maturation and others indicating retardation. One might speculate erroneously that infants born of diabetic mothers will have impaired intelligence because of growth arrest of some biochemical determinants. Yet such is not the case.

ZINC AND PROTEIN ACCRETION

The studies on nutrition in this book have not included the study of trace metals or vitamin deficiency. However, the content of zinc in the cerebrum is discussed in Chapter 5. Zinc is involved in the action of at least 18 metalloenzymes. A relationship is found between the concentration of zinc and carbonic anhydrase. Zinc along with copper and manganese has been of particular interest to our group over the last decade. The demonstration of the changes occurring (per unit DNA of tissue) during kwashiorkor, in hypopituitarism, and in hypothyroidism has been informative. Normal levels of urinary excretion of copper and zinc from infancy to adolescence were documented in our previous book.[4]

Zinc levels may prove to be a valuable index of the rate of protein synthesis in the cerebrum since, under circumstances of reduced protein accretion in the fetal brain (cretinism), the Zn:DNA ratio is reduced while an increased accretion of protein is associated with a rise in the Zn:DNA ratio in the brain (as shown for the infant born of the diabetic mother). Relevant to this is the demonstration of a close relationship between zinc and RNA by our group and the recent demonstration by Sandstead of the relationship of zinc and RNA polymerase.

HORMONES, GROWTH, AND MATURATION

Hormones play an important role in the development of the primate brain. Teaching in pediatrics has emphasized that the cretin should be identified as early as possible in the postnatal period if treatment with thyroid hormone is to prove effective. Such treatment, however, even when given early, often fails to restore the infant to normal mentality. Clearly the concept that thyroid hormone is only necessary for growth after birth needs re-examination. Our work (Chapter 8) indicates that thyroid hormone is necessary for protein synthesis in the brain and for the functional activity of carbonic anhydrase (neuroglial) and of $Na^+K^+ATPase$ (neuronal).

Changes in thyroid hormone levels do not alter cell number or DNA content though the cytoplasm of both neuronal and neuroglial cells appears to be affected. It is recognized that growth hormone has little influence on somatic growth in the primate fetus (Chapter 8). However, the content of growth hormone in the fetal pituitary was reduced in these cretinoid fetuses and the possibility of a role for growth hormone in brain growth cannot be excluded. Thyroid insufficiency in the neonatal rat brain prior to the major growth spurt (9 days) produces similar biochemical changes to those demonstrated in the newly born macaque fetus. Such changes in the rat brain can be reversed to a large extent by the injection of growth hormone prior to the time of the spurt in brain growth. Thus one can ask the question: Does ablation of the thyroid gland in the primate fetus produce a coincidental decrease in functional activity of acidophil cells in the fetal pituitary? Can the changes demonstrated in the macaque brain be completely or partially reversed by the injection of primate growth hormone? These questions remain unanswered.

The changes in brain and somatic growth following interference with beta cells of the fetal pancreas or of the pancreas of the pregnant primate were somewhat unexpected. The injection of streptozotocin is known to ablate beta cells. The data with respect to the fetus illustrated very well the need to assess maturational age. Fetuses receiving streptozotocin during the last third of pregnancy and with a birth weight above the expected normal all had adrenal enlargement and showed a significant advancement in their maturational age when the appropriate equation was applied (Chapter 21). Fetuses with retarded growth or with a weight below the normal and without enlargement of the adrenal gland were retarded in time according to the indices used for assessment of maturational age. Fetuses born of diabetic mothers were shown to be ahead in time when certain criteria were applied.

Thus two effects were obtained when the beta cells of the fetal pancreas were challenged during the last third of pregnancy. These are compatible with the thesis that in the first group with increased weight and adrenal enlargement, progenitor cells of the pancreas may have been stimulated to grow and secrete excessive amounts of insulin. In the second group, without adrenal enlargement decreased insulin secretion produced a failure of overall growth in the fetus. The demonstration by Hill of a human fetus failing to grow in the presence of improper pancreatic development, strengthens the argument (Chapter 18).*

Overgrowth of the fetus in the presence of maternal beta-cell ablation could be explained satisfactorily on the basis that the fluctuations of glucose and amino acids in the mother's circulation would also be reflected in the fetal circulation, resulting in stimulation of the fetal pancreatic cells and excessive secretion of insulin. Not only was excessive cytoplasmic growth demonstrated in the soma (muscle cytoplasm) but also in the brain (cerebrum plus cerebellum). This advancement in maturation was associated with excess protein relative to the DNA in the cerebrum,

---

* See preliminary abstract by Sherwood, W. C., Chance, G. W. and Hill, D. E. A new syndrome of familial pancreatic agenesis: the role of insulin and glucagon in somatic and cell growth. *Pediatric Res.*, **8**: 360, 1974.

cerebellum and muscle. Carbonic anhydrase showed an increase in activity in the brain and other criteria of protein synthesis (Zn:DNA) were found to escalate. Cerebral DNA decreased while cerebellar DNA increased. The reduction in cerebral DNA and phospholipid indicated retarded growth (as discussed earlier). By contrast the reduction of the percentage of water in the brain suggested advanced maturation. Differential effects on growth have been described in other circumstances by other investigators.[5]

Reynolds and Chez (Chapter 19) recognized the general thesis that the fetal pancreas is usually inactive during pregnancy but they point out that if the pregnant macaque is given streptozotocin then the introduction of glucose causes a two- to five-fold increase in fetal insulin. In the placenta there was a trend toward an increased phospholipid and cholesterol concentration, whereas in the brain a reduced concentration of total lipids and of phospholipid was revealed (as is also reported in Chapter 9).

Roux, Chez and Yoshioka (Chapter 19) also investigated tissues from the fetus born of the diabetic macaque to evaluate whether the excess fatness and excess growth were mediated by an increased supply of substrate. Studies were made *in vitro* by introducing labeled glucose and fatty acids into a medium containing tissue from infants born of diabetic mothers. It was found that the concentration of triglycerides was double that of normal in brain, liver, and lung while the conversion of fatty acid to triglyceride was accelerated in several tissues. The production of $^{14}CO_2$ was increased during the metabolism of either palmitate or glucose. Additional insulin added to the incubation medium accelerated these conversions. Although the amount of insulin was excessive physiologically, the data suggest an increased activity of the Krebs cycle and of enzymes concerned with beta oxidation.

The findings from these different experiments support the notion that insulin secretion is important to brain growth and to somatic growth. The finding of an enlarged adrenal gland together with evidence of pancreatic activity leaves one with the impression that the hypothalamus, the pancreas and the adrenal may act as a triad to modify fetal growth, a suggestion consistent with the proposal of Hoet.[6]

The studies in this book have drawn attention to factors and hormones controlling cytoplasmic growth in the cells of the primate fetus. There is no information in this book concerning hormones and cell multiplication in the fetus. Admittedly cell multiplication is retarded when placental blood supply is reduced (Chapter 7), but this is possibly due to hypoxia. Nutritional factors can modify cell multiplication in the fetus. One would seek to know whether somatomedin is released from the placenta or fetal liver for such a purpose. Several factors that have the capacity to stimulate cell multiplication have been described (Chapter 24). These may all belong to a family of peptides. They may all be structural variants of the same factor controlling individual tissues with respect to the increase in cell number. One might also speculate that a balance exists between the stimulation of cell multiplication and an inhibition of cell increase by a family of somatostatins.

An experimental animal with isolated growth hormone deficiency should prove a valuable preparation. The new strain of mouse described by Dr. Eicher at the Jackson Laboratories, Bar Harbor, possesses an isolated growth hormone deficiency. Measurement of cell replication in muscle, escalation of the nuclear class series in liver (polyploidy), and excretion of hydroxyproline relative to creatinine, following the injection of biologically active material, should prove measures of the biological activity of somatomedin.

THE ROLE OF THE HYPOTHALAMUS

In this book studies relating to insulin and pancreatic function have been of particular interest. The whole field concerning neural and hormonal control of the islets of Langerhans has recently been reviewed by Woods and Porte.[7] In this important review they make several major points of importance to the thinking in this book.

1. The islets receive both parasympathetic and sympathetic nerve fibers. The islets contain neurons with neuron terminals together with vesicles that are either cholinergic or adrenergic. The innervation of the islets takes place during fetal growth.

2. Norepinephrine and epinephrine block the release of insulin by stimulation of alpha-adrenergic receptors. Beta-adrenergic receptors, if stimulated, enhance insulin release so the ultimate effect of catecholamines depends on the relative stimulation of alpha- and beta-adrenergic receptors.

3. Epinephrine and norepinephrine stimulate the production of glucagon from alpha cells, probably by activation of the beta-adrenergic receptor.

4. Acetylcholine stimulates secretion of both glucagon and insulin, while vagal stimulation, per se, causes insulin secretion. Stimulation of the splanchnic nerves activates glucagon secretion.

5. Electrical stimulation of the ventrolateral hypothalamic nuclei (VLH) causes insulin secretion and the release of a humoral factor from the VLH which also elicits pancreatic insulin release.

6. Electrical stimulation of the ventromedial hypothalamic nuclei (VMH) causes a decrease in plasma insulin and an increase in plasma glucagon, whereas destruction of the VMH leads to a chronic increase of insulin secretion with hypertrophy and hyperplasia of the beta islet cells.

7. The VMH is a sympathetic center and the VLH is a parasympathetic center. Changes in the availability of glucose in the brain alter the electrical activity of VMH and VLH.

8. The introduction of small amounts of insulin or an elevation in plasma glucose in the brain will stimulate the beta pancreatic cells. Such stimulation is transmitted by humoral factors. A decrease in glucose within the central nervous system causes a reflex increase in peripheral glucose—a response that is mediated in part by the adrenal gland. A neural mechanism must also be present to account for the above findings.

Thus it is clear that the balance between insulin secretion and glucagon secretion is delicate and complicated. Both the autonomic nervous system and humoral factors are involved. Moreover the senses of sight and smell initiate the release of insulin, whereas the presence of glucose and amino acids affect hypothalamic nuclei as well as having a direct effect on pancreatic islet cells.

Conversely, stress or the activation of the sympathetic system can precipitate diabetes mellitus, while the induction of diabetes or the presentation of juvenile diabetes is associated with an elevation of catecholamine release. The VMH which is sympathetic holds a restraining influence on the VLH (parasympathetic). If the VLH is completely released by ablation of the VMH, hyperphagia and obesity develop. These are primarily related to insulin excess per se, since the obesity can be prevented by ablation of the beta cells with streptozotocin.

The hormonal factor from the VLH described by Martin et al.[8, 9] is of central importance, and while insulin secretion is augmented, growth hormone is released as a secondary phenomenon.

That insulin plays an important role in fetal brain growth and in somatic growth is not unexpected. De Gasparo and Hoet[10] reviewed the role of insulin in fetal growth in 1970. They pointed to the insulin:glucose ratio in the umbilical venous blood of normal mothers having a correlation with normal birth weight. It has been known for some years that duration of gestation, birth rank of the infant, maternal stature, maternal weight, and maternal weight gain during pregnancy correlated positively with normal birth weight. The finding that insulin and glucose levels in the fetal circulation are significant is once again a demonstration that genetic factors alone do not govern normal fetal growth—nutritional and hormonal factors are equally important.

In the infants born of the diabetic mother the maternal hyperglycemia and fetal pancreatic hypertrophy correlate with the excess weight of the fetus, while rigid control of maternal hyperglycemia reduces the fetal weight toward normal. Glucose alone is not the only substrate to initiate hyperinsulinemia. Amino acids, especially valine, alanine, and glycine, are present in excessive amounts in the fetal circulation in the infant of the diabetic mother (Chez, personal communication) and may also be expected to play a role.

De Gasparo and Hoet[10] also reviewed the work of Van Assche and others concerning the influence of anencephaly (with and without an intact hypothalamus) on the growth of pancreatic cells. Anencephalic infants born to diabetic mothers have abnormal growth of islet tissue with β cell hyperplasia and hypertrophy, provided the hypothalamus is intact. If the hypothalamus is not intact, no such changes are found and less insulin is present within the pancreas. Moreover in the anencephalic born to the diabetic mothers, the cord blood insulin may reach levels of 64 μU per μl if the hypothalamus is intact, whereas the levels are only 8.8 $\pm$ 2.3 μU per μl if the hypothalamus is not intact. Clearly the hypothalamus is involved in growth. As mentioned previously estrogens stimulate beta cellularity in the pancreas and also enlargement of the adrenal and pituitary glands. Some investigators have shown a positive correlation between estrogen excretion (in mother) and the birth weight of the infant (see ref. 10 for review).

In view of the preceding discussion and the information presented in earlier chapters, it is possible to present an incomplete chart of factors concerned with growth in cell size and cell number in the fetus (Figure 27.2) with the brain being of central importance.

FETAL AGE

The anthropometric and biochemical indices available or obtained in normal fetuses allow the statistician to evaluate the parameters or determinants that best relate to age. Clearly the chapter by Kerr (Chapter 16) indicates the importance of skeletal growth and maturation in the fetus for the prediction or assessment of

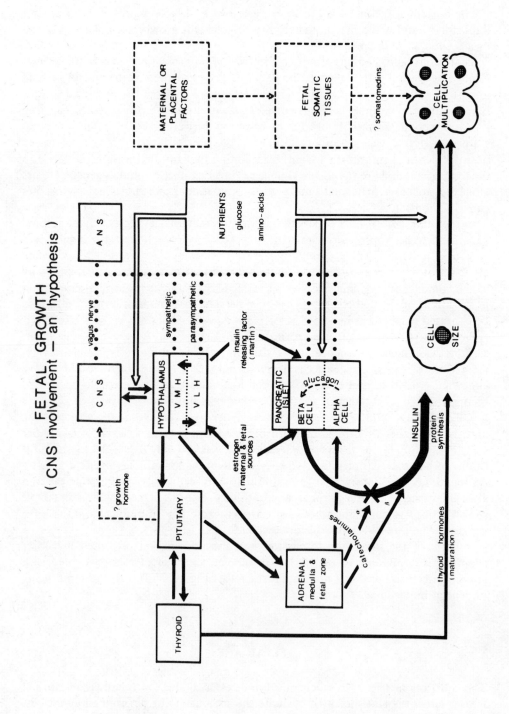

FETAL GROWTH
(CNS involvement — an hypothesis)

484

Fig. 27.3. The figure illustrates the complicated relationship between the brain, autonomic nervous system (ANS) hormone release, and substrate activity in the process of fetal growth. Part of the figure is speculative—especially the role of the somatomedins in fetal cell multiplication or the action of growth hormone on brain growth. On the other hand, a balance in the hypothalamus between the ventromedial nuclei (VMH) and the ventrolateral nuclei of the hypothalamus (VLH) exists. The latter nuclei esculate insulin secretion via a peptide. Estrogens activate VLH and also exert direct effects on the pancreatic beta cells. The pituitary stimulates adrenal development and thyroid development which in turn influence fetal growth. Catecholamines from the adrenal can influence insulin and glucagon secretion—if α-receptors are influenced insulin secretion is decreased, if β receptors are activated insulin secretion is augmented. Both alpha and beta cells of the pancreas are innervated by sympathetic and parasympathetic fibers during fetal development. Stimulation of alpha cells augments glucagon secretion. Nutrients (glucose, amino acids) stimulate receptors in the hypothalamus and in islet cells, as well as acting at the cellular level. A major consequence of all of these mechanisms and their activation is the release of insulin from the pancreatic beta cells which in turn is important to protein synthesis and cytoplasmic growth as is thyroid hormone—a hormone involved also in maturation. In fetal distress one might speculate that catecholamines may block fetal growth by retarding insulin secretion. This figure does not emphasize the balance between glucagon and insulin, especially with respect to protein synthesis. It is thought that in muscle carbon residues plus ammonia form alanine (a strong stimulant to both alpha and beta pancreatic cells) which is transported to the liver and there glucagon stimulates gluconeogenesis and at the same time maintains intracellular glucose levels—an essential facet of protein synthesis according to Wool (for review, see ref. 43). On the other hand, insulin not only stimulates protein synthesis but regulates extracellular glucose levels. However recent evidence indicates that somatostatin reduces the secretion of glucagon and lowers blood glucose concentration.

maturation. As with our previous work with humans,[11] a combination of skeletal assessment with anthropometric and biochemical indices should, in time, provide a sensitive method for the determination of fetal age or fetal maturation.

AMINO ACIDS

As pointed out by Bachmann et al chapters 10 and 20, growth implies protein synthesis. Amino acids are building blocks that traverse both the extracellular and the intracellular fluid. Decreased synthesis can occur with reduced or increased concentrations in either pool, since the mechanisms for protein synthesis may be compromised in several ways. Decreased transport can account for higher levels in the extracellular pool, while alteration in the ratios of essential to nonessential amino acids in either pool can restrict protein accretion.

The concentration of amino acids is up to eight times greater in fetal than in maternal plasma. Fetal tissue amino acid concentrations are greater than those in plasma. At various periods the different somatic tissues (liver, muscle) show different concentrations of amino acids (Chapter 20) and specific patterns can be defined. For example, amino acid concentrations in fetal liver rose steadily and were highest prior to birth. Subsequently they were reduced, rising again 8 weeks after birth. The study of muscle revealed a steady increase in amino acid concentration prior to birth, then a large increase occurred at 60 days postnatally.

While amino acids are involved in protein synthesis they also can act either as neurotransmitters or are important to the synthesis of neurotransmitters (Chapter 10). It is not surprising, therefore, that during protein deprivation changes in neurotransmission occur with, for example, a reduction in serotonin or norepinephrine in the brain stem (Chapters 1 and 6).

The study of normal brain growth during the last half of gestation and in the early postnatal period revealed specific patterns of amino acids at different times. Cerebral tissue had, in general, higher concentrations per unit DNA with a peak in the last third of gestation. Cerebellar tissue had amino acid concentrations reaching a maximum just after birth. Both tissues had concentrations higher than those in plasma.

Experimental procedures caused definite changes in these growth patterns and, for example in cretinism, there was a reversal of the ratio of essential to nonessential amino acids in the cerebrum. The change was due to a reduction in nonessential amino acids. The cerebellum was affected to a relatively slight extent while tryptophan (a precursor of serotonin) was decreased in concentration. With other experimental procedures there were other changes in amino acid concentrations in brain tissue. For example, a challenge to the pancreatic beta cells of mother or fetus (with streptozotocin) resulted in an increase in cerebral glutamine and taurine while other changes in ratios occurred according to the nature of the experiment. A case could be made for the occurrence of increased gluconeogenesis in the brain with increased formation of ammonia and its incorporation into glutamine when fetal beta cells were stimulated. When maternal beta cells were challenged there were elevations of cerebellar glutamine and phenylalanine. The increase in cerebellar methionine and cerebral threonine indicated accelerated transport of these amino acids into the cell with the increased protein synthesis. Possibly insulin enhances this transport. Where the fetal beta cells had been compromised, the levels of amino acids in the plasma were significantly raised suggesting that insufficient circulating insulin could be a responsible factor for poor transport. With maternal beta cell ablation the concentrations of amino acids were all decreased in the liver (Chapter 20) and the change in ratio of essential to nonessential amino acids indicated increased protein synthesis. However, the complete interpretation of results must await further research.

With maternal protein restriction, decreases in amino acid concentrations were found in the cerebrum and cerebellum. Similar findings were made in the cerebellum when calories per se were restricted. In that study increases in concentration of amino acids were detected in the cerebrum. Fetuses subjected to maternal restriction of both calories and protein revealed, in general, an increase of amino acids in the cerebrum and a decrease in the cerebellum. The changes were complex. Variations in calorie and protein intake by the mother can produce different patterns of amino acids in the tissue of fetal cerebrum and cerebellum. This is of considerable interest. Doubtless changes in protein breakdown or protein synthesis and/or changes in amino acid transport are all involved.

When a reduction was made in the placental circulation (Chapter 7), the growth retardation of the fetus was associated with reduced amino acid concentrations in both cerebral and cerebellar tissues as well as in liver and muscle. The concentrations in the plasma tended to rise, indicating that amino acid transport was reduced in the presence of a reduced amino acid supply. Clearly the changes were dissimilar to those encountered when a restriction of maternal diet was implemented.

Thus while certain speculations can be made concerning the nature of the derangements of amino acids, the studies represent a preliminary but new approach to an important problem. Now that the normal patterns of amino acid concentrations are known for the fetal macaque, it is possible to design experiments involving alterations in specific amino acid patterns. The information will be important to the understanding of human growth.

With respect to the fetal lamb, Battaglia (personal communication) has shown that growth will occur if glucose (48%), lactate, threonine, alanine, and glutamine are in sufficient supply. Other substrates are not required.

VISCERAL GROWTH

In Chapter 11 the mathematical relationships between organ growth, gestational age, and postnatal age were considered. Interesting information was revealed, such as the sudden decrease of lung weight at the end of the gestational period when fluid in the alveoli is replaced by air. Other findings, such as the close relationship between the pituitary weight and body length or between pancreatic weight and body weight, may have been fortuitous.

Inspection of the relative growth rates of a particular organ in mammals by using the allometric formula emphasized the similarity in growth between different mammals. Log organ weight was plotted against log body weight. However, the inspection of the adrenal weight relative to body weight in man, macaque and the rat, while demonstrating similar slopes, revealed the presence of different intercepts if the separate lines were projected back to the ordinate.

Earlier in this book it was noted that the relative growth rate of the brain was equal to that of the whole body. In Chapter 11 it was noted that the same relationship also holds for the heart.

The fetal liver (Chapter 12) is of considerable interest as many functions are carried out by one type of parenchymal cell. In other organs single functions are more likely to be carried out by specific cells. The weight of the liver decreased per unit of body weight during fetal development of the mammal. Also the DNA per unit weight decreased from midgestation to birth. When the allometric approach was used it was seen that a similar relationship held for the rat, macaque and man.

Gluck and Kulovich (Chapter 14) considered in detail the development of the human lung according to the glandular, canalicular and alveolar phases. Surfactant is given special consideration in its role of maintaining the stability of the alveolus. It is noted that the structure of the surfactant in the macaque and human is essentially similar. The suggestion is that early detection of changes in the ratio of lecithin to sphingomyelin in amniotic fluid is of diagnostic significance with reference to the respiratory distress syndrome. Of equal interest is the finding that in maternal protein-calorie restriction the surfactant composition of the fetal lung is not changed. However, with either calorie or protein restriction per se, deviations from the normal appear in the fatty acid esters on the β-carbons of lecithins. By contrast the induction of maternal diabetes (with streptozotocin) accelerates the development of lung maturation.

Gluck suggests that glucocorticoids could play an important role in this maturation and of particular interest is Gluck's speculation that the development of phospholipid in the brain may be parallel to its development in the surfactant of the lung. [It will be recalled that infants born of diabetic mothers (Chapters 9 and 19) revealed a reduced cerebral phospholipid content.] The increased incidence of the respiratory distress syndrome in the infant born of the diabetic mother is well established.

PLACENTAL GROWTH

Hill considered the cellular growth of the placenta (Chapter 15). He pointed out that the findings of Winick et al and Weinberg et al indicated that increase in cell number (DNA) of the placenta ceased at the 35th week of gestation, while the studies of Dayton et al indicate that DNA increases linearly with time throughout gestation. The placenta, unlike muscle for example, consists of several cell populations and the method of preparation of the placenta prior to biochemical analysis is very important. The significance of placental DNA is limited because of these factors. In the macaque the DNA content increased linearly throughout gestation as did the RNA. However, the ratio of RNA to DNA decreased with time. Placental weight increased linearly with body weight (or gestational age) during the last third of pregnancy. The noncollagen protein was also related to gestational age in a linear manner ($P < 0.001$). Thus the observations of Dayton for the human agree with our findings. On the other hand the data of Winick regarding RNA and protein changes also agree with our findings.

In sheep Kulhanek et al[12] found that in the last third of gestation total placental DNA remains constant but placental urea permeability per unit DNA rises logarithmically.

SKELETAL AND MYOCARDIAL MUSCLE GROWTH

Initially myoblasts are concerned with the formation of nucleic acids necessary for DNA replication and protein synthesis. After fusion to form myotubes the emphasis is on protein synthesis. The timing of events is related to endocrine function and in particular to the hypothalamic-pituitary axis (Chapter 13). Both insulin and growth hormone *in vitro* enhance the fusion of myoblasts.

We suggest that each nucleus within the myofiber has jurisdiction over a certain volume of cytoplasm (the DNA unit). Measurement of DNA content reveals nuclear number, while the protein: DNA ratio is a measure of the size of the DNA unit. Fiber diameter has little significance with respect to cell growth and metabolism but fiber length may relate to lean body mass.

The satellite cell (described by Mauro) resides between the myotube and the thin membrane surrounding the myofiber. This cell is probably capable of playing a central role in the growth of muscle tissue by acting as a progenitor for new myoblasts, supplying new nuclei to the myotube and forming new myotubes. It may be the locus of action for hormonal and nutritional factors that alter the number of nuclei in the muscle mass or change the ratio of protein to DNA.

In the fetal macaque muscle mass constitutes 20 to 25% of body weight from midgestation to birth. During that time the number of muscle nuclei increases five-fold while the protein: DNA ratio increases by a factor of 2.5. Widdowson has shown for the human that from 30 to 40 weeks of gestation there is a three-fold increase in protein to DNA of muscle.

The heart grows at a similar rate to that of the whole body (Chapter 11). The macaque heart increases from 0.25 to 2.5 g (or ten-fold) from midgestation to birth. Since DNA concentration in the myocardium remains reasonably constant one might expect a ten-fold increase in cell number from midgestation to birth. The increase in protein concentration is from 100 to 150 mg/g. The increase in protein to DNA is not great and is less than that in skeletal muscle. For the human, Widdowson's data suggest a greater rise in the protein/DNA ratio during the last third of pregnancy. Most of the growth of myocardium is accompanied by increase in nuclear number. The accretion of protein proceeds prior to birth in the primate. Growth of the heart is mainly prenatal for the primate but mainly postnatal for the rodent where growth continues up to and past sexual maturation. Miller points out that during the development of the rat heart there is an increase in DNA followed by an escalation of RNA synthesis, and lastly accelerated protein accretion.

While we have pointed to some differences between primate and rodents in the growth of myocardium it is probable that the differences relate mainly to the timing of events (as with the brain). There are similarities. For example, if the nuclear density or the number of nuclei per unit volume is plotted on the ordinate and the weight of the heart on the abscissa, a hyperbolic or "hockey stick" curve is obtained, such that as cell density decreases, cardiac weight increases. Data points from humans, rats and rabbits during growth form a common curve for all three species.[13]

Cardiac muscle, unlike skeletal muscle, exhibits polyploidy Sandritter and Adler,[14] have shown that only about half of the nuclei in ventricular muscle are diploid, the remainder being tetraploid with a small percentage of octaploid. These workers calculated that 2×10^9 nuclei were present in normal human adult hearts. With increasing weight due to pathological processes the degree of ploidy increases and up to 4×10^9 nuclei may be present.

Hypertrophy of the rat myocardium can be produced by partially ligating the aorta. It is of interest that such hypertrophy does not occur in the absence of the pituitary gland.[15,16] Indeed, the whole question of the role of hormones in cardiac growth and/or hypertrophy has received little attention. The fact that an increase in protein relative to DNA occurs in the cardiac muscle of infants born of diabetic mothers suggests that insulin may be important to the cytoplasmic growth of myocardial tissue just as it is of central importance to growth of cytoplasm in skeletal muscle.

The *in vitro* work of Beatty and Bocek (Chapter 13) concerning muscle metabolism in the rhesus monkey is extensive and important. This section gives a brief review of their work. They first established that muscle mass constitutes 20 to 25% of body weight from midgestation to birth. The total number of fibers (myotubes) keeps increasing up to about 90 days of gestation. After 110 days muscle contains only an occasional myotube with a central nucleus.

It is pointed out that muscle in the macaque is ahead in metabolic behavior relative to the human fetus at the same stage of development. Glycogen stores in the musculature are available as an energy source early in gestation. Midway through gestation about half of the lactate originates from glycogen and can be used by peripheral tissue (such as the myocardium, for example). *In vitro* studies revealed that the QO_2 for fetal muscle compared with or exceeded that for adult muscle, indicating that aerobic glycolysis is more active in fetal and neonatal muscle.

In all age groups investigated about 70% of the total CO_2 produced originated from sources other than glucose and glycogen, indicating that energy requirements were obtained from substrates other than carbohydrate. It was found that the pentose cycle was more important to fetal and neonatal muscle than for adult muscle but only a small amount of glucose was metabolized by this route. As early as 100 days of gestation significant amounts of palmitate can be oxidized to CO_2, suggesting that fats may be metabolized by the fetus. Moreover it was clear from further *in vitro* studies that amino acids are also metabolized by muscle. The latter finding is not surprising in view of the work of Smith et al[17] who have shown the rapidity with which human placental tissue takes up and concentrates these amino acids in a remarkable fashion.

CONTEMPORARY INFORMATION

In concluding this review of our own prenatal studies it is pertinent to draw attention briefly to the recent publication, *Size at Birth*— a Ciba symposium. Since a great deal of information was reviewed in this symposium, only some points can be mentioned here.

Widdowson[17a] discussed the variability of fat deposition in different species. Presumably mammals born with body fat quickly utilize their glycogen reserves but have fat available as an energy resource. In some litters (for example pigs) one fetus may be small (runt) and another large. The percentages of fat and glycogen (liver and muscle) are the same in both even though the total amount is less in the small one. While the runt may have smaller and fewer cells the organs are not less competent functionally. Such a thesis is rational. Perhaps only in the endocrine system (pancreas for example) would one express concern if cell number was significantly reduced.

Liggins[17b] discussed a role for the hypothalamus in the growth of the soma of rats since experiments based on aspiration of the fetal rat brain caused a 30% reduction in expected fetal weight. He reviewed the information on anencephaly and found a significant reduction in body growth (allowing for the weight of the brain had this been present). However his conclusion was "that pituitary hormones have at least a small place among the many factors influencing growth of the human fetus."

Thorburn[17c] drew attention to the anephric babies (Potter's Syndrome) and their poor somatic growth. He and his co-workers have removed the kidneys of the fetal lamb (one of twins) during the last third of pregnancy. At term the experimental fetus is smaller with absence of surrounding amniotic fluid. The fetus is about 13 days behind in maturation. A reduction of hemopoietic and osteoblastic tissue was noted. Thorburn considers that the fetal kidney may play a role in fetal homeostasis especially if the placental circulation is compromised. The kidney has an endocrine function. Erythropoietin is secreted and perhaps other hormones or factors important to growth.

With respect to calorie and protein deprivation Young[17d] showed that in the pregnant guinea pig calorie restriction caused a commensurate decrease of fetal and placental size while in protein deprivation the fetus is large relative to placental size, indicating that in this situation some functional adaptation takes place in the placenta. In this direction the work of Beisher and O'Sullivan[17e] is of interest. They infused hypertonic dextrose into pregnant women at rest when their estriol excretion was reduced (suggesting that the well being—or nutrition—of the fetus was poor). The administration of this carbohydrate restored the estriol excretion and fetal growth appeared to improve.

The use of estriol as an index of fetal maturation is unreliable. According to Shearman et al[17f] the study of steroid concentrations in the umbilical artery and venous blood at the time of delivery may offer more meaningful information concerning fetal maturation.

Persson[17g] demonstrated that fetal overgrowth can be normalized by close attention to treatment of the pregnant diabetic mother (keeping the blood sugar at 100 mg/100 ml, for example). The perinatal mortality and morbidity is thereby reduced.

In relation to our own work the small fetal monkeys resulting from a reduced placental circulation and the control fetuses had the same composition in liver or muscle. The total amount of the different components was reduced in the "small for dates" fetuses (Chapter 17).

Our thesis is that the hypothalamus plays a central role in growth and development (Chapter 27). Indeed recent work indicates that the cell multiplying factor(s) somatomedin is secreted or augmented in its action by serotonin from the brain stem but inhibited by melatonin from the pineal body.[17h,17i]

That the kidney may play an important part in fetal growth is of interest and importance. Although we have not studied the problem we have noted the small kidney mass relative to body mass when either protein calorie deprivation is present in the maternal diet or when protein deficiency per se exists (Chapter 17). In this direction the specific but different patterns of amino acids present in tissues, depending on whether calorie or protein deprivation exists, might well result from a change in placental function and/or amino acid transport.

Much of the information in this book surrounds the study of effect of hyperinsulinism (Chapter 9, 18, and 19). The important work of Persson underscores the need to treat the pregnant diabetic mother, since the undesirable effects can be controlled.

POSTNATAL GROWTH

The last section of the text (Part III) summarizes our experience and thinking with respect to studies on postnatal growth in the human. Emphasis is placed on cellular aspects. Only a few major points are re-emphasized here.

The study of cell mass or active tissue mass is of central importance in the human (Chapter 22). This dimension can be assessed by measurement of total body water (which also reflects lean body mass), and the subtraction of extracellular volume to yield intracellular volume. Years of work have been necessary to assess accurately true extracellular volume (see Cheek and Graystone[18,19] for review) and total body water on which measurements of intracellular mass (ICM) are dependent. An alternative is to monitor ^{40}K radiation as a measure of ICM. However, problems exist with respect to that method (See Figure 27.4). The intracellular volume is an index of intracellular mass since the ratio of water to protein in this phase (intracellular phase) of muscle and visceral tissues is considered to be constant. The ICM is related to resting oxygen consumption or to total heat production and

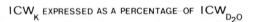

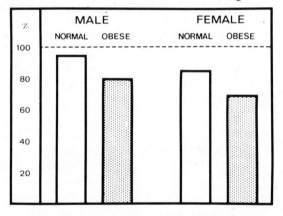

ICW$_K$ EXPRESSED AS A PERCENTAGE OF ICW$_{D_2O}$

Fig. 27.4. Intracellular water (ICW$_{D_2O}$) is shown for normal and obese boys and girls when the correct bromide space (extracellular volume) is subtracted from the deuterium space (total body water). This value is set at 100 per cent. In these subjects the intracellular water (ICW$_K$) can also be calculated by dividing the total body potassium (determined from ^{40}K radiation) by the net concentration of potassium in the intracellular fluid (147 mEq/liter of intracellular water).[40] When this calculation is made, it is found that there is almost agreement for the normal male by the two methods ($p < 0.05$) but there is a significant difference between the two approaches for normal females ($p < 0.001$). In obesity the departures between the two methods for boys and girls are greater. We suspect that ^{40}K radiation is absorbed to a greater or lesser degree by the amount of adipose tissue in the body. This results in an underestimate of total body potassium. The data are derived from the paper by Reba et al.[41]

thus to BMR. It may also be expected to be related to calorie intake. Information with respect to calorie intake is meager.

The fat deposition that occurs in the female at adolescence may obliterate some radiation when ^{40}K is used to measure ICM. During growth ICM is represented more and more by the intracellular phase of muscle (MICM). By adolescence MICM represents 70% of the total. In terms of protein turnover or protein reserves muscle is of prime importance.

The difference between ICM and MICM yields a parameter equivalent to "visceral cell mass" which in turn relates to BMR in a linear fashion from infancy through adolescence. No other parameter holds such a relationship with heat production. Thus heat production of the body at rest is closely linked to visceral cell mass, as has been emphasized by Holliday (Chapter 22). During activity muscle mass of course accounts for a major part of heat production.

The study of body water or of ICM when related to body length (an index of maturational age) indicates that the prepubertal growth spurt occurs at 9 years in the boy and 7 years in the girl (Chapter 22). These ages represent the times (or height ages) at which acceleration of cell mass can be identified. These maturational age limits correspond to the known rise in secretion of male and female sex hormones. The studies of Roche and Davila confirm the thinking. These investigators (Chapter 23) also define the time of cessation of postpubertal growth at 21 years for the male and 17 to 18 years for the female. These ages correspond to those found by Forbes[20] for the cessation of growth in lean body mass for males and females, respectively.

During protein calorie maturation (PCM) one would expect to find a reduction of ICM that would be reflected by a reduction of the BMR. Indeed (Chapter 25) it was shown that the ICM is a sensitive index of protein deprivation. This parameter (ICM) is disproportionately reduced relative to length. Overall body measurements are reduced but the ICM shows the greater reduction. (Animal studies indicate that during calorie deprivation but in the presence of protein sufficiency, the reductions of muscle mass and skeletal mass are proportional, but if protein deficiency is present, muscle mass is reduced to a greater extent.)

Infants with PCM not only have disproportionately reduced ICM (relative to length) but also reveal a failure of "catch-up growth" following some months of rehabilitation. The ICM continues to lag behind the growth of the skeleton. By contrast preadolescent boys with PCM studied in Guatemala (in collaboration with Drs. Habitch and Viteri) when given an adequate diet revealed faster growth of ICM relative to length so that proportionality was soon achieved. Perhaps the failure of infants to increase their ICM in the presence of an adequate diet is due to a failure of adequate insulin secretion and/or imbalance between insulin, growth hormone, and glucagon.

Chapter 24 reviews our information concerning the role of hormones in cellular growth. In muscle tissue the total DNA reflects, for the most part, the total number of nuclei within the myofibers while the ratio of protein to DNA is a measure of a unit akin to a cell (since it is assumed that each nucleus has jurisdiction over a definite volume of cytoplasm).

The increase in muscle nuclei from birth through adolescence is up to 20-fold for the male but less for the female. The ratio of nuclei in the male and female is of the order of 3:2. In the female the accretion of muscle cytoplasm (protein:DNA) is much more remarkable (relative to the male) prior to adolescence. A further expansion of cytoplasm may occur in the male after adolescence (as suggested by rat experiments) but no data are available for men between 18 and 25 years of age. Such changes in muscle growth can be explained on the basis of differential responses to insulin and growth hormone (see Figure 27.5).

Growth hormone (acting through somatomedin) causes multiplication of muscle nuclei while cytoplasmic growth early in postnatal life seems to be under the control of insulin. In early postnatal life thyroid hormone plays a role; and during adolescence androgens may also exert ancillary effects on cytoplasmic growth in the male.

Chapter 26 discusses the subject of overnutrition and adipose tissue growth. In females with obesity, the ICM is excessive (relative to body length as well as to age) and lean body mass and muscle mass are clearly increased. There is an increase in the number of nuclei within the musculature. A lack of sensitivity to the action of insulin in the peripheral circulation is shown by a reduced protein:DNA ratio in muscle.

It is suggested that overnutrition early in life causes excessive stimulation to the hypothalamic-pituitary axis so that excessive multiplication of adipocytes occurs in adipose tissue, and in lean tissues such as muscle, nuclear replication accelerates. In females a lack of estrogens or an excess of androgens is suspected because of the excess number of nuclei within the muscle mass. Indeed it would appear that insufficient estrogen is present. Growth hormone would therefore have an unrestricted effect on nuclear multiplication in muscle.

We find that excess circulating insulin relates closely to the excess fat of the obese individual. In some instances it would appear that the operation of ileal bypass does

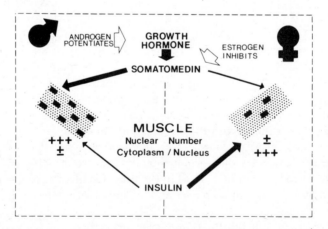

Fig. 27.5. This figure schematically represents in a simplified manner our thinking concerning the balance between insulin and growth hormone and the effects on muscle growth. Growth hormone causes nuclear replication in muscle, and insulin stimulates cytoplasmic growth. The sex difference in the pattern of growth (nuclear number versus the protein:DNA ratio) can be explained on the basis that estrogens inhibit the peripheral action of somatomedin (stimulated by growth hormone), whereas androgens encourage the secretion of growth hormone (and therefore somatomedin). Thus in the female during growth and adolescence the effects of insulin predominate but in the male growth hormone overrides insulin as discussed also elsewhere.[42] Moreover, estrogens in the female favor beta cellularity of the pancreas and insulin release (see ref. 10 for review).

cause a loss of adipocyte cells (fat cell number) and a reduction in the number of nuclei in the muscle mass. Indeed a state of protein-calorie malnutrition can be induced with this surgical procedure, as we reported at the International Congress of Nutrition in Mexico City, 1972.

Finally it is pointed out that while it has long been suspected that nutritional intake is related to longevity, it is not at all clear how diet, exercise, or activity influence cardiovascular status. Appetite, food intake, and hormonal activity all interrelate to influence length of life. It would appear that the life span is not necessarily determined wholly genetically; environmental factors are of great importance. Thus the affluent hypercaloric life may be the pathway to a brief existence due to cardiovascular atheroma, while a strenuous life may be optimal in terms of longevity. The study of negative growth and of senility represents a significant challenge for the investigator of tomorrow. Modern medicine allows many to live to three score years and ten but no new information or research allows this life span to be exceeded.

One can repeat that the time from birth to sexual maturation holds a positive relationship to the time from sexual maturation to senility and death. Aging reveals a lack of peripheral response to insulin and growth hormone. These are the major hormones involved in growth. The question arises as to whether environmental changes will override genetic influences and eventually the life span of man will double as predicted by students of thermodynamics and of biochemical efficiency.[21]

SUMMARY

During the course of our work we have not included any studies relating to the immediate newborn period. We have not investigated the problems of environmental temperature, the effects of acidosis on substrate, nor the metabolism of substrate per se in the early hours of postnatal life. Other investigators have studied these problems, particularly the group at the Karolinska Institute in Stockholm[22-25] and the group in Denver.[26-28] No detailed discussion has been included of the transport functions of the placenta.[29] Workers in Palo Alto have been concerned with the induction and action of enzymes during development and with metabolic aspects of cell multiplication and of pyrimidine nucleotides. Developmental biochemistry of the central nervous system and of visceral tissues have been studied. These papers are listed for the reader.[30-39]

Macaca mulatta has been shown to be a satisfactory model for the study of human fetal growth. Problems concerning maturation of the primate fetus may be better understood by the study of this subhuman primate. If any single lesson comes from this work, the lesson is that small mammals such as rodents, particularly at the fetal stage, are not reliable models for primate growth nor for the study of intellectual development. Nutritional and hormonal influences on fetal growth differ.

The experiments reported in this book make only a small contribution to the understanding of this vast uncharted sea of immaturity, prematurity, malnutrition and teratology, to name but a few of the regions requiring further exploration. The WHO report *Maturation of Fetal Body Systems*[5] crystallizes the thinking, our ignorance, and the sailing orders needed for attack. It is hoped that the preceding chapters describing facets of normal fetal growth in the primate, including brain growth, will form a foundation for further research.

REFERENCES

1. Benjamins, J. A., Guarnieri, M., Sonneborn, M., and McKhann, G.: Lipid metabolism in isolated neurons and oligodendroglia. In: Falkner, F. Kretchmer, N. and Rossi, E. (Eds.): *Modern Problems in Paediatrics*. S. Karger, Basel, 1974, Vol. 13, p. 142.

2. Conde, C., Martinez, M., and Bollabriga, A.: Some chemical aspects of human brain development. I. Neutral glycosphingolipids, sulfatides and sphingomyelin. *Pediatr. Res.*, **8**: 89, 1974.

3. Dobbing, J., and Sands, J.: Quantitative growth and development of human brain. *Arch. Dis. Child.* **48**: 757, 1973.

4. Cheek, D. B.: Cell growth and the possible role of trace metals. In: Cheek, D. B. (Ed.): *Human Growth*, Lea & Febiger, Philadelphia, 1968, Chapter 30, p. 424.

5. Report of WHO. Scientific Group: *Maturation of Fetal Body Systems*. World Health Organization, Technical Report Series No. 540, 1974.

6. Hoet, J. J.: Normal and abnormal foetal weight gain. In: Wolstenholm, G. E. W. (Ed.): *Foetal Autonomy*, a Ciba Foundation Symposium, 1969, p. 186.

7. Woods, S. C., and Porte, D.: Neural control of the endocrine pancreas. *Physiol. Rev.* **54**: 596, 1974.

8. Martin, J. M., Konijnendijk, W., and Bouman, P. D.: Insulin and growth hormone secretion in rats with ventral medial hypothalamic lesions maintained on restricted food intake. *Diabetes* **23**: 203, 1974.

9. Martin, J. M., Mok, C. C., Penfold, J., Howard, N. J., and Crowne, D.: Hypothalamic stimulation of insulin release. *J. Endocrin.* **58**: 681, 1973.

10. de Gasparo, M., and Hoet, J. J.: Normal and abnormal fetal weight gain. Proceedings of the Seventh Congress of the International Diabetes Federation, Buenos Aires. Excerpta medica Internat. Congr. Ser. No. 231, page 667, 1970.

11. Mellits, E. D., Dorst, J. P., and Cheek, D. B.: Bone age: its contribution to the prediction of maturational or biologic age. *Am. J. Phys. Anthrop.* **35**: 381, 1971.

12. Kulhanek, J. F., Meschia, G., Makowski, E. L., and Battaglia, F. C.: Changes in DNA content and urea permeability of the sheep placenta. *Am. J. Physiol.* **226**: 1257, 1974.

13. Black-Schaffer, B., and Turner, M. E.: Hyperplastic infantile cardiomegaly. *Am. J. Pathol.* **34**: 745, 1958.

14. Sandritter, W., and Adler, C. P.: Numerical hyperplasia in human heart hypertrophy. *Experimentia* **27**: 1433, 1971.

15. Beznak, M.: Effect of growth hormone and thyroxin on cardiovascular system of hypophysectomised rats. *Am. J. Physiol.* **204**: 279, 1963.

16. Beznak, M.: The effect of pituitary and growth hormone on the blood pressure and on the ability of the heart to hypertrophy. *J. Physiol.* **116**: 74, 1952.

17. Smith, C. H., Adcock, E. W., Teasdale, F., Meschia, G., and Battaglia, F. C.: Placental amino acid uptake: Tissue preparation, kinetics and preincubation effect. *Am. J. Physiol.* **224**: 558, 1973.

17a. Widdowson, E. M.: Immediate and long term consequences of being large or small at birth: A comparative approach. In: *Size at Birth. Ciba Foundation Symposium 27* (new series). Associated Scientific Publishers, P.O. Box 211, Amsterdam, p. 65.

17b. Liggins, G. C.: The influence of the fetal hypothalamus and pituitary on growth. In: *Size at Birth. Ciba Foundation Symposium 27* (new series). Associated Scientific Publishers, P.O. Box 211, Amsterdam, p. 165.

17c. Thorburn, G. D.: The role of the thyroid gland and kidneys in fetal growth. In: *Size at Birth. Ciba Foundation Symposium 27* (new series). Associated Scientific Publishers, P.O. Box 211, Amsterdam, p. 185.

17d. Young, M.: Pathology of supply line. In: *Size at Birth. Ciba Foundation Symposium 27* (new series). Associated Scientific Publishers, P.O. Box 211, Amsterdam, p. 21.

17e. Beisher, N. A. and O'Sullivan, E. F.: The effect of rest and intravenous infusion of hypertonic dextrose on subnormal extriol excretion in pregnancy. *Am. J. Obstet. Gynecol.* **113**: 771, 1972.

17f. Shearman, R. P., Shutt, D. A. and Smith, I. D.: The assessment and control of human fetal growth. In: *Size at Birth. Ciba Foundation Symposium 27* (new series). Associated Scientific Publishers, P.O. Box 211, Amsterdam, p. 27.

17g. Persson, B.: Assessment of metabolic control in diabetic pregnancy. In: *Size at Birth. Ciba Foundation Symposium 27* (new series). Associated Scientific Publishers, P.O. Box 211, Amsterdam, p. 247.

17h. Smythe, G. A., Brandstater, J. F. and Lazarus, L.: Serotoninergic control of rat growth hormone secretion *Neuroendrinology* (in press, 1975).

17i. Smythe, G. A., Stuart, M. C. and Lazarus, L.: Stimulation and suppression of somatomedin activity by serotonin and melatonin. *Experientia*. **30:** 1356, 1974.

18. Cheek, D. B.: Extracellular volume, its structure and measurement and the influence of age and disease. *J. of Pediatr.* **58:** 103, 1961.

19. Cheek, D. B., and Graystone, J. E.: Intracellular and extracellular volume (and sodium) and exchangeable chloride. In: Cheek, D. B. (Ed.): *Human Growth*, Lea & Febiger, Philadelphia, 1968, Chapter 10, p. 150.

20. Forbes, G. B.: Growth of the lean body mass in man. *Growth* **36:** 325, 1972.

21. Eichhorn, H. L.: The growth reproduction cycle closing phase. *Growth* **24:** 385, 1960.

22. Persson, B., and Tunell, R.: Influence of environmental temperature and acidosis on lipid mobilization in the human infant during the first 2 hours after birth. *Acta Pediat. Scand.* **60:** 385, 1971.

23. Gentz, J., Bengtsson, G., Hakkarainen, J., Hellstrom, R., and Persson, B.: Metabolic effects of starvation during neonatal period in the piglet. *Am. J. Physiol.* **218:** 662, 1970.

24. Persson, B., Starky, G., and Strandvic, B.: Intravenous glucose tolerance in overweight newborn infants and their mothers. *Pediatrics* **45:** 589, 1970.

25. Morris, F. H., Boyd, R. D. H., Makowski, E. L., Meschia, G., and Battaglia, F. C.: Glucose/oxygen quotients across the hind limb of fetal lambs. *Pediatr. Res.* **7:** 794, 1973.

26. James, J. E., Raye, J. R., Gresham, E. L., Makowski, E. L., Meschia, G. M., and Battaglia, F. C.: Fetal oxygen consumption, carbon dioxide production and glucose uptake in a chronic sheep preparation. *Pediatrics* **50:** 361, 1972.

27. Tsoulos, N. C., Schneider, J. M., Colwill, J. R., Meschia, G., Makowski, E. L., and Battaglia, F. C.: Cerebral glucose utilization during aerobic metabolism in fetal sheep. *Pediatr. Res.* **6:** 182, 1972.

28. Boyd, R. D. H., Morris, F. H., Meschia, G., Makowski, E. L., and Battaglia, F. C.: Growth of glucose and oxygen uptakes by fetuses of fed and starved ewes. *Am. J. Physiol.* **225:** 897, 1973.

29. Hagerman, D. A., and Villee, C. A.: Transport functions of the placenta. *Physiol. Res.* **40:** 313, 1960.

30. Levine, R. L., and Kretchmer, N.: Conversion of carbamoyl phosphate to hydroxyurea. An assay for carbamoylphosphate synthetase. *Anal. Biochem.* **42:** 324, 1971.

31. Roux, J. M., Hoogenraad, N. J., and Kretchmer, N.: Biosynthesis of pyrimidine nucleotides in mouse salivary glands stimulated with isoproterenol. *J. Biol. Chem.* **248:** 1196, 1973.

32. Kretchmer, N.: Developmental biochemistry: the central nervous system. *Res. Publ. Assoc. Res. Nerv. Ment. Dis.* **51:** 1, 1973.

33. Henning, S. J., and Kretchmer, N.: Development of interstitial function in mammals. *Enzymology* **15:** 3, 1973.

34. Kretchmer, N., and Bernstein, J.: The dynamic morphology of the nephron: morphogenesis of the protein droplet. *Kidney Int.* **5:** 96, 1974.

35. Levine, R. L., Hoogenraad, N. J., and Kretchmer, N.: Regulation of activity of carbamoyl phosphate synthetase from mouse spleen. *Biochemistry* **10:** 3694, 1971.

36. Lebenthal, E., Sunshine, P., and Kretchmer, N.: Effect of carbohydrate and corticosteroids on activity of glucosidases in intestine of the infant rat. *J. Clin. Invest.* **51:** 1244, 1972.

37. Johnson, J. D., Hurwitz, R., and Kretchmer, N.: Utilization of fat and glycerol for glycogenesis by the neonatal rat. *J. Nutr.* **101:** 299, 1971.

38. Kretchmer, N.: Developmental biochemistry—a relevant endeavor. Borden Award Address. *Pediatrics* **46**: 175, 1970.

39. Kretchmer, N.: Developmental biology. *Amer. J. Dis. Child.* **118**: 836, 1969.

40. Cheek, D. B., West, C. D., and Golden, C. C.: The distribution of sodium and chloride and the extracellular fluid volume in the rat. *J. Clin. Invest.* **36**: 340, 1957.

41. Reba, R. C., Cheek, D. B., and Mellits, E. D.: Body composition studies in pediatrics. In: James, A. E., Wagner, H. H. and Cooke, R. E. (Eds.): *Pediatric Nuclear Medicine.* W. B. Saunders, Philadelphia, 1974, p. 458.

42. Cheek, D. B.: Body composition, hormones, nutrition, and adolescent growth. In: Grumbach, M. M., Grave, G. D. and Mayer, F. E. (Eds.): *Control of Onset of Puberty.* John Wiley & Sons, 1974, Chapter 16, p. 424.

43. Unger, R.H., and Lefebvre, P.J. (Ed.): *Glucagon, Molecular Physiology, Clinical and Therapeutic Implications.* Pergamon Press, New York, 1972, Chapter 15.

APPENDIX I

DISSECTION OF THE FETUS AND INFANT

Macaca mulatta fetuses, newborn and infants, in this study were dissected by the protocol outlined below. The complete procedure, from removal of the fetus and placenta from the uterus to the end of the completion of the protocol, was complete within 35 to 45 minutes, the brain and liver being removed within 10 minutes of exsanguination.

Four people were required to carry out this task within the period of time stated. Two people carried out the actual dissection. A third person manned a precision balance where all critical samples were weighed to 1×10^{-5} g accuracy. This person was also responsible for the recording of all data during the procedure. The final member of the team checked that the samples were placed in the correct weighing vessel, acted as a courier between dissection table and balance bench, and made the less critical weighings on top-loading balances.

Sample sets for each dissection were prepared ahead of time, stored, and were available when required. Each set contained all the preweighed vessels and sample tubes required for a complete dissection. Each vessel was labeled with the same code number and a description of what tissue it would contain. Where more than one sample of a respective tissue was to be taken, the label would include the analysis required. The weight of each preweighed vessel was recorded on a weight record of the same code number. This record sheet and the corresponding sample set was used, respectively, to record all information and store all samples derived from a subsequent dissection.

Procedure

1. (a) The fetus and placenta were delivered by cesarean section and the cord clamped 10 to 15 cm from the fetus. The cord was cut and the fetal blood was collected into heparinized centrifuge tubes. The placenta and membranes were immersed in cold isotonic saline and put aside for further treatment after completion of the fetal dissection. A blood sample was taken from the mother at the time of cesarean section. (b) Newborns born spontaneously, or postnatal infants, were sedated with Sernylan (Parke Davis Co.) and exsanguinated by bleeding from the abdominal aorta into heparinized syringes.

2. The total volume of blood obtained by exsanguination was recorded. This blood was stored on ice until centrifugation. Following centrifugation in a refrigerated centrifuge, the plasma was removed and dispensed into a number of tubes for subsequent analysis of electrolyte, amino acids, hormones, and metabolites. Maternal blood was treated in a similar manner.

3. Following exsanguination (in the case of the fetus the umbilical stump was first removed and the excess amniotic fluid was blotted away with absorbent cotton gauze), the weight (g), crown-heel length (cm), crown-rump length (cm), and head circumference (cm) were determined and recorded. The sex of the animal and the age (in days) were recorded at this time.

4. *Brain.* The skin and periosteum were incised sagitally from nasal bridge to the base of the occiput. This incision was extended to expose the upper cervical muscles. Following incision, the cisterna magnum was tapped using a 21-gauge needle and 2.5-ml syringe and 1 to 2 ml of cerebrospinal fluid (CSF) was aspirated. The CSF was transferred to a glass vial and placed on ice. The brain was exposed by cutting through the parietal-occipital suture line and carefully extending the cut around the skull circumference. The bone flap and dura were removed and placed in a pre-weighed beaker labeled "Carcass." The entire brain was gently elevated at the frontal poles and by proceeding posteriorly the cranial nerves were severed at their origin. The dura was gently stripped from the cerebellum and posterior fossa and the brain was transected at the foramen magnum. Care was taken to remove the brain *in toto* as portions of the cerebellar folliculi were difficult to remove. The brain was then divided quickly and weighed by the following procedure:

(a) The brain stem and cerebellum were separated from the cerebrum by transecting the stem between the superior and inferior colliculi.
(b) The brain stem (pontine) was then dissected from the cerebellum by transecting the cerebellar peduncles at the cerebellar surface.
(c) The cerebellum was divided sagitally in approximately equal halves.
(d) The cerebrum was divided sagitally in approximately equal halves.
(e) Two adjacent samples of occipital cortex were cut from the right cerebral hemisphere. These were taken from the medial aspect at the level of the posterior division of the calcarine fissure.
(f) All the dissected portions were then placed in a preweighed glass vessel, weighed, and the weight recorded.

Each individual brain piece was removed in the following sequence, the vessel being reweighed and the weight recorded after removal of each portion. The weight of each piece was later obtained from the difference in weight between the sequential weighings. The pontine stem was first removed, frozen, and stored, followed by both cerebellar pieces which were placed in another preweighed glass vessel. The occipital cortex samples were then removed, one being frozen and stored for subsequent chemical analysis while the other was snap frozen and embedded in cold liquid paraffin. The intact half of cerebrum was then removed, frozen, and stored for chemical analysis, while the remaining hemisphere from which the occipital cortex samples were taken was subsequently dried at 95°C and reweighed.

The vessel containing the two pieces of cerebellum was then reweighed; one piece was then removed and the remaining half was also subsequently dried at 95°C and reweighed.

5. *Pituitary.* The posterior sella and the lateral aspect of the sella turcica were cut exposing the pituitary. The pituitary was gently removed, transferred to a preweighed vial, weighed, and then stored at −20°C.

6. *Liver.* The abdomen was incised exposing the liver and abdominal viscera. The liver was removed *in toto* and the gallbladder and any visible connective tissue removed. Prior to sequential weighing the liver was apportioned as follows:

(a) Approx. 500 mg (amino acid analysis).
(b) Approx. 50–100 mg (histology).
(c) Approx. 250 mg (nucleic acid analysis).
(d) Approx. 2 g (protein).
(e) Approx. 2–3 g (trace metal analysis).

These were all placed in a preweighed vessel and weighed. The individual specimens were removed sequentially as above and the contents of the vessel reweighed after each removal of liver tissue.

Samples (a), (c), and (d), along with the remaining portion of the liver, were frozen and stored in prelabeled vials at $-20°C$. Sample (e) was transferred to a separate preweighed vessel and reweighed. This was then placed in a 95°C drying oven and subsequently reweighed. Sample (b) was snap frozen and stored in cold liquid paraffin. The remaining liver tissue was also frozen and stored at $-20°C$.

7. *Spleen.* The spleen was removed, excess connective tissue was removed, the tissue weighed directly on a top-loading balance, and the weight recorded to 1×10^{-2} g. The spleen was transferred to a preweighed beaker labeled "Viscera."

8. *Kidneys and Adrenals.* Both kidneys and the adrenals were removed. The tissues were trimmed and the kidneys were weighed on a top-loading balance, the weight recorded to 1×10^{-2} g, and transferred to the beaker labeled "Viscera." The adrenals were transferred to separate preweighed glass vials, weighed, and then stored at $-20°C$.

9. *Pancreas.* The pancreas was carefully dissected from the omentum by beginning at the "tail" and progressing toward the "head." Special attention was placed on complete dissection. Excess fat, lymph nodes, and connective tissue were excised. The dissected pancreas was weighed in a preweighed vessel and stored at $-20°C$. Portions of the pancreas were taken for histology, depending on the particular experiment.

10. *Heart.* The thorax was opened and the heart was dissected free of the pericardium. The heart was then removed from the thoracic cavity by dividing the great vessels at the base of the heart. The heart was divided as follows:

(a) The heart was cut horizontally to divide the auricular tissue from the ventricles.

(b) Cut horizontally to obtain a 50–100-mg sample of the ventricular apex for histology.

(c) Cut horizontally to obtain a 200-mg sample of myocardium for nucleic acids.

These specimens and the remaining myocardial tissue were placed in a preweighed glass weighing vessel and weights were obtained by sequential removal and difference. Specimen (b) was snap frozen for histology. Specimen (c) was frozen and stored at $-20°C$ for later chemical analysis. The remaining myocardial tissue was dried at 95°C and subsequently weighed. The auricular tissue was discarded.

11. *Thymus and lungs.* The thymus and lungs were then removed from the thoracic cavity, divided and trimmed, and weighed individually on a top-loading balance. The weights were recorded and these tissues were transferred to the beaker labeled "Viscera."

12. *Thyroid.* The thyroid gland was dissected out. Most of the gland was located at the side and back of the trachea. A small narrow isthmus was present in most cases. The gland was placed in a preweighed vial, weighed, and stored at $-20°C$.

13. *Muscle sample.* The skin and subcutaneous tissue were dissected off the left thigh region to below knee level and 2 to 3 g of the hamstring muscle removed. This muscle was freed of excess fat, connective tissue, and nerves and was divided into the following aliquots:

(a) Approx. 200 mg (amino acid sample).

(b) Approx. 200–300 mg (nucleic acid analysis).

These pieces and the remaining sample were placed in a preweighed glass weighing vessel and weighed by sequential removal. Muscle pieces (a) and (b) were stored at $-20°C$. The remaining muscle sample was transferred in the weighing bottle to a $95°C$ drying oven and was subsequently weighed.

14. *Bone sample.* The distal end of the femur was cleaned free of adhering tissue and then dislocated at the knee. Approximately 1.0 cm of femur was removed and weighed in a preweighed glass vial. The vessel plus bone sample was dried at $95°C$ and subsequently weighed.

15. *Remaining viscera.* The viscera remaining within the carcass were removed, weighed on a top-loading balance, and then transferred to the beaker labeled "Viscera." The "Viscera" beaker was reweighed and placed in a $95°C$ oven for drying and subsequent fat extraction.

16. *Skin.* The skin and tail were removed *in toto* from the carcass. The tail was removed and discarded. The skin was transferred to a preweighed beaker labeled "Skin" and weighed. The beaker and skin were then dried at $95°C$ for subsequent weighing and fat extraction.

17. *Carcass.* Similarly the carcass was placed in the beaker labeled "Carcass" and weighed. The "Carcass" beaker and its contents were also dried at $95°C$ to be following by weighing and fat extraction. The carcass is essentially muscle and skeleton.

18. *Placenta.* Following the dissection of the fetus, the placenta was freed of blood clots, the membranes were trimmed to the border of the placenta and discarded, and decidua basalis remnants were removed. The cord and surface vessels were also removed. The cleaned, blotted placenta (usually two discs) was then weighed directly on the top-loading balance. One-half of each disc was transferred to a weighed beaker and recorded. This portion was dried at $95°C$, while the remainder was weighed, frozen, and stored in a plastic container at $-20°C$ for later analysis.

PREPARATION OF HOMOGENATES FOR CHEMICAL ANALYSES

1. *Brain.* It became apparent to us early in the program that careful consideration would have to be given to the preparation of the cerebrum and cerebellum homogenates for the following reasons:

    (a)   Accurate estimations of total amount of a component were required.

    (b)   Concentration of the tissue in the homogenate must be suitable for all assays.

    (c)   The possible lability of some components must be taken into account.

    (d)   The practicability of the procedure itself.

Preliminary work indicated that the following precautions be taken during homogenization:

    (a)   Temperature—as near to $0°C$ as possible.

    (b)   All diluents chilled as near to $0°C$ as practical.

    (c)   Thawing of frozen brain samples be carried out as near to $0°C$ as practical.

    (d)   All tissue weighed prior to homogenization to ascertain water loss during storage.

    (e)   All vessels containing diluents be weighed before and after addition.

The following procedure has been devised and used in this study: One frozen cerebral hemisphere or one-half cerebellum is quickly weighed in a preweighed mason jar and returned to the cold room. Chilled water from a preweighed measuring cylinder is added to the mason jar so that there is approximately 10 g of chilled water to 1 g of frozen tissue (homogenate concentration approximately 100 mg/ml). The cylinder is reweighed and the weight of water added to the tissue is recorded. The tissue is first homogenized in the mason jar on a "Lourdes" cutting blade homogenizer in the cold room. This preliminary treatment was always applied to cerebral hemispheres and in cases where the one-half cerebellum weighed in excess of 2.5 g. The preliminary procedure afforded the larger tissues to be handled effectively without the problem of excess local heat production, as is found with "Duall" tissue grinders. Furthermore, the procedure allowed practical homogenization of large volumes (up to 300 ml).

The preliminary homogenate (or the smaller-sized half cerebellum samples) is then homogenized in a 30-ml-capacity "Duall" tissue grinder until all white matter has been disintegrated and the mixture appears homogeneous. The homogenate is transferred to a chilled beaker containing a stirring bar on a magnetic stirrer. After a period of mixing, aliquots for the following analyses were dispensed into pre-labeled tubes or bottles.

(a) Nucleic acids and enzyme aliquots dispensed and stored at 0°C until analyzed (within 24 hours).

(b) Lipid extraction—dispensed into lipid extraction tubes placed in a Virtis "Biodryer" and lyophilized and stored for subsequent extraction and analysis.

(c) Carbonic anhydrase—centrifuged in the cold at 0°C for 30 minutes, the supernatant decanted and stored at 4°C until analyzed (usually within 6 hours).

(d) Amino acids—dispensed and refrozen at −20°C for later analyses.

(e) The excess homogenate is bottled and frozen at −20°C.

Approximately 8 to 10 samples can be handled per day provided two to three people are available to work together, to prepare and subsequently analyze the DNA, RNA, and enzyme components.

2. *Placenta.* Frozen placental samples are prepared like frozen cerebrum.

3. *Muscle, heart, and liver.* The frozen samples of these tissues are prepared by thawing in a cold room at 4° C. The thawed samples are homogenized with chilled water in a "Duall" tissue grinder of appropriate size at a concentration of approximately 30 mg of tissue per milliliter of water.

DESOXYRIBONUCLEIC ACID (DNA)

DNA is determined by a modification of the method of Kissane and Robins.[1] This procedure, which is specific for DNA, is based on the measurement of a fluorescent product from the reaction between 3,5-diaminobenzoic acid (DABA) and deoxyribose following precipitation and lipid extraction. The method is specific for DNA and is not affected by the interfering substances that can yield erroneously high values by some diphenylamine techniques. In previous work, we have applied this method to tissues other than brain. Hinegardner confirms the validity of this application.[2]

Reagents

Analytical reagent chemicals are used throughout the procedure.

1. DNA standards. A *stock* standard is prepared by dissolving 20 mg of a pure DNA preparation (calf thymus DNA—highly polymerized—Worthington Biochemical Corp., Freehold, New Jersey) in 10 ml of 1 N ammonium hydroxide. Aliquots of the stock standard are appropriately diluted with 1 N ammonium hydroxide to obtain a series of working standards ranging from 40 to 200 μg of DNA per milliliter. The standards are stored at 4°C and are stable indefinitely.

2. DABA reagent. One molar DABA (3,5-diaminobenzoic acid dihydrochloride—Aldrich Chemical Co. Inc., Milwaukee, Wisconsin, Catalog No. 11,383-2 gold label) is prepared by dissolving 1.20 g in 5 ml of ion-free water. The solution is treated with approximately 200 mg of activated charcoal (Norit A), mixed, and centrifuged for 10 minutes. The resultant supernatant is sufficient for 60 individual assays.

3. Trichloroacetic acid (TCA)—0.3 and 0.6 N chilled.

4. Perchloric acid (PCA)—0.6 N prepared gravimetrically.

5. Alcoholic potassium acetate—0.1 N. Potassium acetate, 2.5 g, is dissolved in 250 ml of absolute ethanol.

6. Absolute ethanol.

7. Quinine sulfate fluorometric standard—5 μg/ml.

Procedure

1. The tissue to be analyzed, previously homogenized in ice-cold water (see Preparation of Homogenates) at the appropriate concentration shown in column A of the following table, is treated with TCA (columns C and D). This treatment is carried out in 13 × 100-mm tubes in an ice bath.

Tissue	A Homogenate (mg/ml)	B Aliquot of homogenate (ml)	C 0.6 N TCA (ml)	D 0.3 N TCA (ml)	Dilution
Cerebrum	100	1.0	1.0	2.0	1:4
Muscle	30	1.0	1.0	—	1:2
Heart	30	1.0	1.0	2.0	1:4
Liver	30	1.0	1.0	2.0	1:4

The following tissues, which were originally prepared as a 100-mg/ml homogenate, require to be diluted with water 1:5 before proceeding.

Cerebellum	20	1.0	1.0	2.0	1:20
Placenta	20	1.0	1.0	2.0	1:20

Tubes are "vortexed" between each addition and before each transfer as described in the next step. Note that the final concentrations of TCA for each tissue preparation is 0.3 N.

2. Aliquots (0.2 ml) of the TCA-treated homogenate are pipetted into 3-ml centrifuge tubes, each homogenate being analyzed in quadruplicate. Then 0.15 ml

of 0.3 N TCA is added; the tubes are vortexed and centrifuged at 4°C for 10 minutes at 1,500 rpm. After centrifuging, the supernatant is discarded, care being taken not to disturb the precipitate.

3. A volume of 0.6 ml of 0.1 N alcoholic potassium acetate solution is added to each tube. The tubes are vortexed and allowed to sit on ice for 5 to 10 minutes before centrifuging. Again the supernatant is carefully removed and discarded.

4. A volume of 0.6 ml of absolute alcohol is added to each tube, the tubes are vortexed, capped with parafilm, and heated at 60°C in a heating block for 15 minutes. After centrifuging, the supernatant is again carefully removed and discarded. A second alcohol wash is performed. This time 0.6 mls. of absolute alcohol are added, the tubes are vortexed and the supernatant removed after centrifuging. The sample tubes are then placed in a desiccator and dried under vacuum until no visible liquid is observed above the precipitate. It is important that the precipitate remains gelatinous.

5. A 0.08-ml volume of freshly prepared DABA reagent is added to each tube and thoroughly mixed. The tubes are capped and heated at 60°C for 30 minutes in a heating block.

6. A volume of 1.2 ml of 0.6 N PCA is added to each 3-ml centrifuge tube; the contents are mixed thoroughly and centrifuged. Then 2.0 ml of 0.6 N PCA is pipetted into a separate series of labeled 13 × 100-mm tubes—one for each determination. One milliliter of the contents of each 3-ml centrifuge tube is transferred to the appropriate tube containing PCA and thoroughly mixed.

7. Fluorescence is determined in Zeiss PMQ4 spectrophotofluorometer or similar precision instrument using an excitation wavelength of 394 nm and fluorescent wavelength of 510 nm, fluorescence being stable for 2 hours. The spectrophotofluorometer is internally standardized with the quinine sulfate standard.

Standards

Fifty-microliter volumes of the DNA standards (containing 2–10 μg of DNA) are pipetted into identified 3-ml centrifuge tubes in quadruplicate. A series of tubes containing 50 μl of 1 N ammonium hydroxide is prepared as blanks. These tubes are then brought to dryness under dry nitrogen and then treated identically as the tissue samples from step 5 onwards.

Calculation

$$\text{DNA mg/g of tissue} = \frac{\text{fluorescence of sample} - Bl}{m} \times \frac{\text{dilution}}{A} \times \frac{1}{0.2}$$

where m = slope factor (fluorescence/μg DNA)
dilution = see table above
A = mg tissue/ml homogenate
0.2 = sample aliquot (ml)
Bl = fluorescence of blank

Eight to ten tissue samples in quadruplicate can be analyzed by one operator in a working day by this procedure.

RIBONUCLEIC ACID (RNA)

RNA is determined by the modified Schmidt-Thannhauser procedure of Munro and Fleck.[3]

The Schmidt-Thannhauser procedure has been selected as the method of choice because it is least subject to analytical error.[4] In this procedure preliminary acid extraction removes acid-soluble phosphates. Subsequent alkaline hydrolysis is used to extract RNA from the residue. The DNA, being resistant to alkali, is precipitated with acid. The ribose moiety in the RNA is determined by a modified Bial orcinol reaction.

Reagents

Analytical reagent chemicals are used throughout the procedure.

1.   RNA standards. A *stock* standard is prepared by weighing 10 mg of purified RNA (prepared from bakers' yeast by the method of Crestfield et al[5]—Sigma Chemical Co., St. Louis, Missouri—Catalog No. R 6750, Type XI purified) into a 100-ml volumetric flask.

Four milliliters of 0.3 N KOH is added and the contents of the flask mixed thoroughly. The flask is incubated for 1 hour at 37°C. The digest is then cooled on ice and 2.5 ml of 1.2 N perchloric acid is added. Then add 10 ml of 0.6 N perchloric acid, make to volume with ion-free water, and mix thoroughly. The final concentration of one stock standard is 100 μg/ml.

Aliquots of the stock standard are appropriately diluted in 0.1 N perchloric acid to obtain a series of working standards ranging from 8 to 40 μg of RNA per milliliter. The standards are stored at 4°C and are stable for 4 weeks.

2.   Potassium hydroxide (KOH)—0.3 N.

3.   Perchloric acid (PCA)—0.1, 0.2, 0.6, and 1.2 N prepared gravimetrically and chilled at 4°C.

4.   Acid ferric chloride. Stock solution, 10 g anhydrous ferric chloride is dissolved in 100 ml concentrated hydrochloric acid. A working solution is prepared on the day of analysis—0.5 ml of stock solution diluted to 100 ml with concentrated hydrochloric acid.

5.   Orcinol reagent. Take 0.4 g orcinol (methyl rescorcinol—Mathieson, Coleman and Bell) and dissolve in 10 ml of absolute ethanol immediately prior to use.

Procedure

RNA extraction

1.   The tissue to be analyzed, previously homogenized in ice-cold water (see Preparation of Homogenates) at the appropriate concentration shown in column A of the following table, is treated with 0.6 N PCA and water to adjust the final PCA concentration in the tube to 0.2 N (see table). This treatment is carried out in 13 $\times$ 100-mm test tubes in an ice bath.

Tissue	A Homogenate (mg/ml)	B Homogenate volume (ml)	C PCA 0.6 N	D Water
Cerebrum	100	0.5	0.5	0.5
Cerebellum	100	0.5	0.5	0.5
Muscle	30	1.0	0.5	—
Heart	30	1.0	0.5	—
Liver	30	0.5	0.5	0.5
Placenta	100	0.5	0.5	0.5

2.   The tubes are vortexed thoroughly and allowed to stand in ice for 10 minutes. The tubes are then centrifuged at 2,000 rpm for 10 minutes, and the supernatant removed. (*N.B.*   This supernatant can be used for amino acid analysis if required.)

3.   The precipitate is washed with 0.2 N PCA, mixed thoroughly, and recentrifuged at 2,000 rpm for another 10 minutes. The supernatant is decanted and the washing procedure repeated. The tubes are kept on ice during the procedure. The tubes are then inverted on filter paper or convenient absorbant to drain 2 minutes.

4.   A volume of 0.8 ml of 0.3 N KOH is added to the precipitate, the contents are vortexed thoroughly and incubated in a dry heating block at 37°C for 1 hour. During the time of incubation the contents of the tubes are vortexed at approximately 20-minute intervals. At the end of the incubation period each tube is checked for complete hydrolysis.

5.   The tubes are again placed on ice, 0.5 ml of 1.2 N PCA is added, vortexed thoroughly, and allowed to stand for 10 minutes. The tubes are centrifuged at 2,000 rpm for 10 minutes and the supernatant is transferred with a Pasteur pipet to a 5-ml volumetric flask (for muscle or heart) or to a 10-ml volumetric flask (for cerebrum, cerebellum, liver, or placenta).

6.   Rewash the precipitate with 0.5 ml of 0.2 N PCA, followed by mixing and centrifugation for 10 minutes. The washings are added to the appropriate flask. This washing and transfer procedure is repeated.

7.   The 5-ml flasks are made to volume with water while for the 10-ml flasks 5 ml of 0.1 N PCA is added and made to volume with water. This procedure will maintain the PCA concentration at 0.1 N.

8.   The contents of each flask are thoroughly mixed before filtering, which is achieved by using medium-porosity fritted glass filter under positive pressure. The filtrate is collected in identified 25 × 150-mm tubes. (*N.B.*   A filtrate blank is also prepared by passing 5 or 10 ml of 0.1 N PCA through the filter.)

Quantitation

9.   One milliliter of each RNA extract, standard solution, or filtrate blank is pipetted into identified 13 × 100-mm tubes in triplicate. A volume of 1.0 ml of 0.1 N PCA is used as a reagent blank. A volume of 2.0 ml acid ferric chloride (working solution) is added to each tube with a volumetric transfer pipet followed by a volume of 0.2 ml orcinol reagent. The tubes are vortexed thoroughly and placed in a heating block at 100°C for exactly 20 minutes.

10. The tubes are cooled in an ice bath and the optical density (OD) of each tube is determined at 660 nm in a Zeiss spectrophotometer against a reagent blank.

Calculation

$$\text{RNA mg/g} = \frac{\text{OD unknown} - \text{OD filtrate blank}}{m} \times \frac{B}{A} \times \frac{1}{C}$$

where m = slope factor in OD/μg RNA
A = mg tissue/ml homogenate
B = volume in ml of RNA extract (ie, 5 ml—heart, muscle, 10 ml—cerebrum, cerebellum, liver, placenta)
C = volume in ml of homogenate aliquot

Note: The maintenance of the concentration of PCA at 0.2 *N* is optimal and critical during the *whole* process of the extraction of RNA from tissue.[4]

It is essential that all PCA reagents are carefully and accurately prepared and that precision volumetric glassware is used throughout the procedure of extraction. Eight to ten tissue samples can be extracted in duplicate, and each extract can be determined in triplicate by one operator in a working day by this procedure.

PROTEIN

The introduction of the semiautomated micro-Dumas technique for nitrogen has doubled our daily output of protein determinations. As the analysis requires the accurate weighing of the sample as the only manipulative procedure carried out by a technician, technical errors have been greatly reduced.

The apparatus used is a Coleman Nitrogen Analyzer (Model 29) with a modified combustion tube packing that removes the sulfur and halogen components after pyrolysis.

This analysis requires accurate weighing of dried tissue in the 2- to 10-mg range into aluminum "boats." The boat is transferred to a combustion tube, packed with cupric oxide, and inserted into the apparatus. The combustion tube is then purged with high-purity carbon dioxide gas to drive out trapped air in the combustion train. At the end of purging the combustion tube is heated in a series of furnace movements to ensure complete pyrolysis of the sample into its elemental consitutents. The gaseous products formed during pyrolysis are then vented out of the combustion tube by the carrier CO_2 gas and carried over oxidizing and reducing materials leaving only gaseous nitrogen and carbon dioxide. This gaseous mixture is "scrubbed" thoroughly in caustic alkali where all the carbon dioxide is removed. The pure nitrogen remaining is collected and measured in a stainless steel syringe coupled to a precision micrometer. The quantity of nitrogen in the sample is calculated under standard temperature and pressure and this value converted to protein by multiplying by 6.25.

Sequential analysis of different dried tissues demonstrated a coefficient of variation between 0.82 and 1.33%.

BRAIN LIPID EXTRACTION

The brain lipids are quantitatively extracted by a procedure based on the method of Folch and co-workers. [7] This modification allows for a constant water proportion during all stages of the procedure, a critical factor in quantitative extraction and partition of lipids. Large and inconvenient volumes of solvents are not used, and accurate measuring pipets can be employed with conventional centrifugal apparatus.

Eight brain homogenates, each extracted in duplicate, can be processed by one person in one working day.

Reagents

Analytical reagent solvents and chemicals are used throughout the procedure.
1. Chloroform ($CHCl_3$).
2. Methanol (MeOH).
3. Potassium chloride (KCl). 0.015 M KCl in water.

Procedure

1. One- or two-milliliter aliquots of brain tissue homogenates (100 mg/ml) are pipetted into 25-μl screw-capped tissue culture tubes and are lyophilized overnight in a Virtis Biodryer.

2. The lyophilized homogenate is reconstituted with 0.5 ml of ion-free water and dissolved. A 9.5-ml volume of $CHCl_3$: MeOH (2:1) is added, and the tube is sealed with a Teflon sealing screw cap. The contents of the tube are thoroughly vortexed. The total contents were filtered through a medium-porosity fritted glass filter (using nitrogen under pressure) into a similar culture tube labeled "L.P." (lower phase). The sample tube is rinsed with $CHCl_3$: MeOH: water (16:8:1), and the washings passed through the filter and collected in tube L.P.

3. The filtered extract (L.P. tube) is partitioned by the addition of 2.8 ml of water. The L.P. tube is mixed and centrifuged at 4°C for 20 minutes. The upper phase is quantitatively removed and placed in a calibrated 15-ml culture tube labeled "U.P." The interface of the L.P. tube is washed with 2.0 ml of $CHCl_3$: MeOH: H_2O (3:48:47) and the resultant upper phase is added to the U.P. tube.

4. A 2.0 ml volume of $CHCl_3$: MeOH: KCl (3:48:47) is added to the L.P. tube, mixed, and centrifuged for 20 minutes at 4°C. The upper phase is removed and transferred to the U.P. tube. This step is repeated one more time. The U.P. tube is made to 15 ml with ion-free water, capped, and stored at 0°C for subsequent analysis.

5. The contents of the L.P. tube are transferred to a 100-ml round-bottom flask, the L.P. is washed with $CHCl_3$: MeOH: H_2O (86:14:1) a number of times, and the washings added to the round-bottom flask. The contents of this flask are evaporated under vacuum on a rotary evaporator to dryness and the residue taken up in 10.0 ml of $CHCl_3$: MeOH (2:1). This quantitative extract is added to a fresh tube also labeled L.P., capped, and stored for analysis.

The lower phase extract (L.P. tube) is used for the subsequent analysis of cholesterol and phospholipid while the upper phase extract (U.P. tube) is analyzed for lipid N-acetylneuraminic acid (lipid NANA).

BRAIN CHOLESTEROL (TOTAL STEROL)

Free cholesterol (together with the relatively small proportions of cholesterol ester and desmosterol) is determined by the ferric chloride reaction to avoid problems that may arise from different molar extinction coefficients and absorption maxima that are found when estimating these substances with the Liebermann-Buchard reaction.

Initially we used the method of Crawford,[8] an improved Zaltkis procedure, and applied it to dried lower phase lipid extracts. It was found that this procedure was affected with gross gas production (trapped in the viscous acid reagents when these reagents were applied to tissue lipid extract).

Subsequently we have found that the serum cholesterol method described by Franey and Amador[9] was admirably suited to the determination of brain lipids. This method utilizes ethyl acetate as the anhydrous matrix instead of glacial acetic acid. Gas formation is nonexistent, viscosity is low, color development is maximal after a short time period, stable for at least 45 minutes, and is not affected by the photochemical effect exhibited by the Zaltkis-Crawford methods. Absorption spectra and maxima are almost identical and the sensitivity of this method is of an order similar to that of the Zalktis-Crawford procedure.

Reagents

Analytical reagent solvents and chemicals are used throughout the procedure.

1. Cholesterol standards. Source: Cholesterol S.C.W.—Nutritional Biochemical Corporation, Cleveland, Ohio 44128. Stock standard: 200 mg cholesterol dissolved in 100 ml absolute ethanol. Aliquots of stock standard were diluted with absolute ethanol to obtain a series of working standards ranging from 40 to 160 μg of cholesterol per milliliter.

2. Concentrated sulfuric acid. A. R. and anhydrous. Check batch of acid before use.

3. Ferric chloride/ethyl acetate reagent (FCEA). Two hundred milligrams of anhydrous $FeCl_3$ dissolved in 100 ml of absolute ethyl acetate. Stable for at least 6 months.

4. Absolute ethanol. A.R.

Procedure

1. Take 0.2-ml aliquots of lower phase extract and pipet into 16 $\times$ 125-mm tissue culture tubes and dry under nitrogen. The tube is capped and stored until analysis.

2. A volume of 0.5 ml of absolute ethanol is added to each blank or unknown tube (containing dried lower phase extract). Take 0.5 ml of cholesterol working standards and add to the standard tubes.

3. Working with approximately 9 to 12 tubes at a time, add 2.0 ml of FCEA and vortex well. Then add 2.0 ml of concentrated sulfuric acid to each tube while it is being vortexed. Mix to complete homogeneity before proceeding to the next tube.

4. While this group of tubes is cooling, repeat step 3 using a second group of 9 to 12 tubes, and so on.

5. When the second group of tubes is cooling, the absorbances of the first set of tubes are measured in a spectrophotometer. It is essential that all tubes are read within 45 minutes from the time of addition of the acid. Absorbance is determined at 550 nm against a reagent blank. All samples are determined in duplicate.

Calculation

$$\text{Cholesterol mg/g} = \frac{\text{ODu}}{m} \times \frac{1}{A} \times \frac{1}{B} \times \frac{10}{0.2}$$

$$= \frac{\text{ODu}}{m} \times \frac{50}{A} \times \frac{1}{B}$$

where m = slope factor (OD/μg cholesterol)

A = mg tissue/ml homogenate

B = volume of homogenate lyophilized and extracted

10 = volume of lower phase extract

0.2 = aliquot of lower phase extract assayed

ODu = optical density of unknown

BRAIN LIPID NANA

Brain lipid NANA is determined by a modification of the method of Hess and Rolde.[10]

N-Acetylneuraminic acid (NANA) of brain ganglioside is a nine-carbon α-keto-acid. Such compounds readily undergo decarboxylation on treatment with hot mineral acid forming 2 deoxy-4-amino-octose. The 2-deoxy sugars and in general aldehydes of the type $R-CH_2-CHO$ will react with 3,5-diaminobenzoic acid (DABA) to yield highly fluorescent quinaldines. This is the same principle for the fluorometric measurement of DNA.

Hexoses seriously interfere with the quantitation of NANA. Presumably an intermediate in the conversion of hexose to levulinic acid (by hot mineral acid) is hydroxylevulinic aldehyde, an α-methylene aldehyde. However, it has been found that by adjustment of the acid strength and increasing the time of heating and temperature, hexose interference can be reduced to 1.6% on a molar basis. DNA is absent from lipid extracts and therefore cannot interfere with this assay.

Reagents

Analytical reagent chemicals are used throughout the procedure.

1. N-Acetylneuraminic acid (NANA). Source: Calbiochem Corp., La Jolla, California, Catalog No. 110137. Stock standard: 1.0 mg/ml dissolved in water.

Working standard: Aliquots of the stock standard are appropriately diluted with water to obtain a series of working standards from 50 to 200 μg/ml.

2. DABA reagent. Source: Aldrich Chemical Co., Inc., Milwaukee, Wisconsin, Catalog No. 11383-2 (gold label). A solution of 0.005 M DABA 3,5-diamino-benzoic acid dihydrochloride) in 0.125 N HCl is prepared by weighing 30.4 mg of the salt into a 25-ml volumetric flask. Add 3.125 ml of standardized 1 N HCl and make to volume with ion-free water. This reagent is prepared fresh for each assay.

3. Hydrochloric acid—0.05 N.

Procedure

1. The 0.5-ml aliquots of *upper phase* extract are pipetted (in duplicate) into 5-ml ampules (Kimble "color break") using long tip Mohr pipets. Care is taken so that *no* extract is deposited on the stem of the ampule. The 0.1-ml aliquots of NANA working standard are also pipetted into 5-ml ampules (in duplicate) with the same precautions.

2. The contents of the ampules are reduced to dryness under a stream of dry nitrogen in a 40°C water bath.

3. A volume of 1.0 ml DABA reagent is pipetted into each ampule taking care that *no* reagent is deposited on the stem of the ampule. A reagent blank is prepared by adding 1.0 ml of DABA reagent to a clean ampule.

4. Each ampule is sealed with a dual air-acetylene flame, allowed to cool, and the content of each ampule is thoroughly mixed.

5. The ampules are placed in a 100°C hot air oven for 16 hours.

6. After incubation at 100°C, 0.2 ml (or any other convenient volume) is pipetted into identified 13 × 100-mm tubes and 0.05 N HCl is added to make the total volume in the tube 4 ml. The contents of each tube are vortexed.

7. Fluorescence is determined by using an excitation wavelength of 394 nm and a fluorescent wavelength of 510 nm. The spectrophotofluorometer is internally standardized against quinine sulfate solution.

Calculation

$$\text{Lipid NANA mg/g} = \frac{\text{fluorescence unknown} - Bl}{m} \times \frac{1}{A} \times \frac{1}{B} \times \frac{15}{0.5}$$

where m = slope factor (fluorescence/μg NANA)
A = mg tissue/ml homogenate
B = volume of homogenate extracted (ml)
15 = volume of upper phase extract (ml)
0.5 = aliquot of upper phase extract analyzed (ml)
Bl = fluorescence of blank

Note that no attempt was taken to dialyze the upper phase material. Ganglioside NANA amounts to approximately 80% of the lipid NANA value.

BRAIN PHOSPHOLIPID

Nitric acid digestion rapidly liberates inorganic phosphate from the organic lipid combination, is completely volatilized on heating, and leaves no residual acidity. The addition of calcium to the nitric acid digestion mixture prevents the loss of inorganic phosphate. The phosphate is determined spectrophotometrically by the method of Fiske and Subbarow.[11]

Procedure

1. A volume of 0.5 ml of lower phase extract is pipetted (cf lipid extraction procedure) into a 15-ml test tube and evaporated to dryness under dry nitrogen.
2. A volume of 2 ml *concentrated nitric acid* (containing 50 mg anhydrous calcium carbonate in 1 liter of A.R. concentrated nitric acid) is added to the tube together with two glass beads.
3. The solution is boiled to dryness over a Bunsen burner. (When the acid is evaporated almost to dryness, intense yellow fumes appear. Continue heating for a few seconds after all fumes have been expelled to ensure complete elimination of all oxides of nitrogen.) *Fume cupboard procedure.*
4. A volume of 4.3 ml of ion-free water is added to the tube, vortexed, and the inorganic phosphate is determined by the method of Fiske and Subbarow where the blue complex formed is determined spectrophotometrically at 680 nm.

Calculation

$$\text{Lipid phosphorus (mg/g)} = \frac{OD}{m} \times \frac{10}{0.5} \times \frac{1}{A} \times \frac{1}{B}$$

where m = slope factor (OD per microgram of inorganic phosphate standard)
A = mg/ml original homogenate
B = ml of original homogenate extracted

$$\text{Phospholipid (mg/g)} = \text{lipid P} \times 25$$

BRAIN SODIUM POTASSIUM ADENOSINETRIPHOSPHATASE

The method described is adapted from the methods of Samson and Quinn[12] and Abdel-Latif et al.[13]

$$\text{ATP} + H_2O \xrightarrow[\text{Mg}^{2+}\text{Na}^+]{\text{ATPase}} \text{ADP} + \text{Pi} + H^+$$

Na^+K^+ATPase is distinguished from nonspecific ATPase in that it is specific for ATP and is inhibited by low concentrations of cardioactive steroids (eg, ouabain).

Reagents

Stock Solutions

1. Sodium chloride (NaCl)—1.111 *M*.

2. Potassium chloride (KCl)—0.444 *M*.

3. Magnesium chloride ($MgCl_2$)—0.1111 *M*.

4. Tris buffer—0.222 *M* (pH 7.40). Dissolve 27.30 g Certified Primary Standard Tris (hydroxymethyl) aminomethane (Fisher number T395—"THAM") in approximately 500 ml of deionized H_2O. Adjust pH carefully to pH 7.40 (glass electrode) with 10% (v/v) HCl. When adjusted, dilute to 1 liter with deionized H_2O.

5. Ouabain—6 m*M*. Dissolve 109.35 mg ouabain octahydrate (Sigma) in 25 ml deionized H_2O (concentration when added to the final reaction mixture).

6. Trichloroacetic acid (TCA) 20%. Dissolve 100 g TCA in 500 ml of deionized H_2O chilled at 0°C.

Buffered Substrate

Buffered substrate is prepared on the day of assay. Weigh out 273 mg disodium salt-$3H_2O$ adenosine triphosphate (ATP) into a 100-ml volumetric flask. A volume of 10 ml of 1.111 *M* NaCl, 5 ml of 0.444 *M* KCl, and 5 ml of 0.1111 *M* $MgCl_2$ is added to the flask. The flask is made up to volume with Tris buffer 222 mM (pH 7.40). This will make a final reaction mixture composition of 160 mM Tris buffer pH 7.40, 100 mM NaCl, 20 mM KCl, 5 mM $MgCl_2$, 4 mM ATP.

Procedure

No more than 36 to 48 tubes are assayed in each batch.

Stage I

1. Take 12-ml centrifuge tubes and set up in rows of three (or multiples of three if duplicate or triplicate assays are to be done on each sample). (*N.B.* Usually cerebellar homogenates are assayed singularly due to the limited amount of material available.)

2. Each row (or multiples of each row) is identified with a sample number. The first tube of each row is marked "T" (total ATPase activity). The second tube is marked "O" (ouabain containing), and the final tube is marked "BL" (endogenous inorganic phosphate).

3. Buffered substrate, ouabain reagent, and water are added as indicated for stage I in the table below.

4. The tubes are incubated in a water bath at 37°C for 10 minutes prior to the addition of the brain homogenate.

Reaction mixture constituent	T Total ATPase activity	O Mg^{2+}- activated ATPase activity	BL Endogenous inorganic phosphate	Stage
Buffered substrate (ml)	1.8	1.8	1.8	I
Ouabain 6 mM (ml)	—	0.1	—	
H$_2$O (ml)	0.1	—	0.1	
Homogenate (ml) (approx. 100 mg/ml)	0.2	0.2	—	II
Boiled homogenate (ml)	—	—	0.2	

Stage II

1. The homogenates usually have been prepared for this assay ahead of time and have been refrozen prior to use. The homogenates are thawed at 0°C and vortexed. An aliquot is taken (0.5–1.0 ml) from each thawed homogenate and placed in a vigorously boiling water bath for exactly 7 minutes. The boiled homogenates are cooled and 0.2-ml aliquots are added to their respective BL tube. Incubate for 10 minutes. Remove BL tubes, add 1 ml of chilled TCA, vortex, and store on ice.

2. Using a stopwatch or timer with a second hand, the homogenate is added sequentially from an Eppendorff automatic pipet at exactly 30-second intervals. The tube is quickly vortexed and returned to the 37°C water bath. (The homogenate should be vortexed prior to its addition to the reaction mixture.)

3. At exactly 30 minutes from the addition of the homogenate to the first tube in the batch, 1 ml of chilled 20% TCA is added to that tube, vortexed, and the tube placed on ice. This procedure is continued sequentially at exactly 30-second intervals until the whole batch is complete.

4. At the end of the incubation the tubes are centrifuged and 1 ml of supernatant is taken for the assay of inorganic phosphate by the method of Fiske and Subbarow[11] where the inorganic phosphate hydrolyzed by the enzymes is reacted with acid molybdate to form phosphomolybdic acid.

The hexavalent molybdenum of the phosphomolybdic acid is reduced by means of 1,2,3-aminonaphtholsulfonic acid to give a blue complex which is estimated spectrophotometrically by measuring the absorbance (OD) at 680 nm.

Calculation

$$\text{Sodium potassium ATPase activity* } = \frac{\text{OD}_T - \text{OD}_O}{m} \times 3.1 \times 2 \times \frac{1}{0.2} \times \frac{1,000}{A}$$

$$= \frac{\text{OD}_T - \text{OD}_O}{m} \times \frac{31,000}{A}$$

$$\text{Magnesium-activated ATPase activity* } = \frac{\text{OD}_O - \text{OD}_{BL}}{m} \times \frac{31,000}{A}$$

* Activity expressed as micromoles of inorganic phosphate liberated per gram of tissue per hour.

where incubation volume = 3.1 ml

       time of incubation = 30 minutes (activity $\times$ 2 = activity per hour)
       volume of homogenate assayed = 0.2 ml
       conversion to grams = 1,000
       m = slope factor (OD/μM inorganic phosphate)
       A = tissue homogenate concentration (mg/ml)

BRAIN CARBONIC ANHYDRASE

Carbonic anhydrase catalyzes the interconversion of CO_2 gas and carbonic acid.

$$CO_2 + H_2O \rightleftharpoons H_2CO_3 \rightleftharpoons H^+ HCO^-_3$$

In this method, adapted from Maren et al,[14] the rate of change of H^+ is determined by measuring the amount of time taken to neutralize a known amount of alkaline buffer under constant conditions of temperature and CO_2 saturation rate.

Reagents

Analytical reagent chemicals are used in the following procedure.

1.   Carbonic anhydrase. Source: Beef blood preparation based on the method of Keilin and Mann[15] (Worthington Biochemical Corp., Freehold, New Jersey 07728.) Store at 4°C. No loss of activity when stored refrigerated for 1 year. Soluble powder, minimum activity 2,000 units/mg. Stock standard: 1 mg/ml dissolved in water. Working standard: Dilute 2.5 ml stock in 50 ml of water (50 μg/ml). A series of standards is prepared from the working standards to prepare a standard curve, that is, 1 through 15 μg/ml.

     The following solutions should be stored at 4°C and are kept in a constant temperature bath (Forma Model 2073a) during the assay procedure.

2.   Indicator buffer. Phenol red indicator in 0.0026 M sodium bicarbonate. Dissolve 12.5 mg phenol red and 0.218 g $NaHCO_3$ in 1 liter. Filter and store in gas-tight bottle.

3.   Buffer. (a) One liter 1 M sodium carbonate (106.0 g/l). (b) One liter 1 M sodium bicarbonate (84.02 g/l). (c) Mix 300 ml (a) and 206 ml (b) and make to 1 liter. Store each solution in gas-tight bottles. Solution (c) is the buffer used in the determination of carbonic anhydrase.

4.   Chilled distilled/deionized water.

5.   Antifoam A spray—Silicone defoamer (Dow Corning Corp.).

6.   High-purity carbon dioxide (99.999%+).

     Flow rate controlled by low-pressure regulator (Matheson Model 70) and Brooks rotameter (Type R-2-15 A).

Procedure

Sample Preparation

The supernatant of approximately 100 mg/ml cerebrum or cerebellum homogenate is used for assay. A complete assay requires a minimum of 4 ml. A minimum of

2 ml supernatant is deactivated in a tube that has been placed in a beaker of rapidly boiling water for exactly 5 minutes. Cool in an ice bath.

1. Assay vials are prepared as indicated in the table below:

Chilled unboiled supernatant (ml)	Chilled boiled supernatant (ml)	Chilled water (ml)	Chilled indicator buffer (ml
0.2	—	0.8	5.0
0.4	—	0.6	5.0
0.6	—	0.4	5.0
—	0.2	0.8	5.0
—	0.4	0.6	5.0
—	0.6	0.4	5.0
—	—	1.0	5.0

2. Spray lightly with Antifoam A.

3. Cool all assay vials in water bath at 0°C for at least 10 minutes before assaying.

Determination of Activity

4. CO_2 (saturated with water vapor) is adjusted so that a stable flow rate of 600 ml/min is maintained through the assay period.

5. CO_2 is bubbled through the assay vial for exactly 1 minute. The solution in the vial turns yellow during this period.

6. Exactly 1.0 ml of Na_2CO_3/$NaHCO_3$ buffer is injected in a "pulse" into the vial and a stopwatch is started. On the introduction of the buffer the solution in the vial will instantly turn a magenta color and will be mixed almost immediately by the bubbling of the CO_2 gas.

7. The color of the solution in the vial is observed continually until the solution turns an orange-yellow color. At this endpoint the stopwatch is stopped and the time is recorded.

8. The CO_2 introduction tube is washed thoroughly with chilled deionized/distilled water and dried with clean absorbent tissue. A new vial is introduced and steps 5 to 8 are repeated.

Calculation

One unit of carbonic anhydrase activity is defined as the quantity of enzyme that will double the rate of uncatalyzed reaction (water blank or boiled sample) under the specified conditions of temperature, CO_2, flow rate, buffer, and sample volumes.

The unitage is calculated from the following formula:

$$\text{Units/g tissue} = \frac{Td - Ts}{Ts} \times \frac{7000}{A}$$

where Td = time in seconds for boiled supernatant

Ts = time in seconds for untreated supernatant

A = concentration of tissue in homogenate (mg/ml)

Note

The carbonic anhydrase activity of contaminating red cells was found to contribute approximately 1 to 2% of the total activity of brain tissue. This is in agreement with other workers.[16] It should be noted that all the monkeys in the study were exsanguinated before dissection. Carbonic anhydrase activity does not deteriorate in frozen intact brain tissue with time.

The precision of the method determined on the series of aliquots from adult monkey brain and expressed as a coefficient of variation is 9.9 and 9.7%, respectively, for cerebrum and cerebellum. These values are similar to the precision reported by Maren et al.[14]

OTHER METHODS

The methods used to estimate collagen (hydroxyproline), chloride,[17] and cation (eg, zinc) content of tissue and techniques used to determine parameters of body composition are described and evaluated in our previous book.[18]

REFERENCES

1. Kissane, J. M., and Robins, E.: The fluorometric measurement of deoxyribonucleic acid in animal tissues with special reference to the central nervous system. *J. Biol. Chem.* **233**: 184, 1958.

2. Hinegardner, R. T.: An improved fluorometric assay for DNA. *Anal. Biochem.* **39**: 197, 1971.

3. Munro, H. N., and Fleck, A.: Recent developments in the measurement of nucleic acids in biological materials. *Analyst* **91**: 78, 1966.

4. Munro, H. N.: The determination of nucleic acids. In: Glick, D. (Ed.): *Methods of Biochemical Analysis*, Vol. XIV. Wiley, New York, 1966, p. 113.

5. Crestfield, A. M., Smith, K. C., and Allen, F. W.: The preparation and characterization of ribonucleic acids from yeast. *J. Biol. Chem.* **216**: 185, 1955.

6. Gustin, G. M.: Simple, rapid, automatic micro-Dumas apparatus for nitrogen determination. *Microchem. J.* **4**: 43, 1960.

7. Folch, J., Lees, M., and Sloane Stanley, G. H.: Simple method for the isolation and purification of total lipids from animal tissues. *J. Biol. Chem.* **226**: 497, 1957.

8. Crawford, N.: An improved method for the determination of free and total cholesterol using the ferric chloride reaction. *Clin. Chim. Acta* **3**: 357, 1958.

9. Franey, R. S., and Amador, E.: Serum cholesterol measurement based on ethanol extraction and ferric-chloride-sulphuric acid. *Clin. Chim. Acta* **21**: 255, 1968.

10. Hess, H. H., and Rolde, E.: Fluorometric assay of sialic acid in brain gangliosides. *J. Biol. Chem.* **239**: 3215, 1964.

11. Fiske, C. H., and Subbarow, Y.: Colorimetric determination of phosphorus. *J. Biol. Chem.* **66**: 375, 1925.

12. Samson, F. E., Jr., and Quinn, D. J.: Na^+-K^+-activated ATPase in rat brain development. *J. Neurochem.* **14**: 421, 1967.

13. Abdel-Latif, A. A., Brody, J., and Ramahi, H.: Studies on sodium-potassium adenosine triphosphatase of the nerve endings and appearance of electrical activity in developing rat brain. *J. Neurochem.* **14**: 1133, 1967.

14. Maren, T. H., Ash, V. I., and Bailey, E. M., Jr.: Carbonic anhydrase inhibition. II. A method for determination of carbonic anhydrase inhibitors, particularly of Diamox. *Bull. Johns Hopkins Hosp.* **95**: 244, 1954.

15. Keilin, D., and Mann, T.: Carbonic anhydrase purification and nature of the enzyme. *Biochem. J.* **34**: 1163, 1940.
16. Millichap, J. G.: Development of seizure patterns in new born animals. Significance of brain carbonic anhydrase. *Proc. Soc. Exp. Biol. Med.* **96**: 125, 1957.
17. Cotlove, E.: Determination of the true chloride content of biological fluids and tissues—II. *Anal. Chem.* **35**: 101, 1963.
18. Cheek, D. B. (Ed.): *Human Growth.* Lea & Febiger, Philadelphia, 1968.

APPENDIX II

DATA ON NORMAL FETAL AND POSTNATAL MACACA MULATTA

Table

All tables are presented in the same format. Fetal data are arranged in order of increasing gestational age. Postnatal data (including adult data where available) are arranged in increasing age from parturition. Table 1 shows the gestational, postnatal, and conceptual age of each animal. The remaining tables report only the conceptual age of each animal. In Tables 5 through 13, biochemical components of the tissues are generally reported as concentrations. The total amount of a component in a discrete tissue can be calculated as the product of the concentration and the organ weight. The total amount of water in a discrete tissue can be calculated by multiplying the percent water by the organ weight and dividing by 100. Ratios (eg, protein:DNA, RNA:DNA) may also be calculated from these data.

TABLE 1 - NORMAL MONKEYS

MONKEY NO.	SEX	GESTATIONAL AGE (DAYS)	POSTNATAL AGE (DAYS)	CONCEPTUAL AGE (DAYS)	TOTAL BODY WEIGHT(GRMS)	BODY LENGTH (CM)	CROWN RUMP LENGTH(CM)	CIRCUMFERENCE OF HEAD (CM)
FETAL * * *								
34	M	75		75	47.4	13.2	9.7	9.6
36	M	85		85	79.5	15.3	11.7	11.2
41	F	95		95	86.7	17.0	12.1	12.0
35	M	96		96	142.9	19.9	14.1	14.0
40	F	100		100	132.2	19.2	14.3	13.8
32	M	103		103	133.5	18.8	13.8	13.2
33	M	112		112	181.8	22.4	16.0	16.2
8	F	122		122	212.8	24.0	16.5	
9	F	122		122	221.6	24.5	17.0	
10	F	123		123	246.7	24.5	16.5	
11	F	128		128	271.3	26.5	18.5	
17	F	130		130	318.5	27.5	18.5	
12	F	130		130	371.7	27.5	18.5	
14	F	136		136	316.0	28.3	19.5	
13	M	138		138	371.8	29.0	19.5	
15	F	140		140	344.2	28.1	19.5	
18	M	145		145	320.6	27.5	19.5	
17	F	149		149	387.4	29.0	20.5	
21	F	150		150	420.7	28.0	19.7	
37	M	154		154	467.8	30.5		
4	F	154		154	389.6	29.4	20.0	18.5
5	F	155		155	418.7	28.5		
1	M	155		155	397.5	26.6		
6	F	156		156	421.7	30.5		
3	M	158		158	475.9	30.7		
2	M	160		160	417.2	30.5		
POSTNATAL * *								
43	M	171		171	406.4	30.1	20.7	19.4
39	F	161	8	169	459.8	31.4	20.7	19.5
42	F	160	15	175	400.0	29.0	19.9	19.5
16	F	168	30	198	512.0	34.0	23.5	
23	M	169	30	199	578.5	33.8	21.3	
25	M	168	32	200	560.3	33.4	22.8	
28	M	157	60	217	721.4	35.4	23.9	
27	M	163	88	251	987.4	42.0	28.0	
29	M	171	89	260	1057.0	43.3	29.4	22.0
30	M	163	89	252	777.5	40.0	25.5	22.3
26	F	164	117	281	993.5	40.0	28.0	22.3
31	M	176	120	296	954.5	40.0	28.0	22.0
24	M	164	122	286	768.1	39.0	26.0	21.5
38	M	165	299	464	1253.0	45.0	30.8	22.5
ADULT * *								
76	F	165			5680.0			
75	M	165	833	998	2900.0			
71	M	165	901	1066	3700.0			
72	M	165	909	1074	3300.0			
74	M	165	909	1074	4100.0			
73	M	165	941	1106	3400.0			

TABLE 2 — NORMAL MONKEYS — DISSECTION WEIGHTS

	MONKEY NO.	CONCEPTUAL AGE (DAYS)	BODY WGHT (GRAMS)	BRAIN (GRAMS)	CEREBRUM (GRAMS)	CEREBELLUM (GRAMS)	BRAIN STEM (GRAMS)	LIVER (GRAMS)	HEART (GRAMS)
FETAL ***	34	75	47.40	6.22	5.87	0.17	0.18	1.96	0.24
	36	85	79.50	10.04	9.52	0.24	0.28	3.23	0.45
	41	95	86.70	11.91	11.45	0.28	0.19	3.17	0.46
	35	96	142.90	17.86	17.06	0.46	0.37	5.08	0.66
	40	100	132.20	18.99	18.16	0.47	0.33	4.62	0.83
	32	103	133.50	16.65	15.62	0.44	0.60	5.68	0.85
	33	112	101.80	25.03	23.47	0.78	0.78	6.18	0.94
	8	122	212.80	31.36	29.72	1.18	0.46	6.63	1.36
	10	122	221.60	31.70	30.11	1.13	0.46	7.24	1.21
	9	123	246.70	36.75	34.92	1.34	0.49	7.32	1.45
	11	128	271.30	38.71	36.86	1.37	0.49	8.28	1.70
	17	130	318.50	44.70	42.60	1.54	0.56	10.18	2.15
	12	130	371.70	50.87	48.33	1.90	0.65	10.26	2.28
	14	136	316.00	45.92	43.07	2.08	0.77	11.28	1.93
	13	136	371.80	49.73	46.88	2.18	0.66	11.93	2.13
	15	140	344.20	48.87	46.41	2.64	0.82	10.75	2.20
	18	145	320.60	45.27	42.41	2.10	0.76	9.98	1.89
	17	149	307.40	59.67	55.56	3.13	0.98	10.40	1.92
	21	150	420.70	49.09	45.95	2.28	0.86	11.88	2.24
	37	154	467.80		59.09	3.12		13.99	2.45
	2	154	309.60	46.82	42.77	3.26	0.79	13.37	2.07
	4	155	418.70		51.49	2.81		12.41	1.98
	5	155	397.50		54.33	2.78		10.80	2.01
	1	156	421.70		50.78	3.21		12.50	2.39
	6	158	475.90		51.17	3.91		15.85	1.98
	3	160	417.20		48.06	2.71		11.44	1.93
POSTNATAL *	43	171	406.40	53.86	49.55	3.36	0.95	11.84	2.14
	39	169	459.80	60.53	55.67	3.93	0.93	14.91	3.28
	42	175	400.00	59.24	54.54	3.77	0.91	10.71	1.86
	16	199	512.00	66.53	61.15	4.36	1.03	15.68	2.60
	23	199	578.50	65.19	59.18	4.90	1.11	18.31	3.00
	24	200	560.30	59.09	53.42	4.64	1.03	15.30	3.02
	25	217	721.40	83.07	75.40	6.22	1.45	18.33	3.68
	27	251	967.40	77.14	69.44	6.11	1.58	30.84	5.06
	28	260	1057.00	85.51	76.87	7.07	1.58	31.81	4.79
	29	252	778.50	85.13	77.34	6.36	1.44	21.90	3.71
	30	281	993.50	76.12	67.94	6.73	1.46	24.74	4.53
	26	296	954.50	60.84	54.02	5.59	1.23	15.01	4.10
	31	286	708.10	72.03	64.64	6.17	1.21	21.06	3.13
	38	464	1253.00	72.97	64.52	6.64	1.80	30.56	7.13
ADULT ***	76	998	5680.00	66.76	57.69	6.49	2.55	90.88	
	75	1066	2990.00	83.08	71.60	8.95	2.53	67.29	
	71	1074	3700.00	64.67	56.81	6.87	0.99	64.98	
	72	1074	3300.00	81.67	71.67	7.89	2.31	63.52	
	74	1106	4100.00	80.45	70.43	7.97	2.05	92.41	
	73		3400.00	77.22	67.13	7.74	2.35	61.60	

523

TABLE 3 - NORMAL MONKEYS - DISSECTION WEIGHTS

MONKEY NO.	CONCEPTUAL AGE (DAYS)	BODY WGHT (GRAMS)	CARCASS (GRAMS)	SKIN (GRAMS)	TOT VISCERAL WGHT (GRAMS)	LUNG (GRAMS)	KIDNEY (GRAMS)	THYMUS (GRAMS)	SPLEEN (GRAMS)
FETAL ***									
34	75	47.40	24.42	4.59	12.08	1.07	0.34	0.07	0.09
36	85	79.50	41.55	7.92	20.64	2.00	0.60	0.10	0.13
41	95	86.70	43.42	8.46	23.38	2.26	0.71	0.14	0.15
35	96	142.90	74.61	14.49	35.45	3.03	0.78	0.30	0.34
40	100	132.20	68.36	11.43	35.11	3.33	1.05	0.33	0.22
32	103	133.50	68.20	13.92	42.02	2.54	0.88	0.19	0.30
33	112	161.80	91.77	23.95	48.45	4.23	1.51	0.53	0.27
8	122	212.80	107.88		55.86	4.10	1.64	0.82	0.50
10	122	221.60	112.30		59.37	5.32	1.56	0.56	0.45
9	123	246.70	127.25		64.98	5.38	1.34	0.81	0.42
11	128	271.30	141.44		69.79	5.64	1.66	0.61	0.57
17	130	318.50	168.02		80.39	6.30	1.90	1.50	0.42
12	136	371.50	197.32		92.35	8.00	2.39	1.70	0.62
14	138	316.00	177.11		85.32	7.12	1.77	1.11	0.68
15	140	371.80	198.52		93.95	8.06	1.99	1.08	0.59
18	145	344.20	183.06		87.92	7.01	2.32	0.73	0.52
17	149	320.60	165.81		85.98	5.60	2.18	1.10	0.50
21	150	367.40	209.60		104.19	9.68	2.11	0.75	0.71
22	154	420.70	234.50		95.77	9.22	1.80	1.35	
2	154	467.80	254.40						
37	154	388.60	212.76	53.25	98.77	9.54	2.03	1.45	0.71
4	155	416.70	227.14						
5	155	397.50	211.26						0.43
1	156	421.70	223.50						
6	158	475.90	250.82						0.61
3	160	417.20	233.02						
POSTNATAL ***									
43	171	406.40	230.17	56.50	100.07	4.79	1.02	1.36	0.66
39	167	459.80	249.03	71.66	115.89	5.69	2.51	1.35	0.91
42	175	400.00	214.97	58.85	102.62	4.67	2.26	1.61	1.00
16	198	572.00	288.56		128.23	5.08	2.30	1.40	1.30
23	199	576.50	317.88	103.41	145.14	5.25	3.20	3.49	1.15
24	200	560.30	312.66	165.27	124.76	5.09	2.98	4.32	1.07
25	217	721.40	424.31	172.03	156.10	6.73	3.34	3.07	2.02
28	251	1057.00	576.73	119.31	197.48	6.92	4.91	6.00	2.63
27	260	780.50	618.33	176.82	214.48	7.63	4.73	5.60	0.69
29	252	993.50	451.76	146.00	170.38	6.22	4.33	2.48	0.90
30	281	956.50	564.00	102.99	214.00	7.18	6.33	2.69	1.89
26	296	760.10	543.75	105.49	214.62	6.74	6.02	2.21	1.11
31	286		457.75		166.76	5.45	3.35	1.09	1.82
38	464	1225.00	786.61		290.05	9.70	6.72	0.40	

TABLE 4 - NORMAL MONKEYS - DISSECTION WEIGHTS

MONKEY NO.	CONCEPTUAL AGE (DAYS)	BODY WGHT (GRAMS)	PITUITARY (MG)	THYROID (MG)	PANCREAS (MG)	ADRENAL (MG)
FETAL ***						
34	75	47.40	1.69	8.20	31.84	63.33
36	85	79.50	3.55	23.44	65.30	92.61
41	95	86.70	4.50	25.80	82.20	61.90
35	96	142.90	3.52	39.44	88.86	86.29
40	100	132.20	4.20	62.10	87.70	87.70
32	103	133.50	5.66	57.60	96.01	90.19
33	112	161.80	6.75	41.66	97.86	170.47
8	122	212.80	9.90	108.61	114.65	139.90
10	122	221.60	10.45	70.40	99.10	223.96
9	123	240.70	8.91	92.24	162.44	145.71
11	128	271.30	8.86	94.85	120.68	188.24
12	130	316.50	12.61	134.20	162.30	277.30
17	130	371.70	14.40	182.81	197.54	215.34
14	136	316.00	15.31	117.54	156.20	277.19
13	138	371.80	10.78	150.44	136.75	336.00
15	140	344.20	14.74	102.53	181.36	227.20
18	145	326.60	10.44	109.00	216.30	281.33
17	149	387.40	13.94	150.31	226.25	287.41
21	150	420.70	12.46	96.31	166.81	340.24
2	154	467.80		230.00	346.24	241.85
37	154	389.00	10.86	165.31	178.08	221.06
4	155	418.70		167.54	248.85	325.40
5	155	397.50	14.63	145.39	229.28	205.98
1	156	421.70	21.60	243.19	268.95	284.28
6	158	475.90	14.06	212.64	216.23	423.96
3	160	417.20	10.75	165.06	329.79	297.39
POSTNATAL *						
43	171	406.40	14.52	120.40	226.90	682.00
39	169	457.80	20.50	161.90	413.90	296.80
42	175	400.00	18.10	114.70	210.40	201.20
16	198	512.00	17.01	211.80	305.90	286.14
23	199	570.50	17.60	368.23	471.34	250.25
24	200	560.30	15.80	173.74	374.89	385.03
25	217	721.40	27.01	309.64	461.39	283.85
28	251	987.40	28.18	186.00	758.15	485.63
27	260	1057.00	23.09	268.76	1507.62	433.15
29	252	778.50	22.33	306.25	652.78	325.20
30	281	993.50	24.35	394.90	1282.84	304.37
26	296	954.50	26.65	138.00	1240.77	483.17
31	286	768.10	17.13	211.45	867.10	309.59
38	464	1253.00	20.80	172.10	1860.00	494.30

TABLE 5 - NORMAL MONKEYS - CEREBRUM

MONKEY NO.	CONCEPTUAL AGE (DAYS)	CEREBRUM WGHT (GRAMS)	% WATER	D.N.A. MG/G	R.N.A. MG/G	PROTEIN MG/G	P.LIPID MG/G	LIPID NANA MG/G	CHOL MG/G
FETAL ***									
34	75	5.87	90.49	4.73	2.17	62.90	14.09	0.50	4.47
36	85	9.52	89.99	3.90	2.09	65.80	16.17	0.52	5.44
41	95	11.45	90.18	2.76	1.76	63.90	15.86	0.53	5.24
35	96	16.16	90.47	2.46	1.73	60.20	14.37	0.59	5.67
40	100	17.06	90.53	2.95	1.79	61.70	15.12	0.57	5.42
32	103	15.62	90.49	2.66	1.89	60.30	15.18	0.56	5.60
33	112	23.47	90.11	2.28	1.81	61.60	18.62	0.57	6.07
8	112	29.72	89.22	2.09	2.09	70.80	20.58	0.77	6.97
10	122	30.11	89.67	1.79	1.79	61.30	17.11	0.74	6.40
9	123	34.92	89.02	1.70	1.90	67.60	20.54	0.90	6.85
11	128	36.86	89.59	1.80	1.88	65.50	15.65	0.99	6.28
17	130	42.60	89.08	1.32	1.96	67.00	20.14	0.92	6.54
12	130	46.33	89.29	1.49	1.74	67.40	13.62	0.99	6.75
14	136	43.07	88.33	1.59	2.11	71.50	17.26	0.96	7.49
13	138	45.88	89.17	1.34	1.94	68.80	14.86	0.96	6.49
15	140	45.41	88.16	1.31	2.05	73.30	17.46	0.91	7.98
18	145	52.41	87.91	1.44	2.09	71.90	19.03	1.06	7.30
17	149	55.95	87.91	1.26	2.27	71.90	19.57	0.96	8.42
21	150	45.95	86.48	1.22	2.18	84.80	20.77	0.91	9.43
2	154	59.09	87.19	1.20	2.21	78.40	17.89	1.09	9.08
37	154	42.77	86.11	1.35	2.90	86.10	31.90	0.99	10.07
4	155	51.49	86.58	1.42	2.10	84.90	21.25	1.18	9.93
5	155	54.33	87.93	1.18	2.21	71.50	24.19	1.07	8.60
1	156	50.78	86.89	1.32	2.19	81.70	25.99	1.08	9.44
6	158	51.17	85.66	1.24	2.11	90.10	24.06	1.03	11.02
3	160	48.06	86.22	1.36	2.20	87.10	24.41	1.12	10.41
POSTNATAL *									
43	171	49.55	84.66	1.15	2.07	97.70	31.14	1.18	11.55
39	169	55.67	84.05	1.28	2.09	99.40	33.44	1.31	13.12
42	175	60.54	83.71	1.28	2.09	102.40	32.34	1.31	13.06
16	198	61.15	82.39	1.30	2.26	101.40	37.28	1.36	14.18
23	199	59.18	82.73	1.38	2.21	103.40	31.78	1.40	12.94
24	200	53.42	82.07	1.36	2.21	108.90	33.37	1.31	13.37
25	217	75.40	81.09	1.39	1.95	109.90	33.85	1.30	16.95
28	251	69.44	80.36	1.33	2.26	110.40	43.08	1.53	16.58
27	260	76.87	80.91	1.40	2.04	110.70	42.13	1.15	18.55
29	252	77.34	80.97	1.33	1.88	111.90	41.43	1.30	17.57
30	281	67.94	80.75	1.45	1.93	106.50		1.31	17.58
26	296	54.02	80.49	1.44	1.82	113.70	41.24	1.23	18.00
31	286	64.64	80.51	1.42	1.84	111.70	39.18	1.50	18.28
38	464	64.52	80.00	1.31	1.64	113.60	37.79	1.03	19.29
ADULT ***									
76	998	57.69	77.82	1.37	1.78	112.60	57.82	1.23	28.00
75	1060	71.96	76.96	1.22	1.72	121.50	57.47	1.38	22.42
71	1066	56.81	77.54	1.17	1.61	114.20	51.07	1.27	26.08
72	1074	71.67	77.57	1.26	1.86	114.70	49.80	1.33	23.91
74	1074	70.43	77.04	1.28	1.75	117.10	49.85	1.47	25.67
73	1106	67.13	77.76	1.29	1.93	123.00	51.54	1.33	25.68

TABLE 6 — NORMAL MONKEYS — CEREBRUM

MONKEY NO.	CONCEPTUAL AGE (DAYS)	CEREBRUM WGHT (GRAMS)	CARBONIC ANHYDRASE U/G	SOD.POT. ATPASE U/G	CL.SPACE ML/G	NON CL. SPACE,ML/G	ZINC µG/G
FETAL ***							
34	75	5.87	20.30	85.00	0.60	0.30	7.11
36	85	9.52	7.63	77.00			7.38
41	95	11.45	26.18	55.00			5.68
35	96	10.16	13.02	111.00			5.76
40	100	17.06	22.47	54.00	0.64	0.27	6.60
32	103	15.02	13.02	117.00	0.61	0.29	7.09
33	112	23.47	17.43	123.00	0.51	0.39	6.44
8	122	29.72	27.30	114.00	0.51	0.38	6.24
10	122	30.11	30.87	131.00	0.51	0.38	6.37
9	123	34.92	28.21		0.54	0.35	6.39
17	128	36.86	30.94	181.00	0.52	0.38	6.14
11	130	42.60	26.67	185.00			7.06
12	130	46.33	27.44	185.00	0.56	0.34	6.10
14	136	43.07	42.63	191.00	0.44	0.42	7.17
13	138	46.88	24.78	204.00	0.42	0.47	6.66
15	140	45.41	38.64	259.00	0.44	0.44	7.25
18	145	42.41	48.79	213.00	0.38	0.51	7.90
17	149	55.56	42.21	242.00	0.42	0.51	7.05
21	150	45.95	46.76	335.00	0.41	0.46	7.95
37	154	59.09	49.84	278.00	0.43	0.44	7.13
5	155	42.77	31.71	310.00	0.39	0.47	7.95
1	155	51.49	34.09	279.00	0.37	0.49	7.35
6	156	54.33	36.05	277.00	0.46	0.42	8.78
	156	50.78	37.66	213.00	0.42	0.46	8.24
	158	51.17	72.73	434.00	0.40	0.46	8.51
3	160	48.06	56.14	251.00	0.37	0.49	7.86
POSTNATAL ***							
43	171	49.55	58.31	361.00	0.35	0.49	9.84
39	169	55.67	81.76	479.00	0.35	0.49	9.88
42	175	54.54	90.16	435.00	0.33	0.50	10.54
16	198	61.15	138.53	573.00	0.36	0.47	10.43
23	199	54.18	118.16	597.00	0.34	0.49	10.13
24	200	53.42	129.08	503.00	0.31	0.51	12.09
25	217	75.40	111.09	736.00	0.27	0.50	13.41
28	251	69.44	170.17	746.00	0.25	0.53	11.92
27	260	77.87	145.60	669.00	0.27	0.50	12.55
29	252	77.34	164.78	678.00	0.25	0.54	12.93
30	281	67.94	180.88	700.00	0.28	0.55	14.47
26	296	54.02	176.68	656.00	0.26	0.53	12.82
31	286	64.64	190.33	652.00	0.27	0.54	12.64
38	464	64.52	64.12			0.53	10.35
ADULT ***							
76	998	57.69	164.85	679.00	0.26	0.53	14.56
75	1066	56.81	143.99	585.00	0.26	0.52	11.24
71	1074	71.67	242.41	513.00	0.24	0.53	13.10
72	1074	70.43	166.81	669.00	0.28	0.49	13.78
74	1074	67.13	221.55	510.00	0.26	0.52	13.18
73	1106		166.99	451.00			

TABLE 7 - NORMAL MONKEYS - CEREBELLUM

MONKEY NO.	CONCEPTUAL AGE (DAYS)	CEREBELLUM WGHT GRAMS	% WATER	D.N.A MG/G	R.N.A MG/G	PROTEIN MG/G	P.LIPID MG/G	LIPID NANA MG/G	CHOL MG/G
FETAL ***									
34	75	0.17	90.87	3.84	1.49	61.40			
36	85	0.24	91.35	4.30	1.28	60.60			
41	95	0.28	90.86	3.74	2.17	59.80	9.23	0.67	4.75
35	96	0.47	90.79	4.98	1.85	61.20			
40	100	0.46	91.53	3.08	2.72	57.50	11.98	0.48	4.22
32	103	0.44	90.58	5.57	2.35	62.80			
33	112	0.76	90.14	6.96	3.01	66.00			
8	122	1.18	88.02	5.88	3.35	81.90	13.25	0.80	4.49
10	122	1.13	88.76	6.20	2.85	76.70	12.12	0.61	4.58
9	123	1.34	88.29	6.65	3.66	80.90	11.85	0.49	4.46
17	128	1.37	88.09	6.71	2.96	83.30	13.87	0.54	4.53
12	130	1.54	86.92	6.94	3.32	90.40	14.99	0.62	4.05
14	130	1.90	86.89	5.92	3.31	89.50	18.87	0.47	7.09
13	136	2.08	86.02	6.09	2.84	94.40	18.61	0.56	7.13
15	140	2.16	87.25	5.94	3.20	87.80	22.07	0.55	8.15
18	145	2.64	86.09	5.87	3.35	88.70	21.81	0.63	7.46
19	149	2.10	86.32	7.29	3.08	96.00	20.94	0.50	8.50
21	150	3.13	85.92	5.94	2.76	98.90	19.06	0.86	8.72
37	154	2.28	83.92	6.58	2.85	100.80	21.38	0.60	6.25
4	154	3.12	84.99	6.74	2.94	103.30	22.36	0.74	6.50
5	155	3.26	84.18	6.52	3.35	102.50	16.95	0.76	10.79
1	155	2.81	84.47	6.82	3.20	99.10	23.68	0.67	8.49
6	156	2.76	85.54	6.01	3.24	105.00	22.15	0.71	7.22
3	160	3.21	84.45	6.80	3.25	106.70	21.81	0.72	11.69
		3.91	83.81	6.71	3.24	102.80		0.55	11.63
		2.71	84.63	6.47	3.27				
POSTNATAL ***									
43	171	3.36	82.71	6.91	3.03	117.40	35.45	0.84	13.83
39	169	3.93	82.75	6.94	3.03	116.00	30.48	0.68	12.14
42	175	3.77	81.98	7.24	2.79	120.80	32.30	0.76	12.01
16	196	4.36	81.33	6.37	2.47	119.10	27.78	0.87	11.97
23	199	4.90	81.35	5.76	2.48	120.50	25.77	1.06	11.76
24	209	4.64	81.22	7.28	2.82	119.60	38.89	1.14	16.21
25	217	6.22	80.33	6.55	2.61	124.90	40.67	0.79	16.00
28	251	6.11	80.02	6.09	2.40	124.70	39.79	0.95	17.47
27	260	7.07	80.39	5.73	2.29	121.00	33.91	1.03	16.30
29	252	6.36	80.08	5.86	2.15	123.70	34.95	0.99	17.56
30	281	6.73	79.92	5.71	1.96	119.50	31.17	0.76	15.00
26	296	5.59	80.08	6.21	2.08	124.10	35.70	1.13	16.73
31	286	6.17	79.85	6.25	1.69	122.30	35.86	0.84	16.73
38	464	6.64	79.85	5.12	1.57	123.30		0.96	16.29
ADULT ***									
76	998	6.49	77.71	5.51	2.08	120.00	45.28	0.87	29.97
75	1066	8.95	78.87	5.87	1.58	120.80	41.41	0.95	23.66
71	1074	8.87	77.36	5.23	1.66	121.80	39.53	0.97	28.27
72	1074	7.89	78.19	5.40	1.76	119.70	40.22	0.81	24.56
74	1106	7.97	76.48	4.57	1.73	129.40	42.49	0.98	26.72
73		7.74	77.65	5.05	1.60	129.00	38.51		25.90

TABLE 8 - NORMAL MONKEYS - CEREBELLUM

MONKEY NO.	CONCEPTUAL AGE (DAYS)	CEREBELLUM WGHT GRAMS	CARBONIC ANHYDRASE U/G	SOD.POT. ATPASE U/G	CL.SPACE ML/G	NON CL. SPACE.ML/G
FETAL ***						
34	75	0.17		18.00		
36	85	0.24		45.60		
41	95	0.28		5.20	0.58	0.33
35	96	0.47		85.10	0.63	0.29
40	100	0.46		27.90		
32	103	0.44				
33	112	0.78				
8	122	1.18	33.60		0.59	0.32
10	122	1.13	45.64		0.43	0.45
9	123	1.34	34.78	15.80	0.48	0.41
11	126	1.37	18.97	13.50	0.50	0.38
7	130	1.54	16.66		0.50	0.47
12	130	1.90	27.16	20.10	0.41	0.47
14	136	2.08	33.88	47.00	0.40	0.50
13	138	2.18	75.25	8.20	0.37	0.49
15	145	2.64	35.70	45.40	0.37	0.49
18	145	2.10	38.15		0.38	0.49
17	149	3.13	30.52	5.10	0.38	0.49
21	150	2.28	49.63	33.00	0.37	0.50
37	154	3.12	52.15	45.09	0.36	0.51
4	154	3.26	36.12	87.80	0.33	0.51
5	155	2.81	16.66	2.02	0.34	0.50
1	155	2.78	18.76	7.79	0.34	0.52
6	156	3.21	30.24		0.32	0.52
2	158	3.91	58.94	40.81	0.34	0.50
3	160	2.71	35.42	133.00	0.35	0.50
POSTNATAL *						
43	171	3.36	114.17	289.00	0.28	0.54
39	169	3.93	165.55	459.00	0.29	0.54
42	175	3.77	189.07	381.00	0.27	0.55
16	198	4.36	58.80		0.30	0.50
23	199	4.90	131.95		0.32	0.52
24	200	4.64	193.13	346.00	0.28	0.53
25	217	6.22	133.70		0.31	0.49
28	251	6.11	206.78	397.00	0.26	0.54
27	260	7.07	200.76	380.00	0.26	0.55
29	252	6.36	170.94	316.00	0.30	0.50
30	261	6.73	158.76	456.00	0.26	0.54
26	296	5.59	259.98	372.00	0.28	0.52
31	286	6.17	150.29	477.00	0.24	0.56
38	464	6.04	140.70		0.25	0.55
ADULT ***						
76	998	6.49	212.94	237.00	0.25	0.54
75	1066	8.95	134.12	181.00	0.25	0.52
71	1074	6.87	238.91	193.00	0.25	0.55
72	1074	7.89	148.75	278.00	0.23	0.52
74	1074	7.97	143.64	184.00	0.23	0.53
73	1106	7.74	166.95	219.00	0.29	0.49

TABLE 9 - NORMAL MONKEYS - CARCASS AND PLASMA

MONKEY NO.	CONCEPTUAL AGE (DAYS)	CARCASS WGHT (GRAMS)	CARCASS FAT (GRAMS)	% WATER	PLASMA PROTEIN G%	PLASMA U.F. CL MEQ/L
FETAL ***						
34	75	24.42	0.05	86.12	2.40	117.23
36	85	41.55	0.05	85.22	1.80	112.72
41	95	43.42	0.08	84.12	2.30	127.89
35	96	74.61	0.18	83.57	1.80	116.84
40	100	68.36	0.60	82.65	2.00	106.77
32	103	68.20	0.29	82.81	1.80	96.69
33	112	91.77	0.43	79.28	3.40	117.60
8	122	107.88	1.17	75.89	3.50	121.84
10	122	112.30	1.18	76.96	3.50	121.61
9	123	127.25	1.09	76.80	3.60	114.33
11	126	141.44	2.22	76.73	3.15	117.93
7	130	168.02	2.53	74.48	3.70	113.68
12	130	197.32	2.81	75.21	4.10	122.28
14	136	177.11	4.29	72.34	4.35	122.38
13	138	196.52	2.86	75.63	4.20	121.20
15	140	103.06	3.16	74.48	4.40	117.15
18	145	165.81	2.93	74.96	4.10	120.52
17	149	209.60	3.86	74.01	4.20	118.34
21	150	234.50	5.30	71.98	4.00	119.85
2	154	254.40	7.12	72.03	4.50	116.51
37	154	212.76	7.20	71.35	4.90	112.68
4	155	227.14	4.82	73.26	4.75	122.34
5	155	211.26	3.80	73.99	4.00	121.27
1	156	243.50	3.74	72.77	3.85	117.91
6	156	250.82	7.90	72.35	5.00	117.01
3	160	233.02	5.51	73.27	4.10	115.03
POSTNATAL *						
43	171	230.17	4.87	72.18	5.05	125.05
39	169	249.03	17.43	68.40	5.50	122.86
42	175	214.97	5.69	70.19	4.80	124.83
16	198	268.56	10.24	67.94	4.90	117.33
23	199	317.88	13.14	69.40	5.00	118.22
24	200	312.64	19.12	66.92	4.50	123.22
25	217	424.31	19.20	67.55	6.10	128.36
28	251	578.73	42.97	65.09	6.60	127.01
27	260	618.33	42.84	66.01	5.80	126.72
29	252	451.76	27.96	64.64	6.90	130.02
30	281	564.00	38.30	66.15	6.90	122.00
26	296	543.75	46.93	62.75	6.60	133.09
31	286	457.75	18.58	66.43	5.30	129.49
38	464	766.61	23.59	69.30	5.60	119.20

TABLE 10 - NORMAL MONKEYS - MUSCLE (# = FAT FREE FRESH MUSCLE).

MONKEY NO.	CONCEPTUAL AGE (DAYS)	%WATER	% FAT	D.N.A. MG/G #	R.N.A. MG/G #	PROTEIN MG/G #	CL.SPACE ML/G #	I.C.W. ML/G #	ZINC µG/G #
FETAL *									
34	75	88.34	0.07	2.59	3.19	85.30	0.52	0.36	
36	85	86.29	0.25	3.41	3.09	87.10	0.64	0.25	
41	95	87.09	0.31	2.58	2.58	98.60	0.39	0.48	
35	96	87.20	0.64	3.00	2.49	96.50	0.52	0.35	
40	100	86.96	0.21	2.58	2.47	101.71	0.56	0.31	
32	103	86.91	0.54	3.27	2.81	98.90	0.62	0.25	
33	112	84.36	0.70	1.88	2.83	117.50	0.39	0.46	
8	122	82.13	0.72	2.62	3.31	135.80			
10	122	82.03	0.74	2.17	3.13	131.60	0.24	0.58	20.35
9	123	80.92	0.51	2.38	3.17	140.10	0.27	0.55	24.04
11	128	81.42	1.32	2.38	2.89	141.40	0.29	0.53	24.75
12	130	81.12	0.63	2.81	2.93	142.80	0.24	0.56	27.57
14	136	80.77	0.72	2.14	2.73	149.80	0.23	0.57	23.37
13	138	79.28	1.38	2.28	2.74	154.20	0.26	0.55	26.42
15	145	79.79	0.74	2.59	2.64	151.00	0.28	0.54	34.20
18	149	80.36	1.80	2.35	2.73	145.70	0.21	0.59	28.27
17	154	79.96	0.69	2.01	2.43	148.70	0.20	0.60	23.75
21	154	79.24	0.87	2.27	2.44	174.00	0.22	0.58	25.05
37	155	78.86	0.95	2.15	2.81	175.60	0.22	0.57	32.09
4	155	79.38	1.24	2.14	2.69	167.80	0.26	0.58	30.20
5	156	78.55	0.80	2.38	1.93	172.70	0.17	0.55	37.96
1	158	79.34	1.03	2.03	2.62	163.60	0.22	0.62	29.34
6	160	80.71	1.13	2.54	2.54	152.80		0.58	26.11
3		75.73	0.61	2.07	2.89	161.00			27.48
		77.75		2.45	2.46	185.20			32.81
		79.35		2.26	2.70	170.70			26.15
POSTNATAL *									
43	171	77.81	0.37	2.36	1.69	195.13	0.18	0.60	33.44
39	169	77.38	1.24	2.06	1.72	202.11	0.20	0.59	45.95
42	175	77.94	1.23	2.20	1.57	201.07	0.19	0.60	44.53
16	198	78.11	1.34	2.12	1.49	187.90	0.21	0.59	48.60
23	199	77.17	1.90	1.92	2.49	189.60	0.20	0.59	43.29
24	200	77.01	2.28	2.23	2.20	199.40	0.16	0.63	41.99
25	217	76.94	1.78	2.15	1.47	203.60	0.18	0.61	37.52
28	251	76.11	1.67	1.53	1.62	211.70	0.13	0.64	34.79
29	260	75.88	1.74	1.42	1.56	214.70	0.12	0.65	31.24
30	252	75.40	3.14	1.56	1.70	213.80	0.19	0.59	42.50
26	281	77.00	1.18	1.54	1.55	209.20	0.11	0.67	34.68
31	296	74.68	0.82	0.99	1.05	222.60	0.10	0.65	34.46
38	286	77.31	0.81	1.93	1.26	206.70	0.11	0.67	43.65
	464	81.03	0.52	1.27	1.58	159.32	0.22	0.60	18.94

TABLE 11 - NORMAL MONKEYS - LIVER

MONKEY NO.	CONCEPTUAL AGE (DAYS)	LIVER WGHT (GRAMS)	% WATER	D.N.A. MG/G	R.N.A. MG/G	PROTEIN MG/G
FETAL ***						
34	75	1.96	77.66	8.17	11.36	164.90
36	85	3.23	79.78	9.00	12.40	141.90
41	95	3.17	76.77	10.60	8.96	163.17
35	96	5.06	75.68	8.02	9.80	153.90
40	100	4.62	75.28	9.93	8.88	159.65
32	103	5.68	76.23	7.56	9.64	138.30
33	112	6.16	75.25	7.76	9.20	157.90
8	122	6.63	74.67	4.94	7.56	157.60
10	122	7.24	75.61	6.95	8.44	141.30
9	123	7.32	75.34	6.40	7.61	159.30
117	128	8.28	74.80	5.08	7.62	148.00
17	130	10.18	73.53	3.97	7.43	162.40
12	130	10.26	74.54	4.01	7.89	133.00
14	136	11.28	74.07	4.05	6.71	130.10
13	136	11.93	72.26	3.94	6.13	141.00
15	140	9.98	74.78	4.59	7.38	123.50
18	145	10.40	73.67	3.70	7.28	116.00
17	147	11.88	73.70	3.31	6.49	137.00
21	150	13.99	72.32	3.33	5.58	136.20
2	154	13.37	76.02	4.33	6.42	136.60
37	154	12.41	73.30	4.04	8.31	149.90
4	155	10.80	75.50	5.60	6.43	150.10
5	155	12.50	74.25	4.18	7.85	124.10
1	158	15.85	72.29	5.50	7.00	129.20
6	158		74.01	4.15	6.01	
3	160	11.44			6.57	
POSTNATAL *						
43	171	11.84	76.07	3.37	6.18	139.63
39	169	14.91	72.09	4.02	6.07	160.21
42	175	10.71	71.45	4.53	7.34	173.56
16	190	15.68	71.30	3.10	6.45	155.60
23	199	18.31	71.16	3.63	7.48	165.80
24	200	15.30	72.55	4.46	8.54	197.60
25	217	16.33	71.23	4.41	8.62	193.60
28	251	30.84	69.85	3.91	7.30	187.80
27	260	31.81	71.19	3.97	7.36	194.50
29	252	21.90	69.42	4.54	9.13	201.20
30	281	24.74	71.37	4.53	7.83	222.50
26	296	15.01	68.86	3.16	5.94	159.10
31	286	21.06	71.46	4.37	6.33	198.60
38	464	30.56	71.98	1.90	4.60	179.65
ADULT ***						
76	998	90.89	70.77	4.12	7.32	216.60
75	1060	87.29	71.40	3.74	7.76	197.10
71	1074	64.98	72.33	4.99	8.23	228.00
72	1074	63.52	70.48	4.87	8.16	229.40
74	1074	92.41	71.16	3.31	5.97	226.30
73	1106	61.60	71.17	6.71	10.11	218.20

TABLE 12 - NORMAL MONKEYS - HEART

MONKEY NO.	CONCEPTUAL AGE (DAYS)	HEART WGHT (GRAMS)	% WATER	D.N.A. MG/G	R.N.A. MG/G	PROTEIN MG/G
FETAL ***						
34	75	0.24	86.26	4.40	3.45	94.10
36	85	0.45	87.14	3.78	4.09	91.70
41	95	0.46	86.43	4.53	3.03	102.20
35	96	0.66	85.26	4.85	3.54	10.58
40	100	0.83	86.51	4.33	3.14	100.90
32	103	0.85	86.66			99.40
33	112	0.94	85.49	5.46	3.35	111.70
8	122	1.36	84.91	5.44	3.22	117.10
10	122	1.21	83.99	4.93	3.23	118.00
9	123	1.45	85.17	4.03	2.81	117.30
11	128	1.70	85.46	4.76	2.84	115.40
7	130	2.15	84.27	4.28	2.83	123.80
12	130	2.28	84.38	4.83	2.85	122.50
14	136	1.93	83.50	4.50	3.31	135.60
13	136	2.13	84.02	4.00	2.64	124.20
15	140	2.09	83.42	4.20	2.62	129.00
18	145	1.89	83.09	4.76	3.00	130.70
17	149	1.92	83.01	5.34	3.22	129.50
21	150	2.24	81.73	4.54	3.13	135.90
2	154	2.45	81.27	6.18	2.95	139.70
37	154	2.07	82.41	3.76	2.37	132.10
4	155	1.92	81.31	6.09	2.67	141.10
5	155	2.01	84.32	5.56	2.77	122.30
1	156	2.39	83.36	5.33	2.70	128.30
6	158	1.98	80.37	4.64	2.92	150.60
3	160	1.93	82.24	5.54	3.16	134.60
POSTNATAL *						
43	171	2.14	81.64	4.68	2.36	145.80
39	169	3.28	82.28	3.24	3.08	145.90
42	175	1.86	82.59	4.11	2.68	136.80
16	198	2.60	80.46	4.00	2.57	149.50
23	199	3.00	78.19	4.70	2.98	161.40
24	200	3.02	79.68	5.97	2.07	155.70
25	217	3.66	79.94	4.53	2.72	160.10
28	251	5.08	79.92	2.74	2.28	166.50
27	260	4.79	80.46	2.88	2.05	154.40
29	252	3.71	79.20	3.87	2.14	171.40
30	281	4.53	81.06	4.02	1.91	150.80
26	296	4.10	81.79	2.39	2.08	150.80
31	286	3.13	81.09	4.04	1.79	150.50
38	464	7.13	78.68	1.75	2.32	194.00

TABLE 13 - NORMAL MONKEYS - PLACENTA

MONKEY NO.	CONCEPTUAL AGE (DAYS)	PLACENTA WGHT (GRAMS)	% WATER	% FAT	D.N.A MG/G	R.N.A MG/G	PROTEIN MG/G	COLLAGEN MG/G
FETAL ***								
34	75	33.01	85.07	0.48	3.87	3.92	118.60	11.80
36	85	51.08	84.31	0.33	3.99	3.45	127.50	16.00
41	95	37.30	84.11	0.20	4.12	4.17	133.70	12.80
35	96	51.55	83.73	0.08	4.90	3.88	134.80	13.90
40	100	64.12	83.75	0.29	3.38	3.46	131.50	12.60
32	103	53.27	84.24	0.00	4.15	3.40	127.80	12.20
33	112	59.67	82.86	0.00	3.76	3.63	141.70	13.80
8	122	63.95	82.86	0.06	4.07	3.44	139.20	13.20
109	122	65.40	83.83	0.12	3.99	4.08	128.40	18.80
9	123	60.60	83.80	0.15	3.43	3.71	134.70	10.70
11	128	61.10	83.46	0.12	3.94	3.64	138.10	11.40
17	130	71.30	83.30	0.09	4.43	3.31	137.40	11.50
12	130	93.50	82.52	0.16	4.28	3.71	142.60	9.90
14	136	82.60	82.94	0.17	3.83	3.21	138.10	8.70
13	138	73.18	84.11	0.20	4.45	3.53	121.20	6.80
15	140	71.85	82.89	0.23	4.83	3.65	138.90	11.70
18	145	58.53	82.60	0.20	4.54	3.44	140.50	11.10
17	149	72.39	84.67	0.20	3.91	2.85	122.50	14.40
21	150	76.95	83.57	0.22	4.05	2.22	126.30	10.30
22	154	110.14	83.58	0.00	3.15	2.52	135.30	10.10
37	154	78.07	82.87	0.41	4.77	3.36	144.90	9.50
4	155	89.53	83.60	0.13	3.28	2.95	136.00	8.00
5	155	87.52	84.21	0.17	4.09	3.20	130.40	11.50
1	156	106.59	85.93	0.34	3.58	2.91	113.50	10.80
6	158	101.25	84.09	0.20	3.85	2.33	126.80	8.30
3	160	106.61	84.04	0.11	4.05	2.51	132.20	4.60

Index